D1318878

# NURSING

# NURSING
## A Human Needs Approach

**Second Edition**

**Janice Rider Ellis,** R.N., M.N.
**Elizabeth Ann Nowlis,** R.N., M.N.
Shoreline Community College

**Houghton Mifflin Company**    Boston
Dallas    Geneva, Illinois    Hopewell, New Jersey    Palo Alto    London

Part-opening photographs are courtesy of the following people: Lynn McLaren (Parts One, Three, Four, and Five); Chris Morrow/Stock, Boston (Part Two); Danbury Hospital/Russ Kinne/Photo Researchers (Part Six); and Bruce Roberts/Photo Researchers (Part Seven). Chapter-opening photographs used in Parts One, Two, and Five are courtesy of New England Deaconess Hospital.

Printed in the U.S.A.

Library of Congress Catalog Card Number: 80-82841

ISBN: 0-395-29642-0

Houghton Mifflin offers two other books for introductory nursing, which can be used either in conjunction with the present volume or independently. Together these books provide a comprehensive introduction to nursing.

Ellis/Nowlis/Bentz: Modules for Basic Nursing Skills, Second Edition, Volume 1, contains the following skill topics: Assessment; Charting; Medical Asepsis; Basic Body Mechanics; Feeding Adult Patients; Bedmaking; Assisting with Elimination and Perineal Care; Hygiene; Basic Infant Care; Admission and Discharge; Intake and Output; Moving the Patient in Bed and Positioning; Applying Restraints; Range-of-Motion Exercises; Transfer; Ambulation; Postmortem Care; Collecting Specimens; Administering Enemas; Temperature, Pulse, and Respiration; Blood Pressure; Isolation Technique; Assisting with Examinations and Procedures; Applying Bandages and Binders; Applying Heat and Cold; and Cardiopulmonary Resuscitation.

Ellis/Nowlis/Bentz: Modules for Basic Nursing Skills, Second Edition, Volume 2, contains the following skill topics: Common Laboratory Tests; Gastric Intubation; Tube Feeding; Ostomy Care; Administering Oxygen; Inspection, Palpation, Auscultation, and Percussion; Respiratory Care Procedures; Preoperative Care; Postoperative Care; Sterile Technique; Surgical Asepsis (Scrubbing, Gowning, and Gloving); Irrigations; Catheterization; Sterile Dressings; Oral and Nasopharyngeal Suctioning; Tracheostomy Care and Suctioning; Administering Oral Medications; Administering Topical Medications; Giving Injections; Preparing and Maintaining Intravenous Infusions; Administering Intravenous Medications; and Starting Intravenous Infusions.

A **Test Bank,** containing suggested objective test items for Ellis/Nowlis: *Nursing: A Human Needs Approach,* Second Edition and Ellis/Nowlis/Bentz: *Modules for Basic Nursing Skills,* Second Edition, Volumes 1 and 2, and an **Instructor's Manual,** are also available.

# List of Chapters

# Contents

# Part Two
# Understanding the Person   32

# Chapter 3

# Homeostasis and Human Needs   34

# Chapter 4

# The Life Cycle   44

## Chapter 5

# Social, Cultural, and Ethnic Diversity 71

## Chapter 6

# Understanding Groups 89

# Part Four
# Theory and Practice of Nursing  132

## Chapter 9

## The Nursing Process  134

## Chapter 10

## Direct-Care Skills  148

## Chapter 11

## Asepsis and Infection Control  166

# Chapter 12

# Communication   184

# Chapter 13

# Health Teaching   200

# Chapter 14

# Coordination of Care   215

# Part Five
# Psychosocial Needs of the Person 234

## Chapter 15

## Mental Health 236

## Chapter 16

## Spiritual Needs 255

## Chapter 17

## Sexuality 268

# Part Six
# Physiological Needs of the Person 284

## Chapter 18

## Hygiene 286

## Chapter 19

## Activity and Rest 304

## Chapter 20

## Sleep 327

## Chapter 21

## Nutrition 340

## Chapter 22

## Elimination 361

# Chapter 23

# Oxygenation 384

# Chapter 24

# Circulation 402

# Chapter 25

# Neurological Function    435

# Part Seven
# Major Challenges in Patient Care 458

## Chapter 29

## Disturbances of Body Image Integrity   508

## Chapter 30

## The Fragile Older Adult   521

# Preface

*Nursing: A Human Needs Approach*, Second Edition, is the central text in a complete package of books for courses in the fundamentals of nursing. *Nursing: A Human Needs Approach*, Second Edition, presents the theory and rationale that underlie nursing practice and is intended for the lecture portion of the course. It is coordinated with two softcover volumes, Ellis/Nowlis/Bentz: *Modules for Basic Nursing Skills*, Second Edition, Volumes 1 and 2, that teach skilled nursing tasks in a thorough, step-by-step, self-instructional format. The *Modules* are designed for use in the clinical practice laboratory portion of fundamentals of nursing courses. Our separation of the treatments of nursing theory and nursing skills into convenient, independent volumes was one of the most popular features of the first edition of our package, and we are pleased to continue it in this expanded second edition. In this edition we also offer a separate *Test Bank*, consisting of more than 1,000 class-tested multiple-choice test items covering the contents of all three volumes. The *Test Bank* comes in a specially designed book with perforated pages to permit instructors to tear out the test items they choose to use. An *Instructor's Manual* is also available.

## Coverage and The Human Needs Approach

We have retained the human needs approach to nursing that users of our first edition found so useful. The human needs approach provides a clear framework that enables the student to develop an understanding of the self as well as of the person who becomes a patient. This approach, which prepares the student to use the nursing process, adapts easily to a variety of conceptual frameworks for nursing education and has proved successful in constructing a sound foundation for nursing students. We have also continued the corresponding emphasis on psychosocial aspects of patient care throughout the presentation of skilled tasks in *Modules for Basic Nursing Skills*, Second Edition, Volumes 1 and 2.

Our major goal in revising *Nursing: A Human Needs Approach* has been to add depth and detail to our coverage of nursing theory. Scientific and psychosocial topics have been treated comprehensively throughout the book. We also offer greater depth in the presentation of the rationale for nursing actions. This edition includes seven new chapters: Chapter 5, "Social, Cultural, and Ethnic Diversity"; Chapter 6, "Understanding Groups"; Chapter 8, "Stress"; Chapter 14, "Coordination of Care"; Chapter 23, "Oxygenation"; Chapter 24, "Circulation"; and Chapter 25, "Neurological Function."

The book is divided into seven parts. Part One, "Becoming a Nurse," introduces the student to the health care setting. Those students with prior backgrounds in health care may be able to cover some of this material rapidly. But many entering nursing students have had no health-related experience. It is our belief that on the very first contact with a patient, students must see themselves in the role of nurse. Furthermore, we believe that the patient has a right to expect the practitioner, whatever his or her role, to fit into the total plan for care in a meaningful way. To do this, the student needs an understanding of the total health care situation.

In the first part we explore the specific professional, legal, and ethical issues that confront nursing. A definition of nursing based on Henderson's statement is presented. In addition, the role of the nurse is presented as both a direct care provider (instrumental role) and a communicator (expressive role). The nursing process is introduced as the basic methodology of all nursing practice.

The second part, "Understanding the Person," presents concepts related to the person. The human needs framework is introduced. Then the life cycle, social, cultural, and ethnic diversity, and groups are explored to help the student better understand the person who becomes the patient/client.

In the third part, "Understanding Health and Illness," we explore definitions of health and illness. Stress and crisis are introduced as concepts that relate to the entire spectrum of health and illness and not to illness alone.

A fourth part, "Theory and Practice of Nursing," covers in detail the theory that underlies nursing as a science. The nursing process is the focus of Chapter 9 and is then used as a basis for all other presentations. Chapters on direct care skills, asepsis and infection control, communication, health teaching, and coordination of care provide the detail necessary for beginning practice.

Part Five, "Psychosocial Needs of the Person," moves into the specific theoretical material relating to the psychosocial needs of the patient and the ways in which the nurse can be effective in meeting those needs. Awareness of the psychological, spiritual, and sexual needs common to all human beings, and of the differences that may be found, greatly enhances the nurse's ability to help patients cope with illness.

Part Six, "Physiological Needs of the Person," examines the physiological needs of the patient. Because of differing science backgrounds, students will vary in their familiarity with the subjects discussed in this part. We have, therefore, taken pains to define terms and to explain basic processes wherever necessary. Hygiene, activity and rest, sleep, nutrition, elimination, oxygenation, circulation, and neurological function receive thorough treatment in this unit.

Part Seven, "Major Challenges in Patient Care," discusses matters that concern nurses in every setting—pain, loss, sensory disturbance, disturbances of body image integrity, and aging. Though this material is sometimes reserved for a more advanced level of study, these problems are confronted by beginning students as well as by advanced practitioners. We consider it important to provide students with the essential information they will need to recognize and respond to such problems.

In structuring the text as we have, we have tried to use a conceptual framework that not only speaks to the setting in which nursing is practiced and the person who becomes a patient/client but also presents an understanding of health and illness and a theory of nursing practice that includes a definition of nursing, the roles of the nurse, and a methodology for action. We recognize, however, that some instructors will want to reorder topics to fit their own programs, so we have written the text in as flexible a manner as possible. Two alternative sequences are suggested in a section following the preface, but other variations are also possible.

## Readability

We have sought to make *Nursing: A Human Needs Approach*, Second Edition, a book that beginning students can and will read. We have used simple, straightforward language and have taken care to define technical and professional terms. Care studies at the end of many chapters give students the opportunity to apply their knowledge of theory within the context of concrete situations. The situations presented in care studies are ones that might face a beginning nursing student.

## Format

*Nursing: A Human Needs Approach*, Second Edition, is set up to be easy for students to study and to use as a reference. Each chapter contains the following features:

**Objectives** at the beginning of each chapter are intended to guide students in their study. The nature of the objectives varies with the subject under consideration: some are presented in very specific behavioral terms, while others are more general.

**A comprehensive chapter outline** gives students an overview of each chapter.

**An increased number of subheads** breaks the discussion into clear, manageable segments.

**Italic type** indicates important terms.

More than **twice as many illustrations** as in the first edition complement and enhance the prose discussion.

**Exhibits** within the chapter summarize and display important information.

A **conclusion** summarizes the important points in each chapter.

**Care studies** at the end of many chapters show nursing theory applied to real situations in which a beginning nursing student might be involved.

A **list of study terms** at the end of each chapter aids students in review.

**Learning activities** pertinent to the content appear at the end of each chapter.

**Relevant sections in** *Modules for Basic Nursing Skills* are listed at the ends of chapters for the convenience of instructors and students.

**References** suitable for beginning students are listed for each chapter. The references include certain more advanced publications that have become classic in nursing, but we have tried to avoid listing publications that are not available in the usual nursing library.

**Appendices** are included on common abbreviations, abbreviations of medical conditions, combining forms, table of equivalencies, special visual examinations, x-ray examinations, measurement and recording of electrical impulses, miscellaneous tests of specific body functions, tests using radioactive materials, and tests involving the introduction of a large needle into an organ or body cavity.

A **comprehensive glossary** has been added in this edition.

The separate *Modules for Basic Nursing Skills*, Second Edition, Volumes 1 and 2 focus on the student's practice and mastery of nursing skills and procedures. Each module contains step-by-step instructions and carefully chosen photographs and illustrations, along with a main objective, a rationale, a list of prerequisites, a set of learning activities, a vocabulary list, a performance checklist, and a quiz. The two volumes are three-hole punched with perforated pages, so students can tear out pages and hand them in or keep the modules in notebooks.

## Acknowledgments

We are grateful to so many individuals whose suggestions and advice shaped our work in preparing the second edition of *Nursing: A Human Needs Approach*.

## Survey Respondents

We wish to thank the large number of nursing instructors and users of our first edition who responded to the questionnaire survey done by Houghton Mifflin Company in the spring of 1979. Their input was invaluable to us in formulating

plans to make *Nursing: A Human Needs Approach*, Second Edition, a more effective professional reference and classroom teaching tool.

## Reviewers

We are also grateful to the following people for their thoughtful review of manuscript at various stages.

Christine Allen, E.D., R.N.
    Malcolm X College, Chicago

Rosario T. DeGracia, R.N., M.S.
    Seattle University

Patricia Finder-Stone, R.N., M.S.
    Bellin School of Nursing, Green Bay,
    Wisconsin

Hector Hugo Gonzalez, Ph.D., R.N.
    San Antonio College

Sue Petrovich, R.N., M.S.N.
    St. Louis Community College at Meramac,
    St. Louis, Missouri

Joan M. Oustifine, R.N.
    Mt. Auburn Hospital, Cambridge,
    Massachusetts

Marie Ford Reilly, R.N.
    Chairperson, Families-in-Crisis Committee,
    West Suburban Council for Children,
    Newton, Massachusetts

Joan Thrower Timm, Ph.D.

Martha L. Worthington, R.N., M.A.
    St. Petersburg Junior College

Martha Worthington, who read the manuscript in several versions, is due very special thanks.

## Test Bank

For their contributions to the *Test Bank*, we thank Geraldine F. Calder, R.N., B.S., Karine A. Guard, R.N., M.S.N., Celia L. Hartley, R.N., M.N., Geraldine T. Smith, R.N., B.S.N., Stella M. Williamson, R.N., M.S., all of Shoreline Community College.

J.R.E.
E.A.N.

# Alternative Sequences of Topics

The chapters in this text can be covered in various different sequences. The following alternatives are two variations that might be chosen.

**Alternative I**   This alternative sequence may be attractive to programs in which students' clinical experience begins almost immediately. This sequence starts with the general introductory material on nursing, using all or part of Chapter 1, and then moves on to the nursing process. After this, coverage includes direct care skills, the physiological needs, psychosocial needs, and then health care in general. Below is a possible outline for this approach.

Chapter 1    Introduction to Nursing
Chapter 9    The Nursing Process
Chapter 10   Direct Care Skills
Chapter 11   Infection Control
Chapter 18   Hygiene
Chapter 19   Activity and Rest
Chapter 20   Sleep
Chapter 21   Nutrition
Chapter 22   Elimination
Chapter 23   Oxygenation
Chapter 24   Circulation
Chapter 25   Neurological Function
Chapter 26   Pain
Chapter 3    Homeostasis and Human Needs
Chapter 4    The Life Cycle
Chapter 5    Social, Cultural, and Ethnic Diversity
Chapter 6    Groups
Chapter 7    Basic Concepts of Health and Illness
Chapter 8    Stress
Chapter 12   Communication
Chapter 13   Health Teaching
Chapter 15   Mental Health
Chapter 16   Spiritual Needs

Chapter 17   Sexuality
Chapter 27   Loss
Chapter 28   Sensory Disturbance
Chapter 29   Disturbances of Body Image Integrity
Chapter 30   The Fragile Older Adult
Chapter 2    The Health Care System
Chapter 14   Coordination of Care

**Alternative II**   Another alternative sequence begins with the unit on health and illness and then moves to the theory and practice of nursing, the life cycle, physiological needs, psychosocial needs, social, cultural, and ethnic diversity, and groups, and finishes with the information on nursing as a profession. Such an order might be as follows:

Chapter 7    Basic Concepts of Health and Illness
Chapter 8    Stress and Crisis
Chapter 9    The Nursing Process
Chapter 10   Direct Care Skills
Chapter 11   Infection Control
Chapter 12   Communication
Chapter 13   Health Teaching
Chapter 14   Coordination of Care
Chapter 3    Homeostasis and Human Needs
Chapter 4    The Life Cycle
Chapter 18   Hygiene
Chapter 19   Activity and Rest
Chapter 20   Sleep
Chapter 21   Nutrition
Chapter 22   Elimination
Chapter 23   Oxygenation
Chapter 24   Circulation
Chapter 25   Neurological Function
Chapter 26   Pain
Chapter 28   Sensory Disturbance
Chapter 5    Social, Cultural, and Ethnic Diversity

# Part One

## Becoming a Nurse

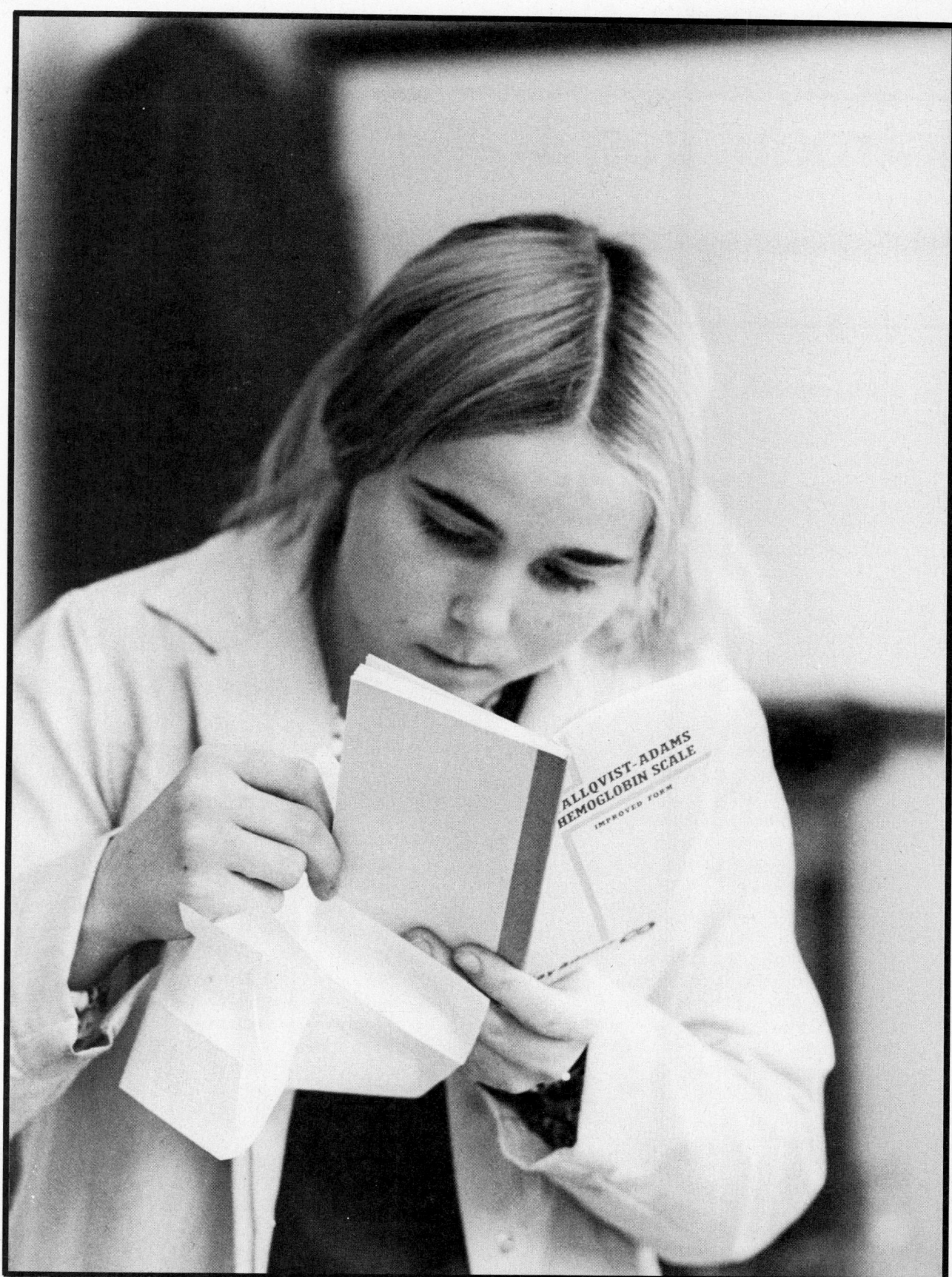

# Chapter 1

# Introduction to Nursing

## Objectives

After completing this chapter, you should be able to:
1. Discuss the definition of nursing and the role of the nurse.
2. Identify the various levels of nursing and the educational pathways to each.
3. Discuss legal and ethical issues in nursing.
4. Discuss consumer rights as a component of health care.
5. List some common legal concerns for nurses.
6. Identify ways you can protect yourself from legal problems in nursing.
7. Identify an appropriate resource to consult on ethical issues.
8. Discuss three contemporary bioethical issues.

## Outline

As you begin the new venture of preparing to become a nurse, you will find that nursing students today are a highly varied group. Among you are recent high-school graduates and experienced individuals embarking on new careers. Your educational attainments may vary from a general equivalency diploma (G.E.D.) acquired through independent study to a baccalaureate degree in another discipline. And your employment experience is also widely varied: some of you have probably had no previous health-related employment while others have worked for years as practical nurses or members of medical corps.

This rich variety of backgrounds is adding depth and breadth to nursing. As an individual, you can contribute to the education of others by sharing your background, knowledge, and experiences with them; and you can learn from those around you.

## Definition of Nursing

Beginning nursing students' views of nursing are undoubtedly as various as their experiences. Many still think of a nurse as a woman in a white uniform who works in a hospital. But nurses today are as diverse in their work settings and roles as in their backgrounds. Nurses practice in industry, in storefront clinics, in rural homes, and in research laboratories. And the number of men in nursing is growing. What then unites nurses? Virginia Henderson's clear definition of nursing (Exhibit 1.1) was adopted by the International Council of Nurses in 1972.

You will note that Henderson's definition does not focus on curing patients of illness but on caring for them in such a way as to enhance their lives. In other words, it embraces health as well as illness. It emphasizes the importance of supporting patients and their families when their lives must end as well as when health can be restored. This definition takes in the full range of an individual's needs—physical, psychological, social, and spiritual—and stresses that nursing involves caring for the whole person. Above all, it underscores the independence and autonomy of the patient/client.

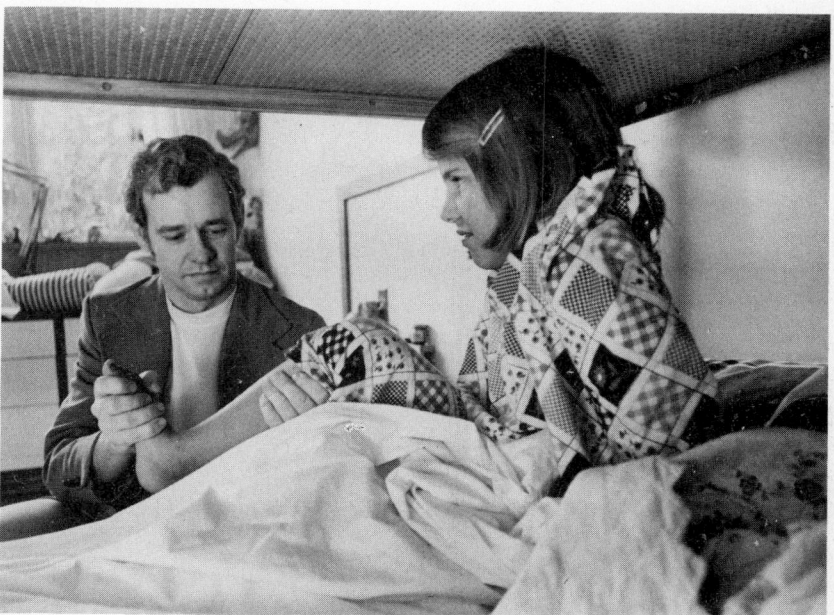

**Figure 1.1**
"Nurses today are as diverse in their work settings and roles as in their backgrounds:" a visiting nurse and patient. (Chris Maynard)

The unique function of the nurse is to assist the individual, sick or well, in the performance of those activities contributing to health or its recovery (or to peaceful death) that he would perform unaided if he had the necessary strength, will, or knowledge. And to do this in such a way as to help him gain independence as rapidly as possible.

. . . The nurse is the authority on basic nursing care— by basic nursing care I mean helping the patient with the following activities or providing conditions under which he can perform them unaided:

1. Breathe normally.
2. Eat and drink adequately.
3. Eliminate body wastes.
4. Move and maintain desirable postures.
5. Sleep and rest.
6. Select suitable clothes—dress and undress.
7. Maintain body temperature within normal range by adjusting clothing and modifying the environment.
8. Keep the body clean and well groomed and protect the integument.
9. Avoid dangers in the environment and avoid injuring others.
10. Communicate with others in expressing emotions, needs, fears, or opinions.
11. Worship according to one's faith.
12. Work in such a way that there is a sense of accomplishment.
13. Play or participate in various forms of recreation.

From Virginia Henderson, *The Nature of Nursing* (New York: Macmillan, 1966), pp. 15–16, and *Basic Principles of Nursing Care*. Revised 1969, International Council of Nurses, Geneva, pp. 4, 12–13. Reprinted with permission.

# The Role of the Nurse

Let us look at how this definition of nursing is realized in nursing practice. When you enter nursing, you will be adopting a new professional role, which requires you to learn new skills, behavior, and ways of relating to others.

## The Social vs. the Professional Role

A positive professional role bears many similarities to a positive social role. At their best, both are based on honesty, which engenders the trust basic to any sound relationship. In both the professional and the social role, one should respect the rights and autonomy of others. Both people in a relationship are responsible for that relationship and its outcomes.

There are, however, major differences between the professional role and the social role (see Figure 1.2). Social relationships may have a variety of purposes, which change as the participants develop and change in relation to one another. Some social relationships have no particular explicit purpose. The professional relationship, however, is purposeful and goal-directed. The participants focus on the goal of the relationship—which is often explicitly stated—and direct their efforts toward accomplishing it.

In social relationships, it is assumed that the needs of all participants are equally important. The focus of a professional relationship with a patient/client, however, is the other person's needs and concerns. Let us examine what this means in a practical way. A nurse who is experiencing stress or a personal crisis might need to talk about such problems with a sympathetic and supportive person. It would be inappropriate, however, to expect the patient/client to meet those needs. A person assumes the role of patient/client because of existing stresses and needs, and it would be inappropriate to introduce more. This does not mean that personal stresses and difficulties do not affect the nurse's functioning; this would be an unrealistic expectation. It means that the nurse should address such difficulties outside the nurse-patient relationship by seeking out a friend, colleague, or professional counselor.

The professional is also expected to bring to the relationship expertise and knowledge beneficial to the patient/client. The patient/client expects the nurse to meet needs he or she is unable to provide for independently.

mechanisms of implementation. Some argue for abolition of one-year practical nursing programs and three-year diploma programs leaving only associate degree and baccalaureate programs with separate licenses. Others foresee retention of the one-year licensed practical nursing programs and establishment of two separately licensed levels of registered nurses: one for associate degree and diploma graduates and another for baccalaureate graduates. Other approaches have also been proposed.

Any change in current licensure requirements will bear on a number of other issues, including the geographically uneven distribution of nurses, the increased cost of more education, provisions for systematic progression from one level of nurs-ing to another, restrictions on mobility if some states change their licensure requirements and others do not, and disagreement among nurses on the best direction for change to take.

In the midst of controversy, a few facts may need clarification. First, no state licensing laws have yet been changed. Second, almost all those who propose changes in the law advocate that nurses licensed at the time of such a change will continue to practice with the same license and that changes in requirements will pertain only to those who graduate after the new law takes effect. Because decisions being made now will shape your future and the future of nursing, it is particularly important to remain informed and let your views be known.

## Legal Concerns in Nursing

Legal issues are those that can be resolved by referring to the law or a court decision. A wide variety of legal matters are of significance to the practice of nursing. After examining the law itself and its implications for nursing practice, we will discuss specific legal issues.

### Nurse Practice Acts

Throughout the United States and in most other countries there is a legal basis for nursing practice. Each state legislature has enacted an official statute called the Nurse Practice Act, which defines nursing, specifies educational standards, assigns the authority to regulate schools of nursing, regulates who can practice nursing, and establishes a state board of nursing.

### Definition of Nursing

In the eyes of the law, nursing entails a specific body of actions and expertise. The law also specifies areas of practice, such as giving medications, which can be undertaken only at the direction of a licensed physician or dentist.

### Educational Standards

The law specifies the minimum education required to apply for licensure as a nurse. All states currently recognize associate degree, diploma, and baccalaureate programs.

### Regulating Schools of Nursing

State law assigns the authority for overseeing schools of nursing within the state to the state board of nursing. Regulation includes setting standards for clinical facilities and faculty and approving curricula.

### Regulating Who Will Practice

In order to regulate who can practice nursing, the law specifies the requirements to obtain and renew a nursing license. It also establishes a mechanism for revoking the license of a person who does not meet or maintain the standards set by the state.

## State Board of Nursing

The state board of nursing is the legal entity with responsibility for implementing the licensure laws, which it does by issuing specific rules and regulations for obtaining a license. It is the state board that conducts hearings on revocation of a license and regulates schools of nursing. Information on the current licensure law in a given state may be obtained by writing directly to the state board of nursing. The addresses of the state boards are published in January and August in the *American Journal of Nursing*, the official publication of the American Nurses Association.

## Continuing Education

More and more states are adding provisions to their licensing laws requiring nurses to pursue continuing education as a prerequisite to renewing their licenses. This is called *mandatory continuing education*. Most leaders in health care believe that, because of the rapid pace of change in health care and the resultant need for providers to renew and expand their knowledge, continuing education will eventually be required of all licensed health-care providers in every state.

In states where continuing education is not mandatory, nurses are urged to pursue *voluntary continuing education* in order to keep their practice up-to-date.

One need not enroll in a degree-granting program to undertake continuing education. Courses are offered by colleges and universities, employers (*in service* or *staff education*) and private agencies, or one may pursue independent study followed by a formal examination.

## Obtaining a Nursing License

An initial nursing license is issued on completion of an educational program approved by the state and a passing grade on a state board licensing examination. The same examination is given in all states on the same day. The test is prepared by the National League for Nursing by contract with the National Association of State Boards of Nursing. Each state has the authority to set its own

standard for passing the examination. All states but one currently designate a score of 350 as passing; Hawaii specifies a slightly higher score. Only applicants who have met all the requirements of the state are entitled to call themselves registered nurses (R.N.).

After initial licensure in one state, it is relatively easy to secure a license in another state. This process is called *licensure by endorsement* or *reciprocity*. Licensure by endorsement is granted on the basis of the candidate's initial educational program and original licensing examination. Some states also require evidence of having practiced nursing since the original licensure and/or evidence of continuing education. If the newcomer has not met these requirements, the state has usually established methods of meeting those standards.

## Understanding the Law

Whenever a legal issue arises, one of the first questions asked is "What does the law say?" Thus it is important to understand what is meant by "the law."

## Statutory Law

There are two primary sources of law. The first and most important is *statutory law*, which consists of the laws enacted by a legislative body, or *enacted law*, and the *rules and regulations* established by governmental bodies to perform their duties under enacted law. Nurse Practice Acts are an example of enacted law; the rules and regulations of the state board of nursing exemplify the other category of statutory law.

## Common Law

The second source of law is *common law*, the collective term for common knowledge, customary procedure, and judicial decisions. For example, a judicial decision on a case involving an applicant denied admission to a particular nursing program would become the law in that situation. Another example is a case in which the court must determine what is correct nursing practice in a given situation. A number of nurses might testify as to correct practice and current nursing journals might be consulted. On the basis of this evidence about customary procedure, a common-law decision is made.

## Crimes and Torts

A violation of a law that threatens society as a whole is called a crime, or a violation of criminal law. An example pertinent to nursing is a violation of the narcotic laws. A violation of a law that injures a private individual but is not a threat to society as a whole, is called a *tort*, or a violation of civil law. Because of their public significance, crimes are prosecuted by the government and guilt is punished by a fine, imprisonment, or some form of restitution. If a tort is committed, redress must be sought in a court by the injured party; if guilt is found, the remedy involves recompensing the wronged individual monetarily or by means of a required action. Most legal cases in which nurses are involved are civil actions brought by an individual, commonly called *suing* or *bringing suit*.

## The Role of Policy and Procedure

The policies of a health-care facility or a school of nursing are established to guide action in a variety of situations. Such policies are based on, among other things, the legal requirements of the locality. Courts often accept hospital policy as evidence of common usage and therefore as the common law. For this and other reasons, you need to learn the policies (or where you can find them) of your school of nursing and the facilities where you practice.

## Personal Legal Responsibility

Nurses are always legally responsible for their own actions. Because of their education, they are expected to know both their own role and the limits of their capability. Under no circumstances can nurses take refuge behind the directions of others. This is a weighty responsibility and must be taken seriously. In order to perform appropriately, then,

a nurse must keep abreast of current practice through education and constant learning on the job.

As a student you have the same legal responsibilities as a practicing nurse. You must know your own abilities and limitations and seek supervision and assistance whenever you need it. If you exceed your competence and make an error, you could be held legally responsible for any untoward effects of that error.

## Personal Involvement in Legal Action

If you are involved in a legal action, you have the right to refer to the patient's written record to help you remember the circumstances. You may be asked to testify under oath, either in a written statement called a *deposition* or orally as a witness in court. In both situations you are expected to recount the facts as you remember them. It is wise to keep your statements brief and concrete. You are expected to answer questions, but you should not introduce topics you have not been asked about. It is appropriate to state that you do not remember, if that is the case, or that "The record shows that I . . ., but I have no personal memory of the situation."

You have a right to legal counsel if you so desire. If you are testifying on behalf of the hospital, you might ask to consult the hospital attorney for guidance and assistance. If you are the defendant in a legal action, you should, of course, have your own attorney.

## Preventing Legal Action

Suits by patients against health-care personnel and facilities are becoming increasingly common. This knowledge need not alarm you, if you let it guide your behavior. The best protection against suit is to provide the very best care of which you are capable. You also need to keep careful and accurate patient records documenting the care provided and the patient's response. Well-written patient records can be the very best defense if a patient decides to take legal action. Finally, try to express awareness of the patient as an individual with special needs and concerns. The patient who feels anonymous, with unmet needs, is the most likely to institute legal action against care givers.

## Professional Liability Insurance

Most registered nurses and student nurses find it highly desirable and prudent to carry professional liability insurance, which pays attorneys' fees, court costs, and any judgment ordered in a lawsuit. Such insurance is available through the American Nurses Association for its members, through the National Student Nurses Association for its members, and from private insurance companies. Some schools of nursing carry group policies for their students. The cost of such insurance coverage is moderate. (For example, the ANA policy cost approximately $30 a year in 1980.)

## Specific Legal Concerns

There are a number of legal concepts and terms of particular pertinence to nursing, and it is wise to be familiar with them. To augment those we will discuss here, you may want to consult a text on the legal aspects of nursing or do some reading in the current literature. See the references at the end of this chapter.

## Negligence and Malpractice

*Negligence* is the legal term for (a) an act that resulted in harm to another person or (b) omission of an act that would have prevented such harm. To be found negligent, one must have failed to act as a "reasonably prudent person" would have acted in a similar situation, and the act or failure to act must have caused harm.

*Malpractice* is a narrower term referring to negligence on the part of a professional person. In the case of a nurse or other professional, the standard of the reasonably prudent person is made specific to the profession. That is, your standard of action is held to be the "reasonably prudent nurse." An understanding of this principle is important to the student nurse. Whenever you perform a nursing procedure, you are subject to the standard of the reasonably prudent *practicing nurse*. You may be

slower or less dextrous, but the outcome for the patient must be the same as would be provided by a practicing nurse. This principle ensures safety and a high standard of care for the patient. It is not reasonable that a patient should suffer for having received care from a student. Malpractice is a civil wrong and is punished by a monetary fine rather than a jail sentence. It is assumed that the harm caused by malpractice was not intentional.

## Informed Consent

Every patient/client has a legal right to be informed about his or her condition and the potential benefits and hazards of the proposed treatment. This information is the basis on which the patient decides whether or not to accept the proposed plan of care. A decision to accept treatment is called *consent*. Consent must be both informed and freely given and can be legally withdrawn at any time. In other words, the patient can change his or her mind.

Consent may be either oral or written. In practice, consent for minor, noninvasive, and temporary treatments is typically oral. Most nursing care measures fall into this category. Consent for major, invasive, and potentially harmful procedures—notably surgery, radiation, and certain diagnostic procedures—should be obtained in writing.

The responsibility for obtaining the patient's consent rests with the person responsible for identifying the problem and determining the appropriate treatment. Thus it is the physician's responsibility to obtain consent for surgery planned by the physician. A nurse is sometimes asked to witness a patient/client's signature on a medical or surgical consent form. Doing so does not transfer to the nurse the legal responsibility for providing information and ascertaining that the consent is informed. The nurse is simply attesting that the person named in the document did indeed sign it freely. The nurse ought to make certain that the form being used is the appropriate one and is filled out correctly. The physician is still legally responsible for ensuring that the consent is informed.

It is the nurse's responsibility to obtain consent for nursing measures. When you give a patient information in order to obtain consent, it is important to make sure he or she understands the information before proceeding. Informed consent may be verbal or implied by an action, such as turning over to receive an injection.

## Who Gives Consent?

Every adult is assumed to be capable of giving personal consent unless a court or other legal authority has determined otherwise. Advanced age is by no means a sufficient justification for assuming a patient is unable to give consent.

The legal age of consent is eighteen in most jurisdictions, but there are several exceptions. An *emancipated minor*—an underage person who is financially independent and does not live in the parent's home—is usually permitted to give consent. A minor who is married is automatically allowed to give personal consent. In most states minors can give consent for care related to reproduction such as birth control, treatment of venereal disease, and pregnancy.

Growing concern for human rights has led to the inclusion of children in decision making about their own care as soon as they seem able to understand. Of course, parental consent must be obtained, but it is also highly desirable to elicit the consent of the child. Children are typically included in decision making by the age of seven or eight.

## Consent in Emergencies

There are alternatives to consent when an immediate threat to life exists and the individual is incapable of giving personal consent. It is wise to have two physicians concur that an emergency exists and that the patient is unable to give consent. Consent is then usually requested from the next of kin. If this proves impossible, the staff will abide by the facility's policy on such situations, which provides for maximum legal protection of the health-care providers and needed care for the patient.

## Assault and Battery

*Assault* is threatening bodily harm (or making a person feel threatened); *battery* is touching or

harming a person without consent. This charge may seem entirely irrelevant to health care, but certain treatment procedures performed without informed consent may constitute battery in the eyes of the law.

## False Imprisonment

Confining a person without consent and without due process is considered false imprisonment. Using restraints without having followed appropriate procedures and documented the circumstances, and refusing to let a competent person leave a health-care facility, are both defined as false imprisonment. It is especially important to follow established policies in regard to such matters as restraints.

## Narcotic Control

In many institutions nurses are responsible for administering and accounting for narcotics and other controlled substances, a responsibility with important legal ramifications. The hospital establishes policies and exact procedures for discharging this responsibility. Altering or falsifying narcotic records is a crime. If you discover an error, you have a responsibility to report it. Established procedure usually entails notifying the unit supervisor and pharmacy personnel as well as filling out a report. By following such procedures carefully, you protect yourself against legal action.

## Wills

Seriously ill hospitalized individuals sometimes decide to prepare wills. Most facilities have policies designating the staff members who can witness such a legal document; usually this responsibility rests with the business office. As a student, it is wise to refrain from signing legal documents. If, as a practicing nurse, your facility's policy allows nurses to witness legal documents, you may feel free to do so.

Your responsibility in such a situation is the same as when you witness a signature on a consent form. You are attesting that the person named in the document is signing it freely and without undue pressure and is competent to make such a decision (that is, not under the influence of drugs or so ill as to be unable to think clearly). In many facilities, the signing of a will is documented in the patient's record, accompanied by a description of the patient's condition at the time.

## Libel and Slander

*Libel* is a damaging written statement that defames a person's character or makes him or her an object of ridicule. *Slander* is an oral statement to the same effect. Statements may be considered libel or slander even when they are true. You should take care what you write in a patient's chart or say about a patient to others. Such statements should be factual and free of opinions and attitudes that might damage a person's reputation. If a nurse reports to other staff members that he or she believes a patient is faking pain, and as a result pain medication is withheld and staff members ignore the patient, the nurse's remarks could be considered slander. If the nurse had instead presented the facts of the situation and discussed the patient's care in a manner that resulted in more individualized attention to the patient's real needs, no damage would have occurred to the patient and slander could not be charged. Slander may also be charged if staff members make indiscreet comments about a patient in a public area of the hospital. In general, statements about a patient should be confined to those involved in his or her case.

## Invasion of Privacy

Every individual has a right to the privacy of his or her own person and belongings. Looking in a patient's suitcase, purse, or wallet, or trying to obtain personal information about him or her by devious means is an invasion of privacy. Consent must thus be obtained before looking through a patient/client's personal effects. When you need information about a patient, be straightforward and honest with him or her about what you need to know and the use to which it will be put. Giving out information about a patient without permission is also an invasion of privacy.

## Child Abuse

Most states now have statutes requiring professionals, including nurses, to report a suspected instance of child abuse to the proper governmental authorities. A professional who fails to do so is guilty of a minor crime. In return, the law protects the professional from suit even if the suspected abuse is not proven or is definitively disproven. The purpose of this law is to provide an added measure of protection for children unable to seek help on their own behalf.

# Ethical Issues in Nursing

Ethical issues are those that have a moral dimension, distinct from but possibly in conjunction with a legal dimension. Needless to say, there may be a variety of opinions on any ethical issue. This does not mean, however, that there is no accepted standard of ethical conduct. Through the American Nurses Association, nurses have developed a set of ethical principles known as the ANA Code for Nurses (see Exhibit 1.3).

## The Code for Nurses

The ANA Code is the general standard by which practicing nurses guide their professional behavior. As an individual, you are free to make your own decisions on ethical questions. However, nursing is a profession with explicit ethical principles, and you must adhere to them in matters that reflect on the profession as a whole. An individual who finds it impossible to comply with the ethical standards of the nursing profession might do well to reconsider a career as a nurse. An interpretation of the Code for Nurses is available from the ANA; the Code is revised periodically to address prevailing issues.

In addition to the Code for Nurses, you will also be guided by your own religious and philosophical beliefs. It would be wise to reflect on and clarify your position on the issues discussed below before you confront them in a clinical situation.

## Confidentiality

*Confidentiality* is protection of the patient's privacy by means of careful written and oral communication. The patient's problems and condition should be discussed only with those who need such information in order to provide or improve his or her care. The patient has a right to decide what information will be shared. In establishing a relationship with a patient, therefore, you may explain that you will share what you are told with your instructor and/or the nurse in charge of the patient's care. The patient can then decide what he or she wants to share with you and others.

You should consider carefully which portion of the patient's remarks are relevant to his or her care, and thus should be shared, and which should be kept confidential. For instance, a patient might confide that she had had a child as an unmarried fourteen-year-old. If the patient were in obstetrics, such information could be important to her care and ought to be shared. If she were being treated for pneumonia or bronchitis, however, such information would not be pertinent. If you are in doubt about the relevance of information a patient has given you, consult your instructor or an experienced nurse before sharing the information more broadly.

Sometimes information about a patient is shared for teaching purposes. In such cases, the identity of the patient is concealed to protect his or her privacy. If you are writing a paper on the care of a particular patient, therefore, you must take care to conceal the patient's identity. In order to maintain privacy and confidentiality, discussions of patients should not be conducted in public places where others may overhear. Even when names are

Exhibit 1.3
**ANA Code for Nurses**

1. The nurse provides services with respect for human dignity and the uniqueness of the client unrestricted by considerations of social or economic status, personal attributes, or the nature of health problems.
2. The nurse safeguards the client's right to privacy by judiciously protecting information of a confidential nature.
3. The nurse acts to safeguard the client and the public when health care and safety are affected by the incompetent, unethical, or illegal practice of any person.
4. The nurse assumes responsibility and accountability for individual nursing judgments and actions.
5. The nurse maintains competence in nursing.
6. The nurse exercises informed judgment and uses individual competence and qualifications as criteria in seeking consultation, accepting responsibilities, and delegating nursing activities to others.
7. The nurse participates in activities that contribute to the ongoing development of the profession's body of knowledge.
8. The nurse participates in the profession's efforts to implement and improve standards of nursing.
9. The nurse participates in the profession's efforts to establish and maintain conditions of employment conducive to high quality nursing care.
10. The nurse participates in the profession's effort to protect the public from misinformation and misrepresentation and to maintain the integrity of nursing.
11. The nurse collaborates with members of the health professions and other citizens in promoting community and national efforts to meet the health needs of the public.

*Source:* American Nurses' Association, 1976. ANA Publication Code No. G56R25M 4/77. Reprinted with permission.

not used, personal characteristics may be mentioned, and rumors—false or true—may result.

Confidentiality of written records is preserved by allowing access only to those who need such information in order to enhance the patient's welfare. In general, the law requires the patient's written permission for the record to be viewed by anyone uninvolved in his or her care. Even within the health-care team, however, there may be those who are simply curious. Reading a patient's record simply to satisfy curiosity is considered unethical.

## Personal Behavior

Behavior at work is also a matter of ethics. What you do as a student nurse reflects not only upon yourself but also upon all other student nurses. There is, however, considerable difference of opinion as to what constitutes correct and incorrect behavior. A useful guideline is to consider whether particular behavior will enhance or impair your ability to work effectively with the patient. For example, seductive or flirtatious behavior toward a patient is considered unethical because it may inhibit your ability to care for that patient effectively.

Nurses and student nurses are responsible for matters of life and death, and their behavior must reflect recognition of the importance and seriousness of their tasks. As a nurse you are obliged not to treat serious matters frivolously, to take patients' requests for help seriously, and to put the patient's well-being before your own.

## Accepting Attitudes

Nonjudgmental attitudes reflecting acceptance of the patient as a person, regardless of your opinion of his or her behavior and life style, are an obligation of health-care professionals. The man wounded in a gun battle with the police and the policeman wounded in the same incident deserve the same quality of care. On a less spectacular level, the patient who fails to follow medical directions and thus causes his or her own problems is still entitled to acceptance and care. Nurses need not be "super-people" lacking feelings about such situations, but they must display nonjudgmental attitudes toward the patient and express their feelings elsewhere. If you find this impossible in the case of a particular patient, you have an obligation to withdraw from the patient's care so as not to increase his or her problems.

## Bioethics

*Bioethics* is the field of study that addresses moral problems that have arisen due to modern health-care technology. In brief, bioethics considers questions of human life. When should maximum life-supportive measures be used? Is it ever ethical to withhold maximum life support or to withdraw it once begun? If care is available for only a few, how and by whom should those few be chosen? How is death defined? The list of such questions is vir-

tually endless, and none have universally accepted answers. The thrust of bioethics is to promote acknowledgment that these issues are ethical and moral, not solely scientific, and to emphasize the need for all citizens—not just the health-care and legal communities—to become involved in such decisions. Let us examine a few bioethical issues you may encounter as a nurse.

## Definition of Death

The definition of death is both a legal and an ethical issue. The growing feasibility of organ transplants has tended to promote a definition of death as potentially occurring before all bodily tissues are dead, in order to allow for transplants. Life-support machines raise serious ethical questions about the maintenance of lives that could not otherwise continue. When should life-support measures be taken? If we *can* prolong a life, should we always do so? At all costs? Who decides? On what basis? Does a patient have the "right to die"?

## Sterilization

Although attitudes toward sterilization differ, most people acknowledge that adults have the right to make their own decisions about it. A more controversial issue is sterilization of individuals who cannot make such decisions for themselves, such as those certified mentally incompetent. Courts are involved in deciding such questions.

## Abortion

Another bioethical issue that nurses frequently confront is abortion. Some nurses consider elective abortion ethically defensible, and they participate in the procedure itself and in the care of the patient. Others who consider the procedure unethical refuse in good conscience to participate in any phase of care. Still others decline to participate in the abortion but consider it ethical to care for the patient after the abortion. Each is an individual ethical decision to be respected and honored even if one disagrees.

You may work in settings where these questions arise. In order to function comfortably as a

## Exhibit 1.4
## Health Consumer Bill of Rights

Access to the highest quality of care that can be provided is a pervading right of each citizen of the state unrestricted by any personal circumstances. Consistent with a purpose of WSNA to foster high standards of nursing practice to the end that all people may have better nursing care, the 1972 WSNA House of Delegates hereby adopts the following Bill of Rights for patients:

The patient has a right to:

**1.** Services which respect the dignity and worth of man, unrestricted by consideration of nationality, race, creed, color, status, age or sex.

**2.** Maximum self-determination in health care situations, consistent with his well-being or health status. Maximum self-determination includes making informed decisions about such things as:

  **a.** Total care planning that is in accord with his value system

  **b.** Refusal to accept aspects of his care with which he is not in accord after receiving adequate information or teaching

  **c.** Determination of the extent to which his family is involved in his care

  **d.** Right to die in dignity consistent with his personal values

**3.** Information and knowledge about his health status and related care.

**4.** Be well informed as to what constitutes quality health care and what mechanism may be used for obtaining action, when, in his opinion, quality care is not given.

**5.** Expect a health care advocate to speak on his behalf when his care and safety are affected by incompetent, unethical or illegal conduct of any person.

**6.** Individualized care related to his unique needs and life style regardless of nationality, race, creed, color, status, age or sex.

**7.** Privacy by having information of a confidential nature judiciously protected, sharing only that information relevant to his care.

**8.** Be taught self-care consistent with his capabilities.

*Source*: Adopted by the Washington State Nurses Association House of Delegates, 1972. (Currently being revised.)

---

nurse, you will need to consider your own beliefs and make ethical decisions. Building your own system of ethics can be a lifelong process.

## Consumers' Rights in Health Care

The rights of health-care consumers are attracting increasing attention, in conjunction with the growth of consumer movements in other areas of life.

The first statement of patients' rights was formulated in 1959 by the National League for Nursing, but it was not widely published or known outside the League. Then, in 1973, the American Hospital Association published a "Patients' Bill of Rights." Because of the AHA's size and influence, and because the public had meanwhile become interested in consumer issues, this document elicited widespread discussion.

As a result, other groups formulated bills of rights, state nurses' associations among them. The Health Consumer Bill of Rights (Exhibit 1.4), enacted by the Washington State Nurses Association, was formulated with particular reference to the role of the nurse.

More recently, the Michigan legislature passed a legally binding Patients' Bill of Rights. Its substance is somewhat less specific than private organizations' statements, which have only ethical—not legal—force. The Michigan law has not been in effect long enough to determine whether it will bring about changes in health care.

## Conclusion

To become a student nurse is to adopt a new role in life, a role that involves both learning and providing for patients' needs. Your conduct in this role is governed by both legal and ethical restraints. The rules governing your behavior as a student nurse are the same ones that will eventually govern you as a registered nurse. Your learning cannot and should not take precedence over the well-being of the patient. While legal decisions are made for you by others, you must make ethical decisions for yourself. Nursing is not an easy road, but it is rich in rewards.

## Study Terms

assault
associate degree
  programs
baccalaureate programs
battery
bioethics
certification
common law
confidentiality
consent
continuing education
deposition
diploma programs
entry into practice
ethics
expressive role
false imprisonment
informed consent
instrumental role
ladder concept

liability insurance
libel
licensure by
  endorsement
licensed practical nurse
  (L.P.N.)
licensure law
malpractice
negligence
Nurse Practice Act
patients' rights
reasonably prudent
  nurse
registered nurse (R.N.)
role
slander
state board of nursing
statutory law
tort

## Learning Activities

1. Research the ways in which an associate degree graduate could obtain a baccalaureate degree in your community or area. Report your findings to the class, or write a one-page summary of them.

2. Find a copy of the American Hospital Association's Patient's Bill of Rights. Compare it with the Health Consumer Bill of Rights in the text.

3. Obtain a copy of an incident report from a clinical facility affiliated with your school. Review the information requested in the form.

4. Learn the policy of the clinical facility with regard to access to patient records. Who has access to current records? To records from previous hospitalizations? What are the regulations regarding photocopying?

5. Investigate sources of malpractice insurance for student nurses. If the school requires an insurance policy, investigate the coverage it provides (amount of coverage, situations covered, and so on).

6. Obtain a copy of your state's nurse practice act from a library. Report on the definition of nursing and the regulations that pertain to obtaining a license.

## References

Bachand, M. "Wanted: A Definition of Nursing Practice." *Canadian Nurse* 70 (May 1970): 26–29.

Bandman, E. L. "The Dilemma of Life and Death: Should We Let Them Die?" *Nursing Forum* 17, no. 2 (1978): 118–132.

Barritt, E. R. "Florence Nightingale's Values and Modern Nursing Education." *Nursing Forum* 12, no. 1 (1973): 6–47.

"Bill of Rights for Patients." *Nursing Outlook* 21 (February 1973): 82.

Creighton, H. "Ten Commandments in Nursing." *Nursing* 73 (January 1973): 7–8.

"Ethics." *American Journal of Nursing* 77 (May 1977): 845–876.

"Facing a Grand Jury." *American Journal of Nursing* 76 (March 1976): 398–400.

Judge, D. "The New Nurse: A Sense of Duty and Destiny." *Nursing Digest* 3, no. 6 (November-December 1975): 20–24.

Kelly, L. Y. "Keeping Up With Your Legal Responsibilities." *Nursing* 76 (March 1976): 81–93.

———. "Nursing Practice Acts." *American Journal of Nursing* 74 (July 1974): 1309–1310.

Lenburg, C. B. "The External Degree in Nursing: The Promise Fulfilled." *Nursing Outlook* 24 (July 1976): 422–429.

Michelmore, E. "Distinguishing Between AD and BS Education." *Nursing Outlook* 25 (August 1977): 506–510.

Partridge, K. B. "Nursing Values in a Changing Society." *Nursing Outlook* 26 (June 1978): 356–360.

Rabb, J. D. "Implications of Moral and Ethical Issues for Nurses." *Nursing Forum* 15, no. 2 (1976): 168–179.

Trandel-Korenchuk, D. M., *et al.* "How State Laws Recognize Nursing Practice." *Nursing Outlook* 26 (November 1978): 713–719.

Wood, L. "Proposal: A Career Plan for Nursing." *American Journal of Nursing* 73 (May 1973): 532–535.

# Chapter 2

# The Health-Care Team

## Objectives

After completing this chapter, you should be able to:

1. Describe health care as a system.
2. Discuss the role in the health-care system of government agencies, third-party payers, health maintenance organizations, independent and institutional providers of health care, community agencies, and voluntary associations.

3. Define the health-care team and discuss its scope.
4. Discuss the strengths and weaknesses of the team approach to health care.
5. Explain the various ways individuals can function within the health-care team.

## Outline

Health-care providers employ a sizable segment of the United States' working population. And, in turn, both individual families and the nation as a whole allocate a significant proportion of their total annual expenditures to health care. Since World War II, health care has experienced extraordinary growth in both size and complexity. Although advances in health care are almost invariably welcomed, concern runs high about how health care is delivered and about the high cost of such care. To help you better understand the vast system you are entering, let us take a look at its components and how they function.

## Health Care as a System

The delivery of health care in the United States may be usefully viewed as a *system*. In other words, it is composed of interrelated parts that act together to form the whole. A familiar analogy is a school system, whose components may be roughly defined as: buildings; personnel, who teach, clean, administer, and perform other tasks; a school board, elected to set policy; the curriculum; and supplies. Lacking any of these components, the schools would be unable to perform their overall task, to educate children.

The extent of a system depends partly on how it is defined. Just as we could focus on the public school system of the entire United States or that of, say, Detroit, we can limit our scope to the health-care system of a particular locality or enlarge it to encompass that of the whole nation. Whatever the case, any system may be analyzed in terms of input and output.

*Input* consists of all the information and material that enter the system. Input may or may not be used by the system. For example, input into the school system includes the tax revenues appropriated to run the schools, which are invariably used; it also includes opinions expressed and information provided to the school board at a meeting, which may or may not be used in decision making. Input into the health-care system includes patients entering the system, money used to support the system, new ideas and techniques, and the like.

*Output* is whatever is produced by the system. The output of a school system is children with increased knowledge. Similarly, the output of a health-care system is people whose health-care needs have been met. Output also includes those who have left the system without having had their needs met.

If a system is to operate correctly, continuous *evaluation* is a necessity. Evaluation must examine not only the system's output but also the means used to produce that output. Evaluation should consider both such clear-cut characteristics as efficiency and economy and more abstract matters like personal satisfaction.

The health-care system is an *open system*. In other words, there is continuing interaction between the system itself and the environment outside the system. New patients and new practitioners enter the system continually. The openness of the health-care system also results from the introduction of new technology, the approaches and attitudes of those within the system, and the influence of organizations and government agencies.

## Major Components of the Health-Care System

### Government Agencies

Government at the local, state, and federal levels is deeply involved in health care. Agencies that provide direct care include city and county hospitals, state public health agencies, and the Veterans Administration. Other government agencies fund programs and projects, such as *Medicare* (health care for those over 65) and *Medicaid* (health care for those with low incomes or disabilities). In addition, government agencies regulate other health-care providers. Such agencies include boards that license individual practitioners, hospitals and other institutions, and agencies that must approve the expansion of a facility or the acquisition of certain equipment. Recent federal legislation created *Health Systems Agencies (HSAs)* and State Health Coordinating Councils (SHCCs) to help plan changes in a community's health-care delivery system. Nurses practice in a wide variety of positions in these agencies.

Thus government is deeply involved in health care. It is impossible to overstress the importance of staying informed about government activity that relates to health care and becoming an active participant in decision making by government bodies. In general, your input through nursing organizations and other political groups has a much more profound effect on health care than any individual action might have.

## Third-Party Payers

Many people have some outside source that pays all or part of their health-care costs. This is often referred to as "third-party payment." As mentioned, some governmental agencies fund medical programs and thus may be considered third-party payers. But more frequently the role is filled by private insurance companies.

In response to rising costs and consumer demands, insurance companies have moved from being passive payers to active participants in the health-care field. Many insurance companies now require second opinions before costly surgery is done; they conduct *utilization reviews* by looking at patient records to determine whether or not facilities and treatments were used appropriately; and they are supporting health education projects aimed at decreasing preventable illnesses. Insurance companies employ many nurses to review claims and patient records, provide health-care screening, and participate in health education.

## Health Maintenance Organizations (HMOs)

*Health maintenance organizations* provide full health-care services to their members for a fixed prepaid fee. Because the HMO's income is fixed, and all needed care is provided without additional cost to

the client, an incentive exists to contain costs. Thus HMOs emphasize the prevention of illness and early treatment before costly hospital treatment is required. Some HMOs own their own hospitals, while others contract for inpatient care with other hospitals in the community. Though a few HMOs have been in existence since the 1930s, they have recently surged in number as a result of federal legislation creating special incentives for the founding of new HMOs.

## Primary Health-Care Providers

*Primary health care* is the level at which a person first contacts the health-care system. It consists of routine checkups, including well-child examinations, and care for episodes of illness. The primary health-care provider may in turn refer a patient to a specialist or a facility better equipped to meet the patient's needs; this level of care is called *secondary health care*. Primary health-care providers may function independently on a fee-for-service basis or they may be employed by an institution that provides health care.

Physicians, dentists, and psychiatrists have all traditionally provided primary care. Primary health care is also provided by *nurse practitioners*, nurses with advanced education and clinical expertise in a broad range of diagnostic and curative services as well as the supportive and educational services ambulatory patients need. *Physician's assistants* are a relatively new group of primary care providers who typically have a health background, such as the military medical corps, and who have completed a specialized program of study in a university. Physician's assistants work with individual physicians. They provide basic health-screening examinations and care for routine health problems. They may also prescribe some medications.

## Institutional Providers of Health Care

### Acute-Care Hospitals

Of the many types of institutions and organizations that provide health care, the best known is the *acute-care hospital*. All such hospitals are not alike. Small community hospitals provide routine

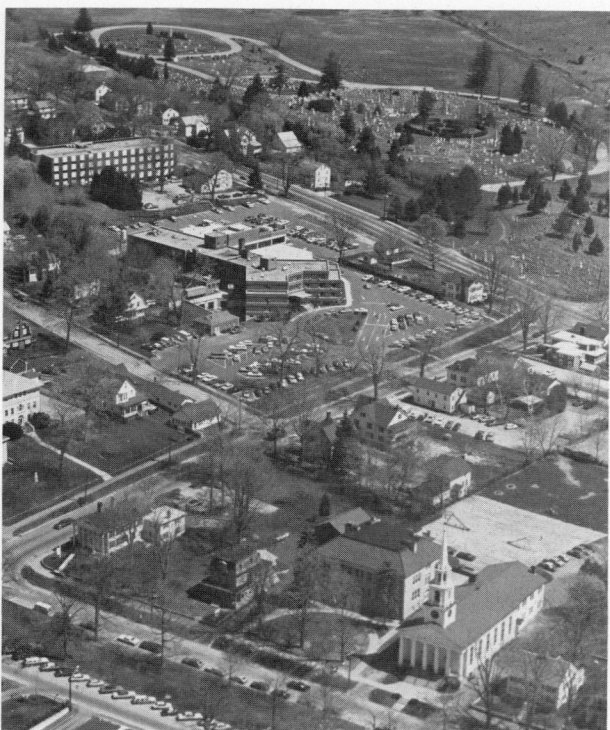

**Figure 2.1**
A small community hospital provides general health-care services. (Russ Kinne/Photo Researchers, Inc.)

tered care includes facilities for those with mild to moderate mental or physical handicaps. Some long-term facilities care for patients not expected to improve but in need of total continued care. The term "custodial care," once widely used to describe such facilities, is falling into disuse because it does not acknowledge the creativity such care requires. A new concept of care is the *hospice*, which provides care to terminally ill patients and supportive services for their families. Hospice care may be provided in inpatient or outpatient settings or a combination of the two. (See Chapter 27 for a further discussion of the hospice concept.)

A single institution may provide several types of long-term care, each on a different unit. Other institutions provide only one type of long-term care. The terminology used to describe various types of long-term care is subject to change. Some terms derive from legislation defining the types of care that will be supported financially by Medicare or other government programs. Medicare legislation, for example, defines a *skilled-nursing facility* (SNF) in terms of types of procedures performed,

**Figure 2.2**
Rehabilitation centers seek to restore function and autonomy. (Dan Bernstein)

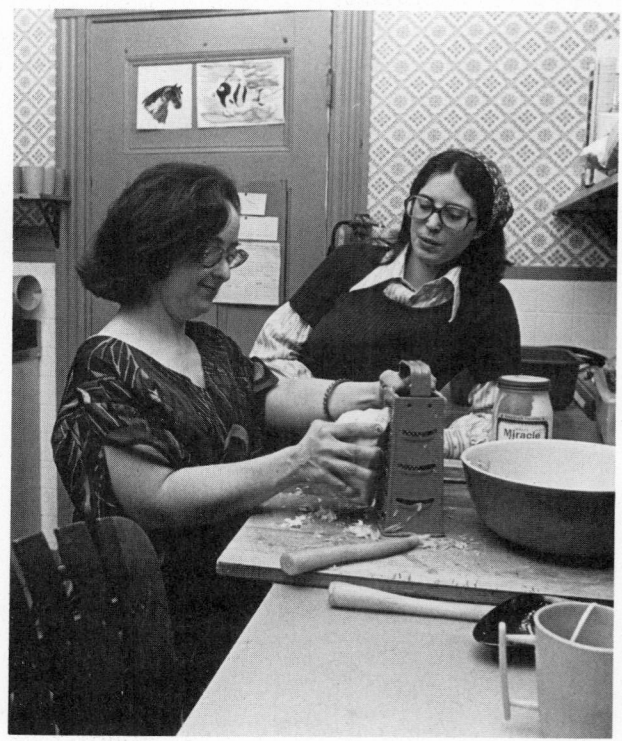

care, such as childbirth and common surgeries and illnesses, while larger institutions with specialized facilities care for more critically ill patients and/or less commonplace problems. Severely burned patients, for example, are treated in specialized burn centers. (These larger facilities may also provide care for commonly occurring problems.) The most specialized facilities, those that pursue research and extensive teaching, are usually associated with large universities or medical centers. Each type of hospital has a place in the overall system, and all employ nurses in direct care and administration.

## Long-Term Care Facilities

*Long-term care* facilities provide care for weeks, months, and even years. Some provide *rehabilitation* for patients whose functioning and autonomy can be restored. Others offer *sheltered care* for those who have reached their maximum level of functioning but still require supportive services. Shel-

staff qualifications, and expected outcomes for the patients. If you encounter an unfamiliar term involving long-term care, it is best to inquire about the overall purpose or goal of such care.

## Community Health Agencies

Community health agencies include both facilities and clinics that patients visit and *outreach* health-care workers who visit patients' homes to provide a wide variety of health-care and supportive services. Their focus is care of the person with a chronic condition who can live independently. Community health agencies are winning recognition for the effectiveness of their supportive services in maintaining people's independence by minimizing the need for institutional care. Such agencies include those that provide homemaking services, therapies of various types, nutritional counseling, and nursing services.

## Voluntary Associations

The United States has a long tradition of private support for health-related causes, which has taken the form of organizations focusing on specific diseases or groups of diseases. The funds they raise from public contributions and corporate and foundation grants support research, specialized professional education, efforts to promote public awareness and understanding of the disease, and

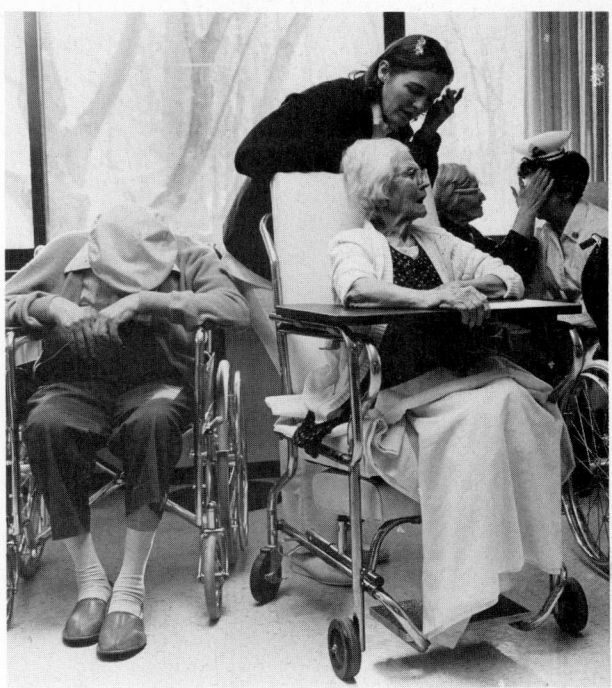

**Figure 2.3**
Nursing homes provide total continued care.

sometimes direct patient services. People with a particular illness may derive valuable psychological support from meeting their counterparts, formally or informally, through these voluntary organizations. As a nurse you may decide to refer patients and their families to appropriate voluntary organizations.

# Specific Health-Care Occupations

The increasing complexity of health care makes it impossible for an individual working independently to provide total care to a patient. This circumstance has given rise to an ever-growing number of health-care occupations, each with a specific area of expertise and responsibility. Any of these individuals who has a direct or indirect impact on the patient's care is considered a member of the health-care team in the broadest sense of the term. And the patient, too, must be a central member of

this team if it is to accomplish its goal of optimum health care.

Some of the occupations that compose the health-care team, such as medicine and nursing, are well known. Others—such as the orthotics technician, who makes braces and prosthetic appliances—are familiar only to specialists. Many of the newer and less well-known occupations administer new diagnostic or treatment techniques or assist more extensively prepared professionals.

## Exhibit 2.1
## Some Health-Care Occupations

**Child care**
  Pediatrician
  Pediatric nurse
    practitioner
**Dental care**
  Dentist
  Dental hygienist
  Dental assistant
  Dental laboratory
    technician
**Drug therapy**
  Pharmacist
  Pharmacy technician
  Pharmacologist
**Eye care**
  Ophthalmologist
  Optometrist
  Oculist
**Laboratory testing**
  Pathologist
  Cytologist
  Medical technologist
  Medical laboratory
    technician

Certified laboratory
  assistant
EEG (electro-
  encephalographic)
  technician
ECG (electro-
  cardiographic)
  technician
**Nursing**
  Registered nurse
  Licensed practical
    (vocational) nurse
  Nursing assistant (aide
    or orderly)
**Medicine**
  Physician (many
    specialties, some
    listed in specific
    categories)
  Resident
  Intern
  Extern
  Physician's assistant

**Mental health**
  Psychiatrist
  Psychologist
  Psychiatric social
    worker
  Mental health technician
**Physical medicine and
    rehabilitation**
  Physiatrist
  Physical therapy
    technician
  Registered physical
    therapist
  Registered occupational
    therapist
  Occupational therapy
    technician
**Radiation and radiology**
  Radiologist
  X-ray technician
  Radioisotope technician
**Recordkeeping**
  Medical records
    administrator

Medical records
  technician
Medical records
  secretary
**Respiratory care**
  Respiratory therapist
  Inhalation therapist
  Respiratory technician
**Social work**
  Medical social worker
  Caseworker
  Community liaison
    worker
**Speech and hearing**
  Otolaryngologist
  Audiologist
  Speech therapist
**Surgery**
  Surgeon
  Operating room nurse
  Operating room
    technician
  Anesthesiologist
  Nurse anesthetist

Exhibit 2.1 lists a number of health-care occupations you may encounter. You may find that some of these occupations are not represented in your locality. Some may have different titles, and certain of these occupations may have overlapping functions. It is important, nevertheless, that you understand these occupations and their areas of responsibility. If you are unfamiliar with some,

look them up in a medical dictionary. As you meet fellow workers in the health-care setting, you may want to inquire about their roles on the health team. It will also be one of your responsibilities as a nurse to interpret to patients the function of those who participate in their care. Thus your own perceptions need to be clear.

## Differences in Preparation for Health-Care Roles

Educational preparation for health-care careers differs greatly. The longest preparation is typically that of the physician who chooses a specialty or subspecialty. Each move into a more specialized level of practice increases the length of the physician's preparation. In contrast, preparation for some health careers consists entirely of on-the-job training, such as that received by some nursing assistants.

Educational preparation may also vary within

a single occupational group. Nursing, as we have seen, provides three pathways to registration: a diploma, associate degree, or baccalaureate degree. However, nursing education programs are subject to approval by state boards of nursing, which tend to have a standardizing effect.

Some health-care workers with identical titles may have had vastly different amounts of preparation, because there are as yet no laws governing their training. One such field is inhalation therapy:

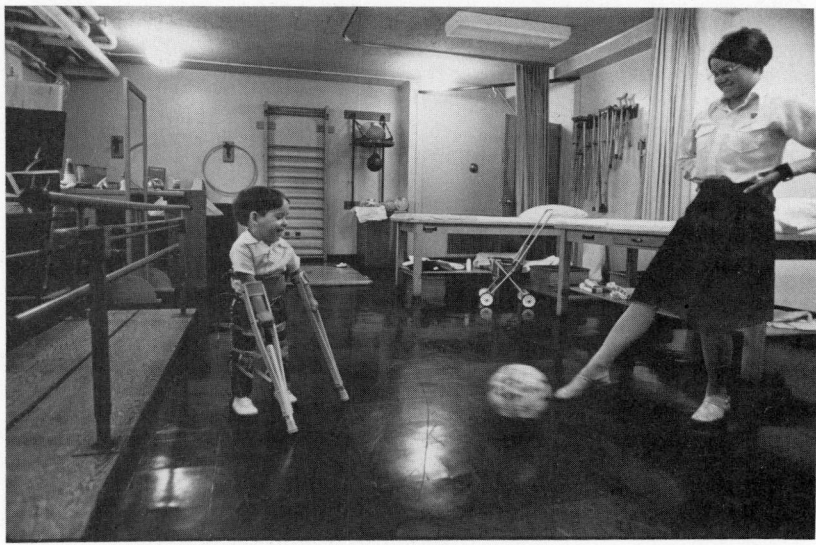

**Figure 2.4**
The physical therapist is one member of the health-care team. (Chris Maynard)

some inhalation therapists have formal educational backgrounds of considerable depth, while others have received only on-the-job training.

Recognition of such differences is important when you are responsible for delegating tasks or sharing them with others. A licensed practical nurse can be expected to observe a patient more knowledgeably than would an orderly. If a patient is in need of close observation and your team consists of an L.P.N. and an orderly, you would thus delegate this task to the L.P.N. It is also necessary to know the range and limits of others' expertise. For instance, a respiratory therapist with a thorough background in respiratory physiology might help you to understand a particular patient's problem, while an inhalation therapist with on-the-job training would be unable to do so. During your orientation to a new facility, you might inquire about the educational backgrounds of staff members with whose occupations you are unfamiliar.

## Credentials for Practice

Just as educational preparation differs, so do the credentials necessary for practice. The standards for registration as a nurse are relatively uniform throughout the country and serve to certify minimum ability to practice safely. Registration is *mandatory* in most places. Medicine, dentistry, and some other health-care occupations have similar standards.

For other categories of workers, registration is not mandatory but *permissive*. This means that one may be licensed but may also practice without licensure. In some states, registration of practical (vocational) nurses falls into this category.

Some professional organizations provide *certification* for practitioners of their specialty. Competence is determined by tests and other criteria, and certification is completely controlled by the profession itself. Physicians are certified as specialists in this fashion. Nurses are being certified in specialized fields by the same kind of mechanism.

In the United States, laws governing health-care occupations are made at the state level. The resulting local variations may limit the mobility of individuals in certain occupations.

All these variables make it difficult for the beginning nurse to know "who's who." It is, of course, far more difficult for patients, who usually turn to a familiar figure for interpretation and guidance as they move through the modern health-care system. The nurse is often that familiar figure and thus must be capable of interpreting the roles of other members of the health-care team to the public.

## Problems in the Delivery of Health Care

A coordinated health-care team in which each person functions optimally is the ideal toward which we should all be striving. However, many problems stand in the way of its realization. We shall discuss some of these problems here, and you may encounter others in your particular work setting.

Certain geographical areas are subject to shortages of personnel in some occupational fields. In such situations, less well-prepared people are often hired, which can result in a lower level of care for the patient and job dissatisfaction on the part of the inadequately prepared workers.

Another problem is that the advent of new types of health-care workers sometimes causes overlapping responsibilities. Such overlap arouses feelings of competition and occasional antagonism.

As health care has grown more complex, certain occupational groups (including nursing) have had to upgrade their skills and relinquish tasks requiring less skill. This circumstance has sometimes been perceived as threatening to experienced nurses, who thus tend to resist change because they feel threatened.

One of the most complex problems is communication. As more people become involved in a particular patient's care, communication among them becomes both more important and more difficult. Communication can and does break down. The result is fragmented care, which causes patients to feel that no one sees them as whole individuals and some of their needs are neither recognized nor met.

In the face of all these problems, what can you do as a nursing student—and later as a practicing nurse—to further progress toward the ideal of a functioning, coordinated health-care team? You can act effectively both as a nurse and as a concerned citizen.

If insufficiently prepared individuals have been given responsibilities that exceed their competence, you can be active in promoting on-the-job educational opportunities for them and in lobbying the power structure to upgrade its hiring criteria.

If individuals with overlapping areas of responsibility are competing, you can promote and participate in negotiations to establish policies—or even laws—that protect workers' rights but maintain a high level of care. You can demonstrate your readiness to compromise with others when appropriate and your commitment to the goal of optimal patient care.

You can keep abreast of current practice through reading, continuing education, and attention to your patients so that you are able to meet and adapt to change.

You can strive to make your communication with other members of the health-care team more complete and more direct. You can ask questions and encourage the establishment of routines and procedures that improve communication. Through such actions, you will be making the health-care team more effective.

## Functioning Within the Health-Care Team

An individual member of a health-care team may, at different times, function dependently, independently, or interdependently. Each mode of functioning has its place and needs to be understood in light of the efforts of the team as a whole.

### Dependent Functioning

Often the person with the most extensive preparation and/or experience in a given area of health care makes decisions to be carried out by others whose backgrounds do not qualify them for such decision making. This practice makes the expertise of one individual available to a large number of patients. Most people are familiar with the practice whereby the physician writes *orders* to be carried out by others. In the past, health-team personnel functioned dependently only in response to the physician's orders. This is no longer true. Today various people may make decisions for others to carry out. The nurse in charge of a patient's care may write *nursing orders* to be carried out by other nurses and by aides and orderlies. The physical therapist may write a *prescription* for the patient's exercises, to be carried out by the assistant or by nursing personnel. The person who carries out such orders is functioning in a dependent role.

It must be clearly understood that dependent functioning does not relieve an individual of responsibility for his or her own actions. It means that directions or orders must be obtained before acting and that the person who gives the order is responsible for his or her own decision making process. When acting in a dependent mode, it is your responsibility to make sure you understand the directions clearly, perform the task skillfully, evaluate the results of what you do, and recognize potential *contraindications* to that action. You must also be aware of the expected result of a given action so that it can be discontinued if an unexpected result occurs. You can be held legally liable for damage resulting from lack of skill, performance of an action when clear contraindications are present, or failure to stop when an unexpected or adverse result occurs. As you can see, dependent functioning does not absolve you of responsibility.

## Independent Functioning

An individual functions independently when working within his or her own area of expertise. Within that sphere, he or she ascertains what needs to be done and initiates action. Others may or may not be consulted, but the final decision is the individual's. Throughout this text, we will point out areas in which it is appropriate for registered nurses to function independently.

A type of nursing in which independent functioning is the dominant model is *primary nursing care*. In this situation, one nurse has complete re-

sponsibility for the patient's nursing care—supportive care, hygiene, and all other nursing needs—while he or she is on duty and, in addition, plans for ongoing care. Of course, the nurse in such a setting works cooperatively with other personnel and performs some dependent functions related to the physician's medical plan of care, but he or she is fully and exclusively responsible for all nursing functions. This approach minimizes communication problems, enhances continuity of care, and often makes patients feel that they are being seen as whole people. The major drawbacks to primary nursing care are its high cost and the shortage of registered nurses in some areas of the country.

Independent functioning may take a different form for nurses with specialized educational preparation. Those with backgrounds in such areas as coronary care and anesthesia function independently in ways beyond the scope of the general staff nurse. They make judgments that were once considered the physician's responsibility. Nurse practitioners in such fields as pediatrics, obstetrics, and family practice also exercise expanded independence justified by their superior education and skill.

## Interdependent Functioning

Interdependent functioning means that decisions are made jointly by those involved in the care of a specific patient. One common occasion for interdependent functioning is the team approach to certain long-term health problems, such as rehabilitation after spinal-cord injury. The physician, the nurse, the occupational and physical therapist, and others involved in the patient's care meet to discuss the patient's problems and determine overall priorities and goals. Increasingly, the patient and his or her family also participate in such efforts. After general priorities and goals have been established by the team, its individual members may work together on some problems and independently on others. This method of making decisions is quite time-consuming but can result in care of exceptionally high quality.

Nurses probably function interdependently most frequently when they engage in *team nursing*. Team nursing is an effort to make the most effec-

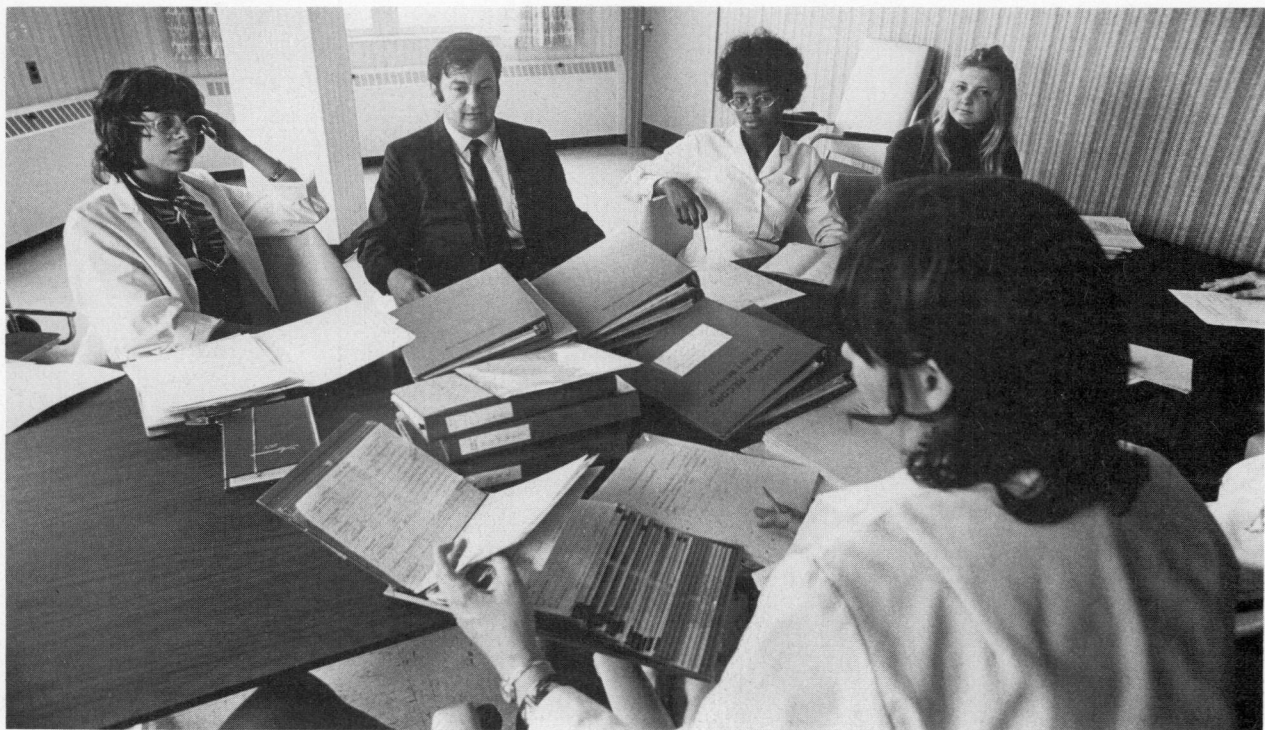

**Figure 2.5   A team conference**
Dan Bernstein

tive use of various types of personnel and to provide the most effective nursing care through joint
decision making. The team leader is usually a registered nurse with the background and ability to
organize and plan care for a group of patients.
Members of the team may be other registered
nurses, licensed practical nurses, student nurses,
and nursing assistants.

The core of the team-nursing concept is team
planning of care. At a daily *team conference*, care is
planned and problems are considered. Of course,
some aspects of care are best dealt with by a single
individual, for the sake of both efficient use of time

and the patient's needs, and need not be considered by the entire team. Conferences usually consider difficult problems or overall direction and
guidance of the patient's care. Specific aspects of
care are then assigned to different team members
for implementation. Herein lies one drawback of
team nursing: because different team members
perform different tasks, the patient encounters
many individuals in the course of his or her care
and may not know where to turn with a given
question or request. The patient may also feel that
he or she is perceived in a fragmented way. Communication is the solution to this problem.

## Conclusion

The complex modern health-care team can be be-
wildering to patient and worker alike. New occupations are emerging rapidly. Familiarity with the
various occupations will make you a more effec-

tive nurse, and understanding of their interrela-
tionships will enhance your ability to work effectively with them to improve total health care.

## Study Terms

acute care
certification
contraindications
credential
dependent functioning
evaluation
health-care team
health maintenance
    organization (HMO)
Health Systems
    Agency (HSA)
hospice
independent
    functioning
input
interdependent
    functioning
licensure
long-term care
mandatory licensure
Medicaid
Medicare

nurse practitioner
nursing orders
open system
orders
output
outreach
patient-care
    coordinator
permissive licensure
physician's assistant
prescription
primary care
rehabilitation
secondary care
sheltered care
skilled-nursing facility
system
team conference
team nursing
third-party payer
utilization review
voluntary association

## Learning Activities

**1.** Identify a community-based health resource or agency and find out (1) the services provided, (2) the qualifications of the care providers, (3) the method by which clients can obtain this service, and (4) the cost to the client.
**2.** Choose a health-care occupation about which you know very little. Research the educational preparation needed and the customary responsi-bilities of the position. (Make sure everyone in your class chooses a different occupation. Then, hold a conference in which information is shared.)
**3.** Identify the nearest comprehensive health-care facility that conducts major research and provides education as well as serves patients with unusual, difficult, or complex care needs.

## References

"Consumer Speaks Out About Hospital Care." *American Journal of Nursing* 76 (September 1976): 1443–1444.

Epstein, C. "Breaking the Barriers to Communication on the Health Care Team." *Nursing '74* 4 (September 1974): 65–68.

Golden, A. S., *et al.* "Non-Physician Family Health Teams." *Nursing Digest* 11 (September 1974): 49–54.

Kelly, L. Y. "Credentialing of Health Care Personnel." *Nursing Outlook* 25 (September 1977): 562–569.

Lee, I. M. "Cope With Resistance to Change." *Nursing '73* 3 (March 1973): 6–7.

Linn, L. S. "A Survey of the Care-Cure Attitudes of Physicians, Nurses, and Students." *Nursing Forum* 64, no. 2 (1975): 145–159.

Mauksch, I. G. "On National Health Insurance." *American Journal of Nursing* 78 (August 1978): 1322–1327.

Roemer, M. I. "Health Care Financing and Delivery Around the World." *American Journal of Nursing* 71 (June 1971):1158–1163.

Wilson, C. "The Health Care Team." *Canadian Hospitals* 50 (March 1973): 27–28.

# Part Two
## Understanding the Person

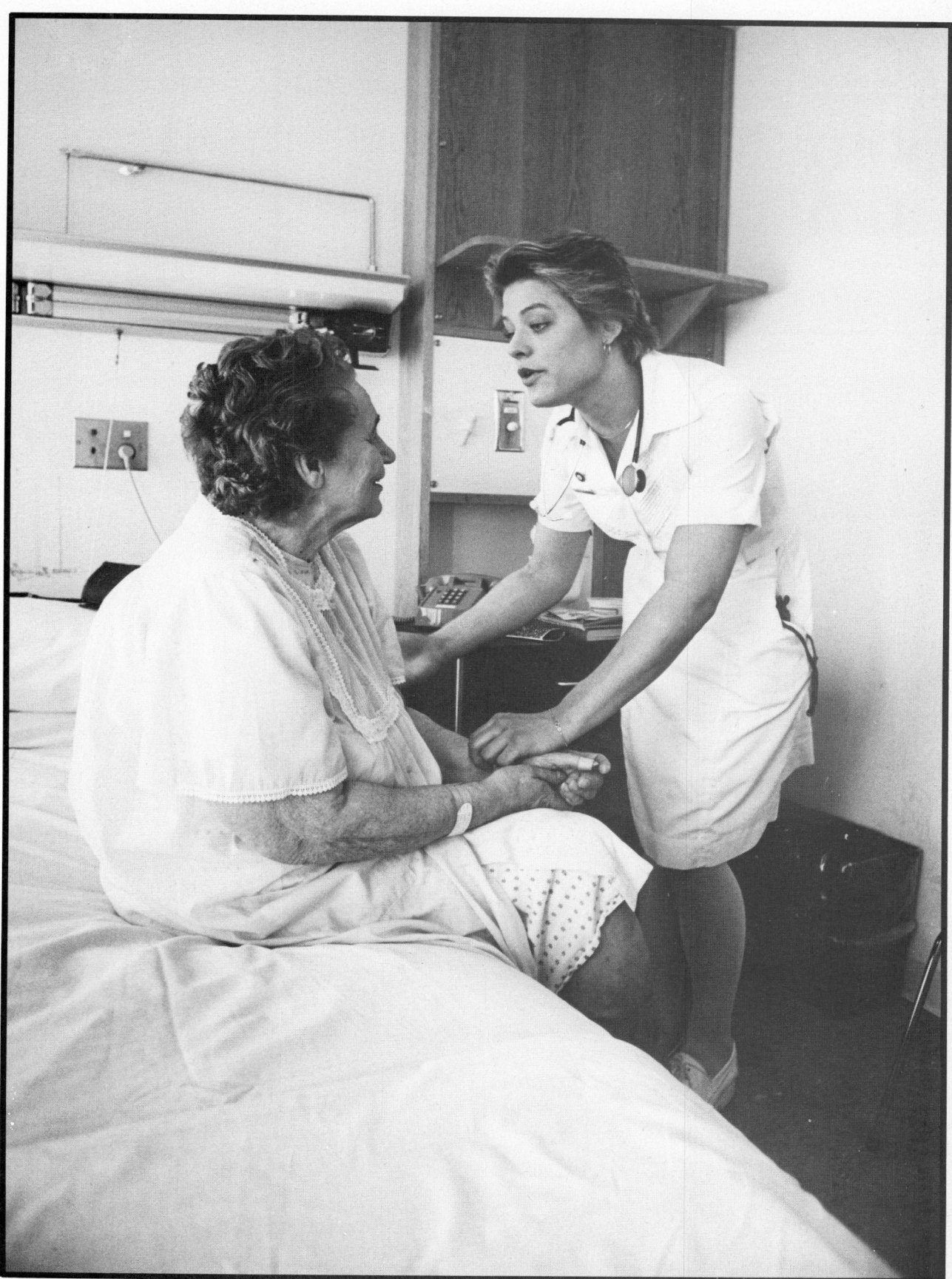

# Chapter 3

# Homeostasis and Human Needs

## Objectives

After completing this chapter, you should be able to:
1. Define *homeostasis*.
2. Explain the relationship of homeostasis to assessment of the patient and the plan for care.
3. List, in ascending order, the seven levels of Maslow's hierarchy of needs.
4. Distinguish between a need and a problem.
5. Define an adaptive force.
6. Name two internal physiological and two internal psychological adaptive forces.
7. Name two external physiological and two external psychological adaptive forces.
8. Briefly describe how the nurse functions as an adaptive force.

## Outline

Fundamental to understanding the person is the determination of what needs we share as humans and to what degree those needs are met. Some human needs are matters of survival; others are a matter of enriching our lives. Identifying and meeting others' needs is basic to nursing, and nursing care is in turn guided by the concept of homeostasis.

## Homeostasis

W. B. Cannon, an endocrinologist, coined the term *homeostasis* in 1926 to describe the ability of primarily physiological processes of the body to maintain a steady state. More recently, the term has been applied to psychological processes as well. For our purposes, homeostasis is the tendency of all living tissue to restore and maintain itself in a condition of balance or equilibrium. Emotional life, evolving as it does from the composition of the brain, is included in the concept of "all living tissue."

Though it may appear to mean "stillness," homeostasis is actually a relative state of balance maintained by the body's constant dynamic shifting and adaptation to threat. The process can be compared to the motion of a gyroscope. Standing on its point, the gyroscope appears to be still—but only because its spinning center keeps it upright (see Figure 3.1). When the movement stops, the balance is lost. So the human being, with the help of the body's internal spinnings, holds to a homeostatic balance.

In *Nature and Human Nature*, Lawrence K. Frank speaks of homeostasis as an orchestra, each organ sensitively responding to the rest to create stability. "The internal environment is like the external environment—it is continually changing, maintaining a dynamic equilibrium by larger or smaller

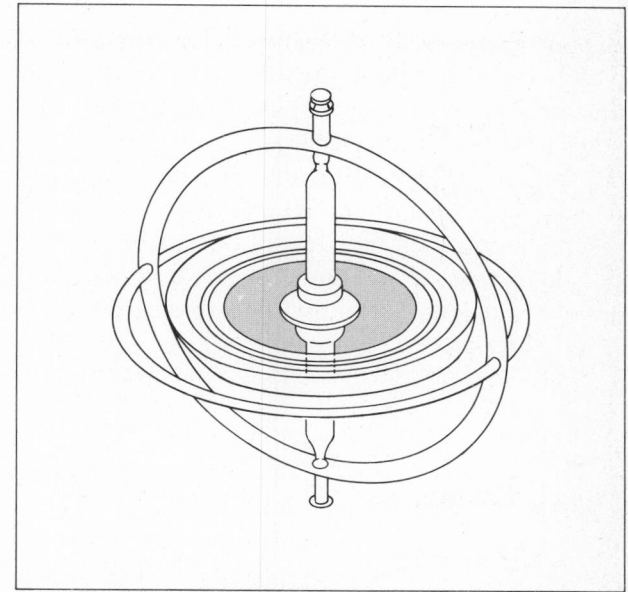

**Figure 3.1  Homeostatic balance**
Like the balance of a gyroscope, human physiological balance is maintained by the steady functioning of all parts of the body. If any of the physiological processes stops, the balance is lost.

fluctuations and sometimes by violent alterations as it continues to oscillate between the limits of living existence" (Frank, 1951).

## Homeostasis and Nursing

The concept of homeostasis is no mere academic formulation. It is directly applicable in day-to-day nursing. When you observe a patient for signs and symptoms of distress—circulatory, respiratory, psychological, and the like—you are in fact looking for signs of disequilibrium, or lack of homeostatic balance. It also becomes important when we see ourselves in relationship to homeostasis.

On an imaginary axis whose end-points are complete homeostatic imbalance (death) and perfect balance (an impossibility), you and most of your patients would register somewhere near the center (though the patient's disequilibrium would usually be greater). Both you and the patient are always in the process of attempting to correct your own homeostatic imbalances. Perhaps the essence of nursing is that you as a nurse have at your command direct and indirect ways to help restore the patient's homeostatic balance. The patient with a fever may be given medication and/or an alcohol sponging to lower body temperature. A patient in shock will probably be given blood products to promote vascular distribution and kept warm and flat to facilitate blood circulation.

With an understanding of homeostasis, you will begin to see that a patient who is in a state of disequilibrium has needs that are not being met. But do all individuals have the same needs? And are some needs more important than others to a given individual?

The human life stretches from birth to death, and we call this the *life span*. We experience an integrated life, that is, one that is made up of physical, social, sexual, cognitive, and moral components (see Chapter 4, "The Life Cycle"). Clearly, the physical homeostasis of which Cannon wrote exists, but so, too, do social, sexual, cognitive, and moral homeostasis. Homeostasis is a fluctuating balance, so that life is an ongoing effort to gain a sense of balance in each of these areas. The aim is to function optimally as individuals in life, keeping each part of our being as near homeostatic balance as possible at any particular time.

This chapter will examine universal human needs and the problems that can arise if these needs are not met. We will then consider the adaptive forces that can help a person regain homeostasis. The nurse is one of the adaptive forces.

## Human Needs

Abraham Maslow, a renowned psychologist, developed a conceptual *hierarchy of human needs* in 1943. This hierarchy is a ranking of needs, primary or physiological needs at the bottom and secondary or nonphysiological needs at the top (see Figure 3.2).

Fulfillment of basic or physiological needs is essential to survival. Only when these needs have been met can a person give attention to fulfilling such higher needs as esteem, self-actualization, knowledge, and aesthetic pleasure. For example, a patient experiencing severe difficulty in breathing invariably shows little interest in reading a favorite book. The basic need for oxygen is foremost, and not until it is met can the patient pay attention to a book. The nurse is integral to meeting patients' needs and helping them, through health teaching, emotional support, and other means, to meet their own needs.

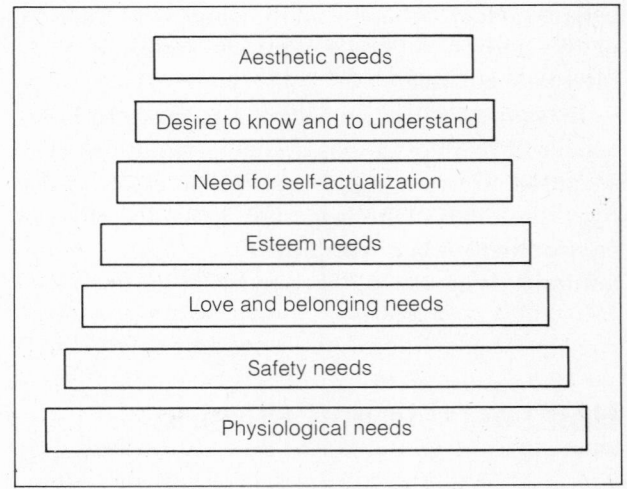

Figure 3.2  Maslow's hierarchy of needs

## Physiological Needs

Physiological needs are the physical needs inherent in all human beings, among them the needs for oxygen, food, fluids, sleep, and procreation to assure the continuation of human existence. Physiological needs are sometimes referred to as basic needs. The effects of their denial are both obvious and measurable. Physiological needs must be met at least minimally for life to continue. Below the level of subsistence, death occurs. However, even physiological needs are variable and somewhat subject to mental manipulation. For example, starving prisoners of war survived against all odds by remembering passages of literature or working mathematical problems; they were, in effect, satisfying intellectual and aesthetic needs in place of a physiological need. More commonly, people experiencing stress overeat not because the need for food is greater at a particular time but because food serves as a "reward" and partial substitute for emotional safety (Biehler, 1972).

## Safety Needs

According to Maslow, the need for safety is subordinate only to basic physiological needs. Safety is both physiological and psychological. The infant experiences safety when held securely and lovingly in the arms of a parent. A playpen too can convey physical safety and limit-setting; for a time, most young children play contentedly within such confinement. Only gradually does the child feel it is safe to venture out and explore further, and even then a perceived threat, such as the greeting of a stranger, can send the child running back to the safety of the parent.

Safety remains important to adults. We need not only a safe physical environment, a shelter, but also the feeling of psychological safety. Individuals also need to feel that their community is safe. Studies of communities threatened by disaster, such as earthquakes, fires, or nuclear accidents, have found both psychological disruption and family discord to result from threats to community safety. In order to feel psychologically safe, most of us need relatively structured lives and definite social expectations for our own be-

havior and that of others. We need freedom from separation, quarreling, disorder, and the sense of loss. To feel safe, we need regular contact with people we trust and feel close to. These people function as a system of support.

## Love and Belonging Needs

The security we gain from love and belonging enhances the feeling of safety. We also learn about ourselves from the responses of those around us. We learn what in our behavior is acceptable and what unacceptable. Our feeling of structure and security is reinforced when we know where we are in relation to others, and who we are to them. This reflection of ourselves in the eyes of others—

**Figure 3.3**
Self-esteem: serving family, job, or profession with competence. (John Goodman)

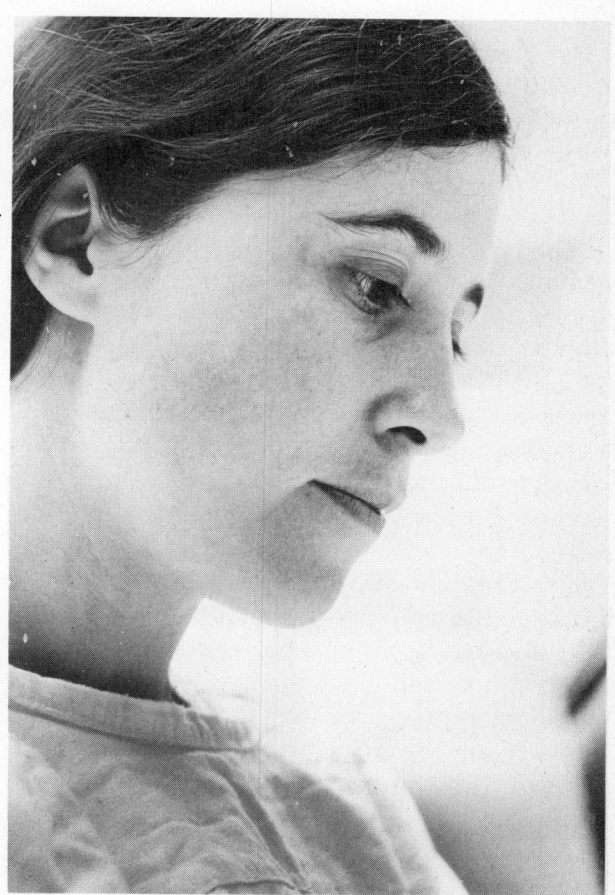

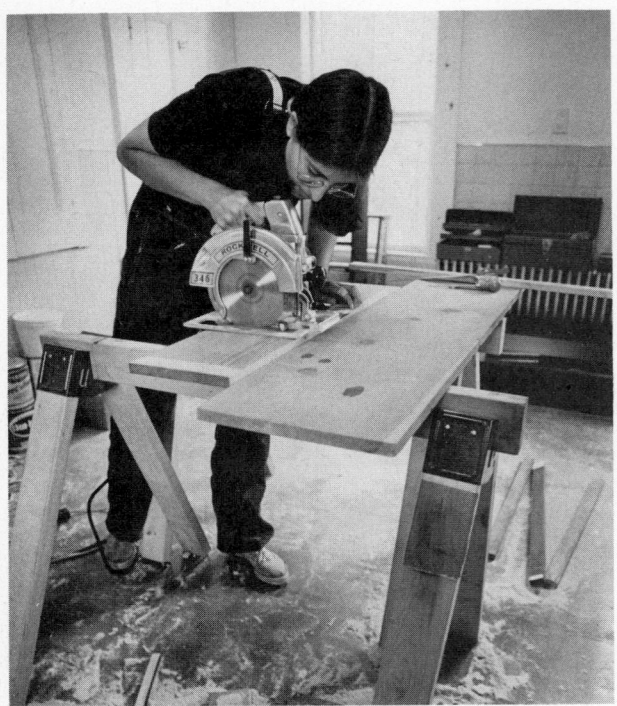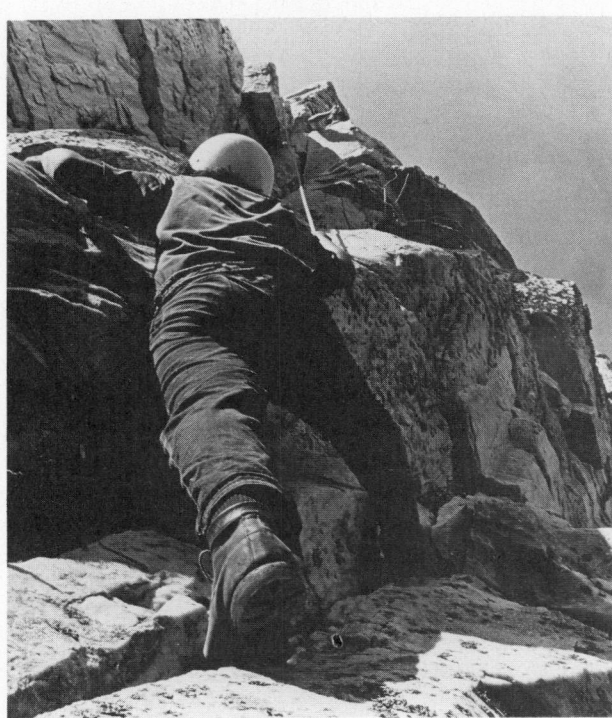

**Figure 3.4**
Self-actualization: to do in life, with joy, what one both wants and is suited to do. (*Left:* Donald C. Dietz/Stock, Boston; *right:* J. Berndt/Stock, Boston)

as well as our ability to interpret other people's selves to them—is the essence of belongingness. We all need mutually meaningful relationships with other people.

The love of which Maslow speaks is not, by definition, sexual. For some people it may be not just love of another person but devotion to a group or even a cause. For an infant or young child, on the other hand, the need for love from a mother figure is at the more elementary or physiological level. René Spitz's classic study of two groups of infants and children demonstrates this. Each group received the same high-quality physical care, but one group was talked to, fondled, and caressed, while the other group received little demonstrativeness. Not only did the children who received little love develop signs and symptoms of lassitude, withdrawal, physical ailments, and delayed development, but their mortality rate was significantly higher (Spitz, 1945).

Adults who are similarly neglected are often able to sublimate or transfer the fulfillment of their love needs to a pet, an artistic endeavor, or a charitable pursuit. Thus the need for love may be considered to exist on more than one level.

## Esteem Needs

Self-esteem is derived largely from feeling that we are valued by those around us. We feel good about ourselves when the people who are important to us express acceptance and approval. But self-esteem also comes from within; it is related to our assessments of our own adequacy, our performance and capacity in the various arenas of our lives, both personal and professional. Self-approval (that is, liking oneself) is essential.

Some people who achieve great esteem in the eyes of others lack self-esteem and try to compensate by frantically pursuing wider public recognition. Most people gain and maintain self-esteem by performing their jobs competently and contributing to the well-being of their families, professions, and communities. Some unfortunate people spend their lives in self-doubt and sadness.

## The Need for Self-Actualization

Maslow calls self-actualization "being true to oneself." More precisely, it is the effort to fulfill one's potential; to do in life, with joy, what one both wants and is suited to do. As Maslow writes, "The farmer plants and tends his crops, the nurse nurses." But to be truly self-actualized, a person must grow: the farmer takes increasing pride in the ability to grow plants, and the nurse sharpens his or her skills and experiences growing empathy with the patient. Self-actualization, then, is not confined to what one chooses to *do* in life; it also includes what one *feels*. Philosophy, morality, and religion, honestly explored, can enhance self-actualization. Though few individuals ever achieve full self-actualization, reaching for one's potential enriches life.

## The Need to Know and Understand

The striving for knowledge is an outgrowth of self-actualization. Motivated by curiosity, people seek answers to the secrets of their world. Perhaps it is this need that led us to our great advances in technology and the exploration of outer space. Opportunities for learning are more abundant today than ever before: the media expose us to masses of information, continuing education is available even in small communities, and self-programmed knowledge packets and texts are readily accessible. It is becoming increasingly commonplace for adults to pursue new horizons by returning to school or learning new skills. The need to know and understand is not necessarily related to the gratification of immediate goals; it may be its own reward.

## Aesthetic Needs

The highest level in Maslow's hierarchy of needs is the aesthetic. Highly developed in the creative artist, who creates beauty on paper or canvas, the aesthetic need can also be satisfied by appreciation of others' artistic efforts and by the cultivation of beauty and form in the details of everyday life.

## The Hierarchy of Needs as a Motivational Force

Maslow wrote about the hierarchy of needs as a motivational force, hypothesizing that the satisfaction of lower-level needs allows a person to proceed to the next highest level. Thus only someone whose physiological needs are satisfied, and who is thus in relative homeostatic balance, can pursue self-actualization.

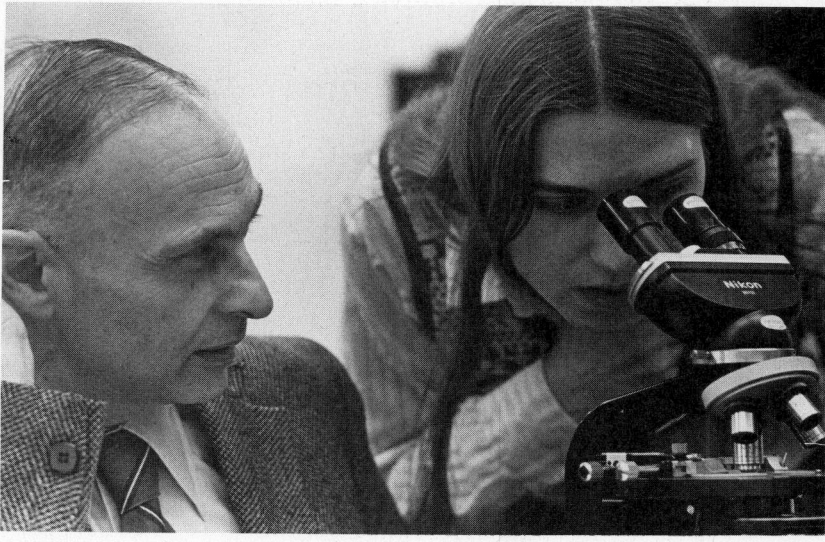

**Figure 3.5**
The striving for knowledge—an extension of self-actualization. (Chris Maynard)

Maslow's theory will be most useful to you as a nurse if you treat it as a flexible set of concepts, not a rigid one. Throughout their lifetimes, people flow up and down through the various levels, often in response to the external world. It is not uncommon for secondary needs to dominate primary physiological needs. You may go without sleep, for example, to study for an exam or finish a gripping book; a mother may go hungry to feed her children, and an artist may willingly live on very little income in order to have time for creative work.

## Needs vs. Problems

Problems are different from needs. If a need is not met, a problem arises. The problem is the situation that develops when a need is not satisfied. Let us say that the water pitcher is inadvertently placed beyond the reach of the debilitated elderly patient. The patient's *need* is for fluid; the *problem* is that the water is not accessible. Lack of water in turn creates such other problems for the patient as dry mouth, flaky skin, and general discomfort. Another example is the nurse who reports to work in the afternoon wearing a sweater, and then shivers all the way home in the evening. The need is for body warmth; the problem is inadequate clothing. When planning care, nurses often confuse needs and problems, causing nursing actions and goals to be poorly defined.

## Meeting Patients' Needs

In nursing, the distinction between needs and problems is particularly applicable to the process of assessment. Keeping in mind that immediate needs must be met before more mature needs (needs of a higher level) can arise (Peplau, 1952) can give direction to nursing care.

The guiding principle in establishing priorities for care is that you must first help the patient meet physiological needs. If a patient is very short of breath, it is not the appropriate time to discuss the importance of keeping an accurate record of intake and output. If a patient is in obvious pain, it would be similarly wise to delay teaching about a therapeutic diet. Helping patients fulfill their basic needs first makes it possible for you to assist in the fulfillment of their higher needs. In this way, you can give real service to the patient. For example, the patient whose basic needs have been met and who is in the state of recovery is ready to be consulted about plans for long-term care and the prevention of recurring illness.

You may also prevent problems by foreseeing when the fulfillment of essential needs may be threatened. Recognizing the need for full oxygenation or lung expansion after surgery, for example, you can teach the patient the techniques of coughing and deep breathing the evening before the scheduled surgery in order to avoid such postoperative problems.

## Adaptive Forces

An adaptive force is *any force, internal or external, that tends to maintain or restore homeostasis.* Those forces that are adaptive, however, can become stressors. For example, a medication meant to be an adaptive force can cause an allergic reaction, thus putting the body out of homeostatic balance.

## Internal Adaptive Forces

Internal adaptive forces are sometimes referred to as compensatory mechanisms—that is, physical or psychological mechanisms capable of bringing about shifts toward greater homeostatic balance.

The vital signs are one reflection of the internal physiologic adaptive process. When body temperature is elevated, respirations increase in an effort to better ventilate and cool the body. Body fluids and chemistries can also undergo alterations in order to compensate for disturbances. Our senses also perform as adaptive forces. As you are probably aware, sightless people usually develop heightened senses of hearing and kinesis (awareness of one's body in relation to space). Virtually all body tissues possess some capacity to help correct imbalance in another organ or body part.

Many internal adaptive forces are psychological in nature. Some are coping mechanisms, such as the ability to problem-solve and reason. For example, a young man paralyzed in an accident may choose to return to school, where he acquires not only knowledge but also self-esteem, self-confidence, and a degree of self-actualization. Mental ability thus compensates in a healthy manner for physical disability.

Various psychological defense mechanisms are internal adaptive forces—some more functional than others—that people use to protect themselves from feelings of shame, anxiety, or loss of self-esteem. These are used in our everyday life in response to our external environment as a way of coping. Two examples with which you may be familiar are denial and rationalization. Defense mechanisms will be considered in detail in Chapter 15.

## External Adaptive Forces

External adaptive forces, too, can be both physiological and psychological. Food, water, oxygen, and medications are examples of external physiological adaptive forces. Giving aspirin to a patient with an elevated temperature, for example, is an application of an external physiologic adaptive force. Meanwhile the patient's internal physiological adaptive forces, such as increased respiration and perspiration, are helping to lower body temperature.

Providing a safe and therapeutic environment for the patient also involves the application or utilization of adaptive forces, such as control of room temperature, lighting, sounds, and odors. Placing the call light within reach of the immobilized patient is a crucial external adaptive force.

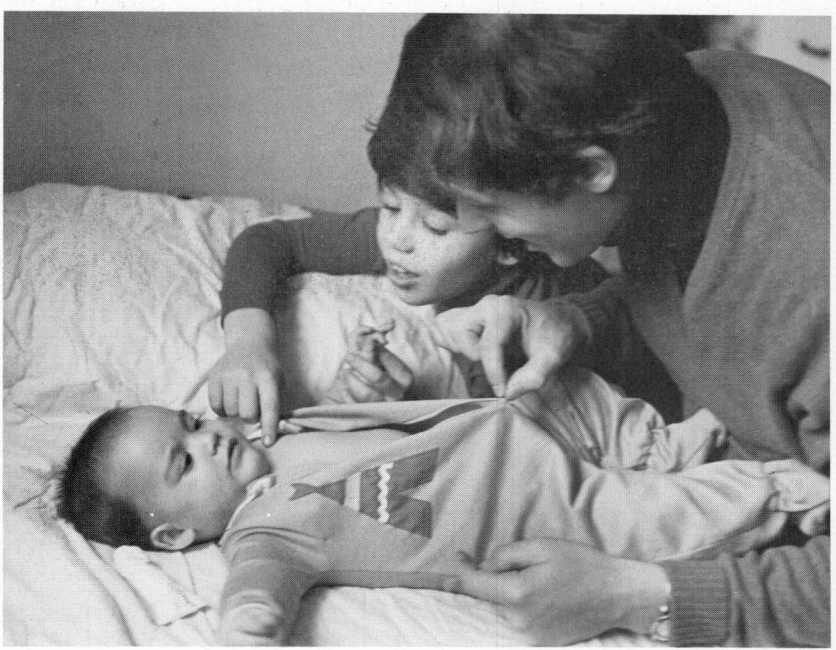

**Figure 3.6  An external adaptive force**
Alice Kandell/Photo Researchers, Inc.

An example of an external adaptive force that is primarily psychological in nature is a caring person who sits quietly and listens to the patient. Groups that provide a safe environment for belonging and personal growth may, in themselves, be an adaptive force. These may be religious or neighborhood groups. Therapy and counseling programs also belong to this category.

## The Nurse as an Adaptive Force

An adaptive force, as we have said, tends to maintain or restore homeostasis. Clearly nursing care is the application of adaptive forces to promote the patient's recovery. We bathe the patient to combat bacteria, administer drugs to bring about a variety of bodily changes, hydrate the patient to prevent fluid loss, and communicate with the patient to offset stress and loneliness. In addition, the nurse can become an adaptive force by his or her approach to the patient. The phenomenon known as the *placebo effect* will shed light on this point (Beecher, 1955).

Though originally applied exclusively to the administering of medications, the concept of the placebo effect has since been broadened in scope. Patients experiencing chronic physiological pain were requesting medication at intervals so frequent as to be dangerous. These patients were having real, physiological pain. Unbeknown to the patient, an inert substance identical in appearance to the prescribed pain medication was sometimes administered, either by mouth or by injection. Though they had received no active substance, a number of patients reported relief of pain. This effect, which evidently has to do with the manner in which the "medication" was delivered and the trust with which it was received, has been termed the placebo effect. Some nurses proved more successful than others at inducing the placebo effect.

In recent years, the increased use of placebos in chronic pain treatment centers has raised ethical issues. Is it right to "fool" patients, even if the results are beneficial? Fortunately, studies show that even with complete disclosure (informing the patient that an active drug will be administered at some times and a placebo at others) placebos are still often effective (Munson, 1979).

The concept of the placebo effect has also been applied to expectations of outcome: patients who are expected to do well, participate in their care, and recover uneventfully often seem to do so, while patients whose outcomes are perceived negatively often respond poorly. This is not to say that health-care providers control the patient's outcome but to underline the power of suggestion (Cousins, 1980). Dr. Albert Schweitzer explained the success of an African witch doctor this way: "The witch doctor succeeds for the same reason all the rest of us succeed. Each patient carries his own doctor inside him. . . . We are at our best when we give the doctor who resides within each patient a chance to go to work" (Cousins, 1980).

## Conclusion

An understanding of homeostasis and human needs is a crucial tool for the nurse. Problems arise from unmet needs, which are the basis of nursing diagnosis and care planning. When the patient's adaptive forces and those of the nurse and other care givers are effectively mobilized, the patient becomes healthier and functions better. Just as no two patients are alike, no condition remains static. Meeting the needs and problems you help define is a challenge you face as a practitioner.

## Study Terms

adaptive forces
  internal adaptive
    forces
  external adaptive
    forces
aesthetic needs
defense mechanisms
esteem needs
hierarchy of needs
homeostasis
love and belonging
  needs
need to know and
  understand
physiological needs
placebo effect
problem

safety needs
self-actualization

## Learning Activities

1. Select a patient in the clinical area as an example. What specific problems do you see as arising from that person's unfulfilled needs? Outline the nursing actions you might undertake to meet those needs.

2. Identify what you see as your primary and secondary needs. Compare these with Maslow's hierarchy of needs. Are they in the same or in a different order?

3. In a clinical or discussion group, have each member select a different age and outline the primary needs of a person at that age. Compare and contrast what each member has identified. Compare the group's views with Maslow's.

## References

Anthony, Catherine Parker, and Thibodeau, Gary A. *Textbook of Anatomy and Physiology*. St. Louis: C. V. Mosby, 1979.

Barach, A. L. "Homeostasis: A Physiologic and Psychologic Function in Man," *Perspectives in Biology and Medicine* 17 (Summer 1974): 522.

Beecher, Henry K. "The Powerful Placebo," *Journal of the American Medical Association* 159, 24 December 1955: 1602–1606.

Biehler, R. F. *Psychology Applied to Teaching: Selected Readings*. Boston: Houghton Mifflin, 1972.

Cannon, W. B. "Some General Features of Endocrine Influence on Metabolism," *American Journal of Medical Science* 171 (1926): 1–20.

Cousins, Norman. *Anatomy of an Illness*. New York: W. W. Norton, 1980.

Frank, L. K. *Nature and Human Nature*. New Brunswick, N.J.: Rutgers University Press, 1951.

Levine, M. E. "Holistic Nursing," *Nursing Clinics of North America* 6 (June 1971): 253.

Maslow, A. H. "A Theory of Human Motivation," *Psychological Review* 50 (1943).

Maslow, A. H. *Motivation and Personality*, 2nd ed. New York: Harper & Row, 1970.

Munson, Ronald. *Intervention and Reflection: Basic Issues in Medical Ethics*. Belmont, Cal.: Wadsworth, 1979.

Peplau, Hildegarde E. *Interpersonal Relations in Nursing*. New York: G. P. Putnam's Sons, 1952.

Spitz, René. "Hospitalism: Inquiry into Genesis of Psychiatric Conditions in Early Childhood." *Psychoanalytic Study of the Child* 1 (1945).

Wu, R. *Behavior and Illness*. Englewood Cliffs, N.J.: Prentice-Hall, 1973.

# Chapter 4
# The Life Cycle

## Objectives

After completing this chapter, you should be able to:
1. Briefly discuss the theories of Erikson, Freud, Piaget, and Kohlberg.
2. Outline the human life cycle, describing (a) physical, (b) psychosocial, (c) psychosexual, (d) cognitive, and (e) moral development at each stage.
3. List four reasons why nurses need a basic knowledge of the life cycle.
4. Describe how responses to illness change at the various stages of the life cycle.

## Outline

Prenatal Influences
Theories of the Life Cycle
    Physical / Psychosocial: Erik Erikson / Psychosexual: Sigmund Freud / Cognitive: Jean Piaget / Moral: Lawrence Kohlberg
Infancy: Birth to One Year
    Physical Development / Psychosocial Development / Psychosexual Development / Cognitive Development / Moral Development
The Toddler: One to Three
    Physical Development / Psychosocial Development / Psychosexual Development / Cognitive Development / Moral Development
Early Childhood: Three to Six
    Physical Development / Psychosocial Development / Psychosexual Development / Cognitive Development / Moral Development
Middle Childhood: Six to Twelve
    Physical Development / Psychosocial Development / Psychosexual Development / Cognitive Development / Moral Development

Adolescence: Twelve to Eighteen
    Physical Development / Psychosocial Development / Psychosexual Development / Cognitive Development / Moral Development
Young Adulthood: Eighteen to Forty
    Physical Development / Psychosocial Development / Psychosexual Development / Cognitive Development / Moral Development
The Middle Years: Forty to Sixty-Five
    Physical Development / Psychosocial Development / Psychosexual Development / Cognitive Development / Moral Development
The Later Years: Over Sixty-Five
    Physical Development / Psychosocial Development / Psychosexual Development / Cognitive Development / Moral Development
The Life Cycle and Nursing Practice
    The Infant / The Toddler / The Preschooler / The School-Age Child / The Adolescent / The Young Adult / The Middle Years / The Later Years

One of the most fascinating aspects of nursing is the variety of patients we care for, from newborns through the very aged. The progression from birth to death is called the *life span* or *life cycle*. In order to understand patients as individuals and to be fully responsive to each patient's needs, the nurse needs thorough familiarity with physical, psychosocial, psychosexual, cognitive, and moral development at the various stages of the life cycle.

*Physical* development is the growth of body systems and tissue and the functioning of the physical self. *Psychosocial* development is the emotional and mental adjustment a person makes to his or her environment and experiences; *psychosexual* development is the emotional development of the sexual instinct. *Cognitive* development involves thinking and other intellectual activity. *Moral* development specifies learning the accepted behavior of the culture in which the person lives.

Just as no two individuals have identical fingerprints, no two human beings develop identically. It is thus more appropriate to speak of *usual* than of *normal* development, since the term *normal* has come to suggest a relatively rigid standard. Knowing what is usual for an age group enables the nurse to identify and assess what is unusual. It is the unusual that may indicate problems.

Many theorists have devoted their attention to tracing particular aspects of individual development, such as the psychosocial. Applied prudently, their insights can contribute usefully to an integrated view of the individual throughout the life cycle.

The work of four researchers in human development has proven particularly enlightening. In the context of a given stage in the life cycle, we shall examine the work of Erik Erikson on psychosocial development, Sigmund Freud on psychosexual development, Jean Piaget on cognitive development, and Lawrence Kohlberg on moral development.

Our presentation of theories of development in terms of age categories is in no way intended to promote rigid expectations with regard to patients' growth and development. It is important to keep in mind, for example, that although most people in their early thirties are involved in an ongoing relationship with another person, and may have small children, others of the same age may be postponing or forgoing such a primary relationship or a family in order to devote their full energies to their careers.

## Prenatal Influences

The life cycle of every individual is influenced by factors determined before birth, or *prenatally*. Some of these factors are understood thoroughly, some only partially, and others remain to be investigated by geneticists.

A newborn infant's inherited characteristics derive from the genetic heritage of both parents. The infant is not a mere mixture of the parents' characteristics; he or she may inherit characteristics the parents do not manifest but that are carried in their genes. Genetic defects can occur in the development of the *fetus*, or unborn child. An example is a condition called *Trisomy 21*, formerly known as Down's syndrome, characterized by low-set ears, skin folds around the eyes, a flattened bridge of the nose, and a degree of mental retardation. Tendencies toward certain diseases can also be inherited; examples are diabetes, heart disease, and hypertension (high blood pressure).

*Congenital* defects are those present at birth but not inherited. Certain viral infections contracted by the mother early in pregnancy can lead to malformation or death of the fetus. An example is rubella (German measles). It has long been recognized that poor nutrition and poor health on the part of the mother affect the health of the infant. Among the other factors now under scrutiny are tobacco, alcohol, and other drugs: babies exposed to these substances through the placenta may tend to be of low birth weight, less vigorous neuromuscularly, and at high risk for cardiac and respiratory problems. Drug and alcohol withdrawal symptoms have been observed in infants of drug- and alcohol-dependent mothers. According to the

National Institute of Drug Abuse, in 1977 alone, 4,742 infants were born to drug-addicted mothers.

The influences on the unborn fetus of such environmental factors as air pollution and toxic chemicals in the parents' workplace are now under investigation. Environmental genetic research is a new field, and there are probably unpleasant surprises ahead with regard to prenatal influence, as well as new discoveries of ways to avoid or minimize birth defects.

# Theories of the Life Cycle

## Physical

Physical changes result from both growth and maturation. The *growth* of a body part or organ is an increase in size and weight, primarily because of cell division. *Maturation*, or development, on the other hand, is refinement or change in the function of a body part or organ. Attaining maturity requires growth, development, and more effective functioning.

Fifty years ago, growth and development were viewed in primarily physical terms, partly because physical measurement was easier than measurement of intellectual and emotional growth. However, the value of such studies was limited because they excluded the social, sexual, cognitive, and moral components of the individual.

More recent studies of growth and development allow for a more inclusive approach. Measurement has become far more sophisticated and flexible. The Denver Developmental Screening Test (Frankenberg and Dodds, 1969), for example, measures the performance of children through the age of six in four areas: personal-social, fine motor adaptive, language, and gross motor. The test notes behavioral responses, such as "responsive smiling" or "hops on one foot." Another excellent measurement tool, designed by the Child Evaluation Clinic of Cedar Rapids, Iowa (Block, 1972), appears as Table 4.1. The test evaluates a child's motor skills, language skills, and personal-social adaptation monthly through the first year, every three months through the second year, and every six-months until the fourth year, ending with usual behavior in the fifth year. A thorough reading of Table 4.1 will provide you with an integrated view of these formative years.

Table 4.1
**Child Development from One Month to Five Years**

### 1 month

*Motor*
1. Moro reflex present.
2. Vigorous sucking reflex present.
3. Lying prone (face down): lifts head briefly so chin is off table.
4. Lying prone: makes crawling movements with legs.
5. Held in sitting position: back is rounded, head held up momentarily only.
6. Hands tightly fisted.
7. Reflex grasp of object with palm.

*Language*
8. Startled by sound; quieted by voice.
9. Small throaty noises or vocalizations.

*Personal-social-adaptive*
10. Ringing bell produces decrease of activity.
11. May follow dangling object with eyes to midline.
12. Lying on back: will briefly look at examiner or change his activity.
13. Reacts with generalized body movements when tissue paper is placed on face.

### 2 months

*Motor*
1. Kicks vigorously.
2. Energetic arm movements.
3. Vigorous head turning.
4. Held in ventral suspension (prone): no head droop.
5. Lying prone: lifts head so face makes an approximate 45° angle with table.
6. Held in sitting position: head erect but bobs.
7. Hand goes to mouth.
8. Hand often open (not clenched)

## Table 4.1
## Child Development from One Month to Five Years (*continued*)

*Language*
9. Is cooing.
10. Vocalizes single vowel sounds, such as: ah-eh-uh.

*Personal-social-adaptive*
11. Head and eyes search for sound.

12. Listens to bell ringing.
13. Follows dangling object past midline.
14. Alert expression.
15. Follows moving person with eyes.
16. Smiles back when talked to.

### 3 months

*Motor*
1. Lying prone: lifts head to 90° angle.
2. Lifts head when lying on back (supine).
3. Moro reflex begins to disappear.
4. Grasp reflex nearly gone.
5. Rolls side to back (3–4 months).

*Language*
6. Chuckling, squealing, grunting, especially when talked to.
7. Listens to music.
8. Vocalizes with two different syllables, such as: a-a, la-la (not distinct), oo-oo.

*Personal-social-adaptive*
9. Reaches for but misses objects.
10. Holds toy with active grasp when put into hand.
11. Sucks and inspects fingers.
12. Pulls at clothes.
13. Follows object (toy) side to side (and 180°).
14. Looks predominantly at examiner.
15. Glances at toy when put into hand.
16. Recognizes mother and bottle.
17. Smiles spontaneously.

### 4 months

*Motor*
1. Sits when well supported.
2. No head lag when pulled to sitting position.
3. Turns head at sound of voice.
4. Lifts head (in supine position) in effort to sit.
5. Lifts head and chest when prone, using hands and forearms.
6. Held erect: pushes feet against table.

*Language*
7. Laughs aloud (4–5 months).

8. Uses sound, such as: m-p-b.
9. Repeats series of same sounds.

*Personal-social-adaptive*
10. Grasps rattle.
11. Plays with own fingers.
12. Reaches for object in front of him with both hands.
13. Transfers object from hand to hand.
14. Pulls dress over face.
15. Smiles spontaneously at people.
16. Regards raisin (or pellet).

### 5 months

*Motor*
1. Moro reflex gone.
2. Rolls side to side.
3. Rolls back to front.
4. Full head control when pulled to or held in sitting position.
5. Briefly supports most of his weight on his legs.
6. Scratches on table top.

*Language*
7. Squeals with high voice.

8. Recognizes familiar voices
9. Coos and/or stops crying on hearing music.

*Personal-social-adaptive*
10. Grasps dangling object.
11. Reaches for toy with both hands.
12. Smiles at mirror image.
13. Turns head deliberately to bell.
14. Obviously enjoys being played with.

### 6 months

*Motor*
1. Supine: lifts head spontaneously.
2. Bounces on feet when held standing.
3. Sits briefly (tripod fashion).
4. Rolls front to back (6–7 months).
5. Grasps foot and plays with toes.
6. Grasps cube with palm.

*Language*
7. Vocalizes at mirror image.
8. Makes four or more different sounds.
9. Localizes source of sound (bell, voice).

10. Vague, formless babble (especially with family members).

*Personal-social-adaptive*
11. Holds one cube in each hand.
12. Puts cube into mouth.
13. Re-secures dropped cube.
14. Transfers cube from hand to hand.
15. Conscious of strange sights and persons.
16. Consistent regard of object or person (6–7 months).
17. Uses raking movement to secure raisin or pellet.
18. Resists having toy taken away from him.
19. Stretches out arms to be taken up (6–8 months).

## Table 4.1
## Child Development from One Month to Five Years (*continued*)

### 8 months

*Motor*

1. Sits alone (6–8 months).
2. Early stepping movements.
3. Tries to crawl.
4. Stands few seconds, holding on to object.
5. Leans forward to get an object.

*Language*

6. Two-syllable babble, such as: a-la, ba-ba, oo-goo, a-ma, mama, dada (8–10 months).
7. Listens to conversation (8–10 months).
8. "Shouts" for attention (8–10 months).

*Personal-social-adaptive*

9. Works to get toy out of reach.
10. Scoops pellet.
11. Rings bell purposely (8–10 months).
12. Drinks from cup.
13. Plays peek-a-boo.
14. Looks for dropped object.
15. Bites and chews toys.
16. Pats mirror image.
17. Bangs spoon on table.
18. Manipulates paper or string.
19. Secures ring by pulling on the string.
20. Feeds self crackers.

### 10 months

*Motor*

1. Gets self into sitting position.
2. Sits steadily (long time).
3. Pulls self to standing position (on bed railing).
4. Crawls on hands and knees.
5. Walks when held or around furniture.
6. Turns around when left on floor.

*Language*

7. Imitates speech sounds.
8. Shakes head for "no."
9. Waves "bye-bye."
10. Responds to name.
11. Vocalizes in varied jargon-patterns (10–12 months).

*Personal-social-adaptive*

12. Plays "pat-a-cake."
13. Picks up pellet with finger and thumb.
14. Bangs toys together.
15. Extends toy to a person.
16. Holds own bottle.
17. Removes cube from cup.
18. Drops one cube to get another.
19. Uses handle to lift cup.
20. Initially shy with strangers.

### 1 year

*Motor*

1. Walks with one hand held.
2. Stands alone (or with support)
3. Secures small object with good pincer grasp.
4. Pivots in sitting position.
5. Grasps two cubes in one hand.

*Language*

6. Uses "mama" or "dada" with specific meaning.
7. "Talks" to toys and people, using fairly long verbal patterns.
8. Has vocabulary of two words besides "mama" and "dada."
9. Babbles to self when alone.
10. Obeys simple requests, such as: "Give me the cup."
11. Reacts to music.

*Personal-social-adaptive*

12. Cooperates with dressing.
13. Plays with cup, spoon, saucer.
14. Points with index finger.
15. Pokes finger (into stethoscope) to explore.
16. Releases toy into your hand.
17. Tries to take cube out of box.
18. Unwraps a cube.
19. Holds cup to drink.
20. Holds crayon.
21. Tries to imitate scribble.
22. Imitates beating two cubes together.
23. Gives affection.

### 15 months

*Motor*

1. Stands alone.
2. Creeps upstairs.
3. Kneels on floor or chair.
4. Gets off floor and walks alone with good balance.
5. Bends over to pick up toy without holding on to furniture.

*Language*

6. May speak four to six words (15–18 months).
7. Uses jargon.
8. Indicates wants by vocalizing.
9. Knows own name.
10. Enjoys rhymes or jingles.

*Personal-social-adaptive*

11. Tilts cup to drink.
12. Uses spoon but spills.
13. Builds tower of two cubes.
14. Drops cubes into cup.
15. Helps turn page in book, pats picture.
16. Shows or offers toy.

Table 4.1
## Child Development from One Month to Five Years (*continued*)

17. Helps pull off clothes.
18. Puts pellet into bottle without demonstration.

19. Opens lid of box.
20. Likes to push wheeled toys.

### 18 months

*Motor*
1. Runs (stiffly).
2. Walks upstairs—one hand held.
3. Walks backwards.
4. Climbs into chair.
5. Hurls ball.

*Language*
6. May say 6 to 10 words (18–21 months).
7. Points to at least one body part.
8. Can say "hello" and "thank you."
9. Carries out two directions (one at a time), for instance: "Get ball from table."—"Give ball to mother."

10. Identifies two objects by pointing (or picking up) such as: cup, spoon, dog, car, chair.

*Personal-social-adaptive*
11. Turns pages.
12. Builds tower of three to four cubes.
13. Puts 10 cubes into cup.
14. Carries or hugs a doll.
15. Takes off shoes and socks.
16. Pulls string toy.
17. Scribbles spontaneously.
18. Dumps raisin from bottle after demonstration.
19. Uses spoon with little spilling.

### 21 months

*Motor*
1. Runs well.
2. Walks downstairs—one hand held.
3. Walks upstairs alone or holding on to rail.
4. Kicks large ball (when demonstrated.)

*Language*
5. May speak 15–20 words (21–24 months).
6. May combine two to three words.
7. Asks for food, drink.
8. Echoes two or more words.
9. Takes three directions (one at a time), for instance:

"Take ball from table." "Give ball to Mommy."—"Put ball on floor."
10. Points to three or more body parts.

*Personal-social-adaptive*
11. Builds tower to five to six cubes.
12. Folds paper once when shown.
13. Helps with simple household tasks (21–24 months).
14. Removes some clothing purposefully (besides hat or socks).
15. Pulls person to show something.

### 2 years

*Motor*
1. Runs without falling.
2. Walks up and down stairs.
3. Kicks large ball (without demonstration).
4. Throws ball overhand.
5. Claps hands.
6. Opens door.
7. Turns pages in book, singly.

*Language*
8. Says simple phrases.
9. Says at least one sentence or phrase of four or more syllables.
10. Can repeat four to five syllables.
11. May reproduce about 5–6 consonant sounds. (Typically: m-p-b-h-w.)

12. Points to four parts of body on command.
13. Asks for things at table by name.
14. Refers to self by name.
15. May use personal pronouns, such as: I-me-you (2–2½ years).

*Personal-social-adaptive*
16. Builds five to seven cube tower.
17. May cut with scissors.
18. Spontaneously dumps raisin from bottle (without demonstration).
19. Throws ball into box.
20. Imitates drawing vertical line from demonstration.
21. Parallel play predominant.

### 2½ years

*Motor*
1. Jumps in place with both feet.
2. Tries standing on one foot (may not be successful).
3. Holds crayon by fingers.
4. Imitates walking on tiptoe.

*Language*
5. Refers to self by pronoun (rather than name).
6. Names common objects when asked (key, penny, shoe, box, book).

7. Repeats two digits (one of three trials).
8. Answers simple questions, such as: "What is this?"— "What does the kitty say?"

*Personal-social-adaptive*
9. Builds tower of eight cubes.
10. Pushes toy with good steering.
11. Helps put things away.

Table 4.1
**Child Development from One Month to Five Years (*continued*)**

12. Can carry breakable objects.
13. Puts on clothing.
14. Washes and dries hands.

15. Eats with fork.
16. Imitates drawing a horizontal line from demonstration.
17. May imitate drawing a circle from demonstration.

### 3 years

1. Stands on one foot for at least one second.
2. Jumps from bottom stair.
3. Alternates feet going upstairs.
4. Pours from a pitcher.
5. Can undo two buttons.
6. Pedals a tricycle.

*Language*

7. Repeats six syllables, for instance: "I have a little dog."
8. Names three or more objects in a picture.
9. Gives sex. ("Are you a boy or a girl?")
10. Gives full name.
11. Repeats three digits (one of three trials).
12. Knows a few rhymes.
13. Gives appropriate answers to: "What: swims-flies-shoots-boils-bites-melts?"

14. Uses plurals.
15. Knows at least one color.
16. Can reply to questions in at least three word sentences.
17. May have vocabulary of 750 to 1,000 words (3–3½ years).

*Personal-social-adaptive*

18. Understands taking turns.
19. Copies a circle (from model, without demonstration).
20. Builds three-block pyramid.
21. Dresses with supervision.
22. Puts 10 pellets into bottle in 30 seconds.
23. Separates easily from mother.
24. Feeds self well.
25. Plays interactive games, such as "tag."

### 4 years

*Motor*

1. Stands on one foot for a least five seconds (two of three trials).
2. Hops at least twice on one foot.
3. Can walk heel-to-toe for four or more steps (with heel one inch or less in front of toe).
4. Can button coat or dress; may lace shoes.

*Language*

4. Repeats ten-word sentences without errors.
6. Counts three objects, pointing correctly.
7. Repeats three to four digits (4–5 years).
8. Comprehends: "What do you do if: you are hungry, sleepy, cold?"
9. Spontaneous sentences, four to five words long.
10. Likes to ask questions.

11. Understands preposition, such as: on-under-behind, etc. ("Put the block *on* the table.")
12. Can point to three out of four colors (red, blue, green, yellow).
13. Speech is now an effective communicative tool.

*Personal-social-adaptive*

14. Copies cross (+) without demonstration.
15. Imitates oblique cross (×).
16. Draws a man with four parts.
17. Cooperates with other children in play.
18. Dresses and undresses self (mostly without supervision).
19. Brushes teeth, washes face.
20. Compares lines: "Which is longer?"
21. Folds paper two to three times.
22. Can select heavier from lighter object.
23. Cares for self at toilet.

### 5 years

*Motor*

1. Balances on one foot for eight to ten seconds.
2. Skips, using feet alternatively.
3. May be able to tie a knot.
4. Catches bounced ball with hands (not arms) in two of three trials.

*Language*

5. Knows age ("How old are you?").
6. Performs three tasks (with one command), for instance: "Put pen on table—close door—bring me the ball."
7. Knows four colors.
8. Defines use for: fork-horse-key-pencil, etc.
9. Identifies by name: nickel-dime-penny.
10. Asks meaning of words.
11. Asks many "why" questions.

12. Relatively few speech errors remain—90% of consonant sounds are made correctly.
13. Counts number of fingers correctly.
14. Counts by rote to 10.
15. Comments on pictures (descriptions and interpretations).

*Personal-social-adaptive*

16. Copies a square.
17. Copies oblique cross (×) without demonstration.
18. May print a few letters (5–5½ years).
19. Draws man with at least six identifiable parts.
20. Builds a six-block pyramid from demonstration.
21. Transports things in a wagon.
22. Plays with coloring set, construction toys, puzzles.
23. Participates well in group play.

Walter M. Block, M.D., and Jean Fitzgerald, Ph.D., Child Evaluation Clinic of Cedar Rapids, Iowa, 1972.

Physical growth and development is uneven. Until about the age of two, neuromuscular motor development proceeds from control of the head gradually downward to the feet. For example, a child can throw a ball from the sitting position before he or she can walk. This sequence is called *cephalocaudal development*. The physical growth of body parts is also disproportionate, or *asynchronous*. By the age of two, the weight of the brain and circumference of the head approximate that of the adult. The skeletal system and muscles grow rapidly from infancy to adulthood, experiencing particularly vigorous growth during adolescence.

All growth and development is characterized by *plateaus*, or periods when change is slow or apparently nonexistent. The pace of growth and development is influenced by genetic background, general health, nutrition, glandular hormones, and psychological well-being.

## Psychosocial: Erik Erikson

In *Childhood and Society* (1950), child psychiatrist Erik H. Erikson describes the human life cycle as composed of eight stages, each accompanied by a characteristic "crisis," with a hoped-for or ex-

Table 4.2
**Stages of the Life Cycle (Erikson)**

| Stage | Age | Crisis | Significant persons | Tasks | Typical response to illness |
|---|---|---|---|---|---|
| **Infancy** | 0–1 | Trust vs. mistrust | Mother or mother substitute | Expressing frustrations. Dependence on mother. | Physiological irritation. Fear of environment. |
| **Toddler** | 1–3 | Autonomy vs. shame and doubt | Parents | Speech. Walking. Assertion of wishes. Beginning the postponement of pleasure. | Fear of threats to the body and painful procedures. Stress of separation from mother. |
| **Early childhood** | 3–6 | Initiative vs. guilt | Entire family | Enlargement of vocabulary. Interaction with total family group. Beginning of peer involvement. | Equation of illness with being bad. Guilt. |
| **Middle childhood** | 6–12 | Industry vs. inferiority | School and neighborhood | Increased physical activity. Competitiveness. Dealing with authority in the school environment. | Anger over restrictions due to illness. Guilt over causing family crisis. |
| **Adolescence** | 12–18 | Identity vs. role confusion | Peers, national leadership models | Independence from family. Strong influence of peer group. Becoming sexually active. Beginning to choose life goals. | Anger over dependency due to illness. |
| **Young adulthood** | 18–40 | Intimacy vs. isolation | Intimates, usually of opposite sex | Carrying out life plans. Choosing a mate. Selecting a life's work. | Fear of possible change in the intimacy relationship. Depression over the interruption of plans. |
| **Middle years** | 40–65 | Generativity vs. stagnation | Expanded family, institutions | Forming ideas and plans for the next generation. Carrying out life goals. Assessment. | Depression over the interruption of work and separation from family. |
| **Later years** | 65– | Integrity vs. despair | Those who promote sense of usefulness | Life review. Finding satisfactions. Setting new goals for retirement. Sharing knowledge with others. | Feelings of no longer being useful. Fear of threat to life. Despair. |

pected outcome or an unfavorable outcome that could result if certain conditions for growth are absent (see Table 4.2). Unlike Freud and Piaget, both of whom treat sexual and cognitive development as virtually complete at puberty, Erikson considers psychosocial development a life-long process. Successful resolution of each crisis is necessary to optimal functioning at later stages. Whether a person experiences a positive or a negative resolution depends primarily, though not exclusively, on interaction with the world in general and with "significant persons." In a sense, then, the subject of Erikson's early writings is what we now call "conflict resolution."

Among the aspects of Erikson's theory with particular pertinence to nursing are his emphasis on the importance of new growth experiences at all ages, the value of the older person sharing skill and knowledge with the young (generativity), and of the effects of caring sensitively for those with whom we interact.

## Psychosexual: Sigmund Freud

Psychosexual development was first systematically described by Sigmund Freud (1856–1939), originally an outstanding neurophysiologist. Freud postulated that much of our mental life occurs outside our awareness, in the part of the mind he called the *unconscious*. The human mind, according to Freud, has three main components: the *id*, motivated by primitive needs and impulses toward gratification and pleasure; the *ego*, the expressive self that consciously controls behavior and pursues goals and interprets reality; and the *superego*, or conscience. The ego is the force that mediates between the id and the superego.

Freud also strongly emphasizes the importance of sexual development, postulating that many adult psychological problems are rooted in failure to resolve sexual conflicts at earlier stages of development (see Table 4.3). Successful resolution allows the individual to achieve a mature sexual identity and a stable emotional life. His writings remain relevant in the area, although they were later modified by colleagues such as Jung and Adler. An unfortunate limitation to Freud's work is that it does not address the sexual development of the later adolescent.

### Table 4.3
### Psychosexual Stages (Freud)

| Age | Stages |
|---|---|
| Birth to 1 year | *Oral Stage* Mouth region provides greatest sensual satisfaction. Unfortunate experiences causing a fixation at this level may lead to greed and possessiveness or verbal aggressiveness. |
| 2–3 years | *Anal Stage* Anal and urethral areas provide greatest sensual satisfaction. Unfortunate experiences causing a fixation at this level may lead to messiness, extreme cleanliness, or frugality. |
| 3–4 years | *Phallic Stage* Genital region provides greatest sensual satisfaction. Unfortunate experiences causing a fixation at this level may lead to inappropriate sex roles. |
| 4–5 years | *Oedipal Stage* Parent of opposite sex is taken as object of sensual satisfaction—which leads to tendency to regard same-sexed parent as a rival. Unfortunate experiences causing a fixation at this level may lead to competitiveness. |
| 6–11 years | *Latency Period* Resolution of Oedipus complex by identifying with parent of opposite sex and satisfying sensual needs vicariously. |
| 11–14 years | *Puberty* Integration of sensual tendencies from previous stages into unitary and overriding genital sexuality. |

Robert F. Biehler, *Psychology Applied to Teaching*, 2nd edition. Copyright © 1974 by Houghton Mifflin Company. Adapted by permission.

## Cognitive: Jean Piaget

*Jean Piaget*, a Swiss educator and psychologist and a contemporary of Erikson, describes the life cycle in terms of cognitive or intellectual processes. Beginning in infancy, according to Piaget, human beings organize information into coherent systems of thought that determine how they interpret and adapt to their environment. The process by which information is absorbed Piaget calls *assimilation*. When new information conflicts with existing perceptions, adjustments or *accommodations* must be made in one's thinking in order to understand both familiar and new information. The process by which such accommodations are made, which Piaget calls *equilibration*, involves making apparently contradictory information consistent and returning to a state of mental comfort. Piaget considers intellectual growth at all ages to be dependent

## Table 4.4
### Stages of Intellectual Development

| Stage and age | Characteristics |
|---|---|
| **Sensorimotor (birth–2 years)** | Learning about properties of things through senses and motor activity. Eventual development of new ways of dealing with situations. |
| **Preoperational (2–7 years)** | Mastery of symbols, permitting mental manipulation of symbols and objects. Acquisition of language that is *egocentric*—words have a unique meaning to each child, which limits ability to consider others' points of view. Gradual acquisition of ability to *decenter* (think of more than one quality at a time) and understand *conservation*. |
| **Concrete operational (7–11 years)** | Ability to conserve, decenter, and reverse, but only with reference to concrete objects. Capacity to mentally manipulate concrete experiences that previously had to be physically manipulated. Ability to deal with *operations*—interiorized actions involving reversibility—but not to generalize beyond actual experience. |
| **Formal operational (11 years and above)** | Ability to think about unseen objects and abstractions. Greater interest in possibilities than realities. Capacity to imagine various future alternatives and of developing hypotheses. |

Robert F. Biehler, *Psychology Applied to Teaching*, 2nd edition. Copyright © 1974 by Houghton Mifflin Company. Adapted by permission.

on these processes by which experience is transformed into concepts (see Table 4.4).

The very young child, age two and under, primarily uses his or her senses to ascertain the properties of objects; by handling a ball, for example, the child experiences roundness. Piaget called this period the *sensorimotor stage*.

Between ages two and seven, the child is at the *preoperational stage*. Piaget describes this stage as characterized by egocentrism and centering. *Egocentrism* is perceiving oneself as the central focus of all experience. At this stage physical objects and other people are seen as directly associated to oneself; for example, the child may expect others to be aware of his or her unexpressed thoughts. *Centering* is inability to see beyond the immediate aspects of a situation. For example, at this age a child

cannot understand that a painful injection will clear up an infection. Rather, the immediate experience is predominant. Egocentrism and centering are natural components of this stage.

Reasoning, imagery, and representation become part of the cognitive process at this stage. The child can mentally picture a ball and compare the letter O to a ball. If an orange is mentioned, the child thinks of its shape.

The *concrete operational stage* usually begins around age seven and continues until eleven or so. The child is able to carry his or her knowledge of the specific ball we have been describing to a state of what Piaget calls *reversibility*. That is, if an orange were cut into pieces, the older child could mentally envision it as it once was, or reverse the image. The child is able to perform acts or "operations" on specific objects in such a way as to begin to understand how the physical environment works.

Finally, at about the age of eleven, the child progresses to the *formal operational stage* of cognitive development. Abstract thought is now possible: for example, the child can think about the roundness of the planets and can understand an analogy comparing the relative sizes of the earth and the sun to the sizes of a cherry and an orange. Piaget offers us as nurses a valuable viewpoint of the evolving intellectual capacity of the individual.

## Moral: Lawrence Kohlberg

On the basis of extensive longitudinal and cross-cultural studies, Lawrence Kohlberg, a developmental psychologist and educator, has distinguished three levels of moral development: *preconventional*, *conventional*, and *postconventional*.

## Table 4.5
### Levels of Moral Development (Kohlberg)

| Level | Characteristics |
|---|---|
| **Preconventional** | Interprets moral situations in terms of consequences to oneself. |
| **Conventional** | Interprets moral situations in terms of acceptance by others and pleasing authority figures. |
| **Postconventional** | Interprets moral situations in terms of general ethics and conscience. |

Each level is further subdivided into stages; though not strictly associated with age, these stages roughly correspond to the levels of intellectual reasoning described by Piaget (see Table 4.5). The reason for the moral decision made is the key to identifying the stage.

At the preconventional level, the child tends to make decisions in light of concrete physical consequences. Fear of punishment and the concerns of the ego mold preconventional decision making. For example, the child of four or five may associate right and wrong with the risk of punishment: "I'd better not do that or my Dad may spank me!"

The conventional level introduces the concepts of acceptance of group values and of pleasing others. A desire for approval guides conventional decision making. Conforming behavior in school or in a religious setting is aimed at bringing about approval of authority figures. However, flouting the rules may also be an expression of conventional morality, if such behavior is approved and encouraged by one's peer group.

The postconventional level takes into account additional ethical considerations which lead to independent thinking and action above and beyond group values. An abstract view of right and wrong guides postconventional decision making. For example, some nurses refuse to participate in abortions because of a belief that abortion is wrong, even though they know another nurse will take their place. Others participate because they believe it is right. The level is identified by the reason for the decision. Many people never reach this level of moral development.

# Infancy: Birth to One Year

## Physical Development

The propulsion of the infant out of the warm, safe, fluid environment of its mother's womb initiates profound bodily changes—or, in Frank's words, "violent alterations" (see Chapter 3)—which contribute to the establishment of physiological homeostasis independent of the mother's body. The infant's first cry expands the countless alveoli, or tiny air sacs, of the lungs, initiating a lifelong dependence on the external environment for oxygen. Structural adaptations begin quickly in the heart to complete the formation of the four chambers. The strong rhythmic pattern of beats, which began in utero, will gradually slow as it persists without interruption for eighty years or more. Peristalsis, the wavelike movements of the intestines, ensues and the gastric juices begin to flow in preparation for the first feeding. Although almost all newborn systems are grossly immature, the infant is virtually immediately responsive to bodily needs and to certain features of the environment: the newborn stretches, startles easily, and blinks at bright light.

The need for nourishment is apparent shortly after birth. Stroking the infant's cheek elicits the rooting reflex, whereby the head turns toward the stroked side in search of the breast. Infants begin early to put their fingers in their mouths and make sucking movements. The *pacifier*, once in disrepute, is now accepted as a device to strengthen and fulfill the sucking reflex. At approximately seven months, the twenty tiny teeth lying dormant within the gums begin to push their way, often painfully, through the surface. Chewing motions take place in preparation for the firm foods soon to be introduced into the diet.

Body movements progress from symmetrical moving of the limbs while lying on the back to rolling over at three to six months. The infant can usually sit upright unsupported at six to nine months and stand briefly or walk with assistance by one year. Birth weight has approximately tripled by one year. Elimination takes place less frequently and more regularly.

## Psychosocial Development

Although physically separated from the mother and thus in a sense independent, the newborn is totally dependent on others for the gratification of

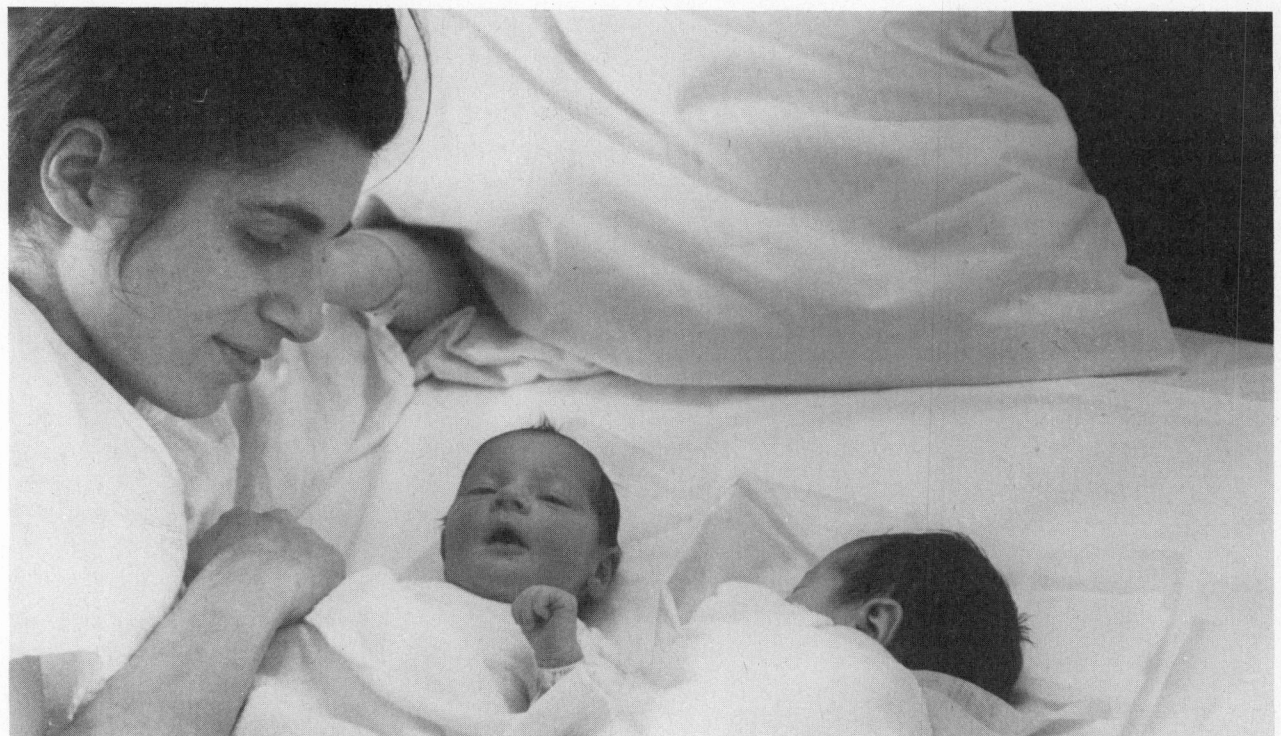

**Figure 4.1** **Newborns, the first stage of life** (Elizabeth Wilcox)

all basic needs: sufficient air of a comfortable temperature, fluids and nutrients, a safe crib, and touch that conveys love.

A wet diaper or hunger contractions of the stomach mucosa (lining) signal distress and elicit a cry for help. The parent hurriedly responds, initiating an emotional as well as a physical dependence that is the most meaningful relationship during the early years of life. Erikson calls this stage *trust vs. mistrust*. If the parent-infant relationship is characterized by consistency and genuine affection, the baby perceives the world as trustworthy, safe, and dependable. If, on the other hand, care of the child is inconsistent or neglectful, the infant displays fear, suspicion, and agitation.

## Psychosexual Development

Although the infant is unaware of sexuality as adults experience it, stimulation of its body parts is pleasurable. Initially the infant's mouth is its primary source of gratification. Freud calls this period the oral stage of sexual development. The young infant may also accidentally explore its genitals and feel pleasure.

Although not pronounced, behavioral differences between the sexes have been noted very early in life. Females appear to be more vocal as infants, and in later life they prove somewhat more adept at verbal skills and less prone to speech difficulties than males. Male infants are superior in motor skills, although fine muscle coordination develops earlier in girls. Thus subtle sexual differences are evident even in the first few months of life.

## Cognitive Development

Piaget describes the infant's cognition as consisting primarily of exploration of the body and immediate surroundings through the senses. Various external stimuli also play an important part in elementary cognition.

The infant initially responds to the internal stimuli of pain and hunger without distinguishing between them. Gradually the infant begins to identify feelings of discomfort that are relieved by food and to distinguish them from other feelings. The same process occurs with all internal stimuli, and the infant gradually learns to trust his or

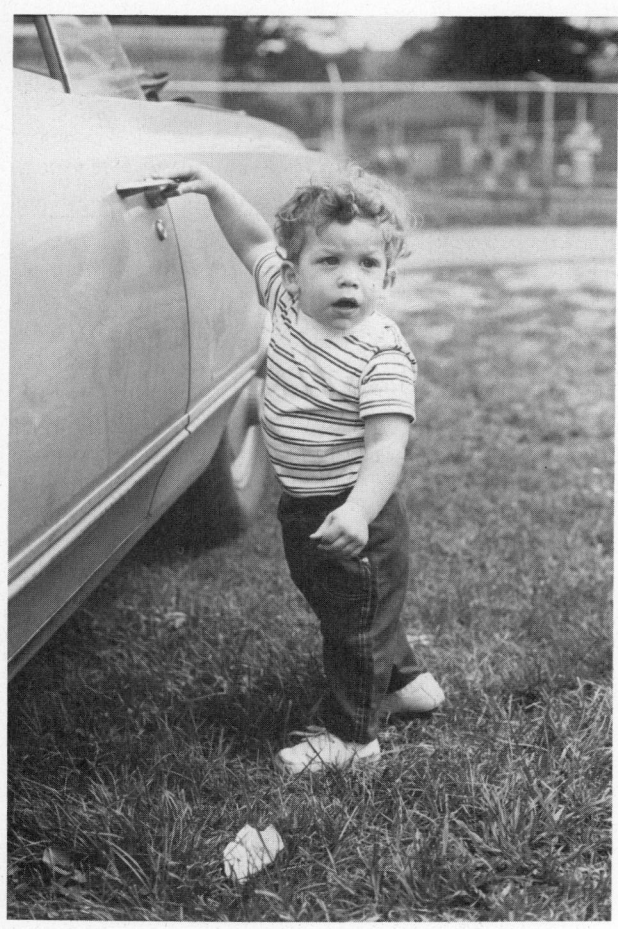

her body and to develop an understanding of its signals.

External stimuli also help infants identify their own bodies. Little babies may cause themselves pain by biting their own toes, since they do not know their own boundaries. The touch of those who care for the infant also helps to differentiate self from nonself.

## Moral Development

Morality is absent in infancy but, since ethical orientation derives in part from the trust engendered by the gratification of one's needs, the infant is beginning to experience feelings that will eventually set the stage for the ethical "give-and-take" of interaction with others.

The first year is characterized by alternating frustration and pleasure, and by inability to postpone gratification. Infants receive pleasure, give nothing consciously in return, and are unaware of the unique pleasure their existence gives their parents.

**Figure 4.2**
**The toddler *is* physically active.** (Bobbi Carrey/The Picture Cube)

# The Toddler: One to Three

## Physical Development

Between the ages of one and three, the child achieves some freedom from total dependence on the parents. Physical freedom results largely from mastery of the art of walking. Everyone knows the wonderful game in which the toddler runs from the pursuing parent with laughter and squeals of delight. If not pursued, the youngster stops, forlorn, only to find reassurance in the welcoming arms of the waiting parent.

The toddler is physically active and characterized by gross body movements. Fine muscular agility has not yet developed well. The body loses some of its "baby fat" and becomes more elongated. Skin texture becomes somewhat coarser. Visual acuity approximates that of the adult. Sphincter control is gradually achieved. The child can now eat with minimal assistance. Language skills are developing rapidly.

## Psychosocial Development

At this age the youngster strives toward psychological independence. "The battle of the potty-chair" can become a confrontation of wills; the parent imposes conformity and the child discovers a new power to manipulate or control. If the rewards exceed the punishments, the child gains pleasure from the parents' approval (love) of the new behavior and from a growing sense of control over the environment. The child begins to understand what is expected and is increasingly aware of being a distinct individual with the ability to affect the surroundings. He or she sees for the first time that pleasure postponed can be pleasure gained. Erikson calls this the stage of *autonomy vs. shame and doubt*.

If allowed to do what he or she is capable of, according to Erikson, the child will develop a lasting sense of confidence and autonomy. If thwarted, the child may develop an unhealthy doubt of his or her own capabilities and, in turn, of other people and the environment.

## Psychosexual Development

New-found control over elimination gives the child a sense of power, which can be used manipulatively at times in relation to the parents. Wanting to please may be translated into using the toilet or potty chair, while anger at the parents may be displayed by refusing to do so. Freud calls this period the *anal* stage of sexual development.

The toddler does not yet have a firm grasp of differences between boys and girls. Young children derive pleasure from touching themselves and from the cuddling and fondling of their parents. In fact, many psychiatrists believe that early childhood is the most crucial period in sexual development, because the child receives open love from the mother and learns—or fails to learn—to love and give to another. Some unfortunate children are punished for touching their genitals and made to believe that all sexual matters are taboo. Other children become confused about the contradictory reactions of adults, who may convey conflicting messages by promoting sexual attractiveness in the child (coyness, flirtation, "cuteness") but react to overt sexuality with silence and secretiveness.

## Cognitive Development

The thought processes of the toddler center on the immediate physical world, or what is happening right now. Ritual, mimicking, and repetitious movements or words are common. The vocabulary progresses from two- to four-word sentences and contains nouns, verbs, and adjectives (for example, "red ball" or "give drink," "let's go out," or "see the big dog").

## Moral Development

The toddler has not yet reached Kohlberg's preconventional level of morality, though behavior is influenced by parental approval and disapproval. Positive reinforcement from significant persons promotes beginning moral or ethical awarenesss by strengthening the concept of self.

# Early Childhood: Three to Six

## Physical Development

Early childhood is characterized by intense physical and mental activity. Physical growth is slower than during the first three years. The child is continuing to shed "baby fat" and acquiring the lean, tall body build of the school-age child. By age four, the child's weight is approximately double what it was at one year. At approximately five, temporary teeth begin to be replaced by more solidly rooted permanent teeth. Coordination has improved, and the child can now climb steps as an adult does, rather than planting both feet on each step. The child spends a good deal of time dancing, skipping, hopping, and jumping. The child can now dress and use the toilet independently.

## Psychosocial Development

Erikson calls this stage *initiative vs. guilt*. The initiative of which Erikson speaks gives the youngster a feeling of accomplishment and thus diminishes rebelliousness. Children of this age tend toward orderliness and willingly perform such tasks as balancing blocks, putting away toys, and washing and dressing themselves. Successful performance of these tasks offsets feelings of guilt at not meeting parental expectations. The three-year-old begins to demonstrate initiative through saying "no" to parental decisions.

Parental attitudes are crucial at this period. If the parents treat the child's activities and questions as significant, the child is encouraged to grow in response to such positive reinforcement. If the child's questions and explorations are treated flippantly or ridiculed, a sense of guilt may delay or undermine further emotional growth.

## Psychosexual Development

Freud subdivides the preschool years into two stages of sexual development. At age three or four, the child enters the *phallic stage*. This term is somewhat misleading in that phallic refers to the phallus or penis. The phallic stage, however, applies to girls and boys both of whom experience sensual pleasure in their genitals, and they may masturbate during this stage.

Freud's *Oedipal stage*, which occurs at about four or five, is characterized by a heightened attachment to the parent of the opposite sex and identification with the parent of the same sex. For example, children of this age may see themselves as "little adults," the boy pretending to be "like Daddy" and the girl imitating her mother. According to Freud, sexual attraction to the parent of the opposite sex is a conflict resolved only by further emotional development.

Parents tend to encourage children to adopt sexual identities very early. For example, a boy may be given a football, while a girl is given a doll. Boys are often dressed in very masculine clothing, and girls in dresses, long before apparel has much meaning to youngsters. In recent years, parents have been widely encouraged to minimize the sexual patterning of children's behavior in order to

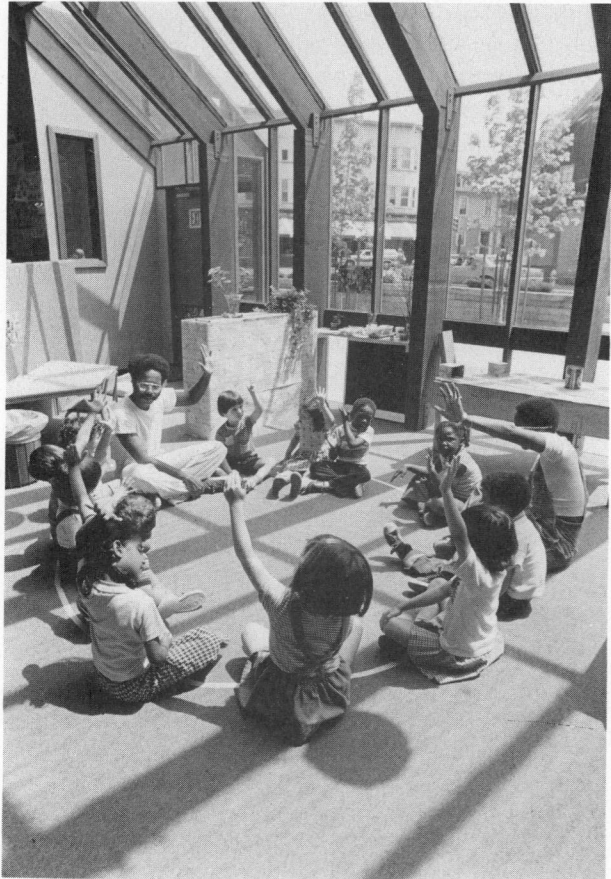

**Figure 4.3 The three- to six-year-old**
Elizabeth Hamlin/Stock, Boston

allow for the development of individual interests and ability.

The three- to six-year-old has a natural curiosity about his or her body, and soon discovers that boys and girls are differently constructed. The proximity of the genitals to the organs of elimination, as well as the attitudes of adults, may cause the child to think of the sexual organs as dirty. Learning that nudity is not generally accepted in our culture may further mystify the child about sex.

## Cognitive Development

Early childhood is a period of intense activity, both physically and mentally. The outstanding cognitive feature of this stage is the child's rapidly growing command of speech. This phenomenon, which has both physical and mental components, affords the child even more independence. A vocabulary of five thousand or more words is typical by the age of six. One has only to observe the extreme depression and frustration of the stroke patient suffering aphasia (loss of the ability to use language appropriately) to realize how essential is the power of speech. Among four- and five-year-olds, "No!" is a very popular response to parental decisions, allowing the child verbal initiative in decision making.

The child's sentences develop from three to four words to several phrases. Fantasy play typifies this age. The child begins learning to count and to ask such questions about the physical world as "Where does the sun go at night?" Books, pictures, and television are interesting diversions for the preschooler. Piaget refers to cognitive development at this age as preoperational; the child is developing the ability to deal with symbols, such as the letters of the alphabet.

## Moral Development

The preschooler reasons on the preconventional level: fear of punishment molds behavior. Pleasing parents is important not for its own sake but to bring about desirable consequences.

# Middle Childhood: Six to Twelve

## Physical Development

The physical growth rate of the child from six to twelve is steady except for a spurt just before puberty. Girls are frequently taller and more developed than boys by age twelve. The brain reaches adult size by age twelve, and the vital signs are close to the adult range. Except for the second molars, the permanent teeth (except for wisdom teeth) have all appeared. The face begins to take on adult characteristics. Coordination improves, and some children seek out competitive sports. Nutritional needs increase to accommodate continuing physical growth.

## Psychosocial Development

Erikson defines these years as devoted to resolving the *industry vs. inferiority* conflict. For both boys and girls, friends and other peers assume great importance. Team sports channel the aggression that is common at this age into competitive agility. Fighting and wrestling dissipate energy. Girls' groups are usually less aggressively oriented. They do, however, form basketball, soccer, and baseball teams that are highly competitive.

If the child's industry is praised and he or she is allowed to undertake and complete tasks, the

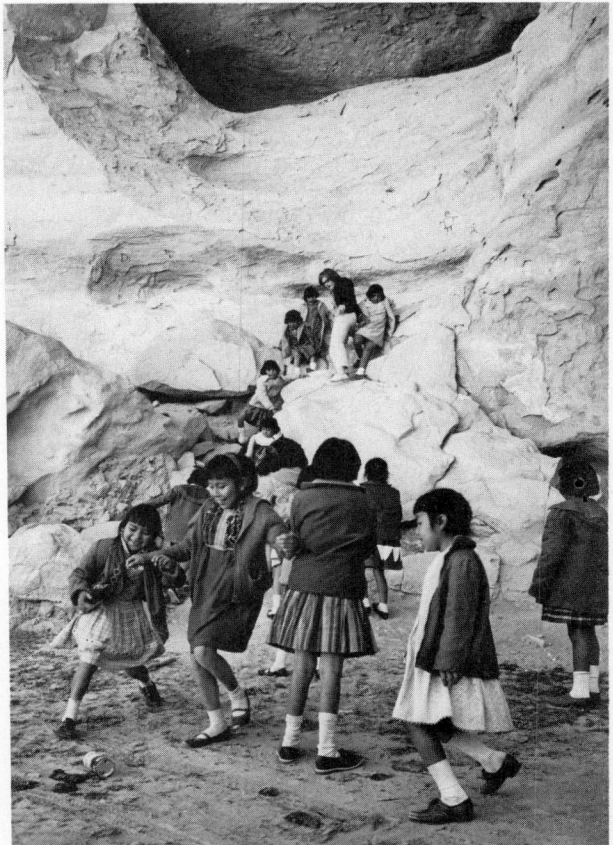

**Figure 4.4   The six- to twelve-year-old**
Paul Conklin

resolution of this stage will be healthy. A child whose efforts are made fun of and criticized becomes discouraged and feels unworthy and inferior.

## Psychosexual Development

Freud calls this stage the latency period. (Latency means quiescence of sexual feelings toward the opposite sex.) The Oedipal conflict has been resolved, and the child aligns with peers and authority figures of the same sex. Boys form all-boy groups and girls socialize only with girls. In spite of such voluntary separation, boys often perform feats of daring and bravery to gain the admiration not only of their male peers but also of girls. Girls in turn are aware of the boys' antics and may express role identification by experimenting with lipstick or asking to learn to sew or cook. It is unclear whether recent trends toward less strictly defined sex roles among adults and the advent of large numbers of women in professions once exclusively male, and to a lesser extent the reverse, is influencing children of this age to identify less exclusively with the parent of the same sex.

## Cognitive Development

Many educators regard the years from six to twelve as the most important period for cognitive development. These are the "doing" years. Teachers share responsibility for the child's development, since the youngster in this age group substitutes the teacher's authority for much of the parents'. The encouragement of a sensitive teacher can have a lasting impact.

Piaget characterizes the cognitive stage of the school-age child as "concrete operational." That is, the child deals best with concrete phenomena and situations but can consider others' ideas and communicate in a controlled, articulate way. He or she understands clear-cut relationships, such as those involving size and location of objects. Questioning and curiosity about life begins, promoting future learning for the youngster. In school skills, preadolescent girls frequently do better than boys of the same age in such areas as reading, spelling, and writing, but boys "catch up" in early adolescence.

## Moral Development

The school years are an important period in ethical development. In general, self-serving motives and avoidance of punishment have been superseded as sources of moral decisions. By the elementary years, conventional-level reasoning begins. Kohlberg (1966) calls this stage the "good-boy morality of maintaining good relations, approval of others." Authority (teachers, parents, the law) is beginning to influence behavior.

# Adolescence: Twelve to Eighteen

Adolescence is usually exciting but unsettling. Today's adolescents are taller, healthier, and more independent than ever before, but their freedom of access to sexual experience, drugs, cars, alcohol, and the like can burden them with choices far beyond the wisdom of their years. Rising divorce rates place additional stress on adolescents. The rise in teenage suicide is of grave concern to community mental health professionals.

## Physical Development

Many physical changes, both overt and internal, are occurring in the adolescent. Physical growth, initially very rapid, ceases in late adolescence, when dreams of what might be must be reconciled with reality. Rapid growth can cause awkwardness and a sense of unfamiliarity with one's body: furniture can be a stumbling block to large feet and uncoordinated legs. Physical activity and exercise can help teenagers overcome these difficulties.

Because of their rapid growth, adolescents have increased nutritional needs. The typical teenage appetite for "junk food" can make obesity as well as skin disturbances a problem.

*Puberty*—the maturing of the sexual organs—takes place during adolescence. Menstruation, or *menses*, begins in girls, often erratically at first but it usually becomes a fairly regular twenty-eight day cycle. Boys typically experience nocturnal emissions, or "wet dreams," during which semen is expelled. Both the onset of menses and nocturnal emissions can cause anxiety, which an understanding parent or other adult can allay.

## Psychosocial Development

Erikson characterizes the adolescent crisis in psychosocial development as *identity vs. role confusion*. A sense of individual identity evolves during these years, setting the stage for adulthood, largely through the process of reconciling one's changing self-image ("Who am I?" "What kind of person am I?") with the image presented to family and friends ("How do other people see me?"). The strengthening of identity is accompanied by a need to separate oneself psychologically from one's family. Family outings become less popular and peer-group activities increasingly important.

Some adolescents express their independence by renouncing the religion they were raised in or adopting a political affiliation different from that of their parents. Such acts can increase the emotional distance between adolescents and their parents. Although teenagers often appear sullen and rebellious in the eyes of their parents, solid parental support remains essential. Limit-setting becomes more difficult but must not be abandoned.

Interest and consideration of a life partner and vocation may begin. Using the reactions of parents and peers as guideposts, the teenager can gradually achieve the security of a valid role identity—that is, a satisfactory self-image congruent with the views of others. If this delicate balance cannot be attained, Erikson tells us, *role confusion* results. Youngsters who fail to establish identity in adolescence typically lack direction and have difficulty making decisions about such important matters as education, work, sexual orientation, and moral values. Adolescents need acceptable role models on whom to pattern themselves. Parents who exercise too much or too little control cannot function as satisfactory role models; as a result, the con-

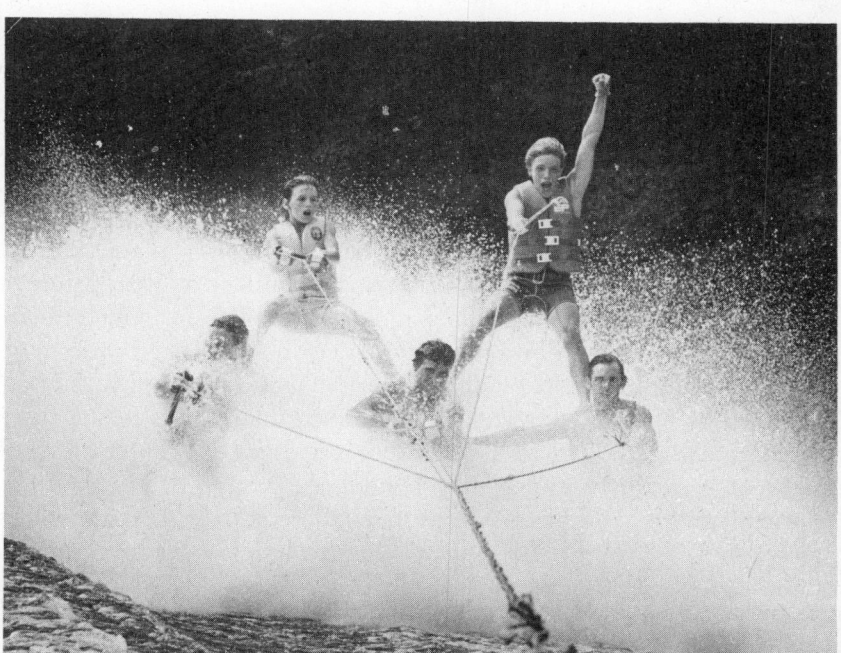

**Figure 4.5  The adolescent**
Anestis Diakopoulous/Stock, Boston

fused young person may grasp at any ready-made identity, such as drug use, sexual precocity, or defiance of authority. Such desperate efforts to "be somebody" can lead to serious problems.

## Psychosexual Development

Freud treats adolescence as synonymous with puberty, which he defines as the conciliation of physical and emotional needs into a sexual identity.

Adolescents tend to be preoccupied with normality and constantly compare the development and the size of their significant body parts, such as breasts and penis, with others'. Facial features take on adult conformation, and it is commonplace for adolescents to be unhappy with their features. Attitudes and values pertaining to appearance are derived from the peer group rather than the family. The adolescent seeks security in handling the responsibilities of intimacy: the desire for sexual activity may be accompanied by fear of its results. As H. S. Sullivan puts it, an adolescent's task is to learn to handle sex without anxiety (Sullivan, 1953).

## Cognitive Development

Piaget attributes to the adolescent the capacity to reason on the formal operational level, characterized by abstract concepts and conjecture about the past and future as well as the present. The potential of the future tends to preoccupy teenagers. Though limited in experience, they tend to think intensely about both personal problems and abstract theories. Adolescents are beginning to adopt behavior patterns based on an understanding of their effects on others.

## Moral Development

In early adolescence, according to Kohlberg, the individual begins to reason on the conventional level of morality. As in the cognitive sphere, ethical decisions may be made on abstract grounds, with a view toward the consequences. The development of a conscience and the desire to be self-governed play a part, as does authority.

# Young Adulthood: Eighteen to Forty

## Physical Development

American society is youth-oriented, and the twenty- to thirty-year-old is typically regarded as the apex of physical attractiveness. Because growth is complete, nutritional needs diminish somewhat. Adult metabolism requires a nutritional range that will maintain both health and recommended body weight. It is highly probable that dietary management at this age can prevent later cardiovascular changes that may lead to serious disease. Some males of forty or younger may experience premature hair loss. Both sexes may begin to have some gray hair. Body changes perceived as signaling the beginning of middle age may cause some anxiety.

## Psychosocial Development

The social options for young adults have changed remarkably over the past decade. It is commonplace for unmarried couples to live together. Shared housing is on the increase in response to rising housing costs. Couples are having fewer children than a decade ago, and many are choosing to have no children. Role and career reversal is taking place, with increasing numbers of women entering formerly male occupations, and men entering traditionally female occupations. No longer is it uncommon to encounter a male telephone operator or nurse or a female engineer or mail carrier. Though the range of alternatives is thus widening, high unemployment continues to restrict young adults in pursuit of their life goals.

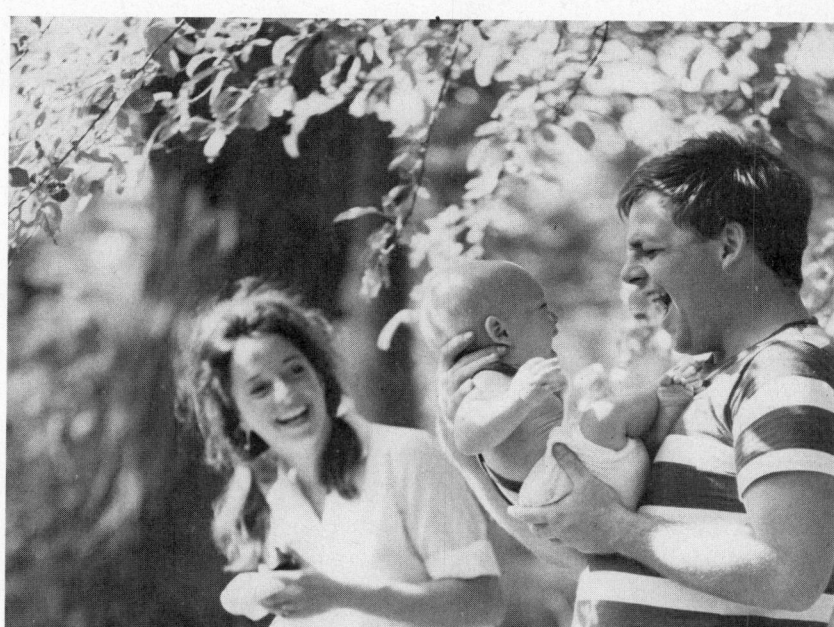

**Figure 4.6  Young adulthood**
Elizabeth Wilcox

During young adulthood, most individuals are pursuing and establishing meaningful long-term relationships. Because today many young adults, for a variety of reasons, do not have families of their own, there may be problems in meeting the need for intimacy. Erikson describes the conflict of young adulthood as *intimacy vs. isolation.*

Although the intimacy desired by the young adult is usually a love relationship with a sexual component, this is not exclusively the case. The basic need is for closeness and real relatedness to another person. Homosexual and bisexual people are finding growing acceptance in the mainstream of society and are increasingly perceived in terms of their individual merits rather than mere sexual orientation.

The attainment of intimacy further enhances the identity first established in the teenage years. The young adult is a competitive, productive, creative person who sees the results—and, one hopes, the rewards—of decision making. Erikson tells us that isolation can occur if "intimacy, competitive and combative relations are experienced with and against the selfsame people." If the individual cannot "fuse" his or her identity with others', self-imposed isolation occurs.

## Psychosexual Development

Young adulthood may be characterized by sexual fulfillment in long-term relationships of satisfying intimacy. However, it has been suggested that many young adults have unrealistic expectations of romantic love and intimacy and find long-term sexual involvement dull and disappointing. Nevertheless, the young adult typically embraces the sexual role and looks for security in a love relationship.

## Cognitive Development

The young adult is typically preoccupied with developing and applying the practical and professional skills necessary to build a satisfying adult life. Completion of schooling and the advent of working life make for financial independence from the parental family. Independence in turn brings responsibilities that require substantial skill at planning, coping, foreseeing problems, and interpreting reality.

Though the slogans and abstractions that often dominate adolescent thought processes may not be forsaken, they are likely to be reinterpreted in terms of the practicalities of life. Ordinary thinking may gradually become more systematic, decisive, and task-oriented. At the same time, thinking, fantasizing, and emotion may become more smoothly integrated than during adolescence.

By this stage in the life cycle, men's and women's overall cognitive abilities are equal, if not precisely identical. Opportunities for women to employ their full capacities in the world of work are growing strikingly, and women are conclusively demonstrating their equal ability to perform. Recent research has indicated that there may be neurophysiological differences between males and females, which may make some types of learning easier for one sex than the other.

By and large, young adults are energetic, forward-looking, and ambitious. However, emotional conflicts about identity, dependence/independence, and other issues of adulthood can interfere with the thrust of cognitive development, and many young adults experience an extended period of indecision, rebellion, and/or relative passivity before resolving such conflicts and wholeheartedly pursuing adult lives.

## Moral Development

Many young adults actively seek an ethical philosophy or religion to adopt and adhere to. Moral certainty and self-righteousness, often accompanied by scorn of divergent beliefs and behavior, usually gives way over time to tolerance and respect for others' convictions. Hypocrisy, however, continues to arouse their outrage. Young adults typically invest a great deal of thought in coming to terms with personal and social ethical issues.

# The Middle Years: Forty to Sixty-Five

## Physical Development

During the middle years the hair grays, body fat is redistributed and may increase, and a deficit in visual and/or hearing acuity may occur. Women stop menstruating, and men somewhat later experience hormonal and psychological changes. Depression is not uncommon in the middle years, perhaps due to realization that one is not going to achieve all the goals of one's youth. Some depression may also be a result of hormonal alterations.

The decreased hormone production that characterizes the middle years brings about changes in one's body and one's feelings. Because of the extreme emphasis on youth in Western culture, many individuals have difficulty facing these changes, and some make massive efforts to continue looking young. Such a person may dress in a youthful manner, use cosmetics to cover signs of aging, and undergo plastic surgery. These activities are not harmful in themselves but may indicate that the person has difficulty accepting body changes. A few individuals react in the opposite way, simply giving up at the first signs of aging: they may refer to themselves as old, wear clothing characteristic of elderly people, and withdraw from physical activity. This response only accelerates the aging process.

## Psychosocial Development

Erikson identifies the middle years as characterized by a crisis of *generativity vs. stagnation*. This may begin as early as age thirty for some people. The individual reviews past accomplishments and assesses what remains to be done, a process that can arouse satisfaction or disappointment. One may make the desirable psychological adjustment of considering one's capacities and accomplishments in light of their value to the younger generation. The development of such a sense of generativity does not require that one have children of one's own; it is more a matter of psychologically "parenting" all youth. Productivity and political and social responsibility in the middle years are ways of striving to help young people grow.

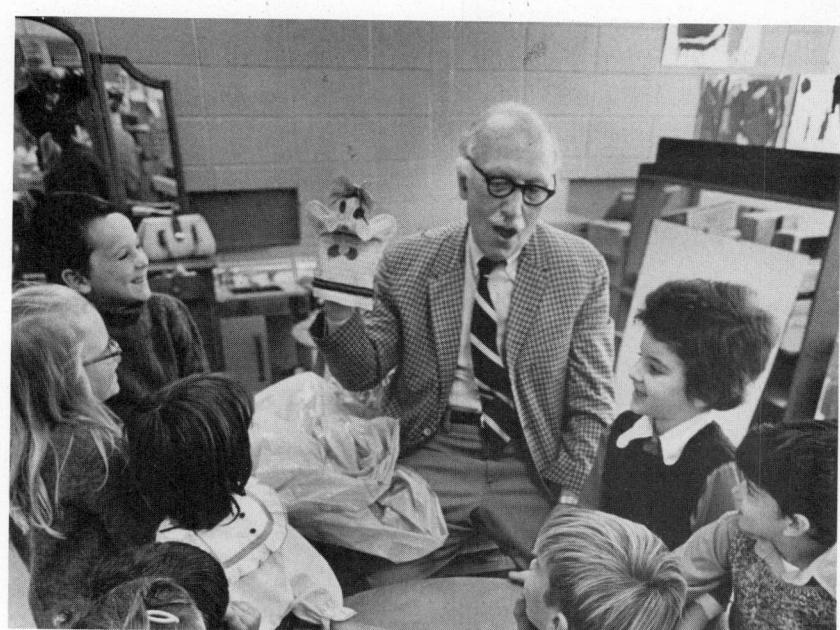

**Figure 4.7 The middle years: A "parenting" of all youth**
Dan Bernstein

If, in the middle of life, one can assess oneself realistically and at the same time concern oneself with the needs of the younger members of society, one can achieve a state of generativity that makes for contentment. If this encompassing view of life is lacking, self-pity, self-interest, and sadness may result.

## Psychosexual Development

Sexual activity can be highly gratifying during the middle years. A woman whose children are reaching adulthood may find new joy in her sexuality. But if she feels unfulfilled and remote from or unappreciated by her partner, sexual pleasure is unlikely to fill emotional voids.

The middle-aged man may experience brief episodes of impotence, usually psychological in origin. The realization that he may not accomplish all he intended can cause him to feel sexually inadequate. If his sexual partner is understanding and supportive, such problems can be fleeting. If they persist, however, professional counseling may be needed.

In spite of the potential problems of middle age, sex may be more satisfying than at any other time in life. When the responsibility of childrearing is past, one has more time to appreciate one's partner.

## Cognitive Development

Cognitive capacity is unimpaired in middle age, and motivation to learn is typically high. Career advancement may require the individual to develop new skills—often administrative or teaching skills—or to apply skills already mastered in a new way. In conjunction with such goal-oriented learning, the wish to enjoy life to the fullest prompts many middle-aged people to make time for more recreational activities: reading, music, art, enjoyable projects, and new interests. Both types of learning experiences can be pursued in continuing education, which many middle-aged people find an extraordinarily rewarding resource.

## Moral Development

Ethical judgments in middle age are typically based on one's past experience and established belief system, which may be either conventional or postconventional. An individual's moral development can progress or regress in response to an emotional crisis. For example, serious illness may elicit a retreat to superstition or an unprecedented maturity and appreciation of life, not to mention possible intermediate reactions.

# The Later Years: Over Sixty-Five

Growing old in Western societies is far from the pleasant experience it appears to be in some Asian countries, where age elicits respect and the young solicit the wisdom of the old. Retirement is often mandatory, and usually unwelcome. However, retirement communities have gained favor as an antidote to the social isolation that plagues the elderly.

## Physical Development

Older people's physical conditions vary markedly. In general, changes occur with age in all body systems. The bones decalcify, which may cause a decrease in body height, and lessened elasticity of lung tissue leads to decreased vital capacity. Peristalsis of the gastrointestinal tract is slowed. The nervous system may undergo changes affecting coordination, balance, and *mentation*, or thought. Loss of hearing is more prevalent than loss of sight, though subtle changes may occur in both senses. Some sclerosis occurs in the vessels, affecting heart action. In fact, cardiovascular disease is the most common life-threatening condition among the elderly.

As old age approaches, the body generally becomes progressively less able to function at previous levels. These reductions in efficiency occur at different rates in different individuals: some people function more slowly, or tire more easily, but can continue in their normal occupations; others age rapidly to the point of dependence on other people.

## Psychosocial Development

The conflict of aging, according to Erikson, is *integrity vs. despair*. Changes that occur with age must be incorporated into the body image, and a realistic adaptation must be made if the elderly person is to participate optimally in life. But lack of trust in one's body, fear of chronic illness, and anxiety about dependence make this a difficult task. Older individuals suffering from ill health, alienation or separation from loved ones, and financial difficulties can understandably succumb to despair. Depression is not uncommon over the age of sixty. As in adolescence, the reactions of others greatly influence how elderly people feel about themselves. The older person who is looked on as useless feels of no use.

By reviewing achievements and disappointments, the older person searches out the meaning of his or her individual life. Many older people make a point of undertaking new ventures and projects, broadening their perspectives and circle of friends. The growth of organizations and programs for the elderly is enhancing the quality of many people's lives. Understanding, respect, and accurate knowledge about aging on the part of health-care providers can promote dignity and integrity.

## Psychosexual Development

In conjunction with changing attitudes toward sexuality, older people now realize that they need not cease sexual activity. A decrease in hormonal activity does not mean absence of *libido* (sexual interest) or the end of intimacy.

The male may produce children well into the later years. The female, although unable to bear children after menopause, retains libido or sexual interest. Although sexual activity may become somewhat less frequent, it can remain pleasurable and meaningful. It is important for nurses to recognize that people remain sexual beings until the end of their lives.

## Cognitive Development

Prior opinion to the contrary, elderly people's minds remain agile, undergoing only slight decline very late in life, unless affected by such phys-

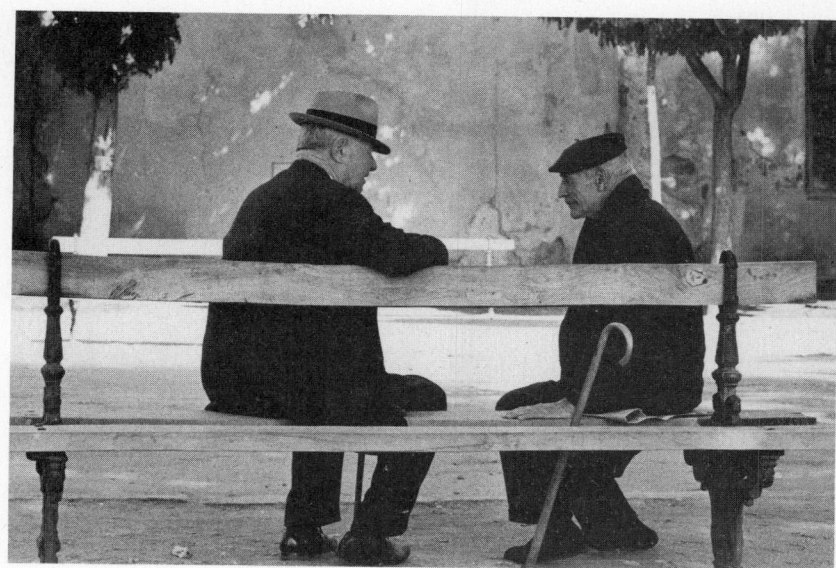

**Figure 4.8 The later years**
Ira Gavrin

iological changes as decreased circulation to the brain due to arteriosclerosis. Any slowing of thought that does occur is often compensated for by problem-solving ability based on life experience. There is some evidence that those older people who have used their minds most actively throughout their lives experience the least diminution of mental ability. And it is clinically demonstrable that intellectual stimulation promotes and maintains alertness.

## Moral Development

A lifetime of moral assessment and experience and observation leads many older adults to ethical clarity and strong convictions without censoriousness. Many achieve Kohlberg's highest level, postconventional ethical thought, and view morality as a matter of individual rights and principles of conscience. Some older people tend to be judgmental about other people's behavior.

## The Life Cycle and Nursing Practice

Thorough familiarity with the life cycle is vastly important to nurses. The changing flow of life provides both challenge and opportunity to those of us who are in the care professions. The integration of an individual's physical, social, sexual, cognitive, and moral components results in a person different from any other individual. In order for care to be maximally effective, it ought to be tailored to the unique characteristics of its recipient.

First, your assessments of the physical and emotional characteristics of the patient are valid or meaningful only if you can make comparisons to what is usual. Notwithstanding the hazards of "putting people in boxes," knowing the norms of

social development will deepen your assessment abilities. For example, if the hospitalized three-year-old cries uncontrollably when the mother must leave the bedside to return home, you can give the child better support and assurance if you know that at this age the mother's presence is all-important and that even brief separation is devastating. Second, knowledge of the developmental stages will give you insight into what is important to the patient, and how he or she might respond to care. Knowing this, you can design care that will meet the unique needs of the ill individual.

## The Infant

The nurse can best care for an infant by providing a physically safe environment free of startling noises or bright lights and by touching, speaking to, and fondling the infant. Nursery-room nurses commonly talk and sing to the infants in their charge. The infant may be irritable, fearful, and anxious. Even without the ability to understand illness, the infant feels systemically unwell and expresses this feeling in behavior. Illness changes the normal "happy" baby into an "unhappy" baby. It is important for you to observe and record such behavior; by doing so, you directly contribute to an assessment of the infant's physical status.

## The Toddler

The toddler who is sick has a special need to know that feeling sick is unrelated to having done something bad. Understanding is very limited at this age, but the child is very sensitive to the surroundings. In addition to guilt over imagined wrongdoing, the primary stress is separation from the mother at a time when the child most needs maternal attention. Hospitals are becoming increasingly aware of the importance of this need and, unless it becomes too tiring for her, the mother is usually allowed to remain with the child almost continually. Since it relieves some of the child's anxiety, this kind of arrangement is usually welcomed by the child, the mother, and the staff.

Medical procedures, particularly painful ones, pose a threat to the body in the mind of the young child. Simple explanations can be offered to the three-year-old. Lying to any child—or to any patient, for that matter—is inappropriate and counterproductive because it destroys trust. If the mother cannot or should not be present, a nurse who relates well to the youngster can give needed physical and emotional support during medical procedures. (The parent should be considered as well as the child: if the procedure is painful or upsetting to watch, the mother may not wish to be present and should not be encouraged to do so.)

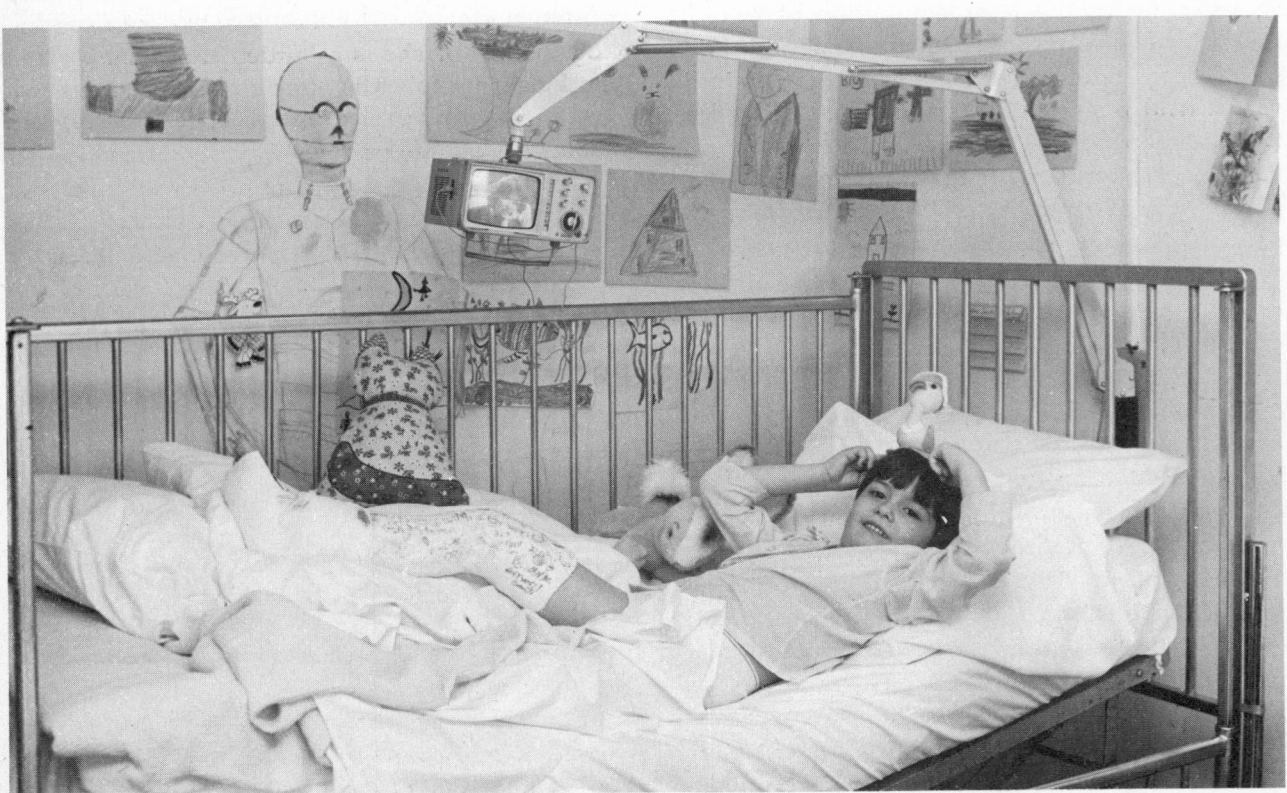

**Figure 4.9**
The room of the hospitalized child can be furnished to look like home. (Russ Kinne/Danbury Hospital/Photo Researchers, Inc.)

## The Preschooler

Guilt over illness persists in the preschooler, who may readily associate it with wrongdoing. Preschool-age patients may relate painful procedures to punishment unless they have been adequately prepared for such experiences.

## The School-Aged Child

The ill school-age youngster keenly resents the restrictive atmosphere of the hospital and the limitations it places on exploratory activities, a major need of this age group. The less understanding nurse may find the school-age child a demanding and boisterous patient. It is important to make time to allow the child to talk about the frustration he or she feels. Such attention and sympathy can help the child become not only less rebellious but also a cooperative participant in the management of his or her illness.

## The Adolescent

Illness is particularly threatening in adolescence, since it imposes ill-timed dependence on an individual who is striving toward independence. The teenager can be a very unwilling and angry patient. Separation from friends and their activities places considerable stress on the adolescent patient. The inventive nurse can help channel such anger into constructive feelings that can aid recovery.

## The Young Adult

The young adult, when ill, may feel most acutely the consequent interruption in productivity. Many also fear change in the quality or character of the intimacy relationship. The nurse's recognition of resulting depression, and acknowledgment of such feelings when they occur, helps the patient work through the experience of illness.

## The Middle Years

Adulthood is an especially difficult time to become ill, since the ideas and plans so essential at this age must be put aside in deference to the illness. Illness may be interpreted as deterioration due to age, thus causing both depression and fear. Ventilating and sharing these feelings is usually helpful to the patient, and the nurse can facilitate this process.

## The Later Years

Illness in an elderly person can undermine the dignity so vital to maturity. Dependence on others may be interpreted by the older patient as meaning that he or she is a burden to the family and no longer useful. It is often nurses' attitudes that largely determine whether or not the older patient maintains dignity or gives way to despair.

Understanding of the life cycle will make you comfortable with the responses described above, which might otherwise appear irrational. Planning care thus becomes more realistic, enjoyable, stimulating, and creative.

Finally, a basic understanding of the life cycle and how it influences human behavior will increase your sensitivity not only to patients but also to colleagues.

# Conclusion

Understanding of the human life cycle is still partial. Research continually reveals new findings and undercuts old beliefs. Those of us who interact professionally with people of all ages ought to keep current and informed. We will also benefit by understanding ourselves better as we move through each stage, recognizing our own value and self-worth.

## Study Terms

| | |
|---|---|
| accommodation | integrity |
| adolescent | intimacy |
| anal | isolation |
| assimilation | latency |
| asynchrony | libido |
| autonomy | life style |
| centering | maturation |
| cephalocaudal | menses |
| development | mentation |
| cognitive | mistrust |
| concrete operational | moral |
| congenital | Oedipal conflict |
| conventional | pacifier |
| despair | phallic |
| doubt | physical |
| ego | plateau |
| egocentrism | postconventional |
| equilibration | preconventional |
| fetus | prenatal |
| formal operational | preoperational |
| generativity | psychosexual |
| genetic | psychosocial |
| growth | puberty |
| guilt | role confusion |
| id | sensorimotor |
| identity | superego |
| industry | Trisomy 21 |
| inferiority | trust |
| initiative | unconscious mind |

## Learning Activities

**1.** Make a list of the members of your immediate family. Where is each on the continuum of the life cycle? What are his or her individual needs?
**2.** On a nursing care plan, write a brief analysis of a patient's present life stage, taking into account the stage conflict, body image, and sexual development.
**3.** Repeat Activity 2 for a second patient.
**4.** Compare in writing the needs of the two patients analyzed above. Consider how this information may guide or modify your care of each.

## References

*American Journal of Nursing* 75 (October 1975). Seventy-Fifth Anniversary Issue. (Entire issue devoted to the life cycle.)

Biehler, R. F. *Psychology Applied to Teaching*, 3rd ed. Boston: Houghton Mifflin, 1978.

Carter, F. *Psychosocial Nursing.* New York: Macmillan, 1976.

Erikson, E. H. *Childhood and Society.* New York: W. W. Norton, 1963.

Freud, Sigmund. *The Ego and the Id.* 1923.

Kohlberg, Lawrence. "Moral Education in the Schools: A Developmental View." *School Review* 74 (1966): 1–30.

Kolb, L. C. *Modern Clinical Psychiatry*, 8th ed. Philadelphia: W. B. Saunders, 1973.

Marlow, D. R. *Textbook of Pediatric Nursing*, 4th ed. Philadelphia: W. B. Saunders, 1973.

The Middle Years. *American Journal of Nursing* 75 (June 1975): 997–1024. Special supplement. Part I: Emotional Tasks of the Middle Adult. Part II: The Sexually Active Middle Adult. Part III: The Change of Life. Part IV: The Full Life. Part V: Living Sensibly. Part VI: Coping with Chronic Illness. Part VII: The Mid-Stage Woman. Part VIII: A Faculty Member Remembers.

Murray, Ruth, and Zentner, Judith. *Nursing Assessment and Health Promotion Through the Life Span*, 2nd ed. Englewood Cliffs, N.J.: Prentice-Hall, 1979.

Oremland, E. K., *et al.* How to Care for the "Between-ager." *Nursing '74* 4 (November 1974): 42–51.

Piaget, Jean. *Origins of Intelligence in Children.* New York: W. W. Norton, 1963.

Smith, D. W., and Bierman, E. L. *The Biological Ages of Man.* Philadelphia: W. B. Saunders, 1973.

Sullivan, H. S. *The Interpersonal Theory of Psychiatry.* New York: W. W. Norton, 1953.

Sutterley, D., and Donnelly, G. *Perspectives in Human Development.* Philadelphia, J. B. Lippincott, 1973.

Weiner, I. B., and Elkins, D. *Child Development: A Core Approach.* New York: John Wiley and Sons, 1972.

# Chapter 5

# Social, Cultural, and Ethnic Diversity

## Objectives

After completing this chapter, you should be able to:

1. Define the terms *bias, prejudice, stereotyping*, and *discrimination*.
2. Discuss what *institutional racism* means.
3. Identify three areas of understanding essential to sensitive nursing care of minority patients.
4. Briefly discuss Native Americans, Asian Americans, Black Americans, and Hispanic Americans in terms of the following: (a) health care and incidence of disease, (b) family, (c) territoriality, (d) diet, (e) communication, (f) religion and healing, and (g) death and bereavement.
5. Identify particular health and health-care problems experienced by migrants and the socioeconomically disadvantaged.
6. Summarize the guidelines for care of minority patients.

## Outline

The phrase *human rights* has been widely used over the past fifteen or twenty years. In most states, the law now reads that there shall be no discrimination on the basis of "race, religion, color, national origin, marital status, sex, age, or handicap." In a broader context, human rights means the right of people to live in harmony, regardless of individual or group differences. Fundamental to the philosophy of nursing is the responsibility to care for *all* people, regardless of social, cultural, or ethnic origin.

To be *diverse* means to be varied. Each person is different in some ways from others. Being variant is not negative or bad. Our differences help to make us interesting to one another and tend to broaden our life experiences. People who come from diverse social, cultural, and ethnic groups are often referred to as *minorities*. *Minority* means not of the majority, that is, of a group that is smaller than the main group within a society. In this chapter, we will speak about the nursing care of people who differ from the majority in a variety of ways.

Except for Native Americans, we are an immigrant nation. By and large, the millions of immigrants North America has received have come willingly, even eagerly, for compelling economic, religious, and political reasons. During the European immigration at the turn of the century, the image arose of the United States as a melting pot—a place where diverse nationalities and ethnic groups would "melt" into the established society, losing many of their distinguishing features in the process. To some degree, this image accurately describes what happened to many immigrants: anxious for their children to become American, some families went so far as to forbid the use of their native language in their homes. Far more common was a gradual loosening of emotional and cultural ties to the homeland over the course of three or more generations. This pattern has been paralleled by a tendency for newcomers to crowd together in ethnically homogeneous neighborhoods, usually in older urban areas, and for their children or grandchildren to leave the neighborhood as soon as they could afford to. Changing patterns in employment opportunities have also contributed to mobility.

Not all immigrants came voluntarily: millions of blacks entered our eastern shores as slaves to work the land. Over a century later millions of Asians entered our western shores, not precisely as slaves but as ill-paid unskilled laborers to build the nation's vast network of railroads. More recently large numbers of Hispanics have immigrated to escape severe economic hardship; many of these families have found a livelihood as migrant agricultural laborers, primarily but not exclusively in the Southwest.

In general, opportunities have been more limited for, and prejudice more pronounced toward, nonwhite people and others whose looks distinguish them from the established norms. Particularly earlier in this century, this situation was reflected in such minority groups' prevailing standards of beauty and behavior, and those individuals who most nearly resembled the norms of the dominant culture were most prized. Some individuals denied their ethnic backgrounds in efforts to achieve total assimilation.

The current resurgence of curiosity about and pride in one's "roots"—that is, one's ethnic, cultural, and family heritage—may be attributable to increasing acceptance of diversity and cultural differences. People can afford, emotionally and socially, to value their origins.

## Problems of a Diverse Society

Ignorance of others' life styles and values can arouse suspicion, intolerance, and even fear. The result is perceived competition for jobs and housing, mutual contempt, and sometimes overt clashes.

### Bias and Prejudice

*Bias* and *prejudice* are interchangeable terms for adverse attitudes and opinions unsupported by evidence or understanding. It is crucial for nurses and others who come into frequent and intimate contact with people of backgrounds other than their own to confront and acknowledge their own biases in order to begin ridding themselves of negative attitudes and behavior. It is well documented that the dominant American culture—to which most nurses belong—prizes egalitarianism, pragmatism, individualism, responsibility for one's own actions, conformity, perseverance, honesty, efficiency, effectiveness, and related values. When this internalized system of beliefs comes into conflict (consciously or unconsciously) with another system of values, prejudice results. Awareness of this process in oneself can lead to significant insights.

Often, getting to know another person of a different belief system, life style, or group helps to minimize prejudice. One should be cautious not to make assumptions about an individual or a group without knowledge. Recognizing patients' individuality is essential in providing objective care and establishing relationships. If we allow our prejudices to persist, we will become confined to a narrow outlook, endlessly uncomfortable with whatever differs from the familiar.

## Stereotyping

*Stereotyping* is the presumption that an individual member of a group typifies or conforms to the perceived characteristics of the group. For example, you may think that all Native Americans (American Indians) are quiet and never express what they are thinking. In taking a nursing history, then, you might find yourself prodding the patient inappropriately to reveal information or abbreviating the history-taking in the belief that you will not be able to gather sufficient information. The inaccuracy of much stereotyping undermines objective assessment. It also narrows our thinking

about others. Even more objectionable is the tendency of inaccurate stereotyping to lead to harmful discrimination.

## Discrimination

*Discrimination* is action motivated or influenced by bias, prejudice, or stereotyping. Discriminatory acts may be implied as well as overt. For example, a nurse who repeatedly fails to respond promptly to the call light of a Chicano patient because he or she believes that Chicanos overreact to illness is discriminating on the basis of stereotyping. If, in the staff dining room, white staff members always sit apart from people of color, their behavior could be construed as discriminatory.

## Institutional Racism

*Institutional racism* is any pattern of practices on the part of social institutions, including healthcare facilities, that has tended to promote racism. Consider employment: the practice of filling jobs with individuals recommended by staff members had the effect for many years of perpetuating ethnically homogeneous staffs. The printing of signs, posters, and policies only in English in a hospital much of whose staff speaks another language is a form of racism. In hospitals, ethnic people of color have typically been more numerous in lower-level jobs than in positions with substantial decisionmaking responsibility. The traditional hierarchy has been that housekeeping and maintenance were performed by people of color, while nursing and management were done by whites. Though this pattern is changing, its existence should be recognized. While active recruitment of minorities will offset its effect, we must also resolve not to participate knowingly in the perpetuation of this or any type of racism.

## The Nurse and the Minority Patient

Nurses as a group are far more varied than was the case only a few years ago. Historically, nurses

have come primarily from the middle and lower-middle classes of society; most have been white,

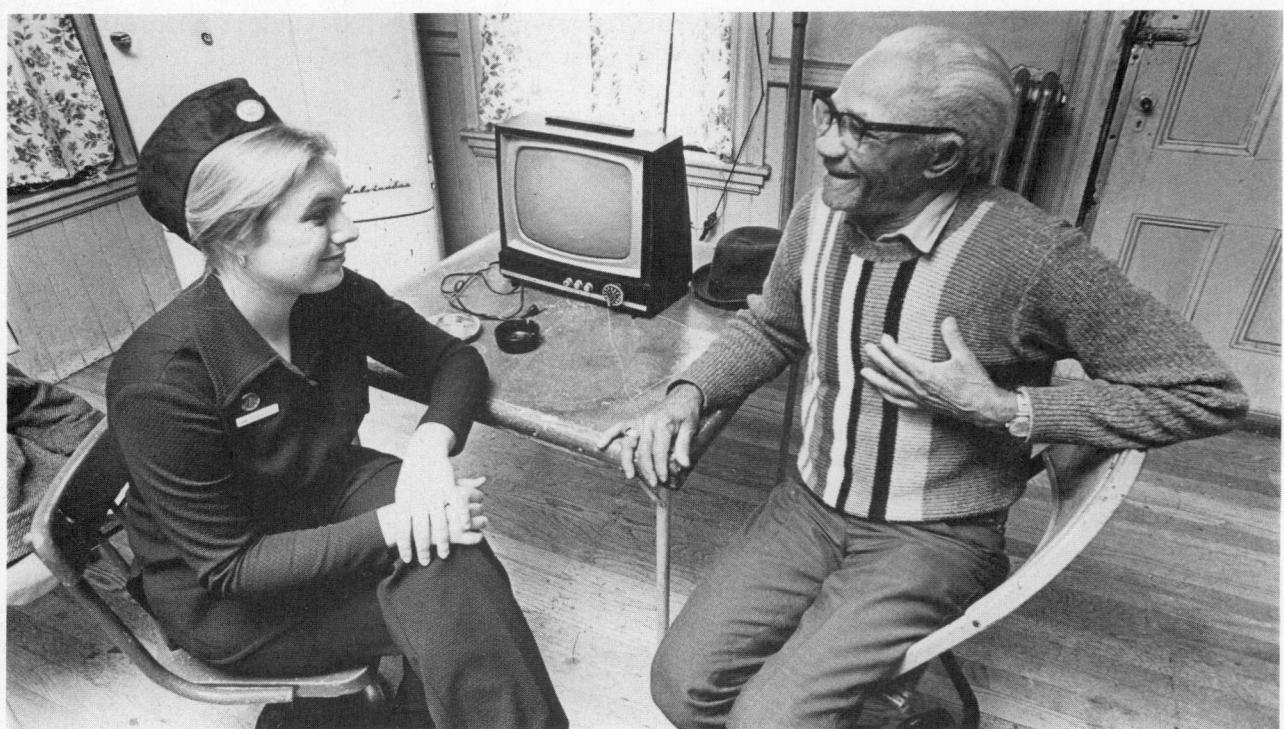

**Figure 5.1**
Smiles are universal! (L. Fleeson/Stock, Boston)

female, and recent high-school graduates. Today substantial numbers of disadvantaged and minority students are entering nursing. At the same time, equal-opportunity hiring practices in hospitals and health-care agencies are making for more social, cultural, and ethnic diversity on their staffs.

Not long ago it was typical for nurses to practice for a number of years in the same setting, caring only for patients much like themselves. Black patients, for example, were cared for in largely black facilities by black nursing staffs. Many Caucasian nurses felt uncomfortable caring for black patients partly because doing so was unfamiliar. Just as the ethnic composition of most facilities' providers has changed, so has that of their patients. Most large health-care facilities' patient populations are highly diverse, which makes it possible for nurses and patients of different backgrounds to learn and care about one another.

To care effectively for patients different from themselves, nurses need to (1) develop self-aware-

ness and understanding, (2) devote time and effort to understanding the group to which the patient belongs, and (3) determine in specific terms what the group means to the patient. Effort in these three areas will enable you to develop an appropriately individualized nursing care plan.

## Self-Awareness and Understanding

To understand yourself, you must examine, with openness and honesty, your feelings toward the group to which your patient belongs. What past experiences have you had with people of this group? Were they positive or negative? How have these experiences affected your attitude? For example, suppose you were very unsatisfied with the Italian auto mechanic who repaired your car; you felt he was uncaring and hostile. You admit you have already transferred some of your consequent hostility to the Italian patient in your care. You must then make a point of seeking out the individual characteristics that distinguish your patient from the auto mechanic, even though they share the same national origin. It may take reminders to yourself, until you know your patient better, that your patient has his or her own value and worth.

## Understanding the Group

Knowledge of the group to which the patient belongs is essential data in patient care. The best way to gain understanding of the patient's group is to spend time reading and talking with other members of that group. Inaccuracies and myths you have long accepted may be dispelled. With a more open and accepting mind, you will be better able to develop an individualized nursing care plan and to relate it to the patient in a therapeutic manner. Keep in mind the effect of recency of immigration: for example, the customs and characteristics of a Chinese immigrant will be more traditional than those of a Chinese person born and reared in the United States who has adopted Caucasian manners and ways of thinking.

## Understanding What the Group Means to the Patient

An interview or informal conversation is the most effective way to learn more about the patient and what the group means to him or her. Such an interchange should be done not in a threatening or probing way but in a manner that conveys genuine interest in the traditions and mores of the group. Simple questions and an accepting, interested attitude will be appreciated by the patient. What you learn may enable you to blend folk or ethnic health care with scientific health care in an appropriate way. For example, an elderly patient may have great faith in the powers of a copper bracelet to lessen the painful symptoms of arthritis. Alternatively, the patient may find your mode of care entirely sufficient and acceptable. Either way, it is valuable to become familiar with the patient's outlook on care.

The opportunity to plan culturally consistent care for the minority patient can be an enriching experience for the nurse.

# Important Factors in Care of Minority Patients

When we consider factors that may modify our care of minority patients, we must again underline that individuals differ more than groups. Nevertheless, it will prove enlightening to look in a general way at aspects of care that may be affected by the patient's background. Some are physical in nature and some psychological.

In every aspect of nursing care, you should consider whether appropriate adaptations should be made for the minority patient. The purpose of any such variation in care is to provide what is needed and meaningful to the patient and thus to strengthen the nurse-patient relationship. At the same time, any modification must adhere to the principles of safe and effective care.

## Assessment

Assessment of the patient, both physical and psychological, must be adapted to the patient's particular way of communicating. Unfamiliar cues are easily missed or misinterpreted. Distributions of such physical characteristics as stature, body weight, skin color, and skin texture vary from one population group to another. Expressions of feeling also differ: distrust, fear, pain, and many other negative feelings may be conveyed in ways unfamiliar to the nurse. When taking the nursing history, it is good to ask specific questions about diet, general care, and religious practices the patient values.

## Facility Policies

Exceptions to standard policy for the purpose of making care minimally disturbing to the minority patient may have to have supervisory approval. For example, the patient may consider "family" to mean not just the nuclear family but also extended family and friends. If the facility's policy is to allow only one or two family members at the bedside at any given time but the patient wants to have the entire family present, difficulties may arise. In such a case, restricting visitors may be detrimental to the patient. Similarly, if the burning or ingestion of incense or herbs conflicts with policy, it may prove best to lift the restriction.

## Diseases and Conditions Common to Minority Groups

Certain diseases and conditions are more prevalent in some population groups than others. Some, such as Tay-Sachs disease, a terminal neurologic disease of Eastern European Jews, are exclusively found in a single population group. Others are not nearly as restricted in prevalence. In general, minority people also suffer from higher incidences of such conditions as hypertension, cirrhosis, respiratory disease, alcoholism, and suicide. For environmental and economic reasons, infant and maternal mortality are higher among several minorities than in the general population.

## Territoriality

*Territoriality* is a person's emotional perception of spatial relationships with other individuals. Many colloquial phrases and metaphors attest to the emotional content of proximity and distance between people: "get off my turf," "I need my own space," "clear out," "we're very close," "let's keep in touch," "you're part of me." Territoriality has a great deal to do with trust. Trust allows for more proximity. Asking probing questions may violate territoriality.

Territoriality is an issue when caring for any patient, but particularly the minority patient. Members of some groups are made uncomfortable and even anxious if the nurse comes very close;

some will interpret standing six feet away to talk as a sign of unfriendliness or haughtiness (Stillman, 1978). The senses of privacy and modesty are essentially aspects of territoriality. Much nursing care may be looked on as an intrusion on privacy, particularly by members of groups that consider the body sacred or sacrosant. Some people will consider a daily bath an excessive and unnecessary affront to modesty.

In some cultures it is considered unwise to talk in an intimate way about others for fear of causing them harm. This outlook might lead you to characterize certain minority people as closed and secretive unless you understand the patient's perception of "safe territory." Finding a way to interact that respects the patient's physical and psychological territoriality is basic to a satisfactory therapeutic relationship. Sensitivity to what makes the patient uncomfortable is essential.

## Diet

The traditional American meat-and-potatoes diet has long since lost its primacy. Recognition that diet plays a central role in health has given rise to a variety of diets, such as low-fat, low-cholesterol, high-protein, high-fiber, and combinations of these. Furthermore, people are becoming more adventurous about the foods of other cultures. Though we as health providers are accustomed to thinking about variations in diet for health reasons, it may be unfamiliar to think about diets in terms of the patient's customs and beliefs.

Some people assign foods not just preventive but also curative power. Some popular foods may be totally unappetizing to a patient or taboo from a religious standpoint. Many Asian and Hispanic people believe in elaborate systems of "hot" and "cold" foods with a direct relationship to wellness-illness; this belief will be discussed later.

Nurses should elicit information from the family and the patient about dietary practices and their relationship to health and religious beliefs.

## Communication

Mutual understanding between patient and nurse is paramount in quality nursing care. Any use of

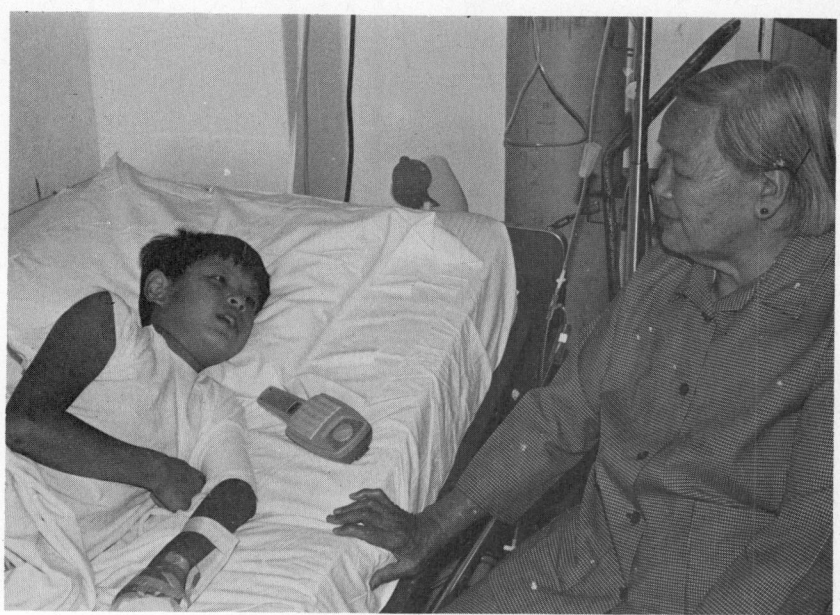

**Figure 5.2**
An elderly aunt or other member of the extended family may be a particularly important visitor for the minority patient.

language that disrupts your relationship with the patient should be carefully examined. Body language too differs from group to group. It goes without saying that the use of derogatory terms for ethnic groups is inexcusable, even outside the patient's hearing. Also offensive are such practices as calling minority patients by their first names without permission, "talking down," or underestimating the patient's skill at English. More subtle but also distressing to the minority patient is the use of so-called trigger words or phrases. Trigger words might appear to be innocuous, but they set off negative emotions in certain individuals. Phrases such as "bury the hatchet" suggest that the Indian is hostile or warlike and may be offensive to the Native American patient. Blacks may react to phrases such as "cotton pickin' hands," which refers to the menial labor once done by slaves. On the other hand, you need not try to speak like the patient; this can prove awkward and contrived. It is more important to convey respect.

Recent immigrants often have trouble with idiomatic English. For instance, a patient admitted for mild head trauma reported he had been struck by a ball; a bystander had suddenly yelled, "DUCK!" and he had looked around for a duck. Try to choose literal, commonly used, straightforward language—the kind you would appreciate if you were learning a new language (see Chapter 12).

## Health Teaching

Some minority patients will have had little or no experience with health teaching and unpleasant and/or limited experience in formal education. The role of learner may seem humiliating or may cause role confusion if the nurse is viewed as a deliverer of physical care rather than a teacher. The process may have to be clearly delineated somewhat more specifically than usual. Visual aids are helpful, particularly if they employ symbols or words familiar to the patient.

## Spiritual Beliefs and Healing

In many minority groups, religion has traditionally pervaded daily life. In particular, religion is viewed as fundamental to the prevention of disease and to healing. Diet, hygiene practices, exercise, rest, and attire may have religious significance. Another outlook shared by people of many backgrounds is the concept of balance: health is seen as a matter of balance between man and na-

Social, Cultural, and Ethnic Diversity    **77**

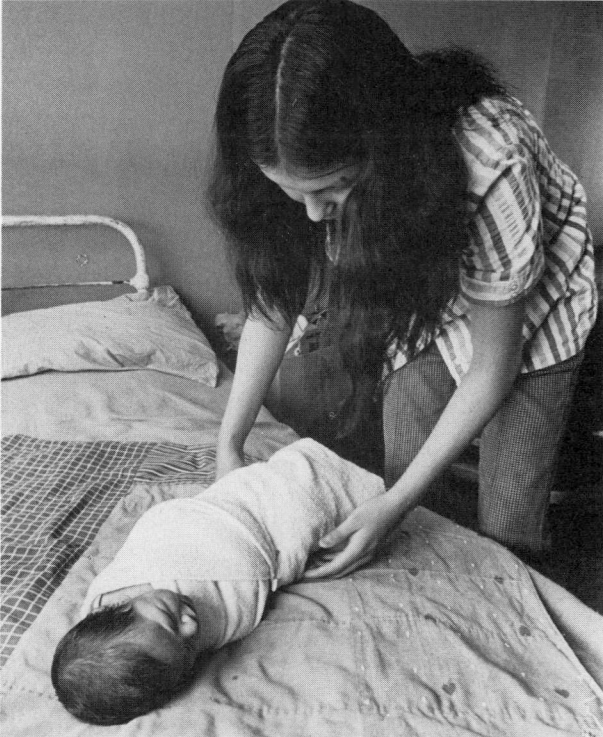

**Figure 5.3**
Attire may reflect traditional beliefs regarding health maintenance. For example, swaddling the infant may be seen as essential to the child's healthy development. (Dan Bernstein)

ture, which is maintained through religion. Because spiritual beliefs are so closely intertwined with health care, it is essential to assess the minority patient's spiritual beliefs as they relate to planning care. By no means will all minority patients, of course, be religious.

The patient may have a religious leader, whether a minister, priest, chief, shaman, or healer. The family may wish to burn or smoke substances at the bedside as part of a ceremony or to bring in foods forbidden by the patient's diet. The nurse should support and try to gain permission, if necessary, for any religious practice that is meaningful to the patient and not injurious.

## Death and Bereavement

Some cultures view death much more realistically than is prevalent in Western society. Death is viewed, particularly if the person's life has been productive, as the natural end of existence. Sudden death may be attributed to outside influences, real or supernatural. The hereafter has varying degrees of importance: some see it as redemptive, with heaven or other sacred abode as the desired goal; other groups consider the hereafter a reuniting with one's ancestors.

Burial practices are expressions of bereavement. It is very important for the nurse to help the family of the deceased prepare for burial according to their customs: conformity to tradition helps greatly to resolve grief. Matters of concern may include sitting with the body in the hospital; prayers, chants, and rituals; cleansing and dressing the body; and whether or not all the body parts are to be released to the family for burial. One must find out the family's specific wishes: assumptions are inappropriate. Hospital policies on death rituals are becoming more liberal.

## Major Cultural and Ethnic Groups

There are over one hundred distinct population groups in the United States. We must of necessity limit ourselves to discussing those that are largest and/or most visible.

There is risk in generalizing any group, since doing so easily suggests stereotyping. It must be repeated that individuals vary more than groups. To assume that every Asian eats rice or that every

black understands and uses Black English is a disservice to the individual.

The following brief portraits are not meant to be taken as definitive. Using other resources including the family, and performing thorough individual assessment are the keys to caring for minority persons.

# Ethnic People of Color

People of color and/or distinctive physical appearance are more recognizable as belonging to a certain ethnic group. It is not uncommon for people of the second and third generations to be taken for recent immigrants. And yet they may know little of the traditions and practices of their heritage.

The main ethnic peoples of color in the United States are Native Americans, Asians, black Americans, and Hispanics.

## Native Americans

*Native Americans*, also called Indians, trace their ancestry to the native people inhabiting the Americas when Europeans arrived. The term Native American refers inclusively to almost one million people, including the Eskimo. It is possible only to sketch general characteristics of Native Americans since there are so many tribal groups. Many Native Americans no longer adhere to Indian or Eskimo tradition and are assimilated into the general population.

### Historical Background

The Bureau of Indian Affairs (BIA) was established by the federal government in 1834 to oversee the affairs of over 250 tribes. For many years there was no Indian representation in the Bureau, and far more effort went into negotiating treaties than into providing good health care, education, and other needed services. In 1955, after years of discontent on the part of Native Americans who believed the BIA was not receptive to them or meeting their needs, the Indian Health Service was organized under the Department of Health, Education and Welfare. This organization has expanded and remains active today.

### Health Care and Incidence of Disease

Native Americans have typically not received quality health care, either preventive or curative.

Though the Indian Health Service is more attentive than its precursor to the needs of Native Americans, the incidence of illness and disease remains high. Infant mortality is twice that of the rest of the population. The average family on a reservation subsists on an income well below the official poverty level. For this reason many aspects of life are substandard, including nutrition. Although accidents remain the prime cause of death, diseases characteristic of the economically disadvantaged have a high incidence among Native Americans: these conditions include alcoholism, pneumonia, gastritis, cirrhosis, and other diseases of the respiratory and intestinal tract. There is also concern regarding the high incidence of homicide and suicide.

### Family

The family is very important in Native American culture and is generally quite broadly defined as consisting of a "community family." All children of the tribe may be conceived of as belonging to all members of the community, and the responsibility of childrearing may be shared. This practice derives from the era when high adult mortality made for many parentless children who were simply transferred to the care of another family. Most Native American children, having learned from the group what is acceptable and unacceptable behavior, need not be constantly reminded to behave.

It is often very important to the Native American patient to have the family—sometimes quite a large group—gather at the bedside. The patient may feel it important to consult with the family on medical treatment before giving consent, and policy may have to be set aside to provide for this.

### Territoriality

A Native American patient may reveal information cautiously, which could lead to the false conclusion that he or she is not interested in care. In-

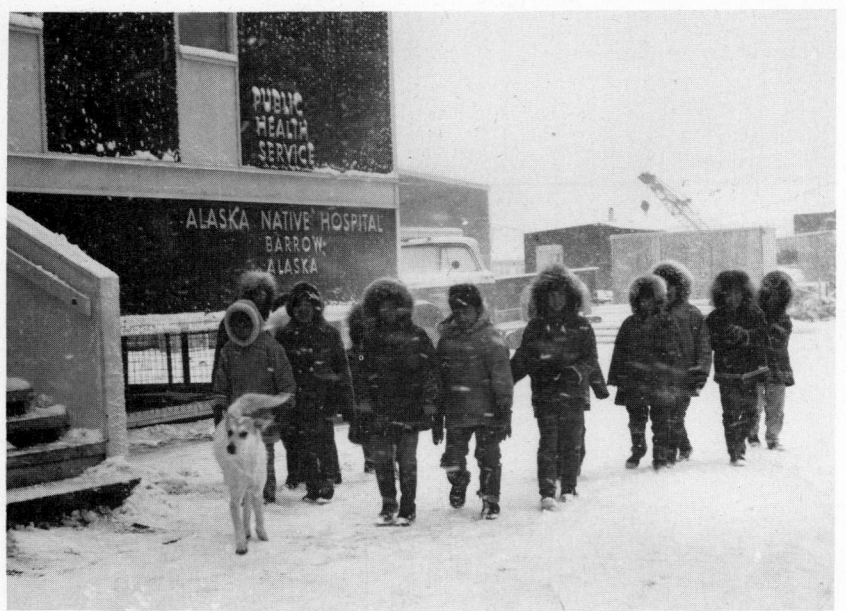

**Figure 5.4**
The Indian Health Service was set up in 1955. (Indian Health Service, U.S.P.H.S., D.H.H.S.)

stead, Native Americans tend to be private people with whom trust is built slowly. The family, however, may prove extremely helpful, offering you information to supplement the nursing history you gather from the patient. Any manipulation or invasion of a body part may be considered a threat to territoriality. A procedure that requires disrobing, for example, should be undertaken only after complete preparation of the patient, including conscientious draping.

## Diet

The diet of Native Americans has traditionally been composed of such natural foods as roots, grains, vegetables, and meats. Food also has a religious significance: for example, cornmeal may be spread around the bedside of the ill to aid recovery; it can be swept up but should not be discarded (Backup, 1979). Native Americans may eat only when hungry, thus may not eat three meals a day at designated times. The nurse's expectations with regard to eating will have to be altered to individualize care. When the government attempted to introduce more protein into the Indian diet by distributing dried milk and cheese, the program proved largely unsuccessful because Native Americans found such food unfamiliar and unappetizing.

## Communication

Native Americans speak many tribal languages and dialects. Most also communicate fluently in standard English, though some idioms may be misunderstood. With non-Indians, the Indian patient may be less verbal than with other Indians. Conversation is often not easily initiated, and eye contact may be avoided since looking into the eyes of a stranger is considered tantamount to looking into the soul. A quiet approach to the patient, combined with genuine interest and acceptance, is the best overture to communication. The nurse should be familiar with traditional forms of address for elders, women, men, youth, and children and should use them accordingly.

## Spiritual Beliefs and Healing

Native Americans traditionally see themselves as part of nature; concomitantly, health is seen as a state of being in balance with nature and illness as an imbalance. Because evil thoughts and deeds are considered possible causes of illness, the ill person may feel punished. Spirits too are perceived as causing illness and needing to be appeased. The medicine man is thus seen as a care giver. The patient may not participate in scientific health care fully or actively, viewing it as essentially unnecessary. Traditional Indian treatments may include exercise, dietary regimens, herbs, "sweating," the use of symbolic amulets, and such rituals as prayers, chants, and dances.

Few Native Americans live "by the clock," which may interfere with the precise schedules we associate with good nursing care. (This equation on the part of nurses is an expression of the dominant culture's preoccupation with efficiency.) The Native American may believe that one sleeps when sleepy and eats when hungry. The patient may not consider it important to have appointments, medications, and meals at any particular time. Minimizing scheduled care and explaining clearly the rationale for procedures that must be done on time is the best approach.

## Death and Bereavement

To the Native American, death is both a mystical experience and the natural end of life. The hereafter is not of overriding importance, though it is consoling that the departed has been united with his or her ancestors. Some groups are very demonstrative in grief; some are silent. Regardless of outward expression, the sense of loss is deeply felt throughout the community.

Burial practices vary widely from one Native American tribe to another. The nurse should carefully inquire about what is customary. Because the body is considered a "whole" of nature, a body part or organ that has been removed may be requested for burial with the body. Some groups bury all the clothes of the deceased so his or her spirit will have no reason to return. All possessions should thus be carefully returned to the family. A few groups still perform ritual wrapping of the body in ceremonial clothes, which may be done in the hospital. Embalming is usually forbidden. The caring nurse will give the bereavement period special attention.

## Asian Americans

The Asian American population is a large, diverse group consisting mainly of Japanese, Chinese, Filipinos, and Koreans. Southeast Asians, such as people from Thailand and Malaysia, have also im-

migrated to North America. In urban areas, second- and third-generation families continue to reside in communities made up largely of members of their own nationality.

## Historical Background

The first Asian immigrants, mostly Chinese, received free passage to the United States in exchange for helping to build the railroads. The trickle of Japanese entering the country soon swelled as the dream of a better life in America became, for some, a reality. By the time the transcontinental railroad was completed in 1869, thousands of Asians had become immigrant Americans. At about the same time, Filipinos were being recruited to work in Hawaiian plantations, Alaskan canneries, and California farmlands. These people received a pittance in pay, and many died of malnutrition and exposure to diseases to which they had no natural immunity. Since the 1950s, many Asian families have immigrated for political and professional reasons, some joining the medical community. Asian immigration is continuing at a rapid rate, the most recent large influx being Vietnamese and Cambodian refugees.

## Health Care and
## Incidence of Disease

Like Native Americans, Asians have often received inadequate health care. The language barrier and adherence to familiar native remedies caused many Asians to forgo modern health care and pursue their traditional medical practice.

Asian Americans appear to be prone to hypertension, tuberculosis, and diseases of the bone. The incidence of heart disease and cancer of the stomach has been lower than in the general population, though both have risen as more Asians adopted Westernized diets. Malnutrition has been reported in the elderly. Health care may consist of a combination of the use of herbs, special foods, acupuncture, and conventional medicine. The dominant concept in Asian medicine is energy. Because energizing the organs and senses is thought to prevent illness, sickness is typically perceived as a lack of energy. Acupuncture has been used for centuries among the Chinese as a method of instilling energy in designated portions of the body and as an analgesic agent. Its use by other Asians as an analgesic agent is relatively recent. Herbal broths are often administered. Among many traditional Chinese and other segments of the Oriental population, harmony with the five elements of nature—fire, earth, metal, water, and wood—is all-important, and these substances are often used in rituals of healing.

## Family

It is typical in Asian families for the elderly to be treated with respect, as having acquired great wisdom. The old and infirm are usually cared for within the family. Children are highly treasured; traditional families may value boys more than girls. In the traditional Japanese home, for example, the males are served meals before the females. Care of the sick is seen as a family and community responsibility.

## Territoriality

Asian patients typically perceive privacy, both physical and emotional, to have well-demarcated boundaries. The stereotype of communal baths to the contrary, Japanese patients tend to be extremely modest. Steps should be taken to provide maximum privacy. It is considered respectful and courteous to ask permission of an Asian patient to perform even routine care, for example, asking permission before opening the patient's bedside stand or closet. It is also important to solicit the patient's participation in decision making.

## Diet

Asians traditionally consider nutrition the most important aspect of keeping in harmony with nature (Branch, 1979). Foods are classified as Yin (cold) and Yang (hot)—on the basis of perceived nature, not temperature. Because one must achieve a balance between the two for optimum health, hot food, such as seasoned bean curd, might be served with a cold food, such as melon. (Some Asian groups, such as Filipinos, do not adhere to this concept.) Some foods are seen as having curative powers in certain illnesses. The powers of food are explained in detail to children. Salads are not typically eaten. Entrails and organs are traditionally considered "blood-building."

## Communication

If there is a language barrier between you and the patient, try to find a bilingual staff member or family member to interpret. Do not assume that anyone from the same country of origin can do so: the Filipinos, for example, speak numerous dialects. Many large cities have language banks that offer free translation services for health-care institutions. More and more hospitals are employing professional medical translators.

## Spiritual Beliefs and Healing

Prevention and healing are central concepts in traditional Asian religion. Fatalism—the belief that what happens is predetermined—may deeply influence the patient's perception of the illness. The family may want to burn incense or leaves and roots thought to have beneficial powers. Amulets are sometimes used to ward off or bring about the exit of evil spirits.

Catholic Asians may wear religious medals or crucifixes around their necks or pinned to their underclothes. A rosary may also be among the patient's most valued belongings. These sources of faith in the healing power of God should not be taken off or misplaced. Vietnamese patients may forbid the drawing of blood, which is thought to cause the good spirit of the body to exit (DeGracia, 1979).

## Death and Bereavement

Death is viewed by most Asians as the process by which one is reunited with one's ancestors and thus as a transcendence to a better life. Weeping may be seen as weakness, particularly on the part of males, though grief is deeply felt. Once again, death practices vary from one group and even one family to another; consult the family. Bells and incense may be used in the death ceremony, particularly by Chinese. Fast and lively music is often played at the funeral to cheer up the survivors. On special occasions during the first year after the death, a place may be set for the deceased at the table. Prayers are said for and to the departed.

## Black Americans

The largest minority in the United States is black Americans. Over 11 percent of the population was black in 1970, and the 1980 census will probably show an increase. Black Americans are predominantly urban; many are confined to ghettos by social and economic pressures. Blacks' visibility has made them particularly vulnerable to discrimination.

### Historical Background

The first black slaves arrived at the ports of New England in the early 1600s to be sold into bondage as commodities. Many whites did not regard blacks as full human beings with feelings like their own. The Quakers were among the first to raise a concerted outcry against inhumane treatment of blacks. The general outlines of subsequent black history in the United States are well known and hardly a source of pride for nonblacks.

Black pride has blossomed over the past two decades, and past discriminatory practices are being redressed by equal-opportunity laws and affirmative-action programs in an effort to correct blacks' economic and educational disadvantages.

### Health Care and Incidence of Disease

The death rate of black infants is twice that of nonblacks, comparable to that of Native Americans. Even more startling, the maternal death rate is eight times that of nonblacks. Other diseases and conditions prevalent among blacks are sickle-cell anemia (a hereditary disease seen largely in blacks), hypertension, diabetes, obesity, heart disease, tuberculosis, and malnutrition. Alcoholism is much more prevalent than among nonblacks.

Black patients may feel suspicious of the predominantly white health-care system. Though there are more black physicians and nurses than ever before, the medical and nursing professions continue to be dominated by whites.

Health may be measured by black patients in terms of ability to work: to have to miss work means one is quite sick. Many blacks do not react to poor health until a crisis situation occurs, such as extreme pain, high fever, or bleeding. Otherwise, they tend to accept poor health as a fact of life. There remains a strong strain of black folk medicine in health and healing practices. Herbs and certain foods are thought to have medicinal powers, and objects may be attributed preventive or curative powers. For example, a copper bracelet may be worn to cure arthritis. Spiritual health and physical health are seen as closely intertwined. Black medicine, which involves beliefs originating in Africa, is still used by a limited number of blacks.

### Family

Black families have felt the impact of poverty and discrimination. Many African societies were matrilineal, tracing descent through the mother (Jacques, 1979). For this and a complex of other reasons, including greater employment discrimination against black men, many black families are headed by women. Children are often strongly encouraged to do well in school so they can live better lives.

### Territoriality

Blacks, whose territoriality has often been brutally ignored, tend to have mixed feelings about privacy. Until trust is built, a black patient may act aloof and suspicious of nonblacks. When trust has been established, however, the same patient may be open, verbal, and generous. Physical closeness and touching are common when trust has been established.

## Diet

The traditional black diet shows the influence of poverty. Grits, a porridge made from coarsely ground cornmeal, is served with most meals in the South, along with cooked greens and potatoes. Lard and fats are prevalent in the black diet, which may contribute to the high incidence of obesity and heart disease among blacks.

## Communication

Because black patients and nonblack care providers both speak English, one might assume communication would present no problems. However, communication is far more than mere words, and even the words we use may cause lapses of communication. Many economically disadvantaged blacks speak Black English, a variation of English with unique inflections, sentence constructions, and vocabulary. For example, the sentence "She be sick" is not incorrect standard English; it conforms to the grammatical rules of Black English. Much standard slang originates in Black English and spreads to the dominant culture.

Mutual suspicion and awkwardness can attend communication between blacks and whites. If the nurse is straightforward, honest, and caring, most communication problems can be overcome.

## Spiritual Beliefs and Healing

Most blacks are Christians, for whom Jesus is the important religious figure. Prevalent attitudes toward illness invoke God's will and redemption through suffering. This outlook sometimes coexists with the age-old view that one must be in harmony with nature to be physically and spiritually healthy. Rituals may be performed for preventive as well as curative reasons.

## Death and Bereavement

Death is no stranger to blacks, whose life expectancy is seven to eight years less than that of the white population. Belief in the hereafter is strong, and death is often referred to as "crossing over."

The outlook that death is God's will and leads to a better life "on the other side" may be of great consolation to survivors.

Bereavement may be expressed very emotionally even to the point of prostration. Such behavior may be upsetting to nonblacks who do not understand its significance for the family. Because viewing the body is important, the nurse should take special pains to make this possible in the hospital and to prepare the body for viewing. All possessions should be returned to the family, since they are valued as reminders of the deceased.

## Hispanic Americans

The inclusive term *Hispanic* refers to people whose native language is Spanish or Portuguese, including immigrants from Mexico, Puerto Rico, Cuba, Central and South America, and Spain.

Easily distinguished by language and appearance, Hispanics have suffered from pervasive discrimination and disadvantage. The difficulty of integrating into the general population has caused many second- and third-generation Hispanics to remain in tightly knit communities known as *barrios*.

## Historical Background

By 1620, when the Pilgrims landed at Plymouth Rock, much of the Southwest had been explored, mapped, and colonized by the Spanish. Texas, California, Arizona, and New Mexico were under the Spanish flag long before the American Revolution. Thus Hispanics were in a sense the first immigrants.

Many Mexican-Americans have more recently entered the United States as farm workers. (The term *Chicano*, which refers specifically to Mexican-Americans, is preferred by some but not all Mexican-Americans. Some identify this term with the politically active segment of their group and choose not to use *Chicano*.) In the past, the relatively unguarded southern borders allowed easy, illegal access to the United States. Many Hispanic immigrants entered the ranks of migrant workers, who move from one part of the country to another as crops need harvesting. The United Farm Workers

Union, whose membership is largely Hispanic, successfully brought pressure on farm owners to improve the lives of other farm laborers.

Even more recently, Hispanic political refugees from several countries have sought asylum in the United States. Many are seeking employment in the professions they practiced in their native countries.

## Health Care and Incidence of Disease

Most Hispanics must contend with below-average family incomes and thus are particularly subject to diseases associated with the economically disadvantaged: obesity, diabetes, hypertension, respiratory disease, and gastrointestinal disturbances are prevalent. Language barriers can magnify economic barriers to high-quality health care. Though high suicide rates usually accompany economic disadvantages, this is not the case with Hispanics, probably due to the teaching that suicide is sinful.

Strongly Catholic, most Hispanics tend to interpret health and illness as the "will of God." Many Hispanics regard *machismo* (maleness) and *hembrisma* (femaleness) as related to health. Belief in the "*mal de ojo*" (evil eye) is unique to Hispanic culture. *Brujas* are evil people able to cause illnesses, discomfort, and other problems. Hispanics who believe in such traditional interpretations of illness consider the established health-care system not beneficial for such conditions and thus use home remedies (*remedios*) and consult folk healers (*curanderos*) who derive their powers from God.

Amulets, charms, and other objects used by Hispanic patients should be considered cultural adjuncts to care. If they do not impede or contradict recognized health therapies, they may provide the Hispanic patient and the family a measure of psychological comfort not available from other sources.

## Family

The extended family is important to Hispanics. Children are a source of great pride and are usually very well behaved. The elderly are shown respect and cared for by younger members of the family. Many religious holidays are observed with family gatherings.

## Territoriality

Hispanic culture tends to be both expressive and inclusive. Hispanic patients usually welcome touch and may be offended if a handshake is withheld. Communication is expressive and personal territory is generously shared in trusting relationships. Other patients and care providers who are more exclusively territorial may feel threatened by traditional Hispanic effusiveness.

## Diet

The diet of the Hispanic population tends to be dominated by beans, lentils, corn, rice, and meats. Garlic, once used by Hispanics to fight diphtheria, is now regarded as a general medicinal agent. Hispanics share with Asians an elaborate system relating "hot" foods and "cold" foods to the incidence and cure of disease. Much of the Hispanic diet is highly spiced.

## Communication

Hispanics from different Spanish-speaking countries can usually understand one another. However, a nurse who speaks only English may have a profound communication problem caring for the Hispanic patient who speaks only Spanish or Portuguese. A small pocket dictionary may prove quite helpful to the care provider in routine care. Using a translator is also a viable alternative for developing appropriate communication.

## Spiritual Beliefs and Healing

Nearly all Hispanics are Catholics. The Virgin Mary is the dominant figure, and prayers for health are offered up to her. Pictures of the Virgin are prominent in Hispanic homes, and the patient may keep a crucifix at the bedside. The patient may find the Sacrament of the Sick a comforting ritual, and prayers may be offered to the patient's patron saint.

## Death and Bereavement

Death is viewed as natural and as God's will. The body may be viewed privately by the family and close friends but is usually not viewed at the Mass. Death rituals may be influenced by such cultural traditions as fast and lively music, lighting of candles, and feasting. Grief is expressed openly, and weeping is widely accepted for both males and females. Body parts and organs are sometimes requested for burial.

# Socioeconomically Disadvantaged Groups

Many socially and economically disadvantaged Americans are also the victims of discrimination. Such people, some of whom are Caucasian and elderly, often suffer extreme hardship and stresses that lead to illness. This population's needs and problems must be addressed if we are to equalize access to health care and promote health maintenance.

## The Migrant Population

Migrants in North American society are not always regarded as a minority, since they do not share a common cultural heritage. Thus, although they share many of the problems of other minority groups, they enjoy few of the benefits.

The mere fact of being migrant creates health-care problems, such as unfamiliarity with the health resources of a community. Disease and unhealthy conditions may not be diagnosed promptly because of a lack of nearby facilities. Health records are frequently lacking. And because the life style and cultural orientation of the migrant patient is different from that of the providers of health care, poor communication is likely to result.

These circumstances lead to poor health maintenance, discontinuous and fragmented treatment, and little or no follow-up care. Migrant health agencies are coming to the aid of migrant families in some states, but their capacities are still far too limited to meet the need.

## The Urban and Rural Poor

Though the urban and rural poor are less mobile than the migrant family, they share many of the same deprivations. Health is relative since many diseases and conditions proliferate among the economically disadvantaged.

Living quarters may make health-care practices difficult, if not impossible. Limited education may affect ability to understand illness and participate in care. Poor people may be reluctant to seek health care because they fear they will feel awkward or shabby, and transportation may be difficult. Another factor may be the feeling that "charity" health care is undesirable or an admission that one is poor. Nutrition may be inadequate because of limited income and lack of information about the purchase and use of correct foods.

Health conditions prevalent among the poor include obesity (caused primarily by excessive consumption of high-carbohydrate, high-calorie cheap foods), malnutrition, diabetes, tuberculosis, depression, suicide, and homicide. Infant and maternal mortality rates are above the national average.

Poverty undermines dignity. Many of the poor must still laboriously justify their qualification for care and spend long hours waiting on clinic benches. They may receive sound medical treatment from medical centers associated with universities but find their personal feelings and individuality ignored. This is, in all fairness, not always the case, and socially responsible health-care providers are influencing changes that better serve the needs of disadvantaged patients.

## Guidelines for Care of Minority Patients

Having briefly reviewed the multitude of factors that must be taken into account, let us consider some guidelines to caring for minority patients.

First, make it your responsibility to learn as much as possible about yourself and about the patient. The patient and the family are the most valuable sources of knowledge and information. Learning about what they value can only serve to enhance the relationship. The most difficult aspects of caring for culturally different patients will probably be remaining nonjudgmental and providing culturally consistent nursing care.

Second, adapt your plan of care to the patient's ethnic and cultural needs. You should not expect patients to adapt their practices to fit in more conveniently with your care plan.

Third, devote time and effort to learning more about the adaptations in care we have discussed, keeping in mind that doing so helps us grow personally and professionally. We must also constantly remind ourselves that each patient is an individual and that we should never assume a particular outlook or life style without verification.

## Conclusion

Opportunities for personal growth in nursing are bountiful. One of the richest opportunities nursing offers is contact with people of all faiths, cultures, and races. Such relationships allow for learning more about others and about ourselves as individuals and as care providers. For too long, nurses have treated patients across a barrier erected by the we/they dichotomy. Particularly with minority patients, this attitude can threaten quality care. It is time to work at ridding ourselves of suspicions, ignorance, unfamiliarity, and fears.

## Study Terms

amulets
Asian
assimilation
*barrios*
bereavement
bias
Black English
*brujas*
Caucasian
Chicano
*curanderos*
disadvantaged
discrimination
diverse
equality
Hispanic
institutional racism
*mal de ojo*
melting pot
migrant
minority
Native American
prejudice
shaman
stereotyping
territoriality
Yin and Yang

## Learning Activities

**1.** Using the most recent census report for your community, identify the various ethnic groups represented and the percent of the community belonging to each group. Share your information with your clinical group.
**2.** Visit a food market that caters to a particular ethnic group. List those foods that are also commonly found in supermarkets and those that are particular to that market. Compare the costs for items in this market with those in a supermarket.
**3.** Find out what provisions (if any) your clinical facility makes for assisting a patient/client who does not speak English.
**4.** Does your community have a language bank available for translating? If one exists, gather information on how it can be contacted and the policies regarding its use. Are fees charged for translation services? Who pays those fees?

# References

Arnold, H. M. "I-Thou." *American Journal of Nursing* 70 (December 1970): 2554.

Backup, Ruth Wallis. "Implementing Quality Health Care for the American Indian Patient." *Washington State Journal of Nursing* (Special Supplement) (1979): 20–32.

Bonaparte, B. H. "Ego Defensiveness, Open-Closedmindedness, and Nurses' Attitude Toward Culturally Different Patients." *Nursing Research* 28 (May/June 1979): 116–172.

Branch, Marie Foster, and Paxton, Phyllis Perry. *Providing Safe Nursing Care for Ethnic People of Color*. New York: Appleton Century Crofts, 1976.

Chow, Effie, "Cultural Health Traditions: Asian Perspectives." In *Providing Safe Nursing Care for Ethnic People of Color*, edited by Marie Foster Branch and Phyllis Perry Paxton, pp. 99–114. New York: Appleton-Century-Crofts, 1976.

DeGracia, Rosario T. "Perspectives on the Asian American's Implications for Health Care." *Washington State Journal of Nursing* (Special Supplement) (1979): 9–19.

Dorsey, Pauline Rodriguez, and Jackson, Herlinda Quintero. "Cultural Health Traditions: The Latino/Chicano Perspective." In *Providing Safe Nursing Care for Ethnic People of Color*, edited by Marie Foster Branch and Phyllis Perry Paxton, pp. 41–80. New York: Appleton-Century-Crofts, 1976.

Gonzalez, Hector Hugo. "Health Beliefs of Some Mexican-Americans." In *Becoming Aware of Cultural Differences in Nursing*, pp. 1–2. Kansas City: American Nurses' Association, 1975.

———. "Health Care Needs of the Mexican-American." In *Ethnicity and Health Care*, pp. 21–28. New York: National League for Nursing, 1976.

U.S. Department of Health, Education and Welfare. *Indian Health Trends and Services*, 1974.

James, S. M. "When Your Patient Is Black West Indian." *American Journal of Nursing* 78 (November 1978): 1908–1909.

Jacques, Gladys. "Cultural Health Traditions: A Black Perspective." In *Providing Safe Nursing Care for Ethnic People of Color*, edited by Marie Foster Branch and Phyllis Perry Paxton, pp. 115–124. New York: Appleton-Century-Crofts, 1976.

Joe, Jennie; Gallerito, Cecelia; and Pino, Josephine. "Cultural Health Traditions: American Indian Perspectives." In *Providing Safe Nursing Care for Ethnic People of Color*, edited by Marie Foster Branch and Phyllis Perry Paxton, pp. 81–98. New York: Appleton-Century-Crofts, 1976.

Leininger, Madeleine M. "Becoming Aware of Types of Health Practitioners and Cultural Imposition." In *Becoming Aware of Cultural Differences in Nursing*, pp. 9–15. Kansas City: American Nurses' Association, 1973.

Martinez, Ricardo Arguijo, ed. *Hispanic Culture and Health Care*. St. Louis: C. V. Mosby Co., 1978.

Malhiot, Grete, and Ninan, Mary. "A Seminar for Minority Students." *Nursing Outlook* 27 (July 1979): 473–475.

Miller, M. H. "On Blacks Entering Nursing." *Nursing Forum* 11 (November 1972): 248–263.

Murillo-Rohde, Ildaura. "Cultural Sensitivity in the Care of the Hispanic Patient." *Washington State Journal of Nursing* (Special Supplement) (1979): 25–32.

Pegues, Thelma. "Physical and Psychological Assessment of the Black Patient." *Washington State Journal of Nursing* (Special Supplement) (1979): 4–8.

Pflug, Charlotte Carver; Marsh, Linda; and Hofbauer, Eileen. "Students Meet the Migrants." *American Journal of Nursing* 75 (July 1975): 1166–1167.

Primeaux, M. "Caring for the American Indian Patient." *American Journal of Nursing* 77, no. 1 (January 1977): 91–94.

Robinson, A. M. "Black Nurses Tell You Why So Few Blacks in Nursing." *RN* 35, no. 7 (July 1972): 33–41ff.

Wass, H., *et al.* "United States and Brazilian Childrens' Concepts of Death." *Death Education* 3, no. 1 (September 1979): 41–55.

White, E. H. "Symposium on Cultural and Biological Diversity and Health Care. Giving Health Care to Minority Patients." *Nursing Clinics of North America* 12, no. 3 (March 1977): 27–40.

# Chapter 6
# Understanding Groups

### Objectives

Upon completion of this chapter, you should be able to:
1. Discuss the needs of a group.
2. Name and describe the stages of a group.
3. Explain the factors that affect the functioning of a group.
4. Characterize the various styles of group leadership.
5. Discuss factors that contribute to the effectiveness of a group leader.
6. Define *group content* and *group process*.
7. Discuss effective group participation.

### Outline

Nurses often work with people in groups, including groups of patient/clients, families, and health-care personnel. A basic familiarity with the functioning of groups will help you approach such situations with greater confidence and skill.

A group is not merely a collection of individuals. People gathered together become a group only when they recognize a common goal, and they remain a group only as long as they continue to share a goal. The common *goal* is what ultimately defines the group. A number of people who happen to gather together without a common goal or function are simply an *aggregate*. For example, a large number of students crossing a campus between classes is merely an aggregate. If six of them stop to help someone who is hurt, those six become a group.

## The Needs of a Group

Just as a person has individual needs, a group has collective needs. Meeting the needs of groups is more complex than meeting individuals' needs. In order for group needs to be met, all the individuals in the group must feel that their individual needs are being met. When such needs are met, the group can function with purpose and direction. When they are not met, the group may become dysfunctional and even disintegrate.

Like individuals, groups have both physical and psychosocial needs (see Exhibit 6.1). They too form a hierarchy on which the physical needs are the most basic and the psychosocial needs are higher. As with individuals, meeting a group's basic needs allows it to address its higher-level needs. It is also possible for a group to ignore basic physical needs when its higher needs are particularly cherished.

### The Physical Needs of a Group

A group's physical needs involve time, space, size, and comfort. Time, space, and comfort may be characterized as *environment*. Physical needs are as important to a group as they are to an individual. Size and environment can facilitate or exercise restraints on the ways a group may act.

### Time

A group needs adequate time together in order to function. Inadequate time will frustrate the individual members of the group and prevent the group from functioning effectively. Another important consideration is a mutually satisfactory time to meet. If group meetings conflict with other aspects of members' lives, their performance in the group will be impaired and they might have to withdraw. Meetings ought not to be so prolonged that fatigue sets in, interfering with interest and productivity. For the same reason, it may be more productive to meet early in the day.

### Space

The place where a group meets ought to be both adequate in size for the number of participants and constructed in such a way as to allow the group to function. The arrangement of furniture, acoustics, lighting, and privacy all affect the suitability of the space. Familiarity is also an important factor: a familiar location where group members feel safe may enhance interaction. On the other hand, a new locale may serve to distinguish the

Exhibit 6.1
**The Needs of a Group**

| Physical | Psychosocial |
|----------|--------------|
| Time | Common goal |
| Space | Action |
| Size | Sense of accomplishment |
| Comfort | Personal satisfaction |

group from outsiders and thus help its members to focus on the goal.

## Size

A small group may consist of only three or four people; moderate-sized groups average twenty to thirty and large groups may number a hundred or more. Appropriate size varies with the purpose of the group. In most situations in which you find yourself as a nurse, a relatively small group of three to fifteen (twenty at most) will prove most effective. Optimum size is determined by the group's tasks and the way its members function.

## Comfort

In order for the group to be physically comfortable, such matters as room temperature, comfortable chairs, and lack of distracting noises need to be considered.

## The Psychosocial Needs of a Group

The psychosocial needs of any group include a common goal, action, a sense of accomplishment, and the personal satisfaction of the individual members. When these psychosocial needs are met, the members will be happier with the group and tend to remain in it, and the group will move more effectively toward its goals.

## Common Goals

Every group has some purpose or goal whether or not it is explicitly stated. For example, though some of their other individual goals may vary, the members of a particular college class share the general goal of learning the content of the course.

## Action

A group acts in such a way as to move toward its goals. This action may or may not be successful,

but a group that is not trying to move toward its goals will soon dissolve. If the students enrolled in a course do not participate actively in it, they fail to constitute a real group. Action is essential to the definition and the continued existence of any group.

## Sense of Accomplishment

A sense of accomplishment originates in the members' feeling that the group is making progress toward its goals. Such progress need not be massive or rapid for a sense of accomplishment to develop; the key factor is its significance in the eyes of the group members. This sense of accomplishment is rooted in the work of the group as a whole rather than the contributions of individual members.

## Personal Satisfaction

Personal satisfaction results when the individual members of a group feel that they are valuable contributors to the group. This process is enhanced when the members feel that the group meets some of their personal needs. The degree to which a group meets personal needs may vary considerably, depending on its purpose. The purpose of some groups is such that individual needs must be submerged in the needs and function of the group. If the members accept this as the way the group will function, its work will not suffer. The members must find their personal satisfaction in accomplishing the goals of the group. If an individual expects the group to meet personal needs, such as a need for recognition, and it fails to do so, he or she may not contribute to the group and may even undermine it. Being clear about the expectations of the group for meeting individual needs and discussing them openly will help to resolve this dilemma.

The major purpose of some groups, such as psychotherapy or counseling groups, is to meet the needs of individual members. In such a group, it is appropriate to expect others to help meet one's personal needs. In other groups, such as nursing teams, the primary goal is to meet others' needs. The personal needs of the nursing staff are met only when they coincide with this primary purpose. In most groups both personal needs and group goals are being sought. For example, a nursing goal is to provide excellent individualized care.

An individual nurse's personal need for self-esteem might be met by providing a high standard of care. Thus group goals and individual needs blend.

# The Stages of a Group

As in the life of an individual, there are stages in the life of a group. These stages are, however, not absolute. In fact, different stages may occur simultaneously. A group may also move backward as well as forward, just as a person may regress in life. The group's experience at earlier stages will inevitably affect how well the group functions in the later stages. Familiarity with these stages will enable you to work more effectively in a group.

The stages of a group have been characterized in two different ways. These two systems describe the same process but label it differently. One identifies five stages and the other three stages. We will here describe the five-stage model and explain how it relates to the three-stage model (see Exhibit 6.2).

## Stage I: Orientation

At this stage the group is formed. The members meet, learn one another's names, and begin getting to know one another and developing ways of working together. This period should also provide an opportunity for the members to explore their common purpose as part of the group. This stage may consist of a formal introduction and orientation, or it may simply be an informal and unstructured opportunity for the members to relate to one another in their own ways.

If there is no opportunity for orientation, the members may always feel isolated from one another. Without an orientation period, trust may never develop, and the members may prove reluctant to take risks in the group. Thus orientation ought to be seen as essential to an effective group; it is by no means a waste of time merely because the group is not yet addressing itself to work.

Orientation will recur whenever a new member joins the group. A new person changes the character of the group and thus requires that the other members change. Either a group may try to orient a new member while maintaining the working phase or it may return temporarily to the Orientation Stage. If you recognize its importance, you will be able to facilitate orientation and help others to recognize its importance. If changes in membership are very frequent, the group may never be able to move beyond the orientation stage and may thus be unable to accomplish its work.

## Stage II: Accommodation

Accommodation is the beginning of the process of working together. During this period, the members adjust their behavior in order to work more effectively with others. If, for example, one member has difficulty expressing his or her thoughts, others in the group must learn to give that person time to make a contribution. If the group fails to make such accommodations, some individuals may be shut out of participating. In the long run the group will suffer from this lack of input. As is apparent, accommodation may continue to be necessary whenever new situations arise in the group. The three-stage model of group process treats Orientation and Accommodation as a single stage termed Initiation.

---

Exhibit 6.2
**Two Models of the Stages of a Group**

| | |
|---|---|
| I. Orientation ⎫<br>II. Accommodation ⎬ | I. Initiation |
| III. Negotiation ⎫<br>IV. Operation ⎬ | II. Working |
| V. Dissolution | III. Termination |

---

## Stage III: Negotiation

This is the stage at which decisions are made. In order to do so, a system of decision making needs to be adopted. Groups arrive at decisions in a number of ways, and there is no single correct approach. Instead, it is a matter of finding the one that is most effective for a particular group and its purpose.

### Voting

Sometimes the formal process of presenting ideas as motions and voting on them proves most acceptable to the members of the group. Whenever this system is used, the group must be prepared to work effectively with those who voted on the minority or losing side of a question. Finding ways to prevent discouragement or loss of commitment on the part of those whose views are not adopted is part of the group's task.

### Consensus

Another means of arriving at decisions is consensus: alternatives and compromises are proposed, modified, debated, and discussed until a conclusion is reached that all members of the group support. The process of reaching a consensus can be very time-consuming. Furthermore, it also may fail if some participants in the group are unable or unwilling to compromise. If successful, however, consensus effectively promotes group cohesion and ensures that all members of the group will support its decisions.

### Authority

A third way of making decisions is for a single individual to decide among alternatives suggested by the group. Decisions can be made very rapidly this way. However, group members tend to feel less investment in decisions they did not help to make. If the members all agree with the decision, however, this lessening of commitment may not occur.

## Stage IV: Operation

During the Operation Stage, the goal of the group is translated into action on the basis of the decisions made at Stage III. This is often informally called the group's "action time." If, for example, the nursing team has decided that a class needs to be presented on charting, the planning and carrying out of that class is the Operation Stage.

As its work progresses, the group may be required to make further decisions. To do so is to return temporarily to the Negotiation Stage. The interrelationship between decision and action explains why the three-stage model simply combines Negotiation and Operation and terms the result the Working Stage.

Some groups make few decisions since their work is clear-cut. Thus Negotiation may be almost nonexistent. In other cases, decision making *is* the group's work, and the Operation Stage is consequently limited.

## Stage V: Dissolution

The last stage is identical in the three-stage and five-stage models. Whether it is called Dissolution or *Termination*, it is the process of ending the group—ending one's participation and withdrawing—when its purpose has been accomplished. In some groups, termination occurs at different times for some members than others. In other groups termination occurs for all the members at once. If the group has been highly cohesive, Termination may be a difficult stage. Some groups find termination so unpleasant that they search for a new purpose in order to remain together as a group. A group of nursing students who have worked together for a semester may find their relationships so worthwhile and supportive that they elect to continue as a social group. This effort may be successful if all of them make the transition to the new purpose. If the group's cohesion grew out of its shared purpose, and the new purpose is not strong enough to re-create such cohesion, it may prove disappointing.

Termination is usually worked through more effectively if sufficient attention is paid to it as a necessary stage in the life of the group. If termination has been planned from the beginning to occur at a given time or at the conclusion of certain work, it may be acknowledged or discussed from time to time so the members recognize that it is in the nature of a group to end. When the time comes to end the group, the members may want to have a leave-taking in which to review the function of the group and evaluate its accomplishments. Such an occasion can round out and complete the experience of the group.

## Factors Affecting Group Functioning

Understanding the characteristics of a group will help you understand its functioning (see Figure 6.1). All of the following characteristics are present in some form in every group, though they may be very informal and not explicitly stated. They may also be changed, deliberately or not, which in turn changes how the group functions.

### Norms

Norms are the rules governing behavior within the group. Some groups adopt very formal norms, such as the use of *Roberts' Rules of Order* to conduct official business. Other groups' norms are un-

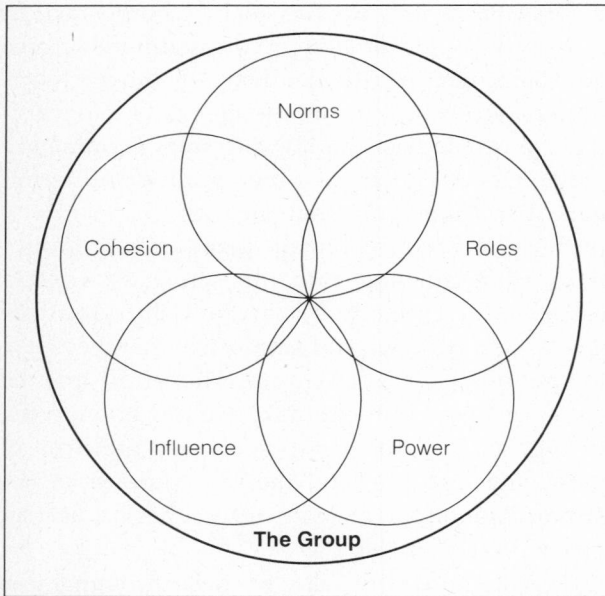

**Figure 6.1**
Factors within a group interact to affect the functioning of the group.

| Exhibit 6.3 | |
|---|---|
| **Roles Taken by Group Members** | |
| Model Member | Exhibits all the characteristics of a positive group member. |
| Eager Beaver | Is unwilling to take time for decision making and discussion; wants to act immediately. |
| Talker | Takes more than a proportionate share of group time. |
| Brilliant One | Offers ability and ideas, but sees own contributions as invariably the best. |
| Emotional One | Invariably reacts strongly, either positively or negatively, to others' ideas. |
| Bored One | Appears uninterested in the group's goal or task. |
| Silent One | Does not talk or contribute. |
| Conformist | Always agrees with others; never voices conflicting ideas. |
| Recognition-Seeker | Draws attention to self and own contributions. |
| Playboy/Playgirl | Socializes instead of focusing on the goal. |
| Suspicious One | Believes that everyone is motivated by self-interest and desire for advancement. |
| Nonconformist | Will do anything to be different and stand out in the group. |
| Politician | Opposes the leader and works to acquire power and influence. |
| Aggressive One | Fights and overrides others to get own ideas accepted. |
| Debunker | Puts down others' ideas but does not contribute. |
| Special Pleader | Has a vested interest in the outcome and tries to direct the group in a personally beneficial direction. |
| Blocker | Tries to keep the group from acting. |

Adapted from William S. Smith, *Group Problem-Solving Through Discussion*, Appendix B. 1965 © by The Bobbs-Merrill Co., Inc. Indianapolis.

stated, and members learn them in the context of the group. Examples of such norms are whether or not it is acceptable to interrupt others when they are speaking and whether or not acceptance requires sustained active participation in the group or allows for discontinuous participation. Unstated norms are usually communicated by members' responses to particular instances of behavior. If a certain kind of behavior is accepted, or even rewarded, it will continue and may spread to other members. If it is punished by negative responses or ignored, it will usually decrease in frequency and eventually cease. Norms may be changed by discussing them and deciding to adopt new norms. Norms may also be changed by the behavior of an influential member.

## Roles

The roles available in groups vary. Some roles are official, such as the officially designated chairperson or leader. Others are informal and not openly acknowledged, such as the person who always raises the problems and difficulties associated with proposed actions, or the peacemaker who helps resolve angry feelings. An individual may persist in one role or may change roles from time to time (see Exhibit 6.3).

## Power

Power is the ability to influence the actions of the *group*. Power may be exercised by individuals within the group or jointly by several individuals. Power can also shift from one person to another in response to a situation. A person who wishes to affect the actions of the group needs to understand where the power in that group lies. Power may be exerted by making or obstructing group

decisions and by furthering or obstructing its actions. Similarly, power can be used to move a group toward or away from its goals.

## Influence

Influence is the ability to affect the decisions and actions of another *individual* in the group. Influence is similar to power, and the same person often possesses both. Influence over others can affect the group as a whole if those being influenced share power in the group. If the person being influenced has little power, however, change may not occur in the group as a whole. Influence may be exerted overtly by openly suggesting that another person behave in a certain way. Influence is also exerted covertly by rewarding desired behavior and ignoring undesired behavior.

## Cohesion

Cohesion results from loyalty, enthusiasm, and involvement on the part of the group's members. For a high degree of cohesion to exist, the group must be important to the individual members. Such feelings prompt them to seek to maintain the existence of the group. If the level of cohesion is low, members of the group might care very little whether the group continues to exist. Cohesion affects individuals' willingness to work toward the aims of the group, as well as their commitment and satisfaction with the group.

Cohesion is enhanced when the members agree on a group's goals and norms, and when they feel they have participated in decision making. It tends to be highest when all participants in the decision-making process are satisfied with the end result. Cohesion is thus a valuable outcome of meeting the group's psychosocial needs.

# Leadership Styles in Groups

There is a variety of styles of group leadership, each of which has strengths and weaknesses. No single leadership style is appropriate for every

group: a leadership style is most effective when it is compatible with the purpose of the group and the feelings of the individual members.

## Autocratic Leadership

Autocratic or authoritarian leadership is centralized and directive (see Figure 6.2). The leader makes decisions for the group and often assigns tasks to individual members. In many instances the nursing team will function in an authoritarian manner. The team leader decides when the group will meet, assigns tasks, and oversees the work of the group. The autocratic leader's position may be based on experience, education, or influence over others. Most of the power in the group is held by the leader, who also establishes group norms. An autocratic leadership style is efficient and tends to be minimally time-consuming, but it has disadvantages. The members of the group may feel little personal satisfaction in the group's accomplishments because little time is typically devoted to meeting personal needs. Cohesion may be lacking if the members do not feel personally committed to or responsible for the group. When decisions are made by an authoritarian leader, the members of the group may feel little commitment to supporting those decisions. Sometimes, though the leader exercises overt power, other group members exert covert influence over him or her.

## Democratic Leadership

A democratic leader shares decision making with the other group members through voting or con-sensus (see Figure 6.3). The leader may be chosen by the group or appointed and subsequently accepted by the group. Democratic leadership tends to be more time-consuming than authoritarian leadership, and decisions may be harder to arrive at. On the other hand, democratic leadership usually produces a wider variety of ideas and options, and creativity is more likely since many individuals are contributing. Group members tend to feel committed to decisions they have shared in making and thus are more willing to work actively toward the group's goal. Power and influence may be widely disseminated throughout the group or concentrated in a few people. Norms are usually based on group decisions, and cohesion tends to be high. The members feel important to and part of the group, which in turn enhances feelings of personal satisfaction.

Democratic leadership is exemplified by a clinical conference group that chooses a different person each time to lead the group's next meeting. Together the group defines the purpose of the upcoming meeting and shares any necessary preparation. At the meeting the leader is responsible for facilitating the process so that all members have an opportunity to share their knowledge and expertise on the patient care problem under discussion. All members of the group act together, by voting or by consensus, to choose a course of action.

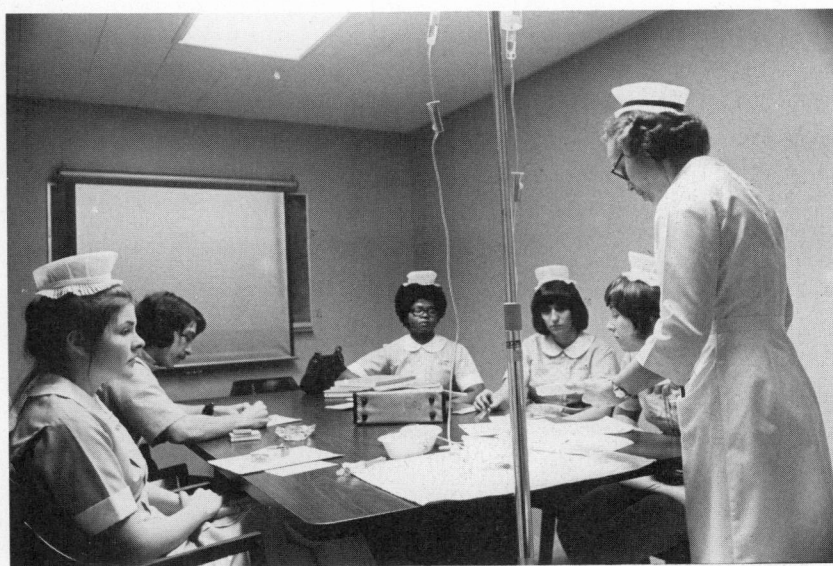

**Figure 6.2**
Autocratic leadership is leader-centered. (Christopher Morrow/Stock, Boston)

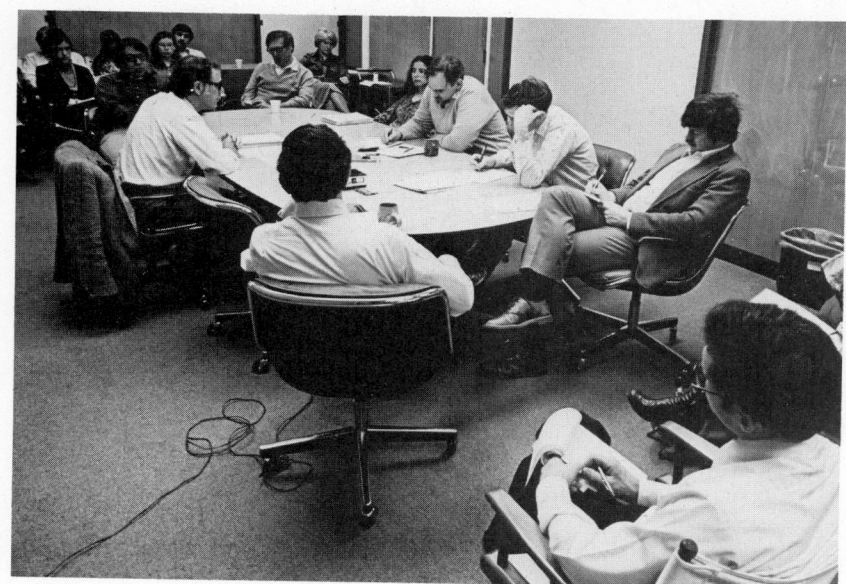

## Laissez-Faire Leadership

Laissez-faire leadership does not reside in any particular individual. Leadership may rotate or the group may operate without an acknowledged leader. Lack of an explicit leader can seriously hamper a group's efforts (see Figure 6.4). A leaderless group tends to have difficulty maintaining its focus on the goal, and there are few norms. Decision making is very difficult, and the group may find itself unable to move in any direction. Such a group's means of decision making is consensus, which may be difficult to attain. A laissez-faire group may be comfortable and unthreatening to some participants, who enjoy its freedom and lack of structure but acutely uncomfortable to others. The latter usually withdraw from laissez-faire groups.

Some clinical conferences operate as laissez-faire groups. Such a group may be composed entirely of people who welcome lack of structure. Though no one directs the group, everyone shares their concerns and ideas. A goal is essential to a laissez-faire group. Without a purposeful focus, one individual with power and influence can easily usurp the group. It is also possible for nothing to happen. Without explicit goals, it is very difficult for a laissez-faire group to be effective.

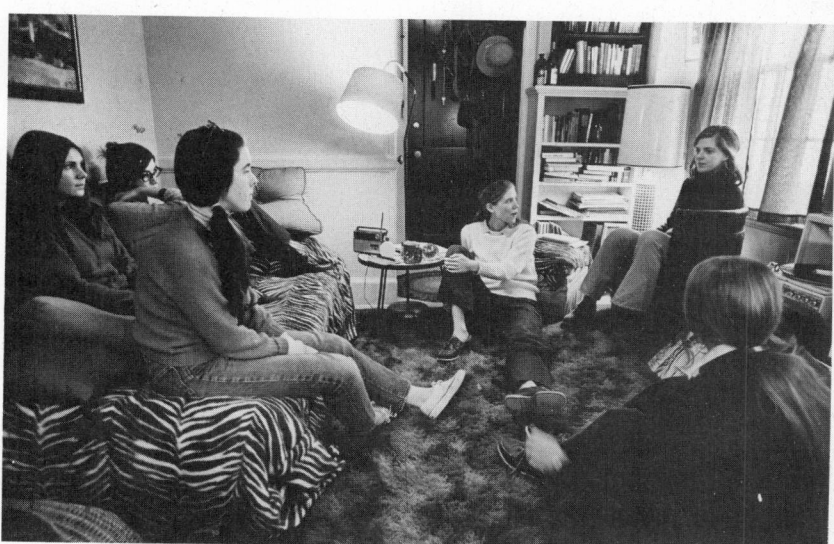

**Figure 6.4**
Laissez-faire leadership may make the group unable to focus on its goal. (Dan Bernstein)

# Leader Effectiveness

There are some characteristics that enhance the effectiveness of any leader. Let us consider them in turn, not so much to prepare you to be a leader as to enhance your understanding of group functioning.

## Orientation to the Individual

A leader who values individuals is usually willing to assist, work with, and listen to the group members. Such a leader also tries to prevent some members from demeaning or undermining others' sense of self-worth. Members who feel respected and taken seriously in turn feel more committed to the group.

## Orientation to Future Goals

In order to help the group move toward its goals, the leader must be able to look beyond the immediate situation toward the continuing concerns of the group. Present actions need to be considered in light of their effect on the future. Such a leader is goal-oriented and helps the group maintain its focus on the goal.

## Ability to Identify and Remedy Group Problems

The effective leader is able to analyze what is happening in a group and to help it adopt more effective patterns of functioning. For example, such a leader might help group members to recognize that their defensive responses to new ideas are inhibiting creative problem-solving.

## Interpersonal Communication Skills

Effective communication with others is critical to sound leadership. The life of the group revolves around the quality of the communication that takes place. The communication skills most important to a group leader will be discussed in detail in Chapter 12.

# Studying Groups

When studying groups, it is useful to distinguish between *content* and *process*. Content consists of the words spoken, decisions made, and actions taken by the group—often called the instrumental functions of the group. The minutes of a meeting are a record of the content of a group interaction.

To evaluate a group in terms of attainment of its goal it is necessary to study content. Studying the written record will enable you to identify the degree to which the goal was reached and the main factors involved in goal attainment.

To study group process is to examine *how* a group functions. Who speaks most? To whom are questions and comments addressed? Who assumes leadership? Who exerts power? Who has influence? What feelings are expressed, verbally and nonverbally?

Process involves communication, individual behavior, and feelings—often called the expressive functions of the group. Studying process can help identify why a particular group is experiencing recurrent problems or why another group is very successful. Understanding group process can help reveal alternative patterns likely to make the group more satisfactory to its members and more effective in its work.

# Participating Effectively in a Group

It is not widely recognized that participation in a group is enhanced by understanding and skill. An effective participant is valuable to all other group members and contributes significantly to the group's ability to meet its goals. In an effort to enhance your skills as a more effective group member, let us examine some of the characteristics that make for effective group membership (see Figure 6.5).

## Understanding the Group

Basic understanding of how groups function, and those factors that facilitate or block effective function, helps the group member participate actively. When you understand the stages through which a group passes, for example, you can participate enthusiastically in orientation, recognizing its importance to the group's eventual success. Similarly, if you understand that the group's leadership style is democratic, you will recognize that you are expected to play a part in the decision-making process. If the group's initial leadership is autocratic and you find yourself uncomfortable with that style, you will be better able to negotiate for shared responsibility if you understand what the alternatives are. In general, the greater your familiarity with all aspects of group life, the greater your ability to work effectively in a group.

## Willingness to Compromise

Because no two individuals can be expected to think identically, groups depend on their mem-

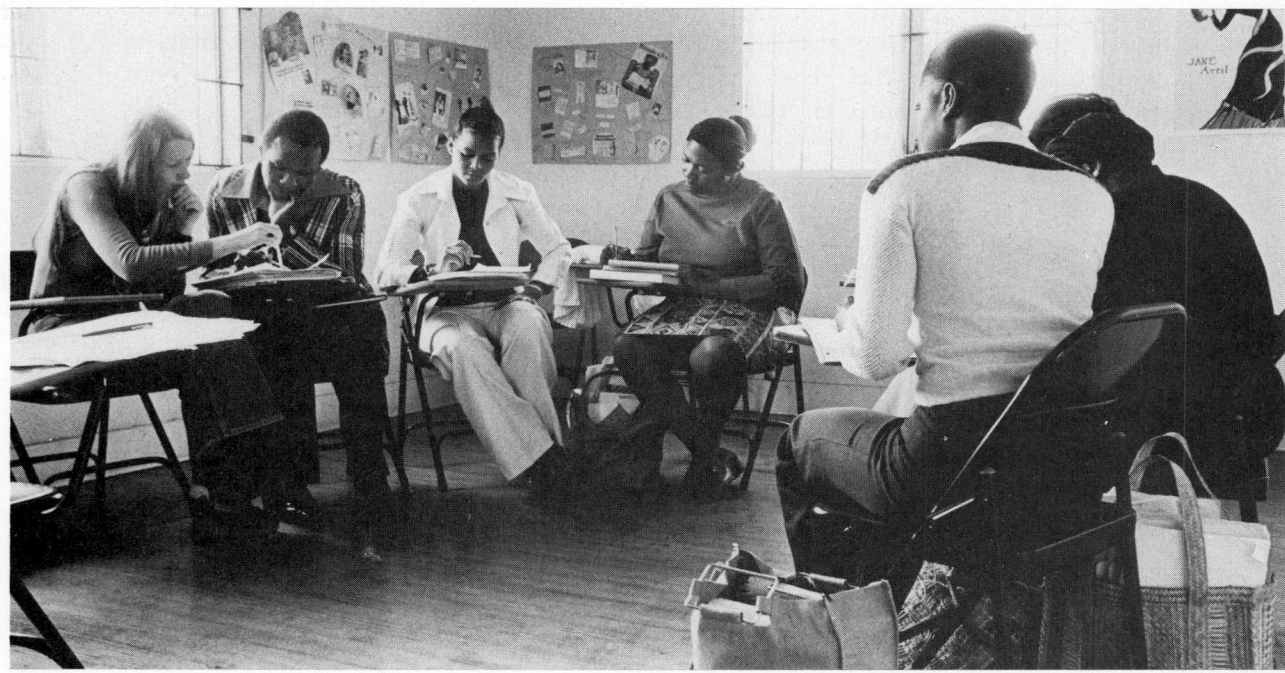

**Figure 6.5**
Are you an effective group member? Are you willing to negotiate and compromise? Are you goal-directed? Are you concerned about others in the group? Are you honest and direct in communication? Do you do your share? Do you understand the group and how it functions? (Bobbi Carray)

bers' willingness to pursue compromise. It can be enlightening to examine your own approach to groups in which you participate. Do you see yourself as a realistic compromiser or do you expect others to adjust to and accept your point of view? However creative and exceptional your viewpoint, it will not be the most effective alternative unless the group as a whole claims ownership of the idea. This cannot happen if you promote its adoption by running roughshod over the ideas and opinions of others. Your willingness to compromise can elicit a similar willingness in others, thus facilitating the work of the group.

## Focus on the Goal

Whether a group's goal is the personal growth and satisfaction of its members or an action-oriented outcome, it is highly desirable to keep that goal in mind as you work with the group. If the goal is personal growth, it will be clear that time devoted to working on interpersonal relationships within the group is well spent. If the goal is to write a procedure for administering medications, you will direct your efforts to that end and not dissipate the energies of the group pursuing other aims. Though working on interpersonal relationships might become necessary in the latter group, it would not be the central focus.

## Concern for Others

Belief in the worth of each individual is a basic ethical principle of the nursing profession (see the *Code for Nurses* in Chapter 1). One way of acting on this belief is to concern yourself with others in the group. Such concern can be expressed by encouraging others to share their thoughts and ideas, accepting their ideas without "putting down" those people with whom you disagree, and striving for the personal satisfaction of all members of the group, not just for yourself.

## Direct and Honest Communication

The functioning of any group is enhanced when the members are direct and honest in their communications. If you are asked for your opinion, state it clearly and briefly. It is false modesty to wait until you are begged to share your views. If you disagree with a certain position, say so. Disagreement can be expressed without personally attacking others. It is very unproductive for the group if you disagree but do not say so and are then reluctant to participate further. Concerns you feel but do not voice can undermine your ability to function and relate to others in the group. Direct and honest praise of others' ideas and contributions is also valuable. Insincere praise tends to be resented, but sincere praise enhances others' self-esteem and thus the group's potential for success. Chapter 12, "Communication," will be of value to you as a participant in groups.

## Sharing the Responsibility

If each member accepts responsibility for an appropriate share of the group's tasks, the goal is more likely to be accomplished. If one or two people become burdened with all the tasks of the group, they may become resentful and eventually withdraw. There is also a danger that overburdened group members will leave tasks undone or do them poorly because of insufficient time and energy.

## Conclusion

Nursing is never a solitary profession. From your first clinical group as a student to eventual participation in health-care teams, studying the groups you are part of will help you to understand them better. And, in turn, the better you understand such groups, the more effective a group member you will be.

## Study Terms

Accommodation Stage
aggregate
authoritarian
  leadership
autocratic leadership
cohesion
consensus
content
democratic leadership
Dissolution Stage
goal
influence
Initiation Stage

laissez-faire leadership
Negotiation Stage
norms
Operation Stage
Orientation Stage
physical needs
power
process
psychosocial needs
roles
Termination Stage
Working Stage
voting

## Learning Activities

**1.** In your clinical or discussion group, appoint one person as process recorder and another as content recorder. After the session is ended (or at the beginning of your next meeting), review the process and content of your group.

**2.** Identify a group to which you belong. What is the leadership style of that group? List all the characteristics of the group that influenced your decision about leadership style.

**3.** In a group meeting, observe the roles filled by group members. What roles discussed in the chapter were present in that group? Identify the roles that were not present.

**4.** Review your own participation in your clinical or discussion group. Compare yourself with the characteristics given in the text for a positive group member. If you identify any areas in which you need growth, plan how you might change your own behavior to enhance the functioning of your group.

## References

Brill, Naomi. *Teamwork: Working Together in the Human Services.* Philadelphia: J. B. Lippincott, 1976.

Donnelly, G. F. "RN's Assertiveness Workbook: How to Face Down a Crowd, Part 7," *RN* 42 (May 1979): 34–37.

Clarke, C. C. "Teaching Nurses Group Concepts: Some Issues and Suggestions." *Nurse Educator* 3 (January/February 1978): 17–20.

Epstein, H. T. "Nominal Group Technique: Psychosocial and Philosophical Bases for a Participative Management Process." *Medical Record News* 49 (August 1970): 39–49.

Jones, I. H., et al. "Group Project." *Nursing Times* 75 (January 1979): 163–166.

Larson, M. L. "How to Become a Better Group Leader." *Nursing '78* 8 (August 1978): 65–72.

Olmstead, Michael. *The Small Group.* New York: Random House, 1979.

Rogers, Carl. "Facilitation Encounter Groups." *American Journal of Nursing* 71 (February 1971): 275–279.

Roseman, E. "Improving Your Interpersonal Skills: Understanding Your Role in Group Dynamics, Part 4." *Medical Laboratory Observer* 10 (July 1978): 47–52.

Samson, E., and Marthas, M. *Group Process for the Health Professions.* New York: John Wiley, 1977.

Smith, William S. *Group Problem-Solving Through Discussion.* New York: Bobbs-Merrill Co., 1965.

# Part Three
## Understanding Health and Illness

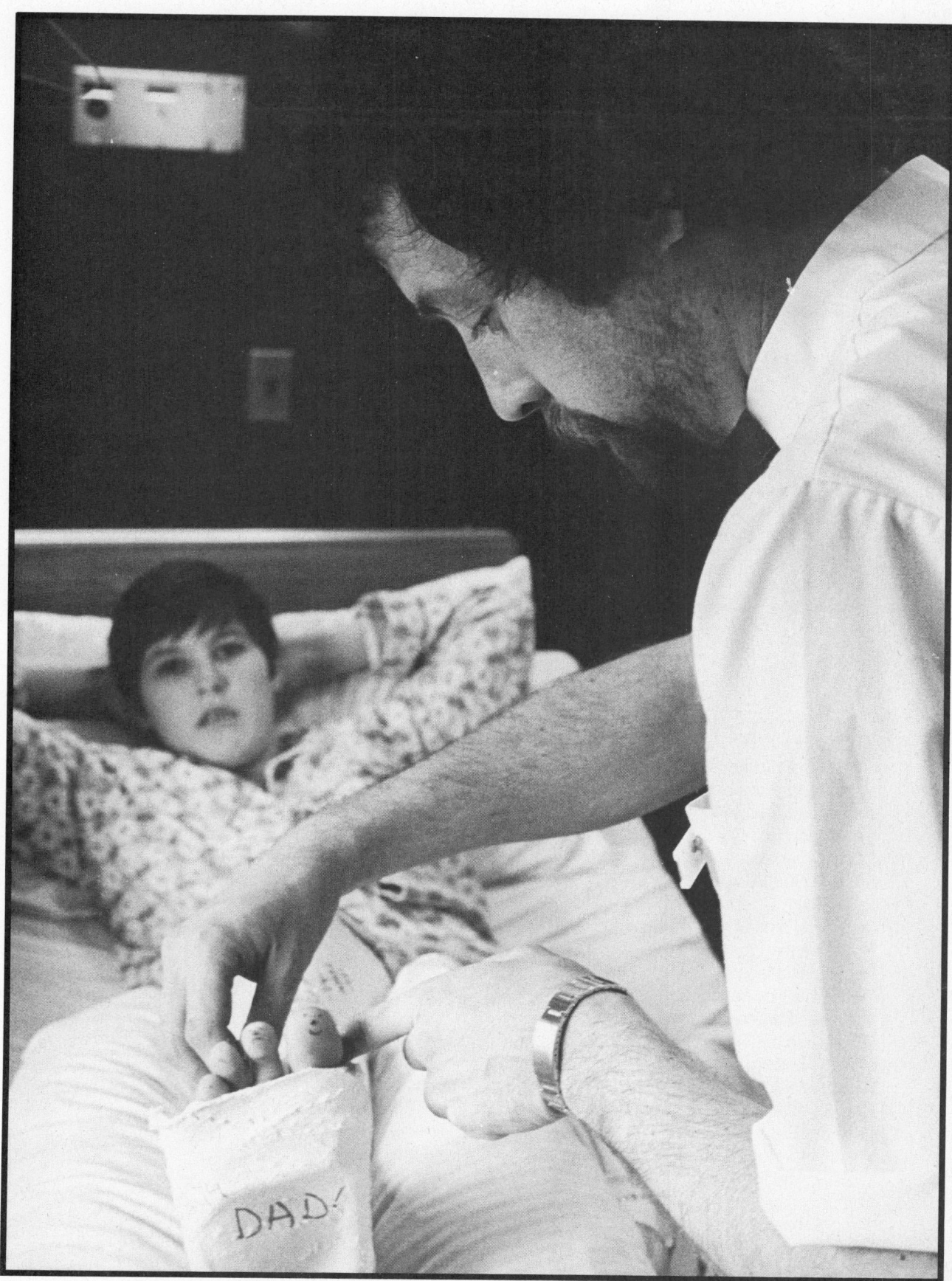

# Chapter 7

# Basic Concepts of Health, Illness, and Healing

## Objectives

After completing this chapter, you should be able to:
1. State three of the five definitions of health.
2. Outline some preventive health measures.
3. Define illness in terms of homeostasis.
4. Name and briefly discuss five causes of illness.
5. Give an example of multiple factors leading to illness.
6. Differentiate between acute and chronic illness.
7. Discuss common perceptions of the ill person.
8. Briefly discuss the impact of dependency on the ill person.
9. Define healing.
10. List the major components of the practice of healing.
11. Explain the meaning of holistic healing.
12. Define rehabilitation.
13. Discuss the importance of rehabilitation throughout illness.

## Outline

A Historical Perspective on Health
Definitions of Health
    High-Level Wellness
    Health and Homeostasis
    Health and Adaptation
    Health and Self-Concept
Health Maintenance
Preventive Health Care
Holistic Health
Definitions of Illness
    Illness as the Opposite of Health
    Illness as Disease
    Illness With Evidence
    Illness as Inability to Function
    Perception of Oneself as Ill
Acute Versus Chronic Illness
    Acute Illness
    Chronic Illness
Causes of Illness
    Invasion of Body Defenses by Pathogens
    Biochemical Imbalances of the Body
    Immunosuppression
    Toxic Substances
    Environmental Conditions
    Injury
    Age
    Genetic Defects
    Congenital Defects
    Inadequate Sleep and Exercise
    Improper Nutrition
    Stress
    Multiple Causes of Illness
Factors That May Reinforce Illness
Common Responses to Illness
    Dependence
    Guilt
    Anxiety
    Fear
    Regression
    Self-Centeredness
    Hostility
The Patient Role
Healing Practices
    Medical Healing
    Surgical Healing
    Holistic Healing
Rehabilitation

Health, illness, and healing are concepts fundamental to understanding the role of the nurse. In preparation for practical application of these concepts to the care of another person, let us examine them closely in this chapter. What is meant by health? What are the needs of a healthy person, and how do these needs change with illness? When is a person considered ill? How do individuals respond to illness? What is healing and how may it be brought about?

Each of these questions may be answered in various ways since health, illness, and healing are all relative. Do you consider yourself healthy right now? What might happen that would make you regard yourself as ill? How would you define healing? We will explore how dramatic changes in prevailing ideas about health and illness have affected the planning and performance of nursing care.

## A Historical Perspective on Health

In technologically unsophisticated cultures, health is defined by the premise that you are healthy if you are able to work. Staying healthy is perceived as requiring adherence to a complicated set of rituals, including avoiding some foods, eating plenty of others, staying out of drafts, wearing warm clothes, and thinking "good" thoughts. Early in the history of our country, youngsters were often routinely "dosed" with laxatives to prevent constipation, rubbed with liniments to prevent congestion, and buttoned into heavy underwear to prevent chilling.

Healing was also largely defined in terms of functioning: if you felt well enough to resume working, you had been healed. Most healing methods were unscientific, such as prescribing of special foods and herbs. A few such remedies were effective: foxglove, for example, was used to alleviate fatigue, water retention, and fast pulse, which were not yet recognized as symptoms of heart disease; foxglove, however, contained digitalis, still used today in treating heart disease. Similarly, isolation of patients was formerly enforced to promote rest since little was known about the transmission of disease. It is now recognized to be an effective way to prevent the spread of organisms. Scientific advances have most significantly influenced our changing ideas about health, illness, and healing.

## Definitions of Health

The most widely accepted definition of health, adopted by the World Health Organization (WHO) in 1947, characterizes health as "the state of complete physical, mental, and social well-being and not merely the absence of disease or infirmity." This definition is noteworthy for its acknowledgment of the nonphysical aspects of health. The word "complete" is somewhat misleading in that it suggests an absolute standard. In actuality, few people who are perceived by themselves and others as healthy have achieved a state of complete and perpetual well-being.

### High-Level Wellness

A broader definition of health—actually more of a description than a definition—is Dunn's concept of "high-level wellness" (1961). Using the term *wellness* for *health* and emphasizing the relationship between wellness and the family, community, environment, and society, Dunn discusses the individual's inner and outer worlds and the need for a balance of energy between them. In other words, according to Dunn, health involves more than the self.

## Health and Homeostasis

We defined homeostasis in Chapter 3 as the tendency of all living tissue to restore and maintain itself in a condition of balance or equilibrium. This definition, broadened to take in the psychological components of the individual, can also serve as a working definition of health. Health, then, may be defined as an optimal state of homeostasis. The three foregoing definitions (the WHO definition, Dunn's description, and the concept of homeostasis) are more similar than not, and each could serve as the basis of a useful model for planning and administering care.

Figure 7.1 illustrates the conceptual relationship between illness and homeostasis. As *stressors* (fac-

tors that require an adaptive response) have an impact on the person, the line of balance is swung off-center. Adaptive forces (psychological and physiological mechanisms of the individual) then take action in an effort to correct the imbalance. Total physical imbalance results in death. Life is characterized by constant dynamic movement through periods of health, crisis, illness, and return to health. This process is more often subtle than critical in nature. There are many types of stressors (see Chapter 8) and many adaptive forces, including the nurse.

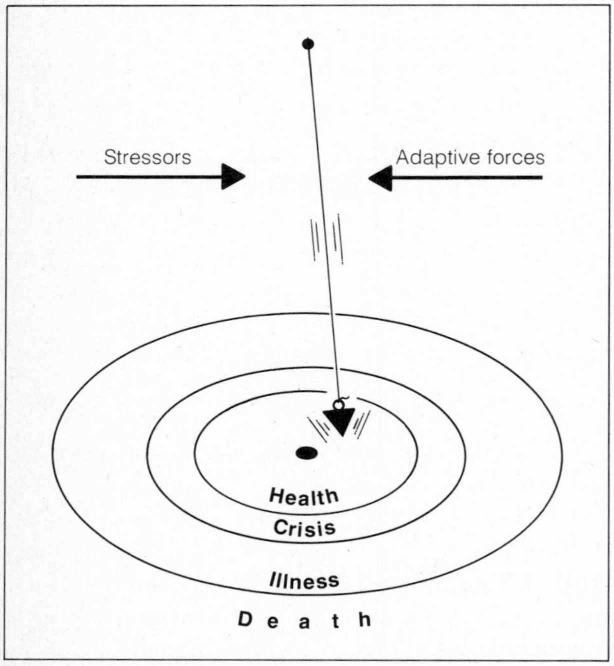

## Health and Adaptation

Sister Callistra Roy's adaptation theory defines health as "man's ability to respond positively, or to adapt" to changes in environment. According to Roy, whether such a change is "a direct assault that causes injury or a subtle variation in psychological nature, man has mechanisms to cope with the changing world" (Roy, 1976).

## Health and Self-Concept

Health is more than the absence of disease. It is also more the subjective feeling of well-being. In some countries, for example, worms in the intestinal tract (helminthiasis) are commonplace throughout the general population. Yet most such people have a sense of well-being and regard themselves as healthy. Similarly, many people with chronic conditions and diseases, such as multiple sclerosis or rheumatoid arthritis, attain a high level of adjustment and would describe themselves as basically healthy. However, the onset of a common cold might prompt these same individuals to describe themselves as ill.

Some people view health as a matter of self-esteem, boasting, "Why, I've never been sick a day in my life" or "I'm as healthy as a horse." Such people are often unsympathetic to others who do not enjoy vigorous health. The traditional definition of health as ability to work still has currency for many people. In summary, perceptions of health are very subjective.

**Figure 7.1   Homeostasis and illness**
Courtesy Nursing Faculty, Shoreline Community College (Seattle, Washington)

## Health Maintenance

As nurses, we ought to pay as much attention to health maintenance of patients as to restoration of health. Wu describes health behavior directed at maintaining optimum health status (Wu, 1972). People's approaches to health maintenance are often very obvious in their behavior. At one end of the spectrum is the patient who carefully assesses the health implications of each item of food eaten, is compulsively clean, never participates in activities involving even minimal risk, and lives a restricted, unvaried life. Such overly conscientious people may be inappropriately apprehensive; some suffer from extreme death anxiety and need counseling. What might appear initially as an overly conscientious degree of health maintenance is, in reality, neurotic or irrational behavior. At the other end of the spectrum, you may know someone who consistently refuses to make any effort at health maintenance even in spite of full knowledge of the dangers of smoking, drinking, overeating, and ignoring signs of illness.

Most people belong somewhere between the two extremes. It is widely recognized that an individual can exercise some control over his or her health by pursuing proper exercise, diet, hygiene, psychological growth, and stress reduction.

## Preventive Health Care

Efforts to prevent illness and injury have a long and spectacular history. Immunization programs have brought about the virtual eradication of such diseases as polio and smallpox in this country. Better sanitation has reduced the incidence of contagious disease in the general population. Occupational health and safety codes, such as those requiring hard hats on construction sites, have reduced the rate of work-related injury and illness.

Medical research is increasingly focusing on environmental and behavioral factors in the etiology of conditions like cancer and heart disease. Perhaps in response to public education about the findings of such research, interest in preventive health care has intensified massively in the past few years. But at present, there are few absolutes in the way of direction. Studies and research are ongoing with the goal of increasing health and decreasing illness for individuals in our society.

## Holistic Health

The *holistic* approach to health emphasizes the functional indivisibility of all aspects of the physical and psychological self. Grant writes that a state of holistic health allows the person "to relate to himself and his world with maximum creativity, efficiency, and responsibility. It is to be in harmony, both physically and emotionally" (Grant, 1978). Defined holistically, then, health involves both optimal functioning of all body systems and psychological well-being. Like Dunn's concept of high-level wellness, the holistic definition of health emphasizes balance with the environment and with individuals who are important to us.

# Definitions of Illness

There are as many ways to define illness as there are to define health. Let us consider five definitions: (1) illness as the opposite of health; (2) illness as disease; (3) illness with evidence; (4) illness as inability to function; and (5) perception of oneself as ill.

## Illness as the Opposite of Health

If we define health and illness as opposites, any state that is not health is illness. Thus, if balance in the sense of homeostasis is health, homeostatic imbalance is illness. This simple definition is widely accepted, but some consider it inadequate, arguing that it is possible to fall short of health without being ill.

## Illness as Disease

Many people, if asked, would assert that illness is the presence of disease. There are difficulties inherent in this definition. What is disease? If you feel healthy and are unaware that you have high blood pressure, are you ill? According to the definition that equates illness with disease, such a person is ill. This definition arouses considerable disagreement.

## Illness With Evidence

Another view of illness holds that there must be demonstrable evidence of an organic nature. This theory differs from the foregoing one in that it defines disease quite specifically and narrowly. That is, a person who feels unwell but has no objective signs of organic illness is not ill. According to this definition, psychological illness can be diagnosed by people skilled at the assessment of normal and aberrant behavior. This view of illness is quite narrow in scope.

## Illness as Inability to Function

We have already briefly mentioned the definition of illness as interference with functioning. The existence of such a condition makes it easier for us to assign the word *illness*. Suppose you sprained your finger playing volleyball yesterday. Though it is tender to the touch and you have applied a finger splint for protection, you are able to take notes in class and pursue your plans for the day without disruption. Although the splint attracts some attention, you do not consider yourself ill. You have a problem condition, but according to this definition you are not ill.

## Perception of Oneself as Ill

Finally, some people argue that illness is present only if a person perceives himself or herself as ill. This too is a very restrictive definition, which excludes the obvious illness of a comatose patient.

# Acute Versus Chronic Illness

## Acute Illness

An *acute illness* is usually characterized by rapid onset. It requires short-term treatment and usually resolves with no apparent residual effects. Uncomplicated influenza is an example of an acute illness.

## Chronic Illness

A *chronic illness* has been defined as one that persists three months or longer, requires medical management, and is characterized by the presence of signs and symptoms (U.S. Department of Health, Education and Welfare, 1976). Some chronic illness is characterized by intermittent episodes of acute symptoms called *exacerbations*, followed by periods of *remission* or abatement of symptoms.

Diabetes, arthritis, and emphysema are chronic illnesses.

## Causes of Illness

Our understanding of the causation of illness has expanded massively over the past several decades due to medical research. Unscientific generalities have been replaced by knowledge of specific causative agents, such as measles virus. Science is beginning to explain how a single illness might have multiple intersecting causes.

### Invasion of Body Defenses by Pathogens

*Pathogens* are disease-producing microorganisms. Many such microorganisms are always present in the human body, but in numbers insufficient to cause illness. If these pathogens multiply enough to threaten homeostasis, illness occurs. The body's defenses against such invasion are discussed in detail in Chapter 8.

In this context, it is essential for us as nurses to understand the theory of "necessary but not sufficient." In order for a certain disease to occur, it is necessary that the pathogen that causes it be present. However, the mere presence of the pathogen may not be sufficient to bring on the illness. For example, it is necessary for the tubercle bacillus to be present for a person to develop tuberculosis. However, the organism alone may not be sufficient to produce the illness, but if the *host* (the person who is carrying the organism) is debilitated, the combination of weakness and the presence of the bacillus could be sufficient for tuberculosis to occur.

### Biochemical Imbalances of the Body

Imbalances of the body's chemical structure and hormones can cause illness, usually of a chronic nature. For example, overproduction of hydrochloric acid in the stomach can produce gastric ulcers.

### Immunosuppression

Some drugs, including those used to combat cancer, cause a decrease in the white cells and platelets of the blood, which are important components of the body's immune system, or defense against pathogens. When this occurs, susceptibility to disease increases and the patient is at a high risk of illness.

### Toxic Substances

*Toxic* substances are those that act as poisons in the body, causing serious damage. Some substances are toxic only in large amounts, over an extended period of time, or in conjunction with other substances or conditions. For example, long-term high intake of alcohol can cause diseases of the liver, pancreas, brain, and other organs. The indiscriminate use of drugs can cause serious physiological and psychological illness. Toxic substances may be absorbed through the skin, inhaled, or ingested orally. Some pesticides used in farming, for example, can be absorbed through the skin or inhaled, and special clothing and/or masks must be worn.

### Environmental Conditions

Health authorities are looking very carefully at environmental factors suspected of causing disease and illness. Among these factors are air pollution, inhalation of certain substances, such as asbestos and silicone, and the handling of certain chemicals. *Carcinogenic* (cancer-producing substances) have been reported in foods, cosmetics, and various household items. Much of the data on these substances is suggestive rather than conclusive. For example, very large amounts of some substances have produced abnormal cells in animals but not humans. Environmental factors will undoubtedly continue to be rigorously scrutinized.

## Injury

Though injury is rarely termed illness, injured people *are* ill by the criteria of interference with functioning and presence of signs or symptoms. Serious injury or trauma is an assault on the body's integrity equivalent in severity to serious medical illness. Furthermore, responses to injury are similar to responses to illness.

## Age

Many people expect illness to accompany aging. *Infirmity*, or general weakening of body systems, is often associated with advanced age. However, gerontologists—those who study the aging process—emphasize that, although the elderly are at high risk of illness, health is an attainable goal for many elderly persons.

Infants, particularly premature newborns, are also susceptible to illness because of their age. The immune system, which protects the body against illness, has not fully developed at birth. Immature body systems are not adept at adjusting to environmental changes, such as minor variations in temperature.

## Genetic Defects

Genetic defects are inherited conditions, caused by errors in genetic makeup and present at birth (Munson, 1979). One of the most common is Trisomy 21, formerly known as Down's syndrome. Although people suffering from genetic defects vary greatly in their capacity for near-normal function, their death rate from illness and injury is higher than average, probably due to accompanying physical and psychological conditions that undermine ability to adapt to disease.

## Congenital Defects

Some congenital defects may be considered illnesses. Such defects are not inherited but are present at birth and caused by "errors that result during the developmental process" within the uterus (Munson, 1979). A common congenital defect is spina bifida, or incomplete closure of the spinal canal. An individual may have more than one congenital defect.

## Inadequate Sleep and Exercise

Inadequate sleep and exercise may lead to a debilitated state that increases the risk of illness. For example, infectious mononucleosis (a viral disease) is common among adolescents and young people who get inadequate sleep. Inadequate physical activity and a sedentary life style increase the risk of cardiovascular disease.

## Improper Nutrition

Obesity can be a contributing or complicating factor in disease, particularly diseases of the heart. Improper nutrition can increase susceptibility to many illnesses. Inadequate protein intake contributes to poor tissue healing. Deficiencies of certain vitamins can cause specific illnesses; for example, insufficient vitamin C leads to a condition called scurvy.

## Stress

Psychological stress has been widely investigated as a contributing factor to illness. Though it remains impossible to measure the damage stress causes a given individual or the quantity of stress

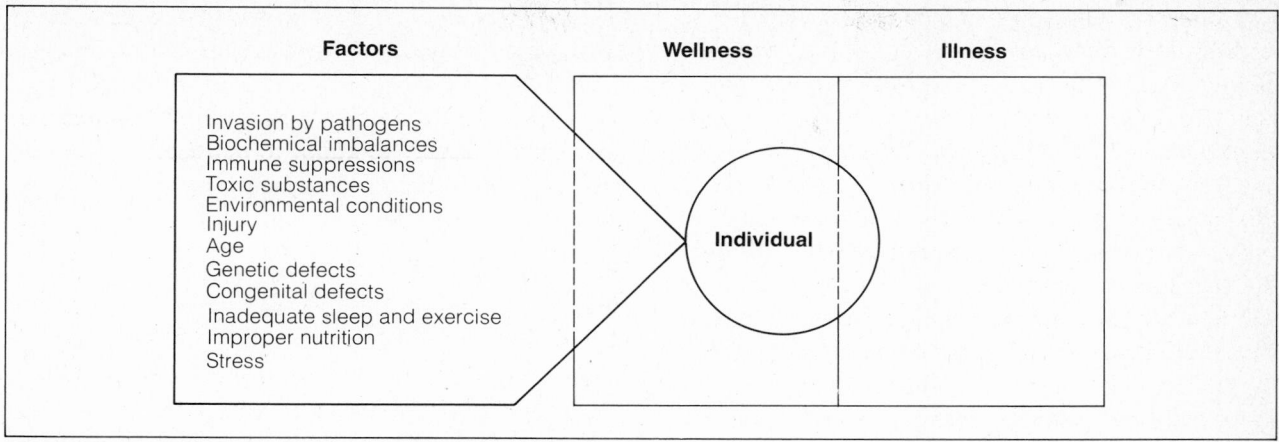

**Figure 7.2   Single or multiple factors that can cause illness.**

that must be imposed to produce illness, some studies appear to show a direct relationship between stress and the onset of illness (Dudley, 1977).

## Multiple Causes of Illness

As we have seen, many different factors can cause illness (see Figure 7.2). It is not uncommon, furthermore, for illness to be brought on by a combination of such factors. Thus a person who does not become ill in response to one such factor may fall ill when a second is imposed. For example, a person paralyzed by a stroke (cerebrovascular accident or CVA) for years may not feel ill until pathogens introduced into the respiratory tract cause pneumonia. Because the stroke-induced immobility increased susceptibility to the pathogens in the respiratory tract, the stroke and the respiratory infection together caused the resulting illness. Stress may also be a factor in such a situation.

## Factors That May Reinforce Illness

Illness may elicit perceptions and attitudes that interfere with recovery. For example, illness may in some circumstances prove rewarding for the patient. The dependence it engenders can be used manipulatively. "Don't you see I'm ill? How can you leave me?" is a plea that can realign relationships in a negative way. It is hard to show anger, regardless of how justified, toward an ill person. Illness also excuses the patient from having to perform tasks or fulfill obligations. Because we tend to protect the ill from added stressors, even the details of everyday life can be temporarily ignored.

A patient who accumulated a great deal of paid sick leave may unconsciously lack motivation to recover. *Malingering* is the conscious exaggeration of symptoms by the patient in order to gain rewards of some type. For example, a patient may feign pain to elicit attention.

If you are tempted to assign one of these behaviors or motives to a patient, you must consider very carefully whether such an assessment is accurate. Judgmental reactions can seriously interfere with your relationship to the patient and the effectiveness of care. Even if such a conclusion is justified, the patient still needs sympathetic care. Good care involves an effort to identify why the patient is behaving in such a way.

# Common Responses to Illness

Most people perceive illness as threatening. Specifically, illness impinges on one of the basic needs in Maslow's hierarchy, safety. The sense that the body is not functioning properly arouses the fear that it may not survive.

Every person responds to the threat of illness in a unique and special way. Individuals develop specific patterns of responding to threat, and the occurrence of illness tends to elicit these responses. A person who usually responds to threat with hostility will probably react this way to illness.

Illness may impose necessary changes on an individual's life style. These changes may affect the person's home, job, or family.

## Dependence

To be *dependent* is to be unable to function satisfactorily without the aid of someone else. Dependence is inherent in the role of the patient and may be very threatening to people who perceive dependence as loss of control.

## Guilt

*Guilt* is a feeling of remorse at having done something wrong. A patient who is the primary wage earner in the family may feel guilty for depriving the family of income. A long-term illness may lower the family's standard of living and possibly incur the resentment of other family members.

Inability to perform household tasks or fulfill social commitments can also arouse guilt, as can the ill person's inability to provide the emotional support or sexual gratification to a loved one.

## Anxiety

*Anxiety* is an ill-defined and disturbing feeling of apprehension. It may take the form of a vague feeling that things are generally not right and that something unknown but unpleasant is going to happen. Lack of understanding of one's illness and its treatment can cause a high level of anxiety, as can simply being ill or being hospitalized and away from one's family.

## Fear

*Fear* is the feeling aroused by danger or threat. Although more acute than anxiety, fear may be easier to deal with in that it is usually more clearly defined. Fear of pain is common, as is fear of the outcome of illness, injury, or surgery. Sometimes fear that an important relationship will change or end because of one's illness can cause psychological suffering. Fear of disability is even more severe than fear of death for some patients.

## Regression

*Regression* is reacting to anxiety by reverting to immature behavior. An ill child who long ago gave up bottle feeding may, for example, demand a bottle at mealtime. Similarly, a sick adult may become whiny or overreact to inconsequential matters. Irritability can be a form of regression.

## Self-Centeredness

The threat posed by illness typically causes patients to become preoccupied with themselves and their health. As the seriousness of an illness increases, even less attention is paid to the outside world or the concerns of others. Sometimes self-centeredness leads to demanding behavior and unreasonable requests for attention.

## Hostility

*Hostility* may be a response to overwhelming anxiety. Patients may occasionally be verbally abusive of the nursing staff. The patient may unconsiously view the nurse as a safer target for pent-up hostility than a family member or other person highly significant to the patient. Such misplaced hostility is difficult for the nurse to manage.

## The Patient Role

Of necessity, patients must conform to the routine of the hospital. For instance, time schedules may have to be different. The patient who habitually awakens at 7:30 a.m., for example, finds that the night nurse appears at 6:00 a.m. to administer early a.m. care.

Patients have traditionally been expected to behave passively and dependently. "Good" patients accepted treatment and care with a minimum of questions and adapted uncomplainingly to the routine of the hospital or institution.

However, the era of the docile patient is past. That the role of the patient is undergoing change is aptly symbolized by the widespread adoption of the Patient's Bill of Rights in health-care facilities (see Chapter 1). Patients and their families are increasingly perceiving themselves as consumers of health care and insisting on their right to quality care. Providers, in turn, are encouraging patients to take an active part in decision making about their own care. In order to participate in such decision making, the patient must be fully informed; thus some facilities allow the patient to see his or her medical record. It has still not been resolved, however, whether the medical record ultimately belongs to the hospital, the physician, or the patient.

A patient concerned about his or her progress may, for example, inquire about a blood-pressure reading. In the past patients were kept relatively uninformed about such matters, and such an inquiry might have elicited a negative response from the nurse. Today the nurse should be prepared to answer such questions straightforwardly or to refer the patient's questions to the physician.

## Healing Practices

*Healing* is restoration to a state of health. In the early days of medicine, the practice of healing was viewed as relatively straightforward: a particular treatment was prescribed for a particular illness. If that treatment proved unsuccessful, alternative methods may have been tried but the variety of treatments was limited by lack of knowledge.

*Spontaneous healing*—that is, healing without treatment—occurs in the case of some illnesses. Usually, however, *intervention* (treatment or therapy) significantly speeds and eases the healing process. Other conditions cannot heal without treatment. Therapy may consist of a combination of methods, medical and/or surgical. Both medical and surgical healing involve tissue restoration.

### Medical Healing

Medical healing is considered to have taken place when signs and symptoms cease. Intervention is aimed at supporting and augmenting the body's own resources. Drugs, rest and/or activity, special diet, inhalation, irrigations, and other measures might be employed, in conjunction with the reduction of psychological stress, to augment the body's own resources.

Infections can be controlled with drugs and by promoting the body's own immune response; rest and diet help restore body tissue. Chemical imbalances are often corrected by the body's homeostatic mechanisms if adequate food and fluids are provided. Patients with more serious diseases such as a bleeding ulcer or a heart attack are typically hospitalized for treatment. Whatever support is given, healing is the gradual restoration of healthy tissue and normal functioning.

### Surgical Healing

Whether performed for surgical reasons or resulting from trauma or injury, wounds heal in two basic ways. If a wound's edges are *approximated* closely together, not raised significantly, and not inflamed, the wound is said to be healing by *first intention.* If the edges are not touching or approximated but healthy tissue is forming in between (granulation), the wound is healing by *second intention.* It is preferable to promote first-intention healing, because it occurs more rapidly and scarring is minimal. The granulation of second-intention healing is often a prolonged process that produces extensive scarring.

Patients who undergo the removal of organs, such as the appendix, gallbladder, or spleen, heal surgically. Surgical healing may also be accompanied by such aspects of medical healing as drugs, rest and/or activity, nutrients, appropriate procedures, and psychological support.

## Holistic Healing

In keeping with the holistic approach to health maintenance, *holistic healing* implies that "all possible avenues of healing must be used (or considered for use) and that no single healing be used to the exclusion of others" (Grant, 1978). This enlargement of the concept of healing beyond the confines of tissue healing allows for any combination of effective healing practices. Meditation, massage, biofeedback, and other approaches (see Chapter 15) may be employed in conjunction with the more traditional methods of promoting healing.

## Rehabilitation

Concepts of rehabilitation are changing. According to a recent redefinition of the concept, "rehabilitation is a creative process that begins with immediate preventive care in the first stage of an accident or illness. It is continued through the restorative phase of care and involves adaptation of the whole being to a new life" (Stryker, 1977). Rehabilitation is therefore essential to anyone who must alter or adapt a normal life to accommodate to the effects of illness or injury.

Rehabilitation was formerly limited to the young and those with obvious potential for improvement. Health professionals typically undertook rehabilitation efforts too late, in the belief that the rehabilitation period began only when the effects of the illness or injury had reached a plateau. According to Stryker, this misconception defeated the goals of rehabilitation.

Nurses are involved in every aspect of rehabilitation. Specific types of rehabilitation in which nurses participate include those involving mobility and immobility, the senses, excretion, and ingestion. Psychological rehabilitation is also an integral part of any such program: for example, in order to adjust to living differently but fully, in spite of necessary limitations, the patient may need help adjusting body image as well. "Rehabilitation is a part of all nursing. Rehabilitation emphasizes the individual's ability rather than disability" (Bertolin, 1977). Texts on rehabilitation nursing outline the specific care to be given in individual cases.

## Conclusion

Nursing is more than helping people recover from illness, though this is a very important component of nursing care. Even more important, perhaps, is helping patients stay well. Understanding the stressors that cause illness and effective ways to minimize them is the essence of preventive health care.

Nursing is a demanding profession, physically and psychologically. With our knowledge of health, illness, and healing, we can become more responsible for our health maintenance. As nurses, maximum health status is essential for giving the best of care to our patients.

Promoting healing and maximum rehabilitation of patients with residual disability is the essence of curative care.

## Study Terms

acute illness
anxiety
approximated
carcinogenic
chronic illness
dependency
fear
guilt
healing
health
health maintenance
high-level wellness
holistic health
host
hostility
illness
immune system
immunosuppression
infirmity

intervention
malingering
medical healing
necessary but not
  sufficient
pathogens
preventive health care
rehabilitation
regression
self-centeredness
self-concept
spontaneous healing
stressors
surgical healing
  first intention
  second intention
toxic
trauma

## Learning Activities

1. Write out your beliefs about health mainte-nance. Discuss these in your small group.

2. Think about the last time you were ill. List your behavioral responses to illness. How were these responses helpful or not helpful to you in resolving your health problem? Discuss this in your small group.

3. Investigate a holistic health-care provider. How does the care provided differ from the standard physician's care? In what ways is it the same? Give a brief report on what you have learned.

4. Interview a patient/client in a health-care facility about that person's view of his or her health. Compare this with your estimate of the person's health status.

## References

Bertolin, Barbara H. *Tidbits of Useful Information in Rehabilitation Nursing.* Tacoma, Washington: Fort Steilacum Community College, 1977.

Dudley, Donald L., and Welke, Elton. *How to Sur-vive Being Alive.* Garden City, N.Y.: Doubleday, 1977.

Dunn, H. *High-Level Wellness.* Arlington, Virginia: R. W. Beatty, 1961.

French, Ruth M. *The Dynamics of Health Care,* 2nd ed. New York: McGraw-Hill, 1974.

Galton, Lawrence. "Questions Patients Ask About Health and How You Can Answer Them." *Nursing '77* 7 (April 1977): 54–59.

Grant, Lillian. *The Holistic Revolution.* Pasadena, Cal.: Ward Ritchie Press, 1978.

Luckmann, J., and Sorenson, K. "What Patients' Actions Tell You About Their Feelings, Fears and Needs." *Nursing '75* 5 (February 1975): 54–61.

Milio, N. "A Framework for Prevention: Changing Health-Damaging to Health-Generating Life Patterns." *American Journal of Public Health* 66 (May 1976): 435–439.

Munson, Ronald. *Intervention and Reflection: Basic Issues in Medical Ethics.* Belmont, Cal.: Wads-worth, 1979.

Oelbaum, C. H. "Hallmarks of Adult Wellness." *American Journal of Nursing* 74 (September 1974): 1623–1625.

Roy, Sister Callista. *Introduction to Nursing: An Ad-aptation Model.* Englewood Cliffs, N.J.: Prentice-Hall, 1976.

Stryker, Ruth P. *Rehabilitative Aspects of Acute and Chronic Nursing Care.* Philadelphia: W. B. Saun-ders, 1977.

Turnbull, J., Sr. "Shifting the Focus to Health." *American Journal of Nursing* 76 (December 1976): 1985–1987.

U.S. Dept. of Health, Education and Welfare, Vital and Health Statistics, 1976.

VanKaam, Adrian L. "The Nurse in the Patient's World." *American Journal of Nursing* 59 (Decem-ber 1959): 1708–1710.

Vincent, Pauline. "The Sick Role in Patient Care." *American Journal of Nursing* 75 (July 1975): 1172–1173.

World Health Organization. *Demographic Year Book 1975.* Department of Economic and Social Af-fairs, United Nations Statistical Office, 1975.

Wu, Ruth. *Behavior and Illness.* Englewood Cliffs, N.J.: Prentice-Hall, 1973.

# Chapter 8
# Stress

Countless newspaper and magazine articles have been written about stress in the past several years. Nevertheless, it is still widely believed—wrongly—that all stress is harmful. As a health professional, you need a clear and accurate understanding of stress and its bearing on health and illness.

## The Nature of Stress

Hans Selye, a Canadian physician and endocrinologist, was one of the first researchers to define and describe stress (Selye, 1956). Whenever a person confronts a threat, according to Selye, the body responds in a predictable way. Furthermore, this response is the same no matter what the nature of the threat. Selye labeled the body's response to stress the *General Adaptation Syndrome* (G.A.S.). This term emphasizes that the response is both generalized and *adaptive*—that is, aimed at neutralizing the threat and restoring the body to homeostasis. Stress, then, is the state in which the body is prepared to act in order to preserve itself.

Selye and other writers have pointed out that stress is both a normal and an essential part of human life. Lacking the ability to respond in this way, the body would be overwhelmed by threats. Selye has also postulated that without threat and accompanying opportunities to respond, development would be inhibited. Stress that is helpful and valuable in this way Selye calls *eustress* (Selye, 1978).

*Distress*, on the other hand, is stress so extreme and/or prolonged as to deplete the body's reserves, induce exhaustion, and contribute to illness and even death. In order to understand how such outcomes could occur, let us examine what happens during stress.

## The General Adaptation Syndrome

The collective response to stress of the many body systems that help prepare the body for action is known as the *General Adaptation Syndrome* (G.A.S.). This neuroendocrine response arises through the *autonomic nervous system*—the branch of the nervous system that governs such involuntary body functions as glandular secretion, heart action, and the activity of smooth muscle in the gastrointestinal tract and the blood vessels. The autonomic nervous system has two components, the *sympathetic* and the *parasympathetic*. It is the sympathetic nervous system that responds to stress.

The primary endocrine glands involved in the stress response are the pituitary, the adrenals, and the thyroid. The *pituitary* is a small gland located at the base of the brain. The anterior portion of the pituitary, often called "the master gland," secretes several hormones that affect the functioning of other endocrine glands. The posterior portion of the pituitary functions separately. It releases antidiuretic hormone (ADH), which causes the kidneys to retain water in the body.

The *adrenal glands* are located on top of the kidneys. They are composed of two sections, the center or *medulla* and the outer layer or *cortex*. The hormones secreted by the cortex, called adrenocorticosteroids, are the most critical in the stress response. Adrenaline (also called epinephrine) secreted by the medulla also plays a role in stress.

The *thyroid* gland is located on the anterior side of the trachea. The thyroid hormone, *thyroxine*, has a major effect on the body's basic *metabolism* (the physical and chemical processes that produce energy). The thyroid gland may have particular significance in long-term stress.

The General Adaptation Syndrome (Exhibit 8.1) has three distinct stages: (1) the alarm reaction, (2) resistance, and (3) exhaustion. The physiological processes are very complex. Figure 8.1 illustrates the neuroendocrine response in the General Adaptation Syndrome.

## The Alarm Reaction

The alarm reaction activates the neuroendocrine response: the sensory nerves receive an external stimulus and relay it to the brain. The brain in turn identifies the stimulus as a threat. In the medulla of the brain are located the centers of the autonomic nervous system. These centers stimulate the sympathetic nervous system to respond. The response generated in this way is often called "the flight-or-fight response" because it prepares the body for both kinds of action. The heart beats more rapidly, the respiratory rate increases, and the peripheral blood vessels constrict (causing a rise in blood pressure). The adrenal medulla is stimulated to secrete epinephrine and norepinephrine, which further increase heart rate and respirations and cause additional vasoconstriction (decrease in the diameter of blood vessels) and higher blood pressure. The kidneys are stimulated to release a hormone (renin) that raises blood pressure even further.

Simultaneously, the stimulation of the central nervous system brings about a response in the hypothalamus (one of the structures of the brain). The hypothalamus activates the anterior pituitary gland, which in turn stimulates the adrenals through adrenocorticotropic hormone (A.C.T.H.) and the thyroid through thyroid stimulating hormone (T.S.H.).

The adrenal cortex increases its production of adrenocorticosteroids, hormones that help to increase glucose in the blood and to retain sodium and water in the body. The thyroid secretes additional thyroid hormone, thyroxine, which increases the body's metabolic rate.

The posterior pituitary increases its release of antidiuretic hormone (ADH), contributing to water retention.

In addition, the adrenocorticosteroids also depress the immune system, the body's ability to wall off organisms through inflammation, and therefore increase the risk of infection.

These complex responses occur very rapidly and require the body to use considerable energy. The overall result is enhanced ability to defend against outside threats and enhanced functioning due to optimum oxygenation and circulation.

## The Stage of Resistance

The body's adaptation to the stressor takes place during the stage of resistance. Having mobilized its abilities, the body neutralizes or destroys the threat. Production of hormones is also decreasing through *negative feedback*. In other words, as the levels of hormones rise, the gland responds by decreasing production. Thus the hormone returns to prestress levels. When the body is successful in its fight against the threat, the General Adaptation Syndrome ends with the stage of resistance.

## The Stage of Exhaustion

If the stage of resistance is not successful, the body may enter a third stage. A prolonged state of preparedness depletes the body's energy stores and eventually its ability to maintain resistance to the threat. Without outside intervention, the outcome of the stage of exhaustion is death. Some external mechanism must be found to support the body and make adaptation possible.

## Signs and Symptoms of Stress

Stress is manifested in a variety of ways, physical, cognitive, emotional, and behavioral. Knowing these signs and symptoms will enable you to recognize stress in yourself and others.

## Physical Signs of Stress

Let us review the physical changes that occur in the major body systems as a result of stress.

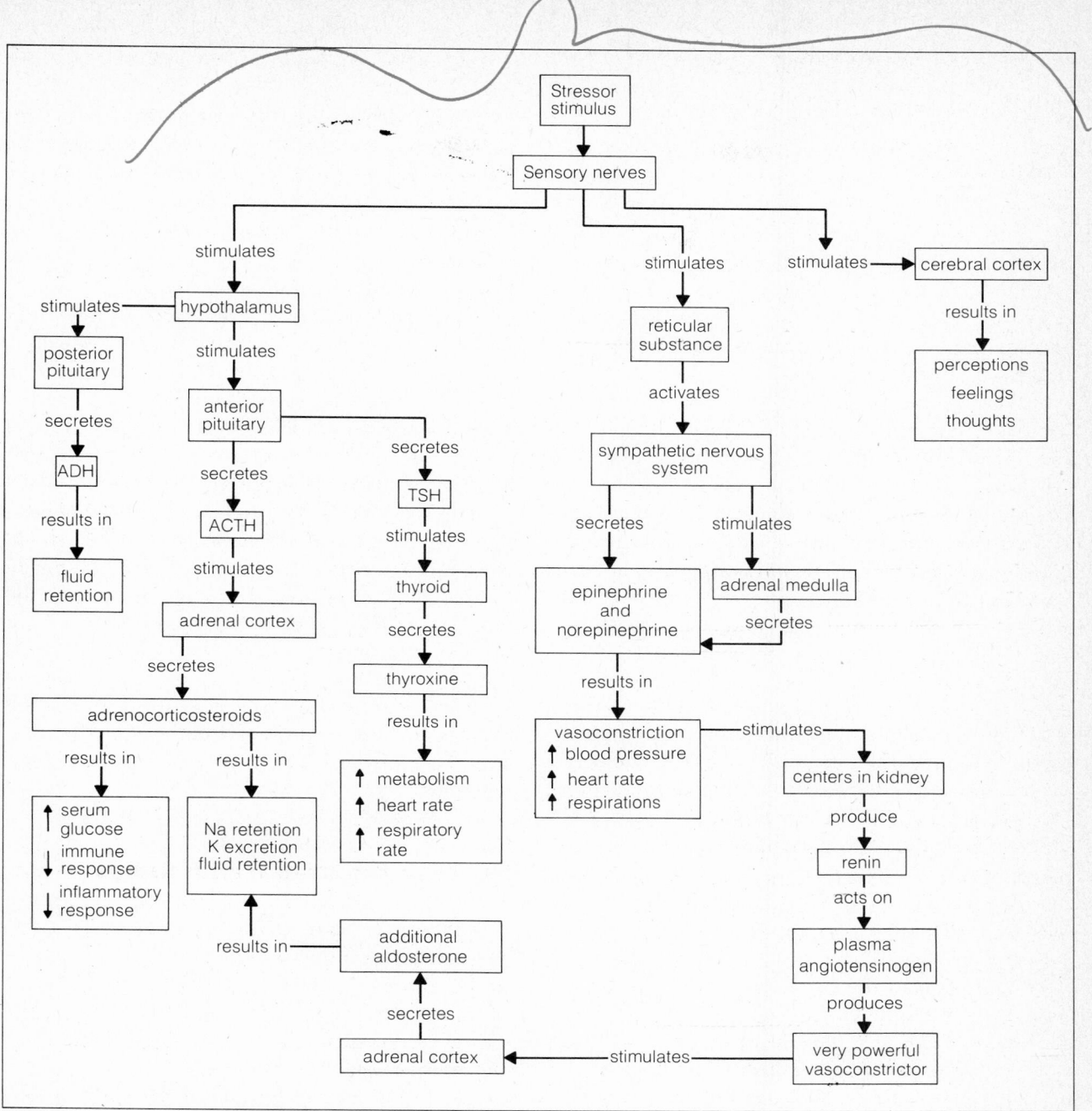

**Figure 8.1  Physiological processes of the General Adaptation Syndrome**

## Circulation

The heart rate increases and blood pressure rises. As circulation speeds up, both blood flow and oxygen to tissue increase, thus preparing the body for action. The peripheral vessels constrict, serving to increase blood supply to the brain and heart. Increased sugar in the blood provides extra energy.

## Respiration

The respiratory rate increases and the bronchial passages in the lungs dilate. Both processes serve to increase the amount of air exchanged in the lungs. Increased red blood-cell production, stimulated by epinephrine, enhances the ability of the blood to carry the oxygen provided by the lungs. Rapid respiration can lead to *hyperventilation*, a condition in which excessive amounts of carbon dioxide are exhaled, upsetting the body's delicate acid-base balance. Faintness, dizziness, tingling of the extremities, and convulsions can result. (See Chapter 24 for a fuller discussion of acid-base problems.)

## Digestion

Because of decreased production of digestive enzymes and decreased peristalsis (muscular contractions that aid digestion), stress can result in anorexia, abdominal distention, nausea, and vomiting. Nutritional needs increase, however, making special attention to diet desirable. Possibly because the lining of the stomach becomes less resistant to acid stomach secretions, heartburn and even ulcers are not uncommon.

## Elimination

Although urine production may decrease, frequency of urination may increase due to autonomic nervous system stimulation of the bladder. Peristalsis usually decreases, causing gas and constipation. In some cases, however, defecation increases in frequency to the point of diarrhea.

## Muscle Tension

Muscle tension in the head, back, and neck is a common symptom of stress. Tension headaches may result from the tensing of scalp and neck muscles. Some people grind their teeth due to tension of the jaw muscle. Backaches are not uncommon. At times muscle tension is clearly visible; even when pain and discomfort are absent muscle tension can sometimes be identified by palpating the muscle.

## Cognitive Changes Due to Stress

*Cognitive* changes are changes that involve thinking. Mild stress typically increases mental alertness and ability to learn, to attend to details, and to solve problems, at least for a while. Energy, ability, and productivity are all likely to increase; the person feels "up."

As stress increases and/or persists, however, the thinking processes function less effectively. Learning becomes more difficult, and even simple instructions may be forgotten. Patients about to undergo surgery, for example, often fail to remember instructions and information they have just received about preparation for surgery.

Severe and/or chronic stress undermines problem-solving ability: the severely stressed person is less able to remember information that would be helpful in problem-solving, and thinking may become so narrowly focused (often called "tunnel vision") that pertinent ideas are not related. Such a person's ability to weigh alternatives and make sound decisions is deficient. Vacillating between different positions is common, as is impulsive, ill-considered decision making. However irrationally arrived at, such a choice may be clung to in the face of conflicting arguments in an effort to minimize feelings of uneasiness.

Stress also typically decreases the number of problems a person can deal with at one time. One problem may be approached successfully, but the advent of further problems is likely to seem overwhelming.

## Feelings Associated With Stress

In addition to changes in cognitive ability, unpleasant emotions also accompany high levels of stress. The most common such feeling is tenseness or anxiety—the nonspecific feeling that something is wrong. Asked the source of these feelings, the person may not know; alternatively, he or she may invoke one or several unconvincing explanations. Irritability and anger in response to inner feelings may be directed at anyone with whom the person comes in contact. When you work with a person undergoing stress, it is helpful to remember that anger directed at you is not fundamentally a response to your behavior or personality.

Stress typically undermines self-esteem and trust in one's own abilities. Loss of self-esteem is in turn often accompanied by self-centeredness and diminished ability to concern oneself with others' feelings and needs. All experiences tend to be interpreted as uniquely significant to oneself.

For example, a patient under stress might suspect routine questions and procedures as signifying that the illness is more serious than he or she has been told. Such a patient might also make unreasonable demands on family members.

As stress persists, malaise—general lack of energy and ability to initiate action—may set in. One may feel purposeless and adrift. Some people become depressed.

## Behavioral Signs of Stress

People's behavior changes under stress in response to the foregoing physiological, cognitive, and emotional changes. Tasks may be left undone or incomplete. Errors become more common. Some people become less active; others take on more and more tasks in an effort to alleviate the feelings they are experiencing. In both cases, actual accomplishment is diminished. Urging a person under severe stress to accept new responsibilities (such as self-care) may precipitate further problems. The focus of conversation tends to be the self. Speech may become more rapid. Conversation may be disjointed due to a tendency to lose one's train of thought and introduce scattered ideas.

Outbursts of anger accompanied by shouting, door-slamming, and other aggressive behavior may occur with relatively little provocation. Random, purposeless movement, such as pacing, jangling keys, and fiddling with one's hair and clothing is common.

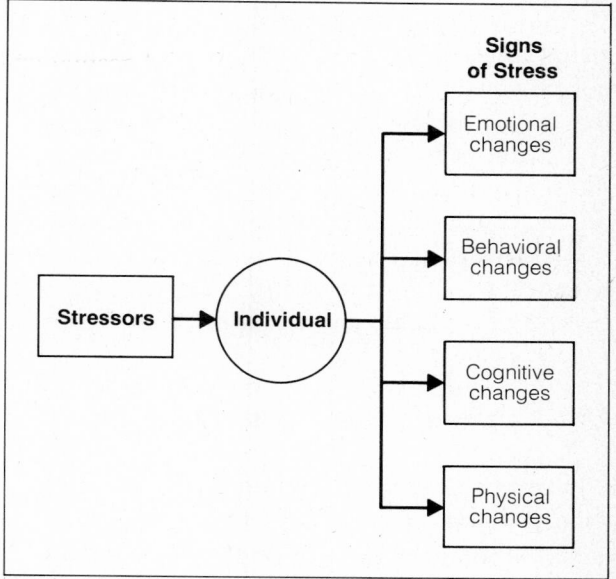

**Figure 8.2**
Stress causes multiple changes

# Stressors

A *stressor* is any agent or stimulus that poses a real or perceived threat to the person. Though the term *stress* is widely used to designate the stimulus as well as the resulting condition, it is preferable to distinguish verbally between the stress (the condition within the person) and the stressor (the external stimulus).

## Origins of Stressors

Some stressors are *internal physiological factors*. For example, the accumulated waste products of fat metabolism can become a stressor: they are acid in nature and pose a threat to the body's acid-base balance. (See Chapter 24 for a further discussion of acid-base balance.) Drugs, disease-causing organisms within the body, and hormonal and metabolic changes may likewise function as stressors.

*External physical factors* may also be stressors. Extreme heat, extreme cold, loud noises, bright lights, and trauma are all physical causes of stress. Although people differ in their ability to withstand physical and physiological stressors, all these factors can cause predictable stress in all individuals and, if extreme enough, may even threaten survival. Much less predictable are internal psychological stressors and external social stressors.

*Internal psychological stressors* are thoughts and

feelings that produce stress. Low self-esteem, loneliness, and hopelessness, for example, can create stress. Even though such feelings may not be based on realistic perceptions, they can pose a threat to a person's integrity.

*External social stressors* are threatening stimuli arising from interactions with other people. Conflict and pressure to perform are common external social stressors. For example, a critical and demanding employer, a spouse who shirks responsibility, or a rebellious child could all threaten a person's stability. Psychological and social stressors are almost always intertwined. Feelings change as a result of interactions with other people, and relationships are altered by our perceptions of ourselves. Change itself is one of the most common social stressors: changes in one's job, home life, responsibilities, relationships, and circumstances require adjustments and can thus produce stress.

## The Nature of Stressors

Whether or not a given stimulus acts as a stressor for an individual depends in some cases on whether he or she *perceives* it as a stressor. If a person perceives something as a stressor, it functions as a stressor for that individual.

Another important characteristic of stressors is their magnitude. For example, cold is a stressor, but different degrees of cold arouse different amounts of stress within an individual. The greater the cold, the greater the stress. Though harder to measure, psychological and social stressors also have magnitude. Individual perception plays a large part in determining the magnitude of a particular stressor for a particular individual. Moving to a new home might be a major stressor for one person and only a moderate stressor for another. Holmes and Rahe (1967) have tried to quantify the magnitude of common social and psychological stressors by assigning them "stress points" on a scale of 1 to 100 (see Table 8.1). The death of one's spouse is assigned the highest stress score; other factors are given proportionate scores. Though this scale is the result of many years of research into stress, it is probably best used as a general guide to a given stressor's magnitude rather than an absolute applicable to any individual.

Stress is also *cumulative*. That is, separate stres-

Table 8.1
**The Social Readjustment Rating Scale**

| Life event | Mean value |
|---|---|
| 1. Death of spouse | 100 |
| 2. Divorce | 73 |
| 3. Marital separation | 65 |
| 4. Jail term | 63 |
| 5. Death of close family member | 63 |
| 6. Personal injury or illness | 53 |
| 7. Marriage | 50 |
| 8. Fired at work | 47 |
| 9. Marital reconciliation | 45 |
| 10. Retirement | 45 |
| 11. Change in health of family member | 44 |
| 12. Pregnancy | 40 |
| 13. Sex difficulties | 39 |
| 14. Gain of new family member | 39 |
| 15. Business readjustment | 39 |
| 16. Change in financial state | 38 |
| 17. Death of close friend | 37 |
| 18. Change to different line of work | 36 |
| 19. Change in number of arguments with spouse | 35 |
| 20. Mortgage over $10,000 (e.g., house or business) | 31 |
| 21. Foreclosure of mortgage or loan | 30 |
| 22. Change in responsibilities at work | 29 |
| 23. Son or daughter leaves home | 29 |
| 24. Trouble with in-laws | 29 |
| 25. Outstanding personal achievement | 28 |
| 26. Spouse begins or stops working | 26 |
| 27. Beginning or end of school | 26 |
| 28. Change in living conditions | 25 |
| 29. Revision of personal habits | 24 |
| 30. Trouble with boss | 23 |
| 31. Change in work hours or conditions | 20 |
| 32. Change in residence | 20 |
| 33. Change in schools | 20 |
| 34. Change in recreation | 19 |
| 35. Change in church activities | 19 |
| 36. Change in social activities | 18 |
| 37. Mortgage or loan less than $10,000 (e.g., car) | 17 |
| 38. Change in sleeping habits | 16 |
| 39. Change in number of family get-togethers | 15 |
| 40. Change in eating habits | 15 |
| 41. Vacation | 13 |
| 42. Christmas | 12 |
| 43. Minor violation of the law | 11 |

Reprinted with permission from *Journal of Psychosomatic Research* 11, T. H. Holmes and R. H. Rahe, "The Social Readjustment Rating Scale," Copyright 1967, Pergamon Press, Ltd., pp. 213–218.

sors experienced simultaneously have a greater effect than does any one of them singly. The stress resulting from two different items in Table 8.1 is thus additive. Holmes and Rahe add together the points associated with the various stressors operating in an individual's life to arrive at a figure representing total stress. It does not matter, they say, whether total stress is a result of many minor factors or one major event; the effect on the person is the same. In this context, let us consider further the relationship between stress and illness.

## Stress and Illness

The role of excessive stress in illness is receiving growing attention from researchers. It is widely believed that constant stress depletes the body's resources, making it more susceptible to additional stressors that may act upon it. This hypothesis helps explain why an individual may develop a cold in one instance but not another when exposed to an identical virus.

Holmes and Rahe state that the likelihood of physical illness increases with an increase in total stress points. Their research has led them to conclude that individuals who score higher than 300 points on the scale have a 90 percent chance of becoming ill within a year. Such illness may be major or minor, and of course its exact nature cannot be predicted. Thus Holmes and Rahe advocate efforts to limit the number of stress-producing changes in one's life at a given time.

Aspects of the stress response itself may also develop into chronic conditions. An example is increased blood pressure. Unremitting stress may produce chronic high blood pressure, which in turn may bring about potentially dangerous illness.

Prolonged stress can also cause body organs or systems to break down. Stress ulcers in the stomach and inflammation in the colon are examples. Although researchers have tried to link specific stressors to specific illnesses, such efforts have not yet met with success. It may be that the specific illness an individual develops is more dependent on basic genetic makeup and physiology than on the nature of the stressor.

When new stressors are superimposed on existing illness, they may interfere with the body's ability to cope with that illness, which may then become more severe or overwhelming.

A constant state of stress may also arouse unpleasant emotions, such as anxiety or depression. If these feelings become severe enough to impair the individual's ability to function, they may require treatment.

Conversely, reducing the number and/or magnitude of stressors may increase the body's ability to cope with existing illness. A stable and supportive emotional life enhances one's ability to cope with physical illness, just as sound physical health enables one to cope better with emotional stressors.

## Stress Management

Many methods have been developed to manage stress so it does not become overwhelming. The success of the various approaches varies. Some can have exceptionally positive effects but only with considerable time and persistence. All require the individual to be an active participant, not a passive recipient of treatment. *Behavior modification* techniques—using reinforcement of desired behavior—appear to be especially well suited to teaching responses that must become semiautomatic in order to be effective, such as relaxing instead of tensing one's back muscles when angry. Some people may find a given technique helpful for moderate stress but less so for severe stress. Each individual needs some mode of individual stress management.

## Eliminating Stressors

The best way of managing stress may be to eliminate the stressor from one's life. Physical causes of stress are commonly handled this way. You protect yourself from the cold, for example, by wearing adequate clothing. You avoid foods to which you are allergic, and you come in out of the rain. But it is usually much more difficult to eliminate psychosocial stressors from our lives. Sometimes this is the result of ambivalence: if a certain situation causes stress, but also has the potential to elicit pleasure or growth, one may be unwilling to abandon it. Sometimes it is impossible to do so. For example, a particular job might be severely stressful but, for a variety of reasons, essential. Willingness to examine the stressors in one's life openly and honestly can be very productive. People under stress often fail to recognize the alternatives available to them. It may be possible, for example, to find a less stressful job, give up an expensive club membership, or stop socializing with a difficult neighbor. Alternatively, one can often eliminate several minor stressors, thus freeing resources to cope with a major stressor that cannot be avoided.

## Increasing Resistance to Stress

Coping with stress requires physical energy. The person who is best equipped physically to handle stress is well nourished, gets adequate rest and regular exercise, and pursues a physically healthful life style. The stress response makes particularly heavy demands on the cardiovascular and respiratory systems. Regular exercise and activity maintain these systems' functioning and ability to respond positively under stress.

It is also possible to become more resistant psychosocially to stress. People who cope effectively with small problems and stressors as they arise develop skills that will prove useful when stress is high. Treating small problems as challenges to learn coping skills can set the stage for handling stress well in the future. One productive way to help others cope with stress is to encourage them to review successful coping methods they have used in the past. Doing so can promote sound problem-solving in the current situation. Stress seems to be more easily tolerated if one feels "in control" of the situation. The sense of control is achieved by making conscious choices and decisions, and undermined by allowing others to direct one's life.

## Physical Activity

In addition to helping the body resist stressors more effectively, physical activity helps prevent the cyclic neurohormone patterns that keep the General Adaptation Syndrome activated when stress occurs. Purposeful physical discharge of accumulated tension acts as negative feedback, preventing the stress response from persisting beyond its usefulness. If you are very tense just before a test, for example, you might benefit more from jogging around the block than from sitting and worrying. Vigorous exercise expends nervous energy and enables you to focus more usefully on the test itself.

## The Relaxation Response

The *relaxation response* recently identified in the human being (Benson *et al.*, 1974)—a state characterized by decreased sympathetic nervous system activity, decreased muscle tone, pupil constriction, decreased blood pressure, decreased heart rate, and decreased respirations—can also counteract the effects of stress (see Exhibit 8.2).

Four conditions must be present to initiate the relaxation response: (1) an environment with minimal stimuli, (2) minimal muscular activity and decreased muscle tone, (3) a mental device to help shift one's thoughts away from the source of stress, and (4) a mentally passive attitude (Benson *et al.*, 1974).

Many different approaches are used to teach people to invoke the relaxation response at will. Most of the following techniques are subject to ongoing research.

### Progressive Relaxation

*Progressive relaxation* is a method of ending muscle tension associated with stress. The first step is to help the person identify tight muscles and evidence of tension. Then he or she is taught to relax these muscles voluntarily. One way of doing so is to alternately tighten and relax specific muscles, beginning with the feet and gradually moving upward until the whole body is relaxed. After learning to relax progressively, some people learn to invoke relaxation of the entire body at will. This response can then be employed in situations of stress (Jacobson, 1938).

## Meditation

Though *meditation* has been practiced for hundreds of years in various Christian mystic and Eastern traditions, it has received widespread popular attention in this country only in the last ten to fifteen years. The meditation method most widespread in the United States is Transcendental Meditation (TM), whose conceptual structure and vocabulary are drawn from Hindu religious thought and religious terminology. Many Americans, however, pursue TM as an aid to life enrichment and stress management rather than a religious experience, and religious beliefs are not essential to the effectiveness of its meditation techniques.

Meditation invokes the relaxation response by helping one structure one's thoughts and actions to shut out stimuli. Meditation is practiced in a quiet, private, pleasant place. The position of the body is one that tends to promote relaxation and decrease muscle tension. Repetition of a word or phrase is used as a mental device to focus one's attention.

Meditation produces definite changes in the brain-wave pattern measured on an electroencephalogram. Sympathetic nervous system activity also appears to be diminished. People who practice meditation regularly report that they feel an increased sense of well-being and are calmer,

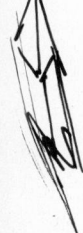

less nervous, and able to function more effectively. Meditation requires a significant investment of time, both to learn and to practice (Wallace and Benson, 1972).

## Autogenic Training

*Autogenic training* is a set of exercises designed to help one focus on physical sensations. Psychosocial stressors are shut out and the relaxation response invoked. The exercises teach systematic concentration on heaviness of the limbs, warmth in limbs, calm regular heartbeat, slow deep breathing, warmth in the abdomen, and coolness of the forehead (Schultz and Luthe, 1959).

## Self-Hypnosis

*Self-hypnosis*—inducing a hypnotic state in oneself at will—is sometimes taught as a stress-management device. A hypnotic state is a form of relaxation response in which external stimuli can be completely shut out.

## Basic Life Skills

Psychosocial stress can arise from inability to manage the day-to-day tasks of adult life, such as organizing one's time, budgeting finances, communicating assertively, and sharing one's feelings with others. Some people handle such daily tasks well but have trouble making sound, well-timed decisions about major changes in their lives. Some individuals need help identifying the skills they lack and deciding where to seek assistance. Learning to manage ordinary tasks well tends to enhance self-image as well as reducing stress. Classes in basic life skills are widely available.

## Maintaining Support Systems

An individual's *support system* is composed of the people who offer him or her emotional support. The members of one's support system may include family members, friends, neighbors, co-workers, and anyone with whom one has a caring relationship.

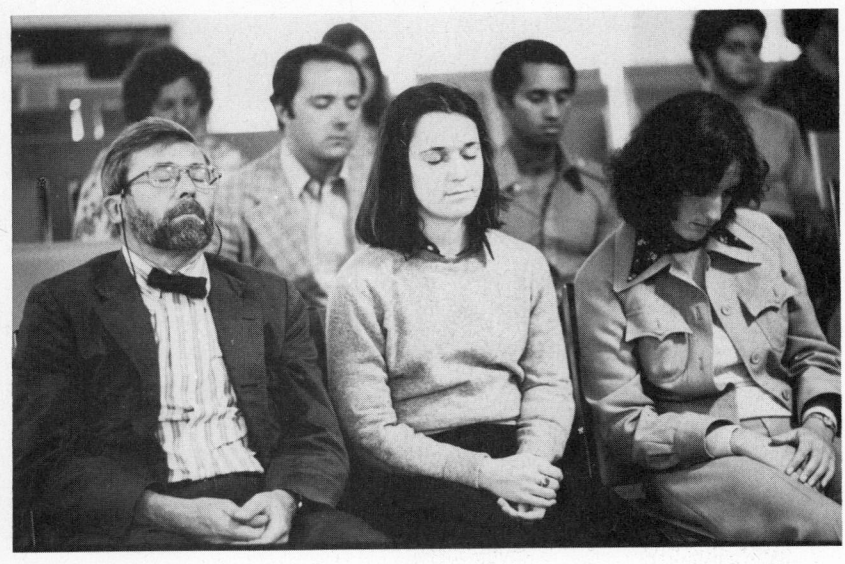

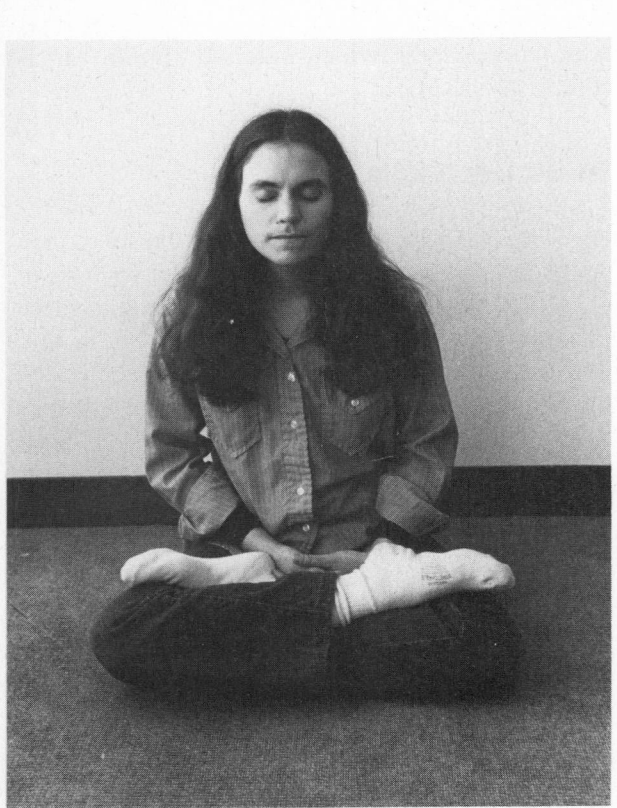

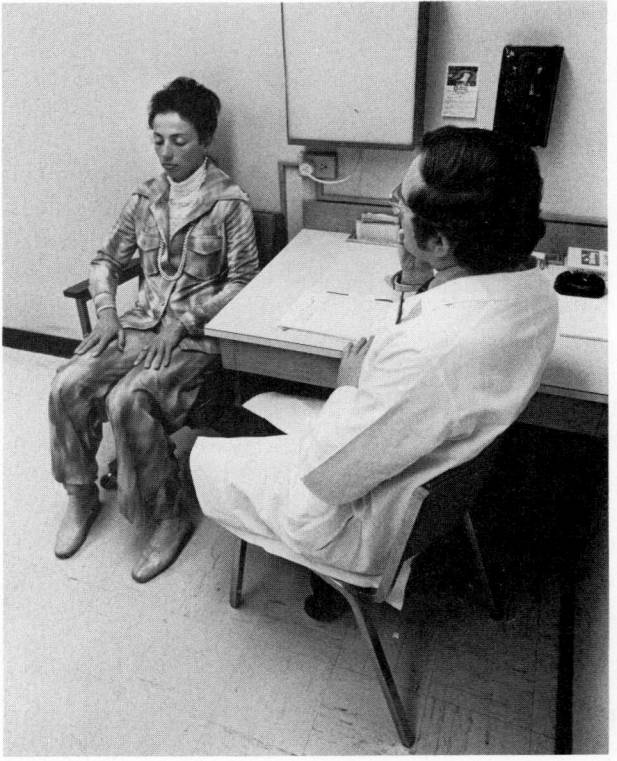

**Figure 8.3**
The relaxation response can be induced in a variety of ways. (*Top:* Arthur Grace/Stock, Boston; *bottom, left and right:* Dan Bernstein)

A sound support system is very important in stress management. Human beings live in community with each other, and concerned and caring people can serve as the solid foundations in one another's lives. Sharing difficulties and concerns often makes them seem less overwhelming and helps identify ways of overcoming them. Occasionally one needs to transfer responsibilities and tasks to someone else temporarily in order to lighten one's load. The concern of others also promotes feelings of self-worth, important in coping successfully with stress.

## Biofeedback

*Biofeedback* is a means of monitoring a body process, such as temperature or blood flow, by machine, and using feedback from the machine in learning to alter that process. Biofeedback may be used in stress management to provide information on circulatory or vascular responses to stressors. By identifying and learning to control an undesirable response, such as rising blood pressure, one may be able to minimize the detrimental effects of stress. Learning to use biofeedback is time-consuming, and refresher courses may be necessary to maintain the skill.

## Psychotherapy and Counseling

Mental-health professionals use a variety of psychotherapeutic techniques to help individuals learn to manage stress. When you study the care of patients with mental-health problems, you will learn about types of therapeutic intervention.

## The Immune Response

In conjunction with the General Adaptation Syndrome, the body employs specific means of promoting adaptation to specific stressors. The *immune response* is one such specific response whereby the body produces specific cells called *antibodies* to destroy specific invading proteins called *antigens*.

When invaded by an antigen, the body initiates the necessary cellular processes to produce the needed antibody. It takes several days to produce a sufficient quantity of the antibody to destroy all the antigen. If other processes destroy the antigen in the meantime, the body simply ceases antibody production. If the same antigen invades the body again, however, immediate production of the antibody is possible. This rapid response allows for all the antigen to be destroyed before the body sustains damage. This process, which protects the body from subsequent episodes of some viral diseases such as measles and mumps, is called *active immunity* (see Table 8.2).

Until the nineteenth century, the only immunity that existed was that which occurred naturally: an invading antigen was destroyed after setting in motion the capacity for rapid antibody production, thus creating an immunity. Science has since developed a variety of ways to induce active immunity without having to suffer the disease. Attenuated (non-disease-producing) virus may be introduced orally (poliomyelitis vaccine), by injection (diphtheria immunization), or by scratching or pricking the skin (smallpox vaccination). All three methods provide for an *artificially acquired* active immunity that lasts all one's life

### Table 8.2
### Types of Immunity

| | Active (Body produces own antibodies) | Passive (Body receives antibodies from external source) |
|---|---|---|
| Naturally acquired | Development of natural antibody in the course of certain viral and bacterial illnesses | Receipt of a specific antibody through the placenta or in mother's milk |
| Artificially acquired | Introduction of a specific antigen | Introduction of a specific antibody |

("boosters" are necessary in the case of some conditions, such as tetanus, to reinvigorate the body's ability to produce antibodies).

Immunity acquired through antibodies not produced by one's own body is called *passive immunity*, since the body is not active in the process. Passive immunity acquired by an infant through the mother's milk is an example of natural acquisition; an injection that contains antibodies, such as gamma globulin, is artificial acquisition. Passive immunity is effective only for a limited time. The body soon destroys the antibodies and, since it has not developed the ability to produce its own antibodies, no residual immunity remains.

## Local Adaptation Syndrome

The body also has several means of responding to localized threats, such as a bacterial invasion. These responses serve to limit the effects of a physiologic stressor and to establish the preconditions for restoration of homeostasis to the affected body part. Selye termed these processes the *Local Adaptation Syndrome* (L.A.S.) to differentiate it from generalized response to stressors. According to Selye, the L.A.S. is also characterized by the three stages of alarm, resistance, and exhaustion. When the stage of exhaustion is reached in the L.A.S., general body responses are called on.

### Inflammation

The inflammatory response is a type of Local Adaptation Syndrome in which the body produces localized tissue changes that serve to confine the injurious agent and prepare the area for destruction of the agent and subsequent healing.

Injury to cells causes the release of *histamine*, a protein produced by the body, and other substances. Histamine in turn results in vasodilatation (expansion of blood vessels), which increases blood supply to the area and results in *redness* and *heat*. Because the other substances released increase the permeability of capillaries, the plasma and white blood cells leaving the capillaries are increased, resulting in the *swelling* of tissue. The released substances irritate the tissues, which, together with swelling, results in localized *pain*. The combined effect of these factors tends to *decrease function* in the involved body part. These five signs are often called the *cardinal signs of inflammation* (Exhibit 8.3).

Inflammation sets the stage for production of a *fibrin* network that confines the injurious agent to the affected area and allows for white blood cells (leukocytes) and antibodies to destroy it. If the inflammatory process persists or spreads, the bone marrow (center of the large bones) releases additional leukocytes, resulting in an increased white–blood-cell count.

### Resolution of Inflammation

Resolution occurs when the white cells have completely destroyed the injurious agent. The stimulus to the inflammatory process is ended, the fluid that caused swelling is reabsorbed, the capillaries return to normal permeability, and vasodilatation ceases. The fibrin network is reabsorbed and normal structure and function are restored.

### Supporting Resolution of Inflammation

In the initial stage of the inflammatory process the use of cold packs causes vasoconstriction, which

---

Exhibit 8.3
**Cardinal Signs of Inflammation**

1. Redness
2. Heat
3. Swelling
4. Pain
5. Decreased function

---

tends to decrease swelling. This process helps minimize pain and loss of function. When capillary permeability has returned to normal (approximately 24 to 48 hours) heat is used to increase circulation, which in turn promotes resolution of the inflammation. Anti-inflammatory drugs may be prescribed by the physician to decrease the inflammatory response.

## The Reticuloendothelial System

The *reticuloendothelial system* is a network of tissues and cells found throughout the body—especially in the blood, general connective tissue, spleen, bone marrow, lymph nodes, and liver (where such cells are also called Kupffer cells)—that plays an important part in the body's adaptive mechanism. Some of the cells are unusually large and capable of engulfing and destroying injurious agents, a process called *phagocytosis*. The macrophage is one type of cell capable of phagocytosis. Such cells may be fixed in one location or mobile and able to wander wherever in the body they are needed. This system of tissues and cells acts to destroy injurious agents that are absorbed from the digestive system or enter the body in other ways. Their routine vigilance prevents more serious problems from developing.

## Interferon

Considerable research is being conducted on *interferon*, a substance produced by cells that protects them from viruses. Ordinarily, the entrance of a virus into a cell causes the cell to replicate the virus. Interferon's interference with this reproductive process is another important adaptive mechanism. Researchers express the hope that a means can be found to increase the body's production of interferon when viral invasion occurs. Also, interferon is being used experimentally in the treatment of cancer and arthritis.

# Conclusion

Stress is a constant in all our lives. An understanding of stress and its potential and actual effects on health will help you understand how nurses can support individuals who are adapting to stress. It is important to keep in mind that people's responses to stressors vary with their perceptions and body makeup.

## Study Terms

active immunity
adaptive response
adrenals
alarm reaction
antibody
antigen
autogenic training
basic life skills
behavior modification
biofeedback
cortex
distress
eustress
fibrin
General Adaptation
  Syndrome (G.A.S.)
histamine
immune response
interferon
leukocyte
life change units
Local Adaptation
  Syndrome (L.A.S.)
meditation
metabolism
negative feedback
passive immunity
phagocytosis
pituitary
progressive relaxation
psychotherapy
relaxation response
reticuloendothelial
  system
self-hypnosis
stage of exhaustion
stage of resistance
stress
stressor
support system
thyroid
vasoconstriction
vasodilatation

## Learning Activities

1. Using the Social Readjustment Rating Scale developed by Holmes and Rahe, assign life change points to your own life. According to Holmes and Rahe, how likely are you to experience an illness?
2. In an interview, determine a patient/client's total life change points. How does this relate to that person's illness?
3. Investigate a specific stress management technique that is taught in your community. Write a brief report that includes information on the time required, the cost, and the numbers of people completing the training.
4. Identify a situation in which you felt a great deal of stress (such as your first day in the nursing program). List all the objective evidence of stress that you exhibited at that time. Compare your own responses to stress with those outlined in the chapter.

## References

Bell, J. M. "Stressful Life Events and Coping Methods in Mental Illness and Wellness Behaviors." *Nursing Research* 26 (March/April 1977): 136–141.

Benson, Herbert; Beary, John F.; and Canol, Mark P. "The Relaxation Response." *Psychiatry* 37 (February 1974): 37–46.

Breeden, Sue, and Kando, Charles. "Using Biofeedback to Reduce Tension." *American Journal of Nursing* 75 (November 1975): 2010–2012.

Engel, G. "Emotional Stress and Sudden Death." *Psychology Today* 11 (November 1977): 114–115.

Gerneroth, S. R. "Stress and Tension Control Lessons as Part of Health Education." *Health Education* 8 (May/June 1977): 20–21.

Golemeir, D., and Schwartz, C. G. "Meditation as an Intervention in Stress Reactivity." *Journal of Consulting and Clinical Psychiatry* 44 (March 1976): 456–466.

Holmes, T. H., and Rahe, R. H. "The Social Readjustment Rating Scale." *Journal of Psychosomatic Research* 11 (1967): 213–218.

Hover, W. "Emotional Stress and How to Respond." *Occupational Health Nursing* 27 (April 1979): 14–16.

Howard, K., and Scott, R. A. "A Proposed Framework for the Analysis of Stress in the Human Organism." *Behavioral Science* 10 (1965): 141–160.

Jacobson, Edmund. *Progressive Relaxation.* Chicago: University of Chicago Press, 1938.

Jones, P. S. "An Adaptation Model for Nursing Practice." *American Journal of Nursing* 78 (November 1978): 1900–1906.

Lazaurus, Richard S. "The Concepts of Stress and Disease." In *Society, Stress, and Disease: The Psychosocial Environment and Psychosomatic Disease,* Lennart, ed. (Oxford: Oxford University Press, 1971): I, 53–58.

Marcinek, M. D. "Stress in the Surgical Patient." *American Journal of Nursing* 77 (November 1977): 1806–1808.

McKay, S. R. "A Review of Student Stress in Nursing Education Programs." *Nursing Forum* 17 (1978): 376–393.

McQuade, W., and Aikman, A. *Stress.* New York: E. P. Dutton, 1974.

Meichenbaum, Donald. "A Self-Instructional Approach to Stress Management." In *Stress and Anxiety,* vol. 1, edited by Sarason and Spielberger. Washington: Hemisphere, 1976.

Pelletier, Kenneth. *Mind as Healer, Mind as Slayer.* New York: Dell, 1977.

Schultz J., and Luthe, W. *Autogenic Training.* New York: Grune & Stratton, 1959.

Selye, Hans. "A Code for Coping with Stress." *AORN Journal* 25 (January 1977): 35–42.

———"Evolution of the Stress Concept." *American Science* 61 (November/December 1973): 692–699.

———. *The Stress of Life.* New York: McGraw-Hill, 1956.

Selye, Hans, *et al.,* "On the Real Benefits of Eustress." *Psychology Today* 11 (March 1978): 60–61.

Shubin, S. "Rx for Stress, Your Stress." *Nursing 79* 9 (January 1979): 52–55.

Sidle, A.; Adams, J.; and Cady, P. "Development of a Coping Scale." *Archives of General Psychiatry* 20 (February 1969): 226–232.

Stephanson, C. A. "The Stress Response: Stress in Critically Ill Patients." *American Journal of Nursing* 77 (November 1977): 1806–1808.

Tamez, E. G., *et al.* "Relaxation Training as a Nursing Intervention Versus Pro Re Nata Medication." *Nursing Research* 27 (May/June 1978): 160–165.

Wallace, R. K. "Physiological Effects of Transcendental Meditation." *Science* 167 (March 27, 1970): 1751–1754.

Wallace, R., and Benson, H. "The Physiology of Meditation." *Scientific American* 226 (October 1972): 84–90.

# Part Four

## Theory and Practice of Nursing

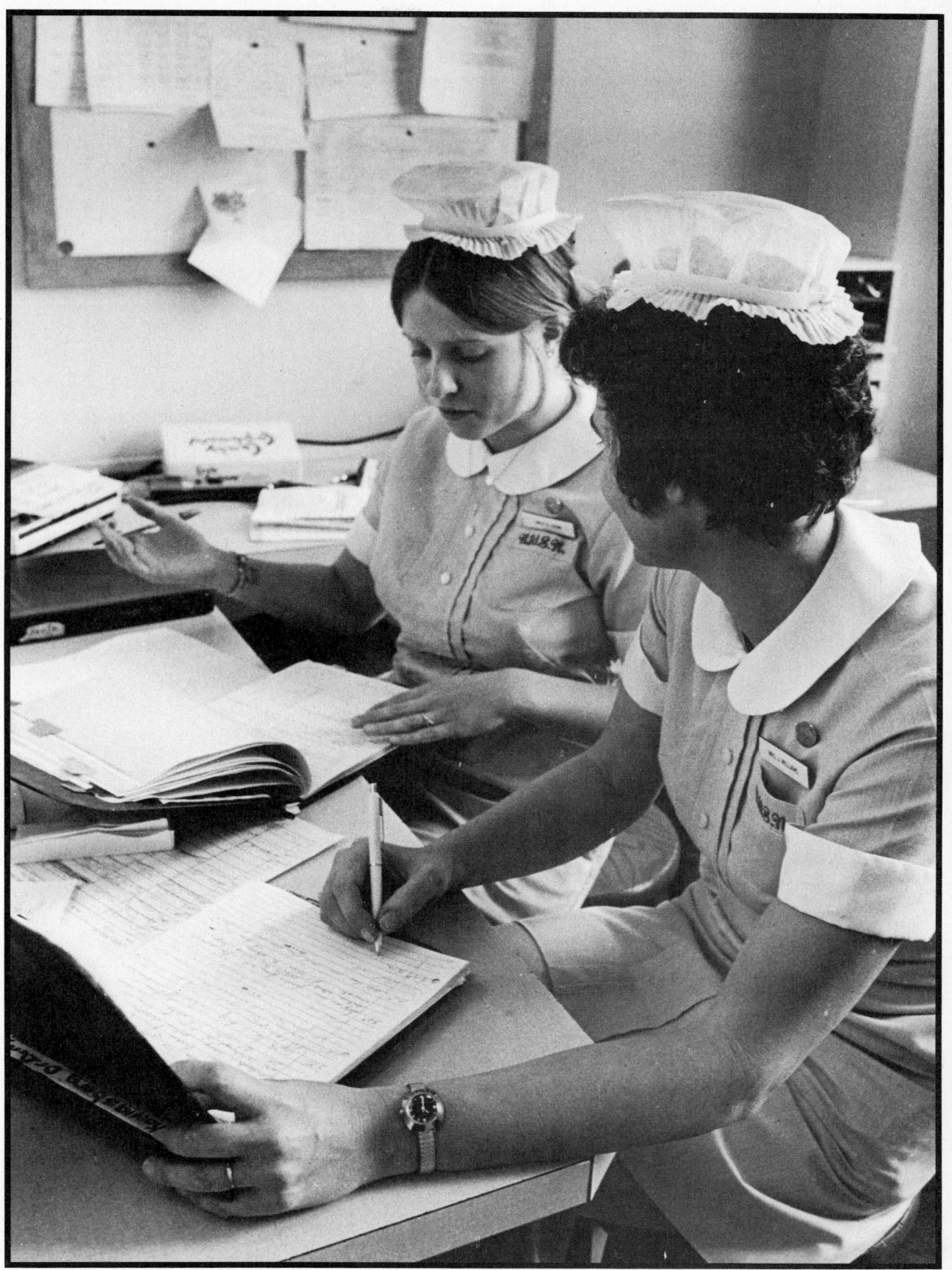

# Chapter 9
# The Nursing Process

## Objectives

After completing this chapter, you should be able to:
1. List the four steps in the nursing process.
2. Discuss how the ANA's Standards of Nursing Practice pertain to the nursing process.
3. Outline the four sources of data on the patient.
4. List three criteria for nursing diagnoses.
5. Explain the five aspects of planning.
6. Discuss implementation as it relates to the nursing process.
7. Describe the use of evaluation to improve the nursing process.

## Outline

Steps in the Nursing Process
Standards of Nursing Practice
Assessment
    Systems of Assessment
    Sources of Assessment Data
        Interview
        Observation
        Physical Examination
        Records
Stating the Problem: The Nursing Diagnosis

Planning
    Goal-Setting
    Collecting Additional Data
    Developing a Plan of Action
    Setting Priorities
    Writing the Plan
Implementation
Evaluating the Results
Care Study: Using the Nursing Process

Only recently did nurses realize that they need a coordinated plan for taking care of each patient. Formerly, each nurse functioned autonomously. As a result, patient care varied from poor to excellent, was often fragmented, and allowed little opportunity for follow-through and evaluation. Since few guidelines existed for planning care, nurses simply did as they had been taught or used trail-and-error to ascertain what should be done.

Today it is generally recognized that the patient receives the best care when a coordinated approach is planned and the results are evaluated. Nursing education consequently emphasizes the *process* of patient care—that is, the method or manner in which the nurse approaches patient care.

## Steps in the Nursing Process

What is the nursing process? What steps ensure completeness and can be applied in a wide variety of nursing situations? Though differences of opinion exist among nurses, most agree that a problem-solving approach is basic to the process. You may find that you have been using a similar approach to problems without labeling or analyzing it. For example, imagine that you will be taking a final examination in a few days. After taking stock of your performance in the class, you decide you need to do well on the test in order to earn the B you want. You then review testable material, what you already know, what references will be useful, and the previous pattern of testing. With all this information in hand, you plan: "I'll review the lecture notes first—that will take an evening. The next day I'll review the text using the lecture outline as a guide. If I have time, I'll review the notes I took on the outside readings." After taking the test, you pat yourself on the back. "I did a great job! I ended up with a B+."

Now reread the above description of your preparation, outlining the steps. There are various ways of analyzing the process, and different people specify different numbers of steps. The following analysis of the process has proven consistently helpful to beginning nursing students and practicing nurses.

First, having assessed your current knowledge, the likely contents of the exam, and your previous performance, you determine that a problem exists: your B grade is in jeopardy. Second, you plan how to solve the problem. In order to do so effectively, you state a concrete and suitable goal—a B in the course. Next you make a precise plan and timetable. Third, you implement your plan, doing exactly what you specified. Fourth, you evaluate the outcome of your activity to determine whether your plan resulted in achievement of your goal (see Figure 9.1).

This, then, is a brief outline of the problem-solving nursing process:

1. Assessment
   a. Collection of information
   b. Statement of the problem
2. Planning
   a. Determination of the goal
   b. Formation of the plan
3. Implementation of the plan
4. Evaluation

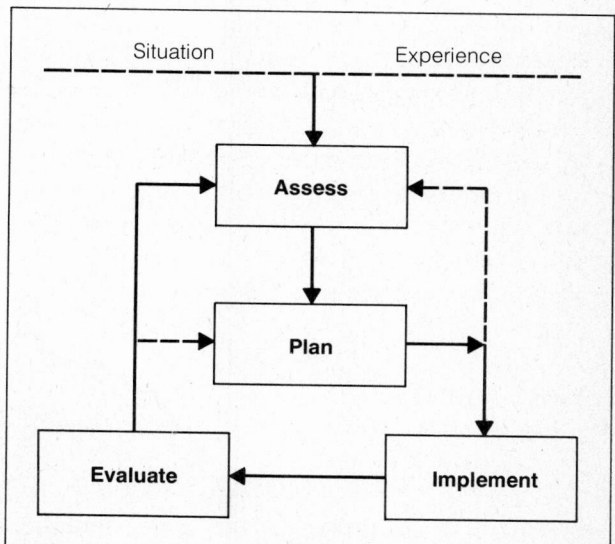

**Figure 9.1   The nursing process**
Courtesy of Nursing Program, Shoreline Community College (Seattle, Washington)

You will notice in Figure 9.1 that in conjunction with the primary direction of flow, there are alternate routes by which the process feeds back into itself. If, during planning, you decide that additional assessment is needed, you can take a detour from the basic direction of flow to return to assessment. If evaluation reveals that additional planning is needed, you may return to that step. New situations and experiences that feed into the process will also have an effect. Thus the nursing process is an ongoing and dynamic approach to nursing care.

## Standards of Nursing Practice

The American Nurses Association has developed standards of nursing care for use as guidelines in evaluating nursing. These standards of practice are based on the nursing-process approach to care (see Exhibit 9.1). They specify, first, that data collection is a basic responsibility of the nurse and that data must be compiled in a usable way. Nursing diagnosis is an outcome of data collection. The standards specify that the plan of care include goals, priorities, and prescribed nursing approaches. Nursing action ought to allow for patient participation and focus on health promotion as well as maintenance and restoration. Evaluation is defined as a means of measuring progress toward the stated goals and, if necessary, redirecting the nursing process.

In addition to the ANA's Standards of Practice, various accrediting bodies are writing criteria for use in evaluating nursing practice. These criteria usually employ the terminology of the nursing process.

If only to comply with standards, then, you need to learn to apply the nursing process. However, there is an even more compelling reason to do so: the nursing process works. You will find that it lends structure to your thought processes, serves as a framework on which to organize information, and guides you to effective action.

Exhibit 9.1
**American Nurses' Association**

Standards of Nursing Practice

**1.** The collection of data about the health status of the client/patient is systematic and continuous. The data are accessible, communicated, and recorded.
**2.** Nursing diagnoses are derived from health status data.
**3.** The plan of nursing care includes goals derived from the nursing diagnoses.
**4.** The plan of nursing care includes priorities and the prescribed nursing approaches or measures to achieve the goals derived from the nursing diagnoses.
**5.** Nursing actions provide for client/patient participation in health promotion, maintenance, and restoration.
**6.** Nursing actions assist the client/patient to maximize his or her health capabilities.
**7.** The client/patient's progress or lack of progress toward goal achievement is determined by the client/patient and the nurse.
**8.** The client/patient's progress or lack of progress toward goal achievement directs reassessment, reordering of priorities, new goal setting, and revision of the plan of nursing care.

Source: American Nurses' Association, Congress for Nursing Practice, Kansas City: ANA, 1973.

## Assessment

Assessment is the process of gathering information and identifying problems. Identification of patients' problems is the foundation of all that the nurse does. It is a skill you will begin developing as a student and never stop refining.

### Systems of Assessment

Many systems and tools for assessing patients have been devised. For many years nurses used Abdellah's "21 Nursing Problems" (1960) as a guide in identifying commonly occurring problems, such as inability to eat and drink normally. Henderson's "Activities of Daily Living" (1966) is a list of activities with which the patient might need help. The list is based on her definition of nursing (see Exhibit 1.1). Dorothy Orem's "Self-Care Concept" (1976) uses identification of deficits in the patient's capacity for self-care as a basis for nursing. Sister Callista Roy's Adaptation Model (1976) defines assessment in terms of identifying effective and ineffective adaptation to stress on the part of the patient.

The conceptual framework with which you approach assessment of the patient is one of the most important aspects of the nursing theory you will learn and use. The theoretical model of patient assessment adopted by your nursing program is part of its total conceptual framework. All such theories have a similar purpose—to provide a systematic and comprehensive framework with which the nurse will be optimally effective at gathering information and identifying the patient's problems.

This book's approach to patient assessment is based on human needs. You will learn to assess patients in light of your understanding of common human needs, such as oxygenation, elimination, and nutrition. The needs that are not being met are the problems with which you will deal. This approach can be adapted and integrated with other approaches (see Module 1, "Assessment").

## Sources of Assessment Data

Whatever conceptual model of assessment one uses, the sources of information are the same.

### Interview

In an interview, one is seeking information that another person possesses. Such information may be sought from the patient, the family, friends, clergy, other health professionals, or anyone else who might have needed data. Interviewing is a complex skill aimed at encouraging another person to talk freely and comprehensively.

The nurse needs to ask the patient/client questions about such matters as appetite, sleep patterns, nausea, pain, fear, dizziness, and the like. The patient's responses constitute subjective data, or information about what he or she sees, hears, feels, and thinks. Such information is essential but should be clearly identified in written records as originating with the patient. Traditionally, subjec-

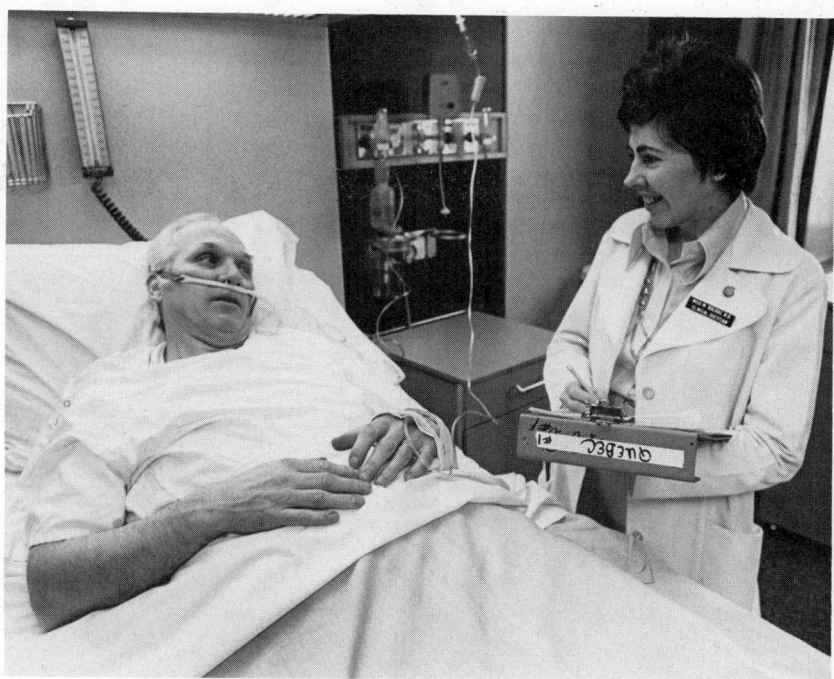

**Figure 9.2**
Making eye contact during the interview encourages the patient to talk freely and comprehensively. (Dan Bernstein)

tive data have simply been called *symptoms*. The term *subjective symptoms*, which clearly identifies their source, is now more commonly used.

In many facilities nursing contact with a patient/ client begins with a *nursing history*. The history is gathered in a planned interview, by asking questions designed to identify commonly occurring patient problems. As a rule, each facility develops its own form, appropriate to the kinds of patients it receives and the services it offers (see Figure 9.3). The nurse who uses such a form should treat it not as an end in itself but as a tool to assist in assessment. Because each patient is an individual with unique problems, the questions you ask may need to vary from those used on the form if you are to discover a given individual's problems.

If you perceive cues to the patient's feelings, they must always be *validated* or checked with the patient to be certain they are correct. For example, the patient, Miss D., appears to be dizzy. You make an objective observation of her stumbling and irregular gait and validate your perception by saying, "You are stumbling. Do you feel dizzy?" By doing so, you solicit subjective information to augment or correct your observation. It may be, for example, that Miss D. merely misplaced her glasses.

A good interviewer is constantly alert, watching and listening carefully for unintentional cues as well as overt statements. Interviewing will be discussed more fully in Chapter 12.

## Observation

Information gathered through observation that can be seen and verified by another person is termed *objective data* or *signs*. General observations about the patient's appearance, stance, facial expressions, and behavior ought to be stated in clearly descriptive language. For example, the notation "appears depressed" is the observer's conclusion, not an objective description. Appropriate descriptive statements might include, for example, "stooped posture," "tears in eyes," and "little facial expression while talking." You should attempt to gather objective data pertinent to the subjective symptoms the patient reports. Table 9.1 lists an assortment of common subjective symptoms and corresponding objective signs.

Table 9.1
**Subjective vs. Objective Data**

| Subjective data (symptoms) | Objective data (signs) |
| --- | --- |
| Heart palpitations | Rapid pulse |
| Feeling of warmth | Elevated temperature |
| Dizziness | Stumbling gait |
| Burning on urination | Cloudy urine |
| Nausea | Emesis |
| Apprehension | Trembling |
| Pain | Wincing on movement |

## Physical Examination

Observation also includes physical examination of the patient. In some settings, nurses perform complete diagnostic physical examinations; this is an advanced skill. However, all nurses must be able to do basic physical examinations. You will first learn to measure blood pressure, temperature, pulse, and respiration. Eventually you will progress to listening to lungs and bowels (auscultation); examining the skin; checking dressings, drainage tubings, and intravenous infusions (inspection); examining body parts by touch (palpation); tapping to identify differences in sound conduction (percussion), and the like (see Modules 20, 21, 23, and 32).

As you observe and listen attentively to what the patient tells you, you must constantly relate the resulting information to your knowledge of such basic sciences as anatomy, physiology, pathology, sociology, and psychology. You will also increasingly relate your observations to your knowledge of nursing theory and practice and gradually become better able to discern when needs are unmet and basic homeostasis is disturbed.

As a beginning practitioner, your skill at observing may develop more rapidly than your understanding of the meaning of your observations. For this reason, you will be communicating your observations and information to other members of the health-care team who can determine their significance. But do not lose sight of your objective, which is to be able to interpret the significance of what you observe. When you have become a registered nurse, nursing assistants, and student

**INITIAL PATIENT INTERVIEW – 3 SOUTH**

Reason for hospitalization  *To have gallbladder surgery.*

Symptoms  *Indigestion -*
*Gall bladder attack 2 mo. ago - really sick - R U Q pain - stabbing*  *Nausea, vomiting,*

**HISTORY**

Infections  *None serious*

Diabetes  *No*
.how long

Heart  *No problems*

Hypertension  *No*

Peripheral
  Vascular disease  *No*

Respiratory  *Usual colds occassionally*
*Seasonal hayfever in May.*
Other problems or illnesses

Previous use of steroids  *None*

G.U.  *No voiding difficulties.*
*Has had 2 bladder infections*
G.B.  *Last one 18 mo. ago,*
  *↳ See above*

G.I.
  constipation ⎫ *No problems*
  diarrhea     ⎭

Special diet
  food allergies  *None*

Tobacco      amt.
Alcohol  ✓ amt.  *occassional wine with*
*dinner and cocktail*
Prior hospitalizations
  *For delivery of babies x 3*
Current meds.
  *Birth control pills - Ortho - Novum*

**BALLARD COMMUNITY HOSPITAL**
SEATTLE, WASHINGTON

**PHYSICAL**
**CIRCULATORY**
Pulse AP  *84*  R  *24*
Rhythm  *regular*
Pedal pulse  *palpable - both feet*
Edema  *none*
Homan's sign  *Neg.*
Calf tenderness  *None*

**RESPIRATORY**
Lung sounds  *Clear*
Dyspnea  *None*
Cough  *None*
Sputum  *None*

**DERMATOLOGY**
Color  *Warm tones - black*
Condition  *Smooth, hydrated, intact*
Lacerations  *None*
Bruises  *1 large on R shin*
Decubiti

**C.N.S.**
Level of
  consciousness  *Alert + oriented*
Pain  *None currently - G.B. pain*
  location  *R U Q*
  type  *stabbing*
  precipitated  *Eating fatty foods*
  by

**G.I.**
Bowel sounds  *Active in all quadrants*
Distention  *No*
Abd. Soft  ✓
  Firm
Palpitation  *No masses*
  tenderness  *None*

**G.U.**
Any problems vd.  *No*
Frequency  *None*
Pain  *No*
Incontinence  *No*
Catheter  *No*
  date inserted

**MUSC. – SKEL.**
Fractures  *None*
Deformities  *none*
Arthritis  *None*
Ambulatory  *Yes*
  Needs assist.  *No*

**PSY. – SOC.**
Anxiety  *Expresses concern re surgery*
Introduce to
  roommates
  and unit  ✓
Pre-op
  teaching  *Begun - See Progress Notes*
Able to Verbalize

**DISCHARGE PLANNING**
Home responsibilities?  *3 children ages 5, 7, & 10.*
Do you live alone?  *No - husband  works parttime as secretary*
Someone to help after discharge?  *for a few days after discharge, Children "very helpful."*
Admitted from SNF or protected care?  *No*

Pre-op teaching  *yes*

Sign  *A. Roberts R.N.*

*Gould, Vera*
*402 - 876 - 935*
*Age 36*
*Dr. O. Lowe*

I 180A  Rev. 10/79

**Figure 9.3  Nursing history interview**
Courtesy Ballard Community Hospital (Seattle, Washington)

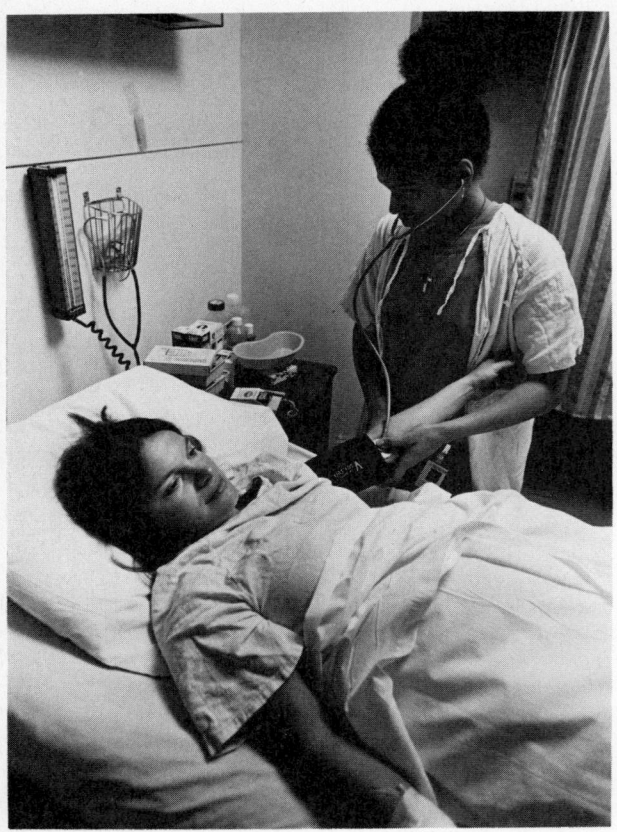

nurses will bring their initial observations to you, and you will be responsible for determining their significance.

## Records

The patient's written record or chart contains information gathered by the physician, laboratory data, and assessments by other members of the health-care team. This information will become increasingly important to you as you learn to interpret its significance.

There may be other written records of potential value to you. These may include a card index (Kardex) used for quick reference to current physician's orders and plans for care, the nursing care plan containing data relevant to care, and any other checklists and forms maintained by the nursing staff.

**Figure 9.4**
Nurses gather information through direct examination of the patient. (Gabor Demjen/Stock, Boston)

## Stating the Problem: The Nursing Diagnosis

*Stating the problem* is so important that some people treat it as a separate step in the nursing process. Some nurses use the term *assessment* to mean only the collection of data, while others use it to refer only to the statement of the problem (Weed, 1969). The terms *nursing diagnosis* and *analysis of data* are also used to refer to the statement of the problem. Historically, nursing has used the term *assessment* to encompass both collection and interpretation of information and statement of the problem; we shall use it that way as well. *Statement of the problem* here is treated as interchangeable with *nursing diagnosis*.

At the current time, nursing diagnoses are not stated uniformly. This lack of uniformity stems from differences in theoretical approach to patient

care and from differing opinions about the usefulness of various ways of stating diagnoses. One such difference involves level of specificity. Some nurses believe that stating the nursing diagnosis in concrete and specific terms facilitates planning. Others believe that stating the diagnosis in narrow terms tends to increase compartmentalization of the patient's care and to interfere with identification of broad syndromes that can be treated as single entities. Instead, they state nursing diagnoses as broad problem areas.

Nurses also differ on the desirability of striving for uniform terminology. The National Group on Classification of Nursing Diagnosis, a group of nursing theorists, is working toward consensus on the terminology of nursing diagnoses in the belief

## Exhibit 9.2
## Accepted Nursing Diagnoses

Anxiety
Body fluids, alteration in
Bowel elimination,
    alteration in
Cardiac output, alteration
    in
Comfort, alterations in
Consciousness, altered
    levels of
Coping patterns,
    maladaptive (individual)
Coping, ineffective family
Digestion, impairment of
Family process,
    inadequate
Fear
Fluid volume deficit
Grieving
Home maintenance
    management, impaired
Injury, potential for
Knowledge, lack of
    (specify)
Manipulation
Mobility, impairment of
Noncompliance (specify)
Nutritional alteration

Parenting, alterations in
Respiratory dysfunction
Role disturbance
Self-care activities,
    alterations in
Self-concept, alterations in
Sensory-perceptual
    alteration
Sexuality, alteration in
    patterns of
Skin integrity, impairment
    of
Sleep-rest activity,
    dysrhythm of
Spirituality, matter of
Social isolation
Suffocation, potential for
Thought processes,
    impaired
Tissue perfusion, chronic
    abnormal
Trauma, potential for
Urinary elimination,
    impairment of
Verbal communication,
    impairment of

Source: National Group on Classification of Nursing Diagnoses, Conferences on Nursing Diagnosis, St. Louis, Missouri, 1973, 1975, 1978.

that the progress of nursing as a science and profession will be facilitated by use of a uniform language. Exhibit 9.2 lists the nursing diagnoses that have been approved by the National Group on Classification of Nursing Diagnoses.

In a very significant book, *Nursing Diagnosis and Intervention* (1978), Claire Campbell outlines a comprehensive system for stating nursing problems. She offers diagnostic statements, the data needed to identify them, and related nursing actions. The present text provides examples of nursing diagnoses to facilitate your ability to understand and state them.

The following three criteria will help you write nursing diagnoses that are clear and understandable to others:

**1.** A nursing diagnosis is a statement of a given patient's actual or potential health problem, and its language should reflect the focus on the patient.

**2.** A nursing diagnosis is a health problem that the nurse is competent to identify and treat by virtue of education and experience.

**3.** Whenever possible, a nursing diagnosis specifies the *etiology* (cause or source) of the problem. In fact, some theorists argue that a statement that does not specify etiology is not a full-fledged nursing diagnosis but only a patient problem.

Such modifiers as *acute, chronic,* and *potential* may be used but are not essential.

A nursing diagnosis related to an open bedsore on a patient's coccyx might be stated in such very specific terms as "decubitus ulcer on coccyx due to immobility." Using the National Conference Group terminology, the statement would read, "impairment of skin integrity; etiology: immobility." Whichever way it is written, this nursing diagnosis identifies an actual health problem of the individual (Criterion 1) and specifies its cause (Criterion 3). The nurse has the education and ability to plan care to relieve this problem (Criterion 2).

The nursing diagnosis related to difficulties in swallowing solids after a cerebral-vascular accident (stroke) might be stated specifically as "unable to swallow solids due to loss of motor nerve control." Using National Conference Group terminology, the diagnosis might be stated as "nutritional alteration, swallowing difficulty; etiology: impaired motor nerve control." This nursing diagnosis identifies a normal ability that the individual lacks (Criterion 1), specifies its etiology (Criterion 3), and the nurse can plan care to alleviate this problem (Criterion 2).

Note that in keeping with Criterion 1, the nursing diagnosis focuses on the patient's health problem, not the nurse's action or the difficulties the nurse encounters in providing care. Specifying the cause (Criterion 3) promotes planning appropriate and specific to the individual's needs. For example, "nutritional alteration, anorexia; etiology: excessive fatigue" requires different planning than would "nutritional alteration, anorexia; etiology: odor of wound drainage." Of course, if the etiology is not currently known, it is appropriate to so indicate ("etiology: unknown").

# Planning

Planning is a complex process with several components: setting goals, gathering additional data, developing a plan, setting priorities, and writing the plan. Let us consider each step in turn.

## Goal-Setting

The first step in planning is to specify the goal. This step is often omitted because it seems to overlap with the statement of the problem, but the problem exists in the present, while the goal is the hoped-for future outcome. At first glance, a goal may be interpreted as a statement of what is optimal, since that is what you hope for. However, skill in nursing requires that the goal be realistic and achievable by the patient—neither so low as to underestimate the patient's potential nor so high as to be unobtainable. This is often a fine line to tread.

It is important that patients be involved in setting their own goals and that they see such goals as appropriate. They will thus participate in their own care to the fullest extent possible. Patients very often enter a health-care setting with predetermined goals, which may or may not accord with those of health-care personnel. It is the nurse's responsibility to find out the patient's goals, communicate the goals the nurse sees as appropriate, and negotiate with the patient a set of goals toward which all can work together.

Goals are stated as *patient outcomes*. In some facilities the term *outcome criteria* is used to refer to specific patient goals. This terminology emphasizes a focus on the desired result for the patient, not on nursing activities themselves. To be most valuable in subsequent steps of the nursing process, goals should consist of statements that are descriptive, measurable, and/or comparable. A goal is also more useful if it includes a deadline when the goal is expected to be reached. For example, a goal for a patient who is not drinking sufficient fluids might be "drinks 3,000 ml. of fluid per day by 8/7/80."

Although long-term goals are valuable for providing overall direction to your planning, they can contribute to frustration on the part of the patient and the care giver alike when progress is slow. In such situations, short-term or intermediate goals are very helpful. A short-term goal might involve only one day or a few days. Student nurses usually feel a greater sense of accomplishment when they set short-term goals and can see the results of their own care rather than merely helping to work toward long-term goals whose attainment they may not be present to see. An example of a short-term goal for the patient described above might be "drinks 500 ml. of fluid during 7–12 a.m. time period today."

Overall goals are sometimes specified for patients with multiple problems. Such goals are often not limited to the nursing diagnosis, encompassing instead the patient's underlying condition and prognosis. Physicians, nurses, and other health-care team members usually collaborate on overall goals, which focus on the expected end of care without giving an exact time for achieving that goal. Examples of overall goals include "a comfortable and pain-free death," "return to self-care within an institutional setting," and "return to self-care and independent living." Overall goals are never substitutes for the specific goals (outcome criteria) written in response to specific nursing diagnoses.

## Collecting Additional Data

At this point in the nursing process, you will have collected some data that will be useful as you plan nursing action. But, before acting, it is essential that more data be obtained on the specific problem in question. Such data generally fall into two broad classes. The first is objective and subjective data about the patient, acquired from observation, interview, and the patient's record. The second type of information is derived from references, resources, and general knowledge, and forms the *rationale*, or reason, for your action. Some practitioners use the term *facts and principles* when discussing the rationale for nursing action. A nursing principle is most often defined as two or more

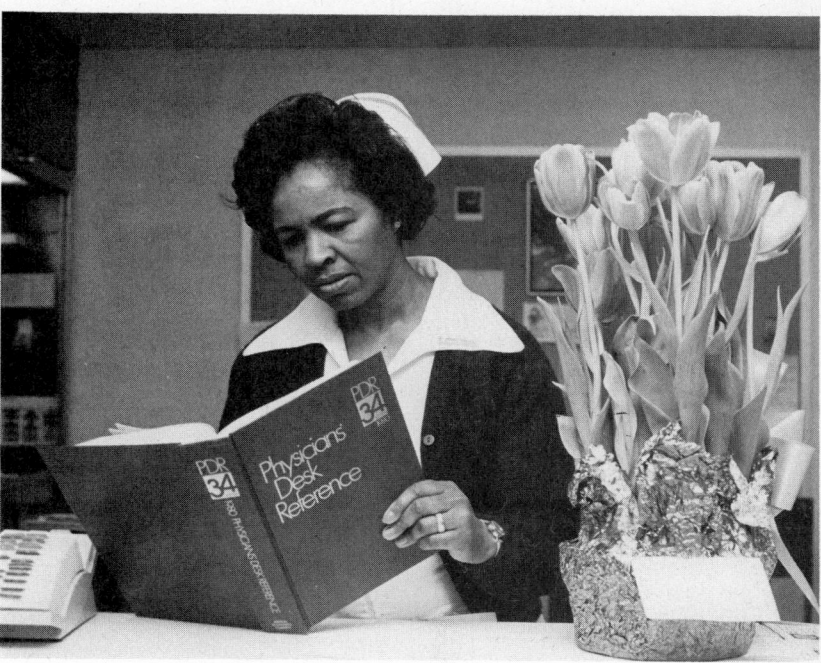

**Figure 9.5**
Nurses must often consult references when planning care. (Russ Kinne/Danbury Hospital/Photo Researchers, Inc.)

facts related by cause-and-effect that directly suggest a given nursing action. We prefer the term *rationale,* which is somewhat broader and encompasses a wide variety of facts, principles, and other information that can be considered together as a basis for action. The very skilled practitioner may carry much of this knowledge in memory. But for the beginning practitioner and the skilled practitioner confronting new or unusual problems, it will be necessary to consult books and periodicals. For example, an experienced nurse faced with a decubitus ulcer due to immobility would know the nursing actions likely to resolve this problem. As a beginning student, you might need to spend some time with your texts in order to identify appropriate nursing actions. Nursing has moved far beyond the era when it was considered necessary only to do and not to think.

## Developing a Plan of Action

After you have set a goal and gathered the information, it is time to construct a plan for action. At this point you will weigh all your data to decide what is relevant and what is not. You will be relating the theory, facts, and principles you have gathered to what you know about this particular patient.

All possible actions must be judged by a variety of criteria. The first, of course, is "Will it work?" Does this action have the potential for solving this problem? The second is "Are the necessary resources available?" Resources are both people and material. If any necessary resource is missing, the proposed action cannot be performed. For example, if there are too few people on duty to move a very obese person to a chair, that action is impractical; if the facility does not have alternating-pressure mattresses, you ought not to plan to use one. The third criterion is acceptability to the patient. It is necessary to consult the patient on the proposed action, interpreting it if necessary and enlisting cooperation.

## Setting Priorities

Setting priorities involves determining which of several problems is the most critical or most in need of attention. When addressing a single problem, the various actions that are planned also need to be given priorities. Questions that might help you set priorities are "If only one of these problems could be attended to today, which would it be?" and "If I had time to perform only one action in response to this problem, which would it be?"

## Writing the Plan

A written plan of action is most effective when each part clearly relates in terms of sequence and timing to every other part (see Figure 14.2). Steps that must be followed in sequence or that depend on the completion of a prior task should be listed in the appropriate order. The degree of detail that is specified depends on who is expected to perform the action—you yourself, nursing assistants, registered nurses, or a variety of other providers.

However detailed the description, the actions outlined are more likely to be performed consistently if a timetable is included. For example, "good skin care" may be interpreted differently by different people, but "turn and rub back q2h (every two hours)—even hours" is unlikely to be misinterpreted or ignored. Your plan might also include checklists or other record-keeping devices to assist those giving care. The card index (Kardex) commonly used in many institutions is a practical device for recording a plan for nursing action.

# Implementation

In order to achieve the goal, the nurse must next perform or delegate performance of the specified actions. Assignment of tasks is not a minor matter, for the nurse must decide on the skills required by the proposed task and by the patient's needs. Even a task that requires elementary skills, such as feeding a patient, might need to be performed by the registered nurse if knowledgeable attention to the patient's respiratory status and fatigue level is required during the feeding process.

It is very important for the person who performs the nursing action to be skillful at it. Skill and confidence in the performance of tasks enhance the patient's trust in the provider of care and thus alleviate anxiety and insecurity. By the same token, hesitancy, clumsiness, and carelessness can arouse such feelings where they did not previously exist.

The actions taken and the patient's response to them must next be recorded and/or communicated orally for the benefit of others on the health-care team.

# Evaluating the Results

Though generally regarded as an essential component of nursing practice, evaluation of nursing care often receives little time and attention. Evaluation is frequently limited to asking whether or not a given action was performed. Other questions that ought to be answered address the result observed in the patient, whether the problem was solved, whether the goal was attained, and whether patient satisfaction was achieved.

If the problem and the goal were originally stated precisely and in detail, evaluation is a relatively easy task. For example, if the problem was that the patient ate too little to provide for healing,

and the goal was for the patient to eat half the food served on the meal tray, it is enough to state "Yes, this was accomplished, the problem is solved, and the plan was a success" or "No, this was not accomplished; therefore the plan was unsuccessful." This is evaluation at its simplest. The criterion—the standard for judging success or failure—is merely success or failure at attaining the goal.

If the problem and the goal were originally stated in general terms, the first step in evaluation is to review criteria. For example, if the goal in the above case was simply for the patient to "eat more" or "eat enough," a decision would have to be made about what constitutes "more" or "enough." Only after a criterion is established can one determine whether it has been met.

Written records facilitate evaluation, since care is typically provided by different nursing personnel at different times. If actions and results are recorded, and if there is a record of the goal and/or criteria being used to measure results, evaluation could be undertaken by someone other than the nurse who made the plan.

More complex evaluation involves subtler questions and determinations. Often the degree of progress made toward the goal must be estimated. If the patient has made progress, the nurse must try to determine whether that progress resulted from the action taken. If so, the nurse must then consider whether the action should be continued or whether the patient would benefit more from a reconsideration of the plan.

So far discussion has focused exclusively on the nurse's evaluation, but the patient's evaluation of care is equally important. Patients need to be encouraged to examine their goals and their progress. The patient's opinion of care should be actively sought. If care is producing the desired result but is not being delivered in an acceptable manner, the patient can very readily evaluate it.

At its simplest, then, evaluation is simply asking whether the criteria have been met and the goal achieved, and answering "yes" or "no." In its more complex form, evaluation requires that the nurse be able to distinguish degrees of progress toward the goal and to identify the reason or reasons for such progress. The patient ought to be involved in the entire evaluation process, and especially in determining the appropriateness of the method of delivering care.

The purpose of evaluation is to enable you to continue the nursing process. If evaluation reveals that your actions are unsuccessful, you must begin again to examine the problem. Your initial definition of the problem may have been inappropriate, or you may have failed to validate your information with the patient. If you acted before collecting sufficient data, the action may have been inappropriate. If so, you repeat the entire process. If evaluation then shows that you were successful, you may proceed to another problem.

## Conclusion

The nursing process outlined in this chapter can be adapted to a wide variety of nursing situations. It may be long and painstaking or it may be performed quickly in an emergency. Wherever you encounter a patient/client—in the hospital, in the outpatient clinic, in the emergency room, or in the mental health center—the nursing process will enable you to determine his or her problems. Only when problems are clearly defined is it possible to begin solving them. Because patients seldom have only one problem, the process will be continuous.

## Care Study  Using the nursing process

Mrs. Sarah Davenport is an eighty-two-year-old widow admitted to the hospital because of severe weight loss. The nurse assigned to care for Mrs. Davenport interviews her, using the unit's nursing-care history form, and makes careful observations as she assists the patient to bed.

Among the nurse's observations are the following:

**1.** Mrs. Davenport's skin is thin and transparent and feels dry.
**2.** All bony prominences are very pronounced, and the skin over them appears taut (stretched).
**3.** There is a reddened area over each elbow.
**4.** Mrs. Davenport stated she "feels tired" and "can scarcely move."

The nurse determines that Mrs. Davenport has beginning skin breakdown over the elbows and might easily incur further skin breakdown. On the nursing care plan she writes, "Beginning skin breakdown over both elbows. Potential skin breakdown over all bony prominences, due to fragile skin and friction on sheets."

The nurse decides that an appropriate goal is "skin over all bony prominences clear and intact with no persisting redness within five days." She then specifies the date on five days hence so there is no question as to when she expects the goal will be reached.

The nurse reviews what she knows about prevention and treatment of skin breakdown. She reads the patient's chart to learn what activity and diet have been ordered. She spends time talking to Mrs. Davenport about her ac-

tivity at home, her eating habits, and her concerns about care. She also checks on the equipment currently available for this patient. As the nurse collects all these data, she sorts out their relevance to Mrs. Davenport's problem. The nurse then formulates the following plan:

**1.** Put foam-rubber "topper" over mattress.
**2.** Use cornstarch on sheets at point of contact with elbows to reduce friction. Replace p.r.n. at least q4h (9-1-5 and so on).
**3.** Help patient change position q2h, odd hours (9-11-1 and so on).
**4.** Visit patient during meals and when nourishment is served to encourage the intake of high-protein, high-calorie foods.

The nurse asks the orderly to get the foam "topper" and, with the assistance of the nurse's aide, to put it on the bed. She gets the cornstarch herself and goes to the patient's bedside to explain what she is going to do and to apply it.

At the end of the fifth day of hospitalization, the nurse reviews all the patient's current problems. She checks Mrs. Davenport's skin during her morning rounds. Her evaluation is charted: "Redness on elbows gone; skin still appears dry and taut; no skin breakdown apparent on any other bony prominences." Reviewing what has been done, the nurse decides that the plan has been generally successful and should be continued, but that something more needs to be done about the dry skin.

## Learning Activities

**1.** Choose a simple patient problem. Write a paper outlining a nursing-process approach to the problem.
**2.** Review the nurse's record on a patient for a twenty-four hour period. Make one list of the subjective data and another of the objective data recorded.
**3.** Obtain a copy of a nursing care plan from your facility. Analyze the plan in light of the criteria given in this chapter. Rewrite the nursing care plan to make it conform to the criteria if it does not.
**4.** Find out who is responsible for writing the initial nursing care plan in your facility. Who is re-

sponsible for updating that care plan during the patient's stay? Discuss with your instructor how you as a student nurse can fit into this ongoing process.

## Study Terms

| | |
|---|---|
| assessment | nursing diagnosis |
| criterion | nursing history |
| data collection | nursing process |
| evaluation | objective data |
| etiology | observation |
| implementation | outcome criteria |
| interviewing | patient outcomes |
| nursing care plan | planning |

principle
priority
problem-solving
    approach
rationale

sign
subjective symptom
symptom
validation

## Relevant Sections in
## Modules for Basic Nursing Skills

| Volume 1 | Module |
|----------|--------|
| Assessment | 1 |

## References

Abdellah, Fay G., *et al. Patient-Centered Approaches to Nursing.* New York: Macmillan, 1960.

Baer, E. D., *et al.* "How to Take a Health History." *American Journal of Nursing* 77 (July 1977): 1190.

Bailit, H., *et al.* "Assessing the Quality of Care." *Nursing Outlook* 23 (March 1975): 153–159.

Barba, M., *et al.* "The Evaluation of Patient Care Through Use of ANA's Standards of Nursing Practice." *Supervisor Nurse* 9 (January 1978): 42.

Berg, H. V. "Nursing Audit and Outcome Criteria." *Nursing Clinics of North America* (June 1974): 331.

Campbell, Claire. *Nursing Diagnosis and Intervention.* New York: John Wiley & Sons, 1978.

Gebbie, Kristine, and Lavin, Mary Ann, eds. *Classification of Nursing Diagnoses.* St. Louis: C. V. Mosby, 1975.

———. "Classifying Nursing Diagnoses." *American Journal of Nursing* 74 (February 1974): 250.

Henderson, V. *The Nature of Nursing.* New York: Macmillan, 1966, pp. 15–16.

House, M. J. "Devising a Care Plan You Can Really Use." *Nursing '75* 5 (July 1975): 1214.

Jarvis, C. M. "Perfecting Physical Assessment: Part 1." *Nursing '77* 7 (May 1977): 28.

———. "Perfecting Physical Assessment: Part 2." *Nursing '77* 7 (June 1977): 38.

Orem, Dorothy E. *Nursing: Concepts of Practice,* 2nd ed. New York: McGraw Hill, 1980.

Roy, Sister Callistra. *Introduction to Nursing: An Adaptation Model.* Englewood Cliffs, N.J.: Prentice-Hall, 1976.

Smith, D. M. "Writing Objectives as a Nursing Practice Skill." *American Journal of Nursing* 71 (February 1971): 319.

Weed, L. L. *Medical Records: Medical Education and Patient Care.* Cleveland: Case Western Reserve University Press, 1969.

Wolff, H., and Erickson, R. "The Assessment Man." *Nursing Outlook* 25 (February 1977): 103.

# Chapter 10
# Direct-Care Skills

## Objectives

After completing this chapter, you should be able to:
1. Discuss the relationship between proficiency in skills and a trust relationship with a patient.
2. Name the primary factors involved in protecting the physical safety of the hospitalized patient.
3. Outline the nurse's responsibility with regard to procedures.
4. Identify the sources of information you need to explain diagnostic and treatment procedures to patients.
5. List the steps in performing any procedure or treatment.
6. Articulate the nurse's responsibility with regard to administering medications.

## Outline

The Nurse's Role in Direct-Care Skills
   Knowledge
   Technical Skill
   Using the Nursing Process
Procedural Checklist
   1. Check the Order
   2. Review the Procedure
   3. Gather the Equipment
   4. Prepare the Patient Psychologically
   5. Prepare the Patient Physically
   6. Perform the Procedure
   7. Evaluate the Results
   8. Make the Patient Comfortable
   9. Care for the Equipment and the Specimen
   10. Record the Data
Assisting with Diagnostic Tests and Procedures

Physical Safety
   Environmental Assessment
   Falls
   Electrical Hazards
   Burns
   Fire
      Reporting Fires
      Fighting Fires
      Evacuation
Administering Drug Therapy
   Knowledge of Drugs
   Knowledge of the Patient's Condition
   The Nurse's Responsibilities
   Routes of Administration
   The Five Rights
   Medication Errors
Care Study: Assisting with a Physical Therapy Treatment

The popular image of a nurse is a person who performs skilled tasks for ill patients. Though this is a limited view of nursing, direct-care skills are an essential component of nursing. Direct-care skills include routine physical tasks performed for the patient, such as bathing, moving, and feeding, as well as such specialized diagnostic and treatment procedures as injections, catheterizations, and dressing changes.

Providing direct care in a skillful and caring way based on sound knowledge enhances the patient's well-being and promotes trust between nurse and patient. The patient who is convinced that his or her care provider is both knowledgeable and skill-ful will be able to relax and focus energy on the central task of regaining health.

Another important outcome of skillful direct care is the therapeutic effect of touch. Nurses have long believed that the touch of caring hands can make a difference in a patient's well-being, but this conviction was unsupported by scientific evidence. Research into the therapeutic effectiveness of touch (Kreiger, 1978) and the role of stress and other psychological states in illness (see Chapter 8) suggests that direct care has extraordinary potential for promoting return to health and well-being.

## The Nurse's Role in Direct-Care Skills

Some direct-care skills are exercised at the discretion of the nurse. These include facilitating all the activities the patient would perform independently if he or she had the necessary "strength, will, or ability" (see Henderson's definition of nursing in Chapter 1), such as bathing, turning, and moving. Throughout this text we will point out circumstances in which nurses may exercise independent judgment with regard to direct-care skills. Other skills, such as giving medications and inserting catheters, are employed only after consultation with the physician. Whether a skill is performed independently or in response to a physician's order, the nurse's responsibilities are considerable.

### Knowledge

First, the nurse is always responsible for personal knowledge of the skill to be performed. You will acquire basic knowledge as a nursing student, but the nurse's knowledge base is growing so rapidly that as a graduate you will inevitably find more and more procedures added to your list of responsibilities. Thus you will need to pursue continuing education to learn new skills, review previously acquired skills, and take advantage of opportunities to learn from nursing colleagues. It is very important to decline to perform skills for which you are not prepared. Even as a student, you must take responsibility for recognizing the limits of your ability and working within them.

Your knowledge must include understanding the reasons why a skill is performed and the desired outcome. You must be familiar with the equipment involved so that you can obtain and use it correctly. You must know how to perform the procedure and what must be done to ensure the patient's safety. To facilitate your teaching of the patient, you will need to know the response expected from the patient. The primary sources of such knowledge are textbooks, professional journals, and continuing education classes.

### Technical Skill

You will need to practice new skills repeatedly until you can perform them with ease. Doing so assures that you can concentrate on the patient, not the equipment, during the procedure. Practice is also necessary to maintain your proficiency at skills you have already acquired but use only occasionally. You will need to ask for supervision when learning new skills, so as to ensure the safety of the patient. Technical skill allows for the procedure to be accomplished quickly, causing the patient less fatigue. Technical skill certainly assuages the patient's anxiety and may also minimize discomfort.

## Using the Nursing Process

Before beginning a procedure and throughout the performance of it, you should be using your assessment skills to gather data and identify problems.

Planning is necessary before you begin in order to proceed in an organized manner. You may also wish to facilitate the planning of future procedures by noting helpful ways to do things. Planning should include setting goals (though they may be very simple) as well as identifying the equipment needed and thinking through the procedure.

Implementation—performance of the procedure itself—is the only part of the process clearly visible to the patient. Often the entire process will be judged by the patient on the basis of implementation alone.

You must always evaluate the effects of any procedure you perform. Was it effective? What was the patient's response? How could I have performed better?

# Procedural Checklist

The checklist that follows lists the ten essential steps in any procedure (see Exhibit 10.1). Some steps involve assessment, some planning, some implementation, and one evaluation. The steps are listed in typical chronological order. However, their order may need to be changed to suit a specific situation. For example, assessment and planning often proceed simultaneously, and assessment typically continues during implementation. Similarly, when a patient must be given time to decide whether or not to consent to a procedure, psychological preparation would precede gathering of the equipment.

Exhibit 10.1
**Procedural Checklist**

1. Check the order.
2. Review the procedure.
3. Gather the equipment.
4. Prepare the patient psychologically.
5. Prepare the patient physically.
6. Perform the procedure.
7. Evaluate the results.
8. Make the patient comfortable.
9. Care for the equipment and the specimen.
10. Record the data.

## 1. Check the Order

If the treatment or procedure requires an order, the order must be checked, verified, and transcribed accurately. Whether the procedure is ordered or independently initiated, you must verify that it is not contraindicated by other orders or by the patient's condition. A *contraindication* is evidence that the treatment or procedure contemplated could cause an adverse response in the particular patient in question. Contraindications are, however, not absolutes. For example, sedatives are contraindicated for patients with severe liver disease because the liver may be unable to metabolize the drug. Nevertheless, a physician may order a sedative for a person with liver disease if the hoped-for benefit outweighs the potential risk. When contraindications are present, you should consult with the physician to clarify the appropriate action and your own responsibilities for careful assessment in order to recognize any problems that arise.

## 2. Review the Procedure

Treatments you perform often will be familiar to you and easily recalled. Any procedure with which you are unfamiliar can be checked out in a procedure book or reference text. Sometimes it is necessary to consult a more experienced nurse to learn the details of a procedure. When a procedure has not been established, you can often design an appropriate one on the basis of the treatment's purpose and your background knowledge of the sciences and nursing theory. If you move to a new area of the country or even to another hospital in the same city, you may find that procedures are performed differently. Review the new procedure in light of the basic principles of care. If these principles are observed, minor variations in procedure are not significant. For example, some facilities use prepackaged disposable sets for changing dressings, which contain some instruments and sterile gloves; others do not use prepackaged materials, and the nurse has to determine what items are needed and arrange to provide them. It is possible to perform a dressing change with excellent sterile technique by both methods.

## 3. Gather the Equipment

Many procedures are now performed with prepackaged disposable equipment, which saves a great deal of time formerly spent gathering supplies. It is important to recognize that sets of equipment differ, and you should study their labels to determine exactly what is contained and what is not. For example, some urinary catheterization sets contain all the equipment necessary for the procedure, including the catheter and the drainage bag. Other sets contain everything except these items. In addition to the prepackaged set, you may need a sheet for draping the patient, a light, and a pencil and paper on which to make notations.

When no prepackaged set is available, the task is more complex. While reviewing the procedure, you might note the equipment needed for each step so that you remember to provide it. The *Modules for Basic Nursing Skills* list the equipment needed for each procedure.

The major reason for organizing equipment ahead of time is to minimize the patient's anxiety. Making numerous trips for forgotten equipment is distressing to the patient and erodes confidence in your ability to perform the procedure correctly.

Organizing your work also saves you steps, prevents fatigue, and enables you to accomplish more in the same amount of time.

## 4. Prepare the Patient Psychologically

People are better able to handle a stressful situation if they have some knowledge and understanding of it. Therefore, you will want to explain to the patient exactly what is to be done. The details you provide should be those needed by the patient and unlikely to arouse undue alarm. Thus patients having bladder irrigations should be told that they may experience some pressure during the procedure. They need not be told all about the sterile technique you will use or the possible adverse consequences of improper techniques. If pain is likely to occur, the patient is usually less frightened if told that discomfort is expected at a certain point in the procedure. Otherwise he or she might fear that something is seriously wrong. On the other hand, a description of the extent and severity of the discomfort might only increase anxiety. Of course, patients' specific questions should always be answered.

In addition to conveying direct information, you should be alert to unarticulated questions and feelings the patient would like to express or work through before the procedure begins. The techniques of therapeutic interaction are used in such instances (see Chapter 11).

In *Modules for Basic Nursing Skills*, the sections on specific skills note concerns patients commonly express and suggest ways to decrease patients' anxiety.

## 5. Prepare the Patient Physically

When the patient understands what is to be done, you may proceed to make physical preparations. These preparations may include ensuring privacy, positioning the patient, changing the position of the bed, moving tables and stands, draping the patient, and providing proper lighting. Sometimes you will give medication for pain or a tranquilizer to prepare the patient for the procedure. Deciding

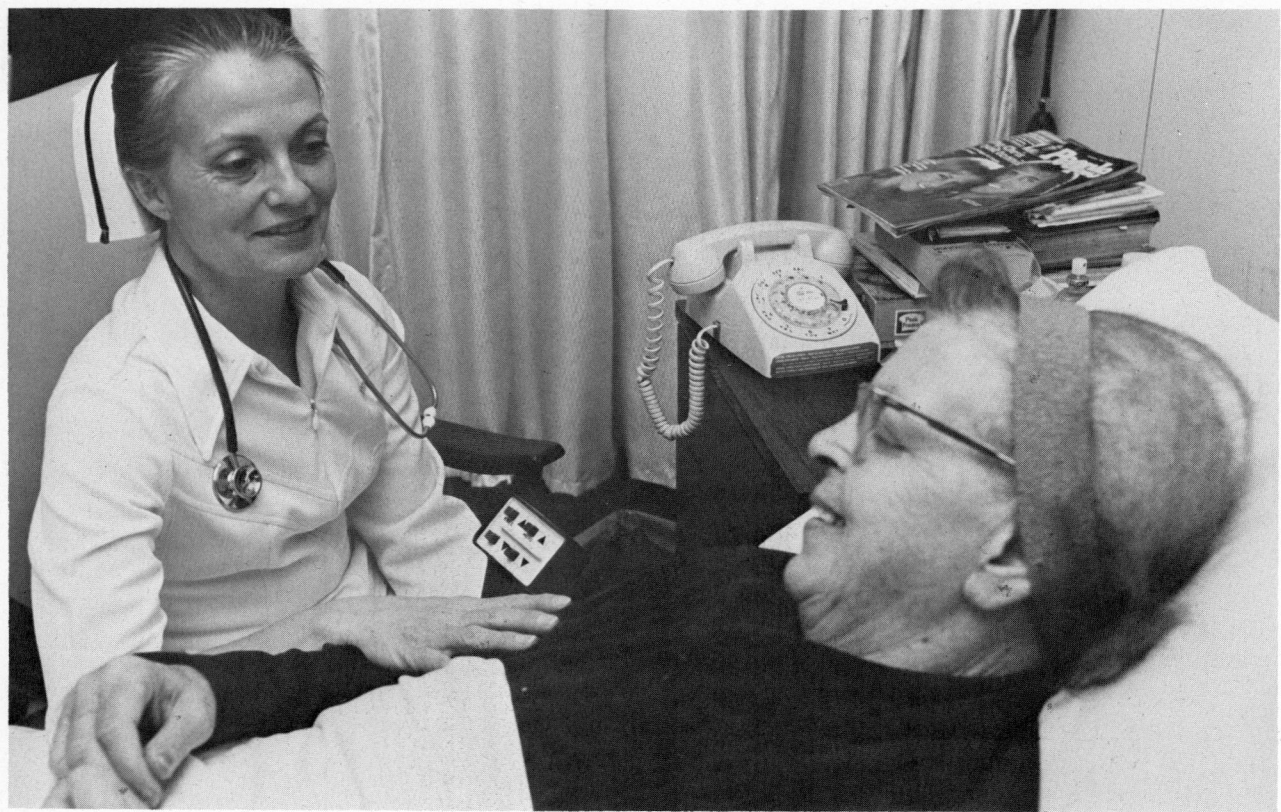

**Figure 10.1 Preparing the patient psychologically for a procedure**
(Russ Kinne/Danbury Hospital/Photo Researchers, Inc.)

when PRN (whenever necessary) medications should be given is an important nursing responsibility.

## 6. Perform the Procedure

Once everything is prepared, you can proceed with the procedure as planned, paying careful attention to detail. It is important that you observe the patient's responses closely. There may be times when the procedure must be changed, delayed, or even halted because of the patient's response. It is a very common trait of inexperienced nurses to become so engrossed in technical details that the patient is neglected.

## 7. Evaluate the Results

Though you will be evaluating your performance and the patient's reaction during the procedure, a more complete evaluation of its effectiveness in accomplishing its goal and the patient's response

is undertaken when you have finished. You may need to talk to the patient to elicit feedback on his or her response. Keep the purpose of the treatment in mind when evaluating it. That is, if a hot pack is used to reduce pain and inflammation of a swollen arm, but the patient experiences no relief from discomfort, the procedure is not considered completely successful even if it is performed correctly. Though evaluation cannot always be completed immediately after the procedure, criteria and a plan for evaluation can be established at that time.

## 8. Make the Patient Comfortable

Before moving on to other tasks, make the patient as comfortable as possible. Doing so may entail rearranging bedding, changing the patient's position, returning tables and stands to positions convenient for the patient, and consulting the patient about any immediate needs. Again, the pa-

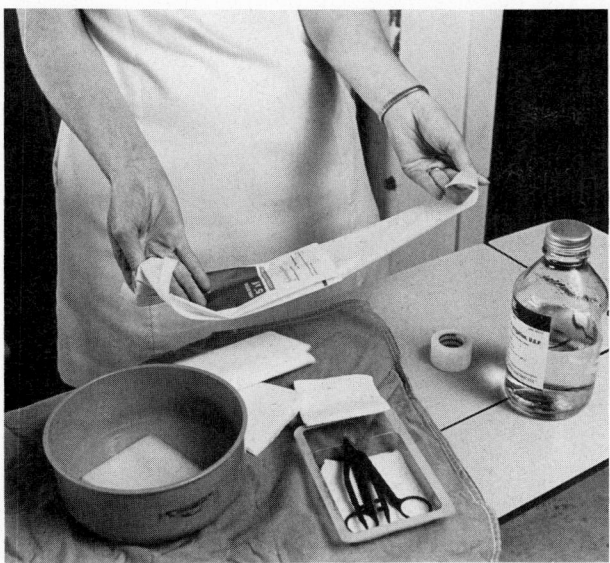

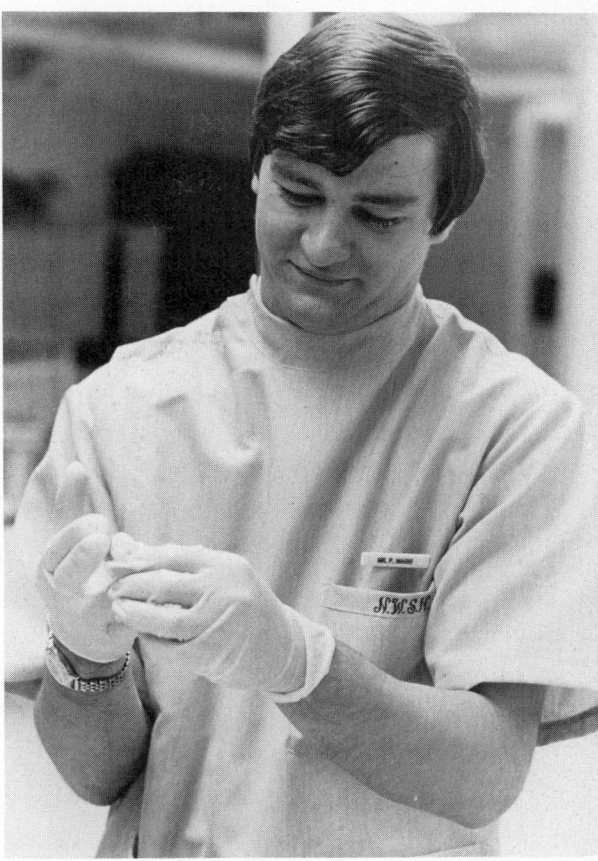

**Figure 10.2 Setting up for a sterile treatment**
*Above:* Dan Bernstein; *right:* Lynn McLaren, courtesy of Newton-Wellesley Hospital

tient's psychological well-being and possible need for pain medication should be considered. The patient may wish to talk about the experience or may prefer quiet and privacy to regain composure if the procedure has been particularly long and/or difficult.

## 9. Care for the Equipment and the Specimen

Equipment and supplies must be cared for in the manner prescribed by the facility. Disposable equipment may need to be thrown away in a particular place to avoid endangering housekeeping staff with needles and sharp instruments. Nondisposable equipment may need to be cleaned according to a particular routine or sent to the department where such cleaning is performed. Nurses are expected to demonstrate care with the many costly pieces of equipment used in the modern health-care setting.

If a specimen (such as a body fluid) was obtained in the course of the procedure, it must be labeled carefully to avoid errors. It is then processed in whatever way is appropriate to prevent deterioration, which would render the specimen useless. In certain instances, for example, a stool specimen must be kept warm so that organisms present in it can be identified in the laboratory; urine must sometimes be refrigerated to slow chemical decomposition. Some specimens must be placed in special preservatives or treated containers. Information on care of a specimen for a specific purpose should be available from the laboratory to which the specimen is being sent or from a laboratory manual (see Module 18, "Collecting Specimens").

## 10. Record the Data

Data on the treatment itself, the patient's response, the effectiveness of the treatment, and the disposition of the specimen (if any) are usually recorded on the patient's medical record. A flow sheet is sometimes used to record repeated treatments in much the same way that medications are charted. In other instances, treatments are recorded on nurses' notes in a narrative fashion. Whatever the format, a clear record is needed.

Each module in *Modules for Basic Nursing Skills* specifies what must be recorded and suggests how to do so.

You will find that these ten steps are easily adaptable to both simple and complex procedures. For a simple procedure, such as taking a temperature, you will perform the steps very rapidly: you might gather your equipment, enter the patient's room, explain your purpose, rearrange the pillow, and take the temperature in less than five minutes. You have simply telescoped the steps, performing some almost simultaneously. For a longer and more complex procedure, you might isolate each step and enter the patient's room twice: once to prepare the patient and again to bring the equipment to the bedside and perform the procedure. Thus, the procedural checklist is a useful tool, not an implacable formula.

## Assisting with Diagnostic Tests and Procedures

The nurse is frequently called on to assist with special tests and procedures performed by the physician or other members of the health-care team. The procedural checklist will also be of value in this situation. In reviewing the various steps, you can clarify which will be performed by others and which will be your responsibility. For a diagnostic study or procedure to be performed in another department, the process may be as follows: (1) Check the order. (2) Review the procedure to determine what you need to do and to prepare yourself to explain it to the patient. (3) Equipment will be taken care of by the other department. (4) Prepare the patient by teaching about and discussing the procedure. (5) Physical preparation may be performed by the other department or by you. (6) The procedure is carried out in the other department. (7) Evaluate the patient on his or her return. (8) The other department will take care of the equipment used. (9) The other department will record its own procedures or treatments, but you will record those portions you have performed. (10) Make the patient comfortable. (See the Care Study on page 164.)

In some situations, such as a diagnostic procedure performed by the physician, you may find that you perform all the steps except the procedure itself. While the physician is performing the procedure, you will assist by making equipment available, positioning the patient, and helping the patient tolerate the procedure. Module 23, "Assisting with Examinations and Procedures," specifies what will be required of you in many different procedures.

Appendices E through J describe some common procedures and tests performed by other members of the health-care team. Specific aspects of these procedures will vary from place to place, and the procedure manual for your institution should be consulted for details. Consult a medical-surgical nursing text for information on understanding the results of the test and providing more skilled care if it is required.

## Physical Safety

Illness can compromise a person's ability to perceive potential hazards and to act independently to secure safety. Thus the nurse is responsible for maintaining a physically safe environment for the patient.

### Environmental Assessment

An environment arranged to meet the patient's needs also promotes safety. The bedside stand and/or overbed table should be within reach so that the patient need not stretch or get out of bed. The call bell too must be within easy reach. Siderails not only protect the patient from falling but also provide support when turning. Equipment should be regularly inspected for proper functioning. When liquid is spilled on the floor, ensuring that it is wiped up promptly may prevent a serious accident to a patient or a staff member. The patient's environment is your responsibility; make a habit of looking at it carefully with safety in mind.

## Falls

Falls are a major cause of injury to the ill. Falls commonly occur when patients faint upon first standing up, remain up longer than they can tolerate, or attempt to function independently before they are physically strong enough to do so. Sometimes patients overreach their capacities because the nurses do not respond to their calls for assistance. Thus an elderly, infirm patient whose call light is not answered may try to go to the bathroom alone rather than be incontinent in the bed. Falls are also common among confused or disoriented patients.

In the course of your basic assessment, you should identify patients who are at risk of falling. Consider the person's stability, strength, and usual level of activity. If you conclude that a patient is at risk, you will need to include protective measures in your nursing care plan. Such measures might include keeping the bed in the low position, using siderails, and/or employing protective devices (restraints) when appropriate. Restraints, the least desirable method of assuring patient safety, should be approved by the physician, though they may be initiated by the nurse in a hazardous situation. Only necessary restraints should be used, and these should be removed for short periods regularly to allow for movement and skin care. Restraints must be checked frequently to make sure they do not impede circulation or cause skin damage (see Module 13, "Applying Restraints").

Correct use of crutches, walkers, and safety belts during *ambulation* (walking) helps prevent falls. After ascertaining what assistance a patient needs to ambulate, make sure the device is available and that it is used correctly.

## Electrical Hazards

Electrical equipment is widely and increasingly used in the care of the acutely ill. Even the bed is usually equipped with electrical controls. Thus steps must be taken to protect patients from electrical hazards.

First, you should care for electrical equipment to ensure that plugs are not pulled loose from cords, cords do not get caught in equipment (which might sever internal wires), and liquids are not spilled on electrical equipment.

Second, inspect electrical appliances for frayed or broken cords before using them. All electrical equipment used in hospitals should be grounded, which requires a three-pronged plug. The third prong should under no circumstances be removed. Discontinue use of faulty equipment and report the problem to the appropriate repair department immediately.

Third, extension cords should not be used unless they have been specifically approved by those responsible for such equipment in your facility. Extension cords often reduce voltage, making the equipment function less well, and the cords themselves may be a hazard if they extend across the floor. Furthermore, many extension cords are not constructed heavily enough to meet the needs of special equipment; they might short out, creating a fire hazard.

When special equipment such as a cardiac monitor is in use, it is the responsibility of the nurses involved to acquaint themselves with the manufacturer's suggestions for safeguarding the patient from electrical shock. When delicate instruments are attached to cardiac monitors, even very low levels of "microshock" may be a hazard.

## Burns

Fortunately, burns are a rare cause of injury in the health-care setting. When they occur, however, they can be a serious hazard. Burns are most likely when heat is being applied therapeutically. In such circumstances, the skin eventually becomes insensitive to heat, thus thwarting the warning mechanism which signals that the heat should be removed. Some elderly people and those with diseases that affect sensation and circulation, such as diabetes, are unable to feel discomfort due to heat.

The nurse must be extremely vigilant to safeguard a patient receiving heat treatments. The temperature should be carefully set, the patient's skin should be monitored, and the duration of treatment should not be excessive.

Hot showers and baths can also cause burns, especially when the skin is very sensitive. The water temperature should be tested before the person gets into the shower or tub.

## Fire

A fire in a health-care facility is often a major crisis since many patients are unable to move by themselves. As a nurse, the most valuable thing you can do with regard to fires is help prevent them. One of the commonest causes of fires is careless use and disposal of cigarettes. Identify patients who should not smoke unattended due to weakness, confusion, or the effects of sedatives and narcotics. Persuading these patients not to smoke would undoubtedly be best for their long-term health, but this suggestion is often not well received. In such instances, smoking must be monitored by a staff member or family member. Sometimes smoking is monitored by designating an area where it is permitted and a staff member is present.

Cigarette stubs must be disposed of carefully. Occasionally a patient will empty an ashtray into a wastebasket, unaware of a stub still hot enough to ignite tissues in the basket. When in doubt, empty a patient's ashtray in the toilet, not the wastebasket.

Care with electrical equipment, described above, also prevents fire. Sparks from broken cords or defective motors can start fires.

Oxygen equipment is a particular hazard since oxygen supports combustion and allows higher temperatures to be reached, thus igniting many substances. When you use oxygen, familiarize yourself with the proper procedures.

Each facility has it own procedure for fire safety. It is your responsibility to learn this procedure thoroughly. The following sections discuss some points that should be covered in every facility's fire policy.

## Reporting Fires

Your first concern when you discover a fire is usually to safeguard anyone in immediate danger. Doing so might require, for example, moving a patient immediately or pulling burning blankets off a bed. Each facility specifies how an alarm is to be raised: by calling a switchboard, activating a fire alarm on the wall, calling a code word to a secretary, or whatever.

All staff members should be clear about their responsibilities when a fire alarm has been sounded. Usually fire and smoke barrier doors are closed. All ordinary windows and doors are closed to decrease air circulation, which could spread the fire. Patients must be reassured of their safety, and someone should be assigned to stay with very upset or anxious people. Often oxygen and/or electrical connections are turned off in the areas affected.

## Fighting Fires

Whether or not you fight a fire is usually a matter of individual judgment. If the fire is small enough to be extinguished with basic fire-stopping techniques—such as smothering with a blanket, pouring a water pitcher on a wastebasket, or using a fire extinguisher—you should attempt to put out the fire after safeguarding others and sounding the alarm. If the fire is not discovered until it is very large, such as a storage room in flames, it is wiser to close the doors to contain the fire, evacuate patients and staff, and leave fire fighting to the professional firefighters.

Read the directions on the fire extinguishers in your area before there is a need for their use. Identify the types of fire extinguishers present and the types of fires each is designed to fight. A Class A extinguisher is to be used only on paper or wood fires, never on electrical or chemical fires. A Class

B extinguisher is to be used on chemicals, grease, and anesthetic agents, as well as wood and paper fires. Only a Class C extinguisher may be used on electrical fires as well as fires of all other types.

## Evacuation

The procedure for evacuation is to move the most physically able patients first. The reason for this policy is to get the greatest number of patients to safety in the shortest time. Some patients will be able to walk safely if directed where to go. It may be necessary for one staff member to accompany a group of ambulatory patients to their destination. The first staff member who leaves should take a card index (Kardex) or notebook that lists all patients, so rescue can be performed systematically.

After the physically independent, patients who can use wheelchairs or walkers are evacuated. The last to be evacuated are completely dependent patients. Stretchers may or may not be available. If not, there are a variety of other ways to carry patients. Two nurses can form a chair of arms to carry a person, or one nurse can use the "fireman's carry"—carrying a person across one's lower back. Since most nurses are women and some are physically small, it may be unrealistic to try to carry all patients. More effective evacuation

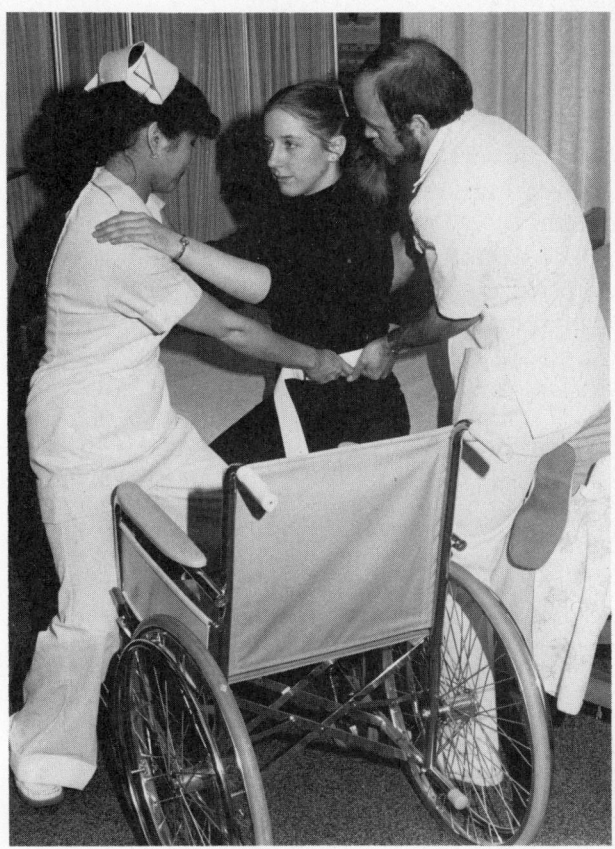

**Figure 10.3  Bed to wheelchair: Two-person maximal assist**
Courtesy Ivan Ellis

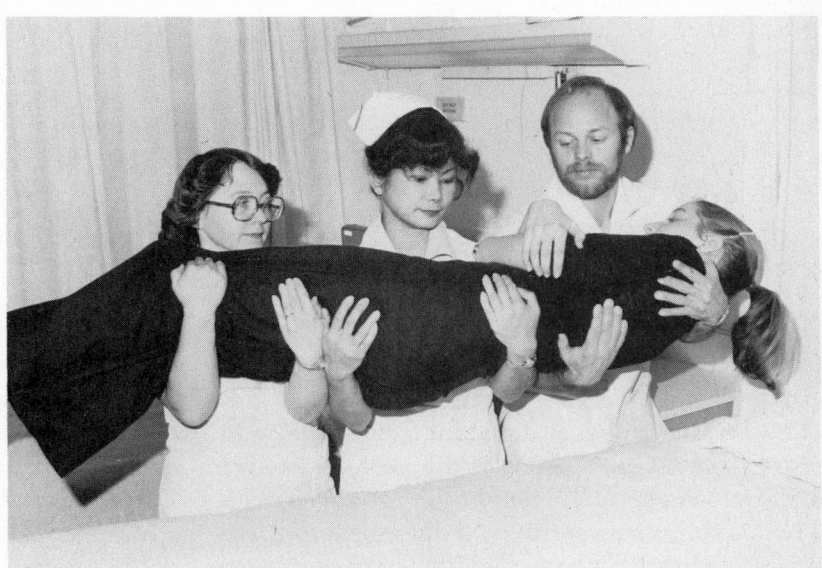

**Figure 10.4  Horizontal lift: Three-person assist**
Courtesy Ivan Ellis

may be accomplished by laying a patient on a heavy blanket or spread on the floor and dragging him or her to safety. (This is not recommended on carpeted floors, however, because of the heat produced by friction.) This is one time when the hazards of microorganisms on the floor can be ignored.

The first step in evacuation is usually to move all patients on a particular floor to the least affected area close to an exit. Next, patients are evacuated to units of the hospital farther from danger. Only as a last resort are patients completely evacuated from the facility since exposure can be a very serious hazard to the ill.

Acquaint yourself with the fire plan of the institution where you will be practicing. Prior preparation is essential to prevent loss of life if a fire does occur.

# Administering Drug Therapy

Implementing drug therapy ordered by the physician involves far more than merely administering medications.

## Knowledge of Drugs

The nurse's first responsibility is to understand the drug itself—its purpose, the way it acts, contraindications to its use, and possible side effects. Acquiring a basic knowledge of drugs takes a great deal of time and effort, and even then the task is not over. Because new drugs are constantly being produced, familiarizing yourself with the drugs you administer is an ongoing responsibility. Such knowledge enables you to consider a given drug's potential and actual effect on an individual patient. Although the physician is responsible for ordering medication, the system is strengthened by the double-checking of a knowledgeable nurse.

## Knowledge of the Patient's Condition

The patient's physical condition, diagnosis, and history should be available to the nurse whenever medications are to be administered. Unless you have this information, you will not be able to make correct judgments about medications or to discern changes caused by drugs.

## The Nurse's Responsibilities

Information about the patient should be considered in conjunction with information about the drug, paying particular attention to contraindications to the drug's use. Attention to possible allergies to medications can prevent unfortunate and sometimes tragic mistakes. If, for example, the medication ordered is contraindicated for patients with glaucoma (an eye disease) and checking reveals that the patient has glaucoma, it is the nurse's responsibility to bring this circumstance to the attention of the physician. If the physician is aware of the conflict, the nurse should request an explanation of the rationale for giving the medication. If, after hearing the rationale, the nurse is still reluctant to give the medication, the nursing supervisor may be contacted for advice and direction. It is the privilege and responsibility of the nurse not to administer a medication he or she firmly believes will be harmful to the patient.

In order to evaluate the effectiveness of medications you administer, you must know the expected reaction and establish criteria for ascertaining its effectiveness. For example, you need to know that codeine is given to reduce pain in order to evaluate its effectiveness for the patient. Knowing how long it takes a medication to become effective also helps you establish specific criteria, such as "pain relief obtained within thirty minutes."

Side effects and allergies to drugs are a common complication of drug therapy. Familiarity with the problems that can result from a given medication will enable the nurse to recognize their presence in a patient. The earlier a problem is recognized, the sooner appropriate action may be taken to combat it. It may be necessary for the physician to lower the dosage, discontinue the medication altogether, or even order other medications to counteract a given reaction.

It is another responsibility of the nurse to know the correct dosage of a medication. Errors can occur because of incorrect transcription of orders from one place to another, poor penmanship, and simple human fallibility. The nurse who knows the correct dosage and checks the order is often able to catch such errors and contact the physician to correct them. This task is particularly important for nurses working with children. Children's dosages are so much smaller than adults' that even slight errors can cause serious problems.

## Routes of Administration

The way in which a medication is applied to or enters the body significantly affects the speed with which it works and the area of the body affected.

*Oral* medications are those that are swallowed. Some medications taken orally are absorbed in the stomach. Liquids are usually absorbed more quickly than solids, which must dissolve before absorption. However, some solids (such as aspirin) dissolve so rapidly that this advantage is not significant. Some oral medications are destroyed by stomach secretions, and must therefore be coated to allow them to pass into the small intestine for absorption. This coating is called *enteric* coating (see Module 43, "Administering Oral Medications").

Some medications are held against the mucous membranes of the mouth, where they dissolve slowly and are absorbed by the mucous membrane. Those held next to the cheek are called *buccal* medications; those held under the tongue are called *sublingual.*

*Topical* preparations, those applied to external surfaces of the body, include powders, lotions, and ointments. Also included in this category are eye (ophthalmic) and ear (otic) preparations. Because a few medications are absorbed from the skin, topical application may have systemic effects

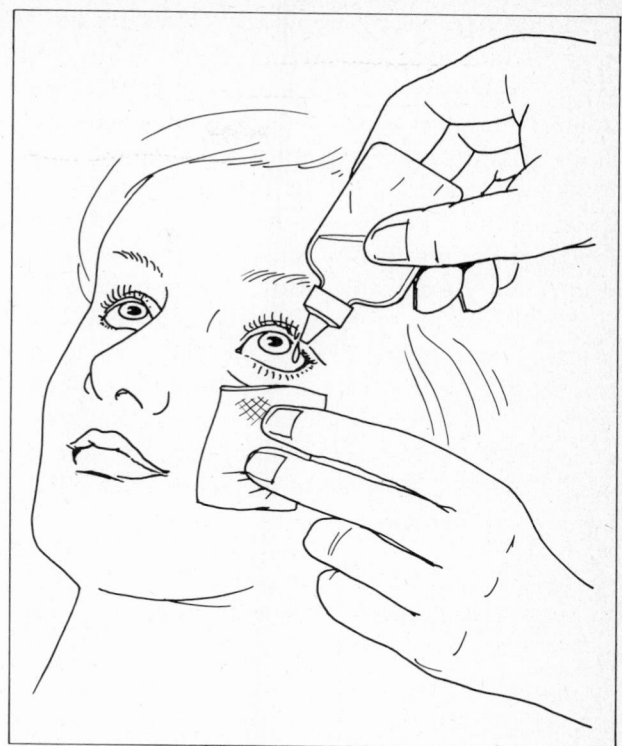

**Figure 10.5   Administering eyedrops**

(see Module 44, "Administering Topical Medications").

Some medications can be administered *rectally.* Many of these are prescribed for local effect on the bowel, but some rectal medications can be absorbed by the mucosa and thus have a systemic effect.

*Parenteral* medications, those injected into body tissue, are categorized according to the tissue into which the medication is injected. *Intradermal* medications are injected into the skin, and *subcutaneous* medications into those tissue layers under the skin that lie over the muscle. *Intramuscular* injections go directly into the muscle tissue. *Intravenous* medications are directed into the bloodstream by way of a vein. *Intra-arterial* injections go into an artery. *Intracardiac* medications are injected directly into the heart (done only with emergency drugs in life-threatening situations). *Intrathecal* injections go directly into the subarachnoid space, to combine with the cerebrospinal fluid, by way of a lumbar puncture (see Module 45, "Giving Injections," and Module 47, "Administering Intravenous Medications").

The faster a medication enters the circulatory system, the sooner a systemic result will occur. Topical medication is the slowest to have a systemic effect since it is absorbed very slowly if at all. Rectal absorption is faster and oral medications faster still. Buccal and sublingual absorption is faster than oral because of the rapidity of absorption from the mouth. As for the parenteral medications, the deeper the tissue, the more vascular and thus quicker to absorb it is. Intravenous is fastest, followed in descending order by intramuscular, subcutaneous, and intradermal. Many intradermal medications are not systemically absorbed at all. Intrathecal medications are administered for local effect in the cerebrospinal fluid, and little absorption occurs.

## The Five Rights

In addition to the foregoing general responsibilities with regard to medications, the nurse must give medications according to very rigid guidelines established to assure that the *right patient* receives the *right medication* at the *right time* in the *right dosage* by the *right route* of administration. These guidelines are sometimes referred to as "the five rights."

The cycle begins when an order for a medication is written by a physician, osteopathic physician, or dentist. A written order is usually required to lessen the possibility of error. In emergency situations, however, verbal orders are given; errors are minimized if the emergency order is repeated exactly before it is carried out. In some settings orders are given to the nurse over the telephone; such an order should be written down as it is given and read back to check for error. Both emergency verbal orders and telephone orders are recorded in the patient record, with a notation of the origin of the order ("Telephone order, A. J. Smith, M.D.") and signed by the person receiving and recording the order ("by J. Jones, R.N."). This written record is checked and countersigned at the earliest opportunity by the physician who gave the order.

A complete drug order should include the following:

1. The patient's name (usually stamped directly on the order sheet in a hospital chart)
2. The date (either on each individual order or stamped on a sheet for each day)
3. The name of the drug
4. The dosage of the drug to be administered
5. Frequency of administration
6. The route by which the drug is to be administered
7. The physician's signature

If any of these seven items is not clear, it is the nurse's responsibility to clarify the order before proceeding.

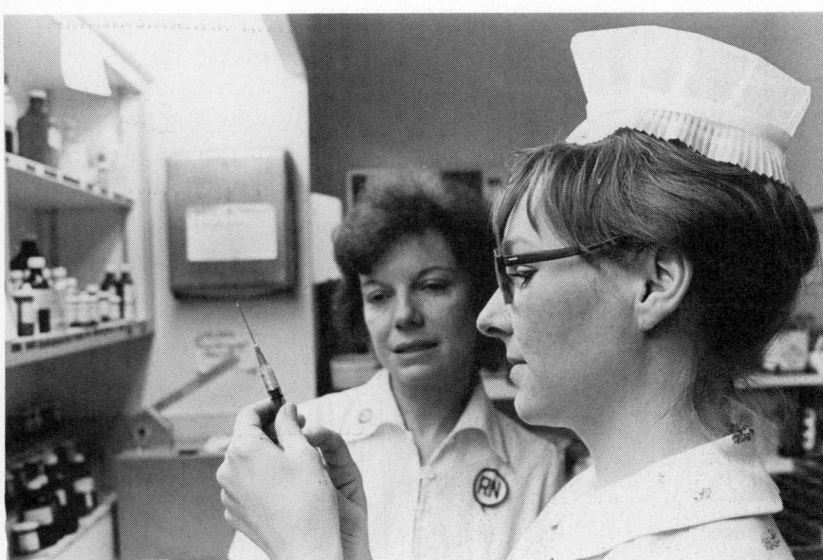

**Figure 10.6 Preparing an injection**
Lynn McLaren, courtesy of Newton-Wellesley Hospital

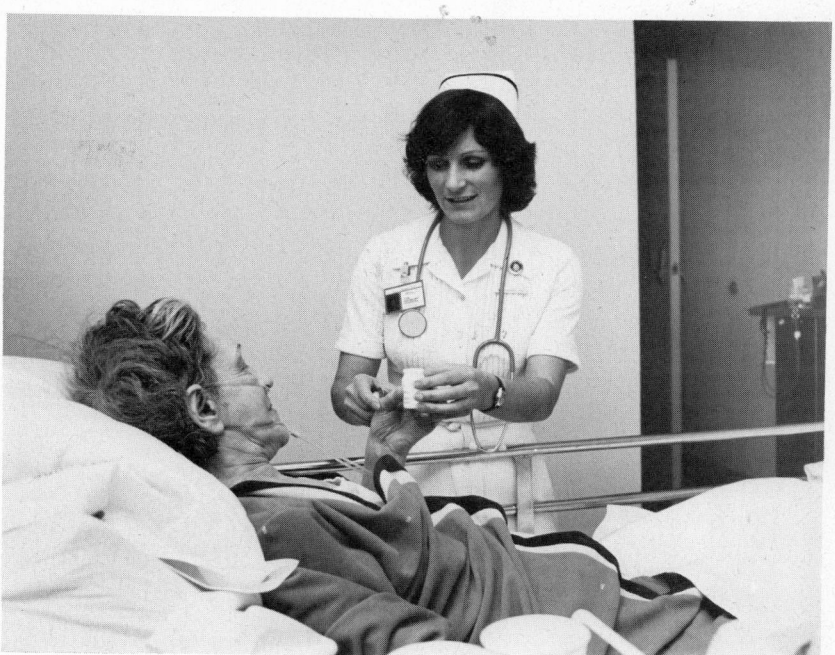

**Figure 10.7  Giving medications**
Russ Kinne/Danbury Hospital/Photo Researchers, Inc.

After receiving the order, the nurse has many further responsibilities with regard to it. The order must be transcribed from the patient record to the card index (Kardex), chart, and/or medication cards consulted when giving medication. In some facilities this step is eliminated by writing the order directly on the record from which the medication is given. In other settings the task of transcribing is assigned to the ward secretary or clerk. Nevertheless, the ultimate responsibility for checking the correctness of the transcription belongs to the nurse.

If the order has previously been transcribed, a routine for checking the accuracy of the duplicate record may have been established. This is especially likely when small cards are used to record each medication for administration. Such cards are easily misplaced, and failure to check them against an original record could result in medication errors.

Once you have ascertained that you have the correct information, you may begin the procedure of administering the medication. Whatever its structure, the system of drug administration is designed to provide the right patient with the right medication in the right dosage, by the right route, at the right time. You will need to learn the exact system or procedure of any facility in which you

are employed. Some systems, such as the Brewer system, have been commercially designed, while others originate in the hospitals that use them. Still others, such as medicine cards, have been in use for so many years that no one may know how they originated. Whatever the system, it is the nurse's responsibility to perform it correctly so that the chances of error are minimized.

After administration of the medication, a record is made of the medication, dosage, time, and route (oral, I.M., I.V., or whatever). This legal record must be signed by the person administering the medication. The importance of accurate recording cannot be overemphasized. Failure to record might result in a patient's receiving an ordered medication twice, with potentially serious effects. Omission of a medication must also be recorded, along with the reasons for omission.

## Medication Errors

Because of the complexity of modern medication regimes, errors do occur. Whenever any *one* of the five rights is not observed, an error has been made. A distinction is made between *errors of commission*, such as giving a wrong medication or an incorrect dosage, and *errors of omission*, such as

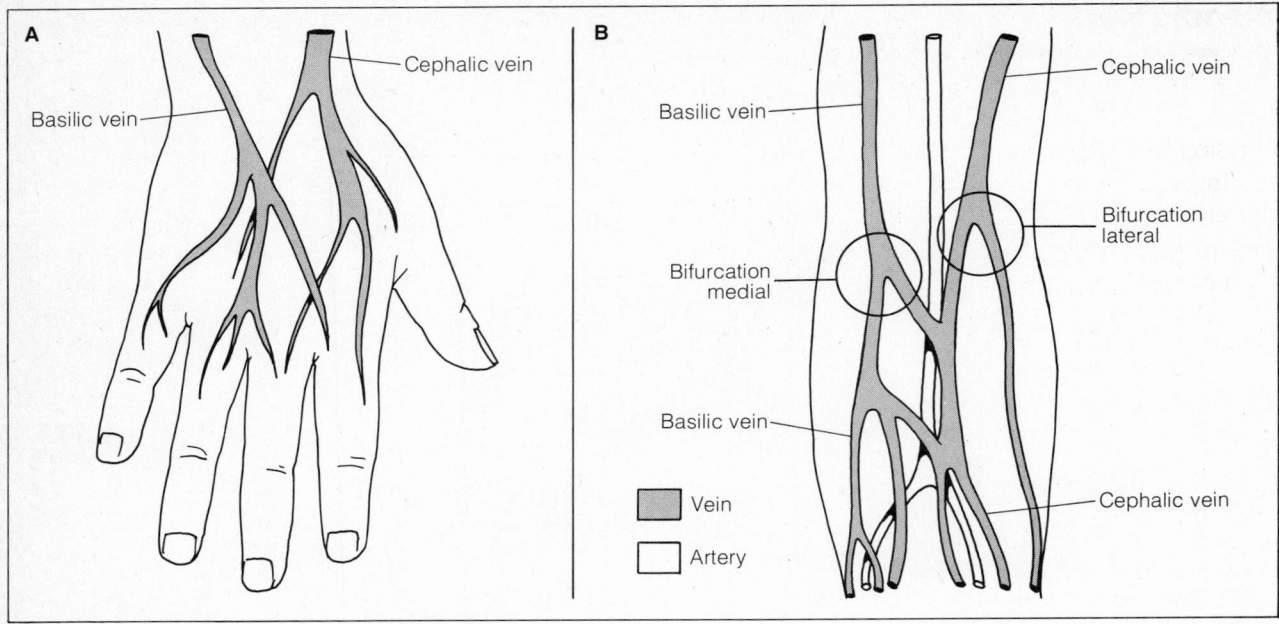

**Figure 10.8   Suitable veins for starting IVs. *A*: Hand; *B*: forearm.**

failure to administer the correct medication.

However a medication error occurs, your immediate concern must be the well-being of the patient. The patient is assessed in light of the nature of the error. If an overdosage was administered, are there signs of adverse reactions? If a medication was omitted, are there possible adverse consequences for the patient? When the patient's immediate status has been assessed, the nurse must plan the course of action. Sometimes immediate measures should be taken. When, for example, a medication to relieve muscle spasm was to have been given at 8:00 a.m., and the nurse discovers at 10:00 a.m. that it was omitted, the nurse elects to give the medication immediately because the patient needs relief. Other errors may require other types of action. It may be sufficient to make a notation on the nursing care plan or card index (Kardex) to alert other nurses to watch for particular problems.

The plan of action must always include notification of the physician. When doing so, the nurse should be prepared to give the physician a complete assessment of the patient's condition and a summary of any action taken and to consult with the physician on further action. If the problem is not serious, notification may be postponed until the physician's next visit. Otherwise, notification should be made immediately. If the physician is not available, the nursing supervisor and another physician may be called.

Another part of the nurse's plan will be to fill out a special incident form for the hospital or facility. The primary purpose of such forms is to gather data on errors so that steps can be taken to eliminate them. They also serve as a legal record for the facility.

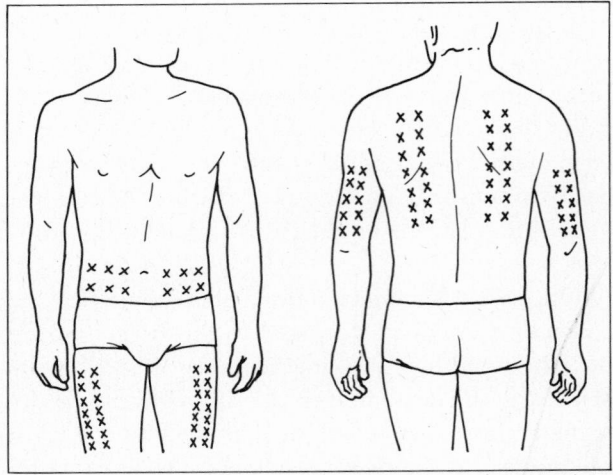

**Figure 10.9   Sites used in rotating insulin injections**

# Conclusion

Nursing is characterized by many modes of functioning and relating to others. As a nurse, you will exercise your decision making ability constantly as you function independently. Working effectively with other health-care team members and carrying out delegated tasks requires the same kind of capable functioning. The nurse cannot simply do as directed. Both the law and those who depend on nurses expect informed, thoughtful action in every situation.

## Care Study  Assisting with a physical therapy treatment

Mrs. Jones, an elderly woman with severe arthritis in both hands, is a newly admitted patient. Mrs. Schultz, the registered nurse, checks the physician's orders (Step 1 on the Procedural Checklist, Exhibit 10.1) and notes that physical therapy treatment involving the application of hot wax to both hands is to take place daily. Mrs. Schultz calls the Physical Therapy Department to arrange appointments for Mrs. Jones, and at the same time inquires about the exact manner in which the procedure will be carried out (Step 2). This is Mrs. Schultz's first experience with such a treatment since her employment at General Hospital.

Mrs. Schultz then goes into Mrs. Jones's room to explain the treatment (Step 4). Mrs. Schultz also plans for morning care to be given to Mrs. Jones after treatment so that the pain relief afforded by the treatment can become effective before Mrs. Jones tries to perform self-care.

The next morning Mrs. Schultz prepares Mrs. Jones to go to the Physical Therapy Department. Assessing Mrs. Jones's abilities, the nurse determines that a wheelchair is the most appropriate means of transportation (Step 5).

The treatment is performed by the physical therapist (Steps 3 and 6), who records complete information on Mrs. Jones's chart (Steps 7 and 9).

When the patient returns to the unit, Mrs. Schultz makes her comfortable (Step 8) and notes her fatigue level. She inquires about the pain relief experienced and watches for any untoward results, such as skin irritation (Step 7). Mrs. Schultz then records her observations on Mrs. Jones's record (Step 10) in the following manner. "Upon return from P.T., appeared pale and exhausted. Stated the hot wax had decreased pain in hands. Skin appears pink and smooth. No irritation of skin noted. H. Schultz, R.N."

## Study Terms

allergy
ambulation
contraindication
diagnostic test
dosage
drug therapy
enteric
error of commission
error of omission
"five rights"
medical plan of care
procedure
routes of
   administration
buccal
intra-arterial
intradermal
intrathecal
intravenous
oral
parenteral
rectal
subcutaneous
sublingual
topical
side effect
treatment

## Learning Activities

**1.** Select a treatment and write a complete procedure for it. Use the procedural checklist in the chapter as a guide.
**2.** Review the medication procedure for your facility.
**3.** Review the fire and disaster plans for your facility.
**4.** In your clinical facility, check and record the exact location of all fire extinguishers and fire alarms on the unit to which you are assigned. Be sure to identify the type of fire extinguisher at each location.

## Relevant Sections in
## Modules for Basic Nursing Skills

| Volume 1 | Module |
|---|---|
| Applying Restraints | 13 |
| Collecting Specimens | 18 |
| Assisting With Examinations and Procedures | 23 |
| Applying Bandages and Binders | 24 |
| Applying Heat and Cold | 25 |

| Volume 2 | |
|---|---|
| Common Laboratory Tests | 27 |
| Inspection, Palpation, Auscultation, and Percussion | 32 |
| Preoperative Care | 34 |
| Postoperative Care | 35 |
| Irrigations | 38 |
| Administering Oral Medications | 43 |
| Administering Topical Medications | 44 |
| Giving Injections | 45 |

## References

Bermock, L. S., *et al.* "Do We Practice What We Teach?" *Nursing '73* 3 (September 1973): 26–32.

Brunner, L. S. "Standards on Policies and Procedures and How to Write Them." *Association of Operating Room Nurses Journal* 13 (1971): 39–55.

Budd, R. "We Changed to Unit Dosage System." *Nursing Outlook* 19 (February 1971): 116–117.

Burkhalter, P. "Medication Errors: Let's Eliminate Them!" *Supervisor Nurse* 3 (November 1972): 58–59.

DelBueno, D. J. "Verifying the Nurse's Knowledge of Pharmacology." *Nursing Outlook* 20 (July 1972): 462–463.

Harmon, M. L., *et al.* "Fiber Optics Photography in the Stomach." *RN* 34 (July 1971): 46–51.

Levine, R. "Breaking Through the Medication Mystique." *American Journal of Nursing* 70 (April 1970): 799.

Kreiger, Doris. "Therapeutic Touch: The Imprimatur of Nursing." *American Journal of Nursing* 75 (May 1975): 784–787.

Newton, Marian, and Newton, David. "Guidelines for Handling Drug Errors." *Nursing '77* (September 1977): 62–68.

Siegler, A. M. "Trends in Laparoscopy." *RN* 34 (November 1971): 1–4.

"Standing Orders and Nursing Judgment." *Regan Reports on Nursing Law* 11 (November 1970): 1.

# Chapter 11

# Asepsis and Infection Control

## Objectives

After completing this chapter, you should be able to:

1. Diagram and explain the movement of pathogens through the infection chain.
2. List and briefly describe the six categories of pathogens.
3. List actions you might take at each link in the infection chain to stop the spread of infection.
4. Describe the practice of asepsis with regard to handwashing, care of linens and equipment, care of the patient's unit, and caring for more than one patient.
5. Name the six methods of cleaning or sterilizing.
6. Briefly discuss the three categories of antimicrobial drugs.
7. Outline the five types of isolation technique.
8. Discuss the potential psychological problems of the isolated patient and possible modes of intervention.
9. Name several resources and agencies whose main purpose is the control of infection.

## Outline

A Brief History of Asepsis and Infection Control
The Origin and Nature of Infection
The Infection Chain
    Infectious Agents
        Bacteria / Viruses / Fungi / Protozoa / Parasitic Worms / Rickettsia
    The Reservoir
    The Portal of Exit
    Means of Transmission
    Portal of Entry
    The Susceptible Host
The Nurse and the Transfer of Infection
    Actions That Can Spread Infection
    Actions That Can Prevent the Spread of Infection
Medical and Surgical Asepsis
    Methods of Maintaining Asepsis
        Handwashing / Care of Linens / Care of Equipment / Arrangement of the Patient's Unit / Caring for More Than One Patient

Methods of Killing or Reducing Infectious Agents
    Soap-and-Water Cleansing / Boiling / Ultraviolet Rays / Antiseptic, Disinfectant, and Bactericidal Agents / Autoclaving / Gas Sterilization
Aseptic Conscience
Control of Infection with Drugs
Nursing Care of Infection
Isolation
    Types of Isolation
        Strict Isolation / Respiratory Isolation / Enteric Isolation / Wound and Skin Precautions / Protective Isolation / Psychological Isolation
The Role of the Nurse in Isolation Technique
Staff and Visitor Acceptance of Isolation
Community Efforts to Control Infection
    Hospitals
    Counties
    States
    The National Center for Disease Control
    The World Health Organization

*Asepsis* is the absence of all disease-producing microorganisms. The concept of asepsis is the key to protecting hospitalized patients from infection and preventing the spread of infection from a patient who is already infected.

Infection poses a serious problem to the hospitalized patient. Many patients are admitted to the hospital because they have contracted an infection. And, more often than we would like, patients who are in the hospital for surgery or treatment of a medical condition develop secondary infections. Thus a major component of nursing care is the prevention, management, and treatment of infection. An understanding of asepsis and infection control is the foundation of the nurse's continuing efforts to prevent transmission of infection.

## A Brief History of Asepsis and Infection Control

Asepsis as a means to prevent and control infection was virtually unknown until the nineteenth century, when the transmission of organisms began to be understood. Even so, it had been observed that previously healthy people who touched or came in contact with the ill often became ill themselves, and isolation of the ill was thus common. Nothing was known of the transmission of organisms.

As long as human beings have existed, their wounds have been accompanied by infection. Though attempts were made to contain it, infection was long thought to be a natural component of healing. The ancient Romans dressed wounds with mixtures of molds and yeasts spread on cloth, called poultices. These mixtures slowed the infection process, though it was not understood why. Not until the twentieth century was it discovered—by Sir Alexander Fleming, an English bacteriologist—that penicillin, a compound derived from a mold, is effective in the treatment of many infections. Penicillin is the most widely used antibiotic in the world today.

In the interim, both effective measures to combat infection and specific knowledge of how infection was transmitted from person to person were lacking. In 1862, Louis Pasteur, a French chemist, proved beyond a doubt the germ theory of disease. About the same time Ignaz Semmelweis, an obstetrician, demonstrated that germs could be transmitted from the hands of one person to another person. Physicians routinely examined pregnant women immediately after examining cadavers, without washing their hands, and Semmelweis observed that these women became infected and often died of what was known as "childbed fever."

Before the advent of aseptic surgical practice, a surgeon might wear the same soiled frock coat for several surgical procedures. Clean gowns came into use in 1880. Ten years later Dr. William Halsted introduced the use of sterile gloves, in a first attempt at asepsis on the part of the operative team (Historical Look at Infection, 1977). Understanding of infection and its control through asepsis thus expanded gradually, eventually giving rise to scientific principles with important implications for the health-care team.

## The Origin and Nature of Infection

Extremely small animals and plants called *microorganisms* exist throughout the human body. Many of these tiny organisms are beneficial, but some are not. Those that are beneficial, called *normal flora*, prevent the growth of disease-producing microorganisms within a particular area of the body, such as the nose, throat, intestinal tract, and vagina. Disease-producing microorganisms are called *pathogens*. When pathogens multiply to the point of causing signs and symptoms, the individual is said to have an *infection*. In other words, all of us carry pathogens, but we remain infection-free unless the pathogens multiply sufficiently to cause disease.

An infection contracted in the hospital is called *nosocomial*. It is these types of infection that are most worrisome to hospital personnel. Despite their appearance, hospitals are not clean places. Many people, from many different environments, are confined to a fairly constricted facility in which contact with one another can hardly be avoided. This exposes patients to a wide variety of strange microbes. Also, patients' other health problems weaken their resistance to infection. Many patients have open wounds, which offer entry for pathogens. Nosocomial infections cost several million dollars in health-care bills each year, not to mention the suffering and lost wages of patients.

## The Infection Chain

To understand how pathogens cause infection, let us look closely at Figure 11.1, which illustrates the chain reaction that spreads infection. The infection chain is the way pathogens pass between human beings.

First of all, an *infectious agent* or pathogen must be present. The pathogen grows in a place, called a *reservoir*, where the conditions for its reproduction are optimal. The pathogen leaves the reservoir through what we call a *portal of exit*. It is then transmitted from the reservoir by some means, or *vehicle*, to a person (*host*) who is susceptible to it. The pathogen enters the host through a *portal of entry*, usually a body opening, and may or may not multiply further. If not extinguished within the host, it may exit through the same or a different portal. For example, an organism taken in through the respiratory tract may exit through the same portal by means of a cough or sneeze. Or the portals of entry and exit may differ: an organism that enters by mouth may exit through the bowel.

Each link is essential to the chain. If the chain is broken at any point, by chance or due to deliberate intervention, the pathogen is inactivated. Let us examine each link in more detail.

## Infectious Agents

There are six types of infectious agents or pathogens. The kind of infection control that is appropriate depends on the type of pathogen causing the infection.

Some strains of the same pathogen are more *virulent* than others. A pathogen's virulence is its potency, or ability to cause disease. In any given person, the strain must be virulent enough to cause an infection.

### Bacteria

The most numerous of all the pathogens, bacteria are one-celled microorganisms. Bacteria that can

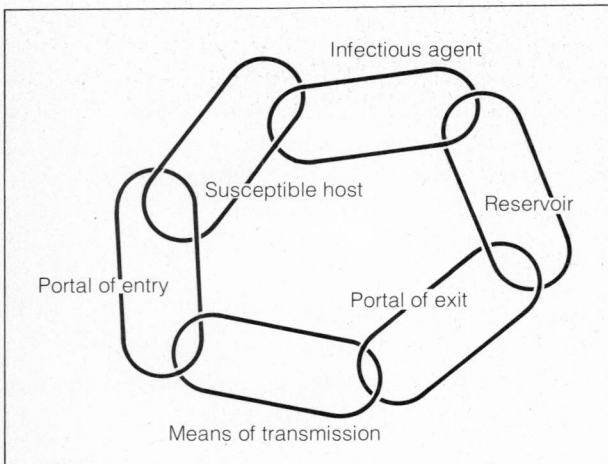

**Figure 11.1   The infection chain**

Infectious agent

Susceptible host

Reservoir

Portal of entry

Portal of exit

Means of transmission

live only in the presence of free oxygen are called *aerobic*. *Anaerobic* bacteria do not multiply in the presence of oxygen. Harmless bacteria far outnumber those that are harmful. Among the human diseases caused by bacteria are food poisoning, tuberculosis, pneumonia, urinary-tract infections, and syphilis. Some bacteria when dormant form *spores* with thick, resistant walls, which make them extremely difficult to kill. Tetanus is caused by spore-forming bacteria.

## Viruses

The smallest of all pathogens, viruses became observable only recently with the advent of powerful electron microscopes. Few viruses are responsive to existing drugs, and many of the infections they cause, such as one type of pneumonia, measles, mumps, influenza, and the common cold, must simply "run their course."

## Fungi

Moldlike pathogens, fungi can also cause difficult-to-subdue infections. Fungi grow best in moist climates, and infections caused by fungi are very prevalent in wet tropical areas. Athlete's foot and ringworm are both fungus infections.

## Protozoa

There are over 15,000 species of protozoa, large single-celled microorganisms that live in fresh or ocean water (particularly stagnant water) and in soil. Malaria is one of the common diseases caused by protozoa.

## Parasitic worms

Parasitic worms are not technically microorganisms but small, disease-causing invertebrate animals that cannot exist unless they feed off a host or microorganism. Infections caused by parasitic worms are called *helminthic* infections. Pinworm and hookworm are caused by parasitic worms.

## Rickettsia

Rickettsia are small bacteria transmitted by blood-sucking parasites such as ticks, lice, and fleas. Rocky Mountain spotted fever is a rickettsic disease.

## The Reservoir

The reservoir is the place where the pathogens multiply. Common reservoirs are water, food, excreta, body tissues, and contaminated objects such as basins, equipment, and dressings.

In order to multiply, microorganisms need one or more of a variety of conditions: the presence or absence of oxygen, light or darkness, compatible temperature, moisture, and some form of nourishment. A pH (acid-base balance) above 5, slightly alkaline, promotes the growth of many pathogens.

## The Portal of Exit

When body tissue harbors the organism, a pathway for pathogens to leave the body, a portal of exit, can be identified. This may be by the orifices of the respiratory tract in the form of secretions, the gastrointestinal tract in the form of vomitus or feces, and the genitourinary tract in the form of urine. Wound drainage and blood can also serve as a portal of exit. If the reservoir is outside the body, the portal of exit is the point at which the organism leaves the food, water, or other substance.

## Means of Transmission

As we shall see, the means of transmission, or means by which pathogens move from one person to another, is the link in the infection chain at which intervention is often most effective. We will discuss this later in relation to isolation technique.

Some pathogens can be transmitted by only one means. Others use more than one means of transmission. In general, there are four routes of transmission (U.S. Department of Health, Education and Welfare, 1975).

*Contact*, the first route, may be *direct* or *indirect*. Direct contact is a means of transmission with particular pertinence for nurses who provide hygienic care or perform procedures. Touching another person is a way to transmit pathogens by direct contact. Transmission of pathogens by *droplet*—the projection of moisture by coughing or sneezing—is also considered direct contact. Indirect contact is transmission of a pathogen on linen or equipment that has been contaminated. Carrying a stethoscope that has not been cleaned between patients is a breach of proper technique (see Figure 11.2).

Pathogens are also transmitted by *vehicles*—substances in or on which they are conveyed. Food and water serve as vehicles for some organisms. "Food poisoning" is an infection caused by the bacteria *staphylococcus* and transmitted by the vehicle of spoiled food. Blood can also serve as a vehicle for the spread of pathogens. An example is the virus that causes hepatitis B or serum hepatitis, which can be transmitted in blood transfusions.

Pathogens can also be *airborne*, carried on dust particles surrounded by moisture and suspended in the air. Pathogens projected by a sneeze can become attached to dust particles and remain airborne.

Finally, pathogens can be transmitted by *vectors*. Common vectors are insects and animals such as birds or rats. Turtles are no longer sold in pet stores because they often carry the infection-producing bacteria *salmonella*. Rat-control measures have greatly reduced the incidence of vector-transmitted infections.

## Portal of Entry

The pathogen enters the body of a susceptible host through a portal of entry. Any of the *orifices* or openings of the body, such as those of the respiratory, gastrointestinal, and genitourinary tracts, can serve as portals of entry. Skin that is no longer intact is an important portal of entry. Even small skin abrasions may serve as portals of entry, as can larger wounds and decubitus ulcers (pressure sores).

## The Susceptible Host

The person in whom the organism is present is called the *host*. In some persons the number of pathogens never reaches a level high enough to cause an active infection but is harbored and can be passed along to someone else. Such a person is called a *carrier*. One famous carrier was a food handler, later nicknamed "Typhoid Mary," who caused numerous cases of typhoid fever in people to whom she served food but never developed the disease herself.

Not only must the strain be virulent to that person, but to become ill, the host must also be susceptible. Some people are more susceptible to infection than others, for one or a number of reasons. Age is a major factor. The very young lack the immune mechanisms developed later in life and may contract infections more easily. Elderly people who are weakened by the infirmities

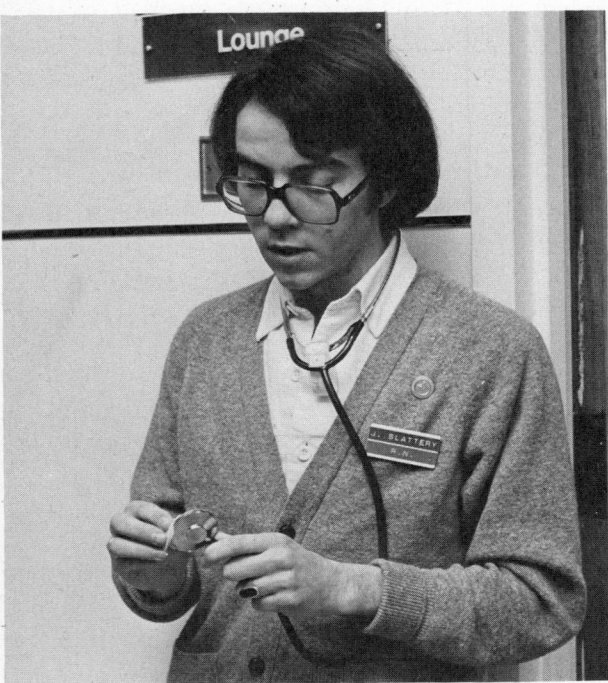

**Figure 11.2**
Equipment that is not cleaned between patients can transmit pathogens. (Russ Kinne/Danbury Hospital/Photo Researchers, Inc.)

of old age have a high incidence of infection. A person's general condition can affect susceptibility, and specific disabilities sometimes contribute to the occurrence of infection. For example, the patient whose bladder does not empty completely may be subject to repeated bladder infections. People who are adequately nourished are less prone to infection than the malnourished. The presence of another disease can allow an infection to develop, as in the case of the patient with chronic obstructive lung disease who contracts pneumonia. Certain medications encourage infection by suppressing the body's immune system. The large class of drugs known as steroids and some chemotherapeutic agents used to treat cancer are examples. The use of such drugs, in conjunction with the patient's already decreased ability to fight infection, make infection an ever-present danger. It is now known that stress also increases the risk of infection, possibly due to the interaction between physical and psychological coping (see Chapter 8).

Familiarity with the contributory factors to infection enables the nurse to determine which of a group of patients are at high risk and should be guarded most closely against infection. If a patient has more than one predisposing factor, the chance of infection multiplies accordingly. All patients should be protected from infection in the hospital, and some should be given special care.

# The Nurse and the Transfer of Infection

## Actions That Can Spread Infection

A clear understanding of the infection chain can prevent the lapses in technique whereby a nurse can unknowingly spread infection from one patient to another.

Let us follow the actions of a nurse caring for a patient with a wound infected with staphylococcus bacteria, informally known as a *staph infection*. Such wounds are usually dressed, both to protect the wound and to help prevent transfer of organisms. The *infectious agent*, the bacteria, is growing in a *reservoir* provided by the wound. Drainage of the wound provides a *portal of exit*, and the bed linen is thus contaminated. After dressing the wound, the nurse cuts the tape with bandage scissors, places the scissors momentarily on the bed, and then puts them in her uniform pocket. The infectious agent has thus carelessly been provided a *means of transmission*. The nurse's pocket is now also contaminated. The nurse then uses the same scissors to cut tape to secure a nasogastric tube to another patient's nose. The tape is placed in close proximity to the nostrils, where the pathogen finds a *portal of entry* through a small abrasion on the nasal mucous membrane. Since the patient is ill and thus a *susceptible host*, signs of infection shortly appear. Thus the actions of a nurse have been instrumental in spreading the infection from one patient to another.

## Actions That Can Prevent the Spread of Infection

By clearly understanding the infection chain, the nurse can identify and perform appropriate nursing actions designed to interrupt the transfer of infectious agents at each link (see Table 11.1). Knowledge of the characteristics of particular organisms is also crucial.

Nurses can encourage and take part in the surveillance of reservoirs of pathogens, both in the community and in the hospital. Supervision of housekeeping activities is often in order. Personal cleanliness is also crucial to reducing reservoirs of pathogens.

The nurse plays an important role in preventing the spread of infection at the portal of exit by properly handling and disposing of secretions and excretions. Special precautions must be taken in han-

## Table 11.1
### Interruption of the Infection Chain

| Link in the infection chain | Nursing action |
| --- | --- |
| Infectious agent | Knowledge of the characteristics of pathogens.<br>Sterilization techniques. |
| Reservoir | Surveillance of reservoirs in the hospital.<br>Handwashing and, when appropriate, surgical asepsis.<br>Personal cleanliness. |
| Transmission | Knowledge of pathogens' routes of transmission.<br>Routine medical asepsis.<br>Isolation, when appropriate. |
| Susceptible host | Knowledge of factors affecting susceptibility.<br>Identification of high-risk patients.<br>Knowledge of pharmacology relative to antibiotics.<br>Clean environment.<br>Support of body's own defenses. |
| Portal of entry | Precautions to ensure food and equipment free of contamination.<br>Measures to keep integument intact.<br>Sterile technique when skin is not intact and for invasive procedures. |
| Portal of exit | Proper handling of secretions and excreta.<br>Special precautions with needles and syringes, when appropriate.<br>Proper disposal of linens and equipment. |

dling needles and syringes if the patient's blood and tissues are thought to be contaminated. Linen and equipment are always disposed of in such a way as to avoid spreading pathogens to clean areas, health personnel, or other patients.

If a patient with a proven infection represents a potential hazard, isolation techniques can be initiated to prevent transmission of the organism. Refer to Module 22, "Isolation." The isolation routine must be conscientiously adhered to by all who care for the patient if it is to be effective. Interrupting the transmission of infectious agents is one of the nurse's most important functions in infection control.

In order to prevent the introduction of pathogens to the body through a portal of entry, the nurse must ensure that all food and equipment that comes into contact with the patient's body is free of contamination. A variety of nursing measures should be taken to protect any breaks in the skin or integument that may invite infection (see Chapter 19).

Using careful assessment, nurses can identify patients at high risk for infection as potentially susceptible hosts. Special attention should then be given to providing a clean environment and supporting the body's own defenses. If there is extreme need for protection, the patient can be isolated. Sometimes antibiotics and vaccines are employed *prophylactically* (preventively) as a safeguard against infection.

## Medical and Surgical Asepsis

Nurses and other health-care team members differentiate between two kinds of asepsis. *Medical asepsis* is designed to reduce the number of pathogens in an area and decrease the likelihood of their transfer. It is often referred to as *clean technique*. Microorganisms may continue to be present, but a threshold of safety has been established. The daily practice of hygiene falls into this category, as does the administration of oral medications, tube feedings, enemas, and many other treatments. The aim of *surgical asepsis*, on the other hand, is not simply to reduce the number of pathogens but to make the object or person free of all microorganisms. Also known as *sterile technique*, it is reserved primarily for such procedures as changing sterile dressings, performing catheterizations, and surgical procedures in the operating room.

## Methods of Maintaining Asepsis

The nurse plays a vital role in asepsis and must accept it as one of the responsibilities inherent in nursing. During a given day, a nurse's hands may touch numerous patients and a variety of equipment, perform various procedures, and attend to personal needs. Each such contact or task represents a potential transfer of microorganisms. Because a nurse must move quickly from patient to patient, it is easy to forget to wash one's hands properly between patients. It is hard but necessary for beginning student nurses to remember. Refer to Module 3, "Medical Asepsis."

## Handwashing

Handwashing, the primary barrier to infection, must always be the last task before going to the patient and the last performed upon leaving. The hands must be washed with flowing warm water over a sink (see Figure 11.3). A good soap or detergent is accompanied by brisk friction. If the hands are dirty, they are rinsed from the wrist downward, the elbows held high to allow microorganisms to be rinsed off the fingers into the sink. This procedure is called *medical asepsis handwashing*. If, on the other hand, the hands are uncontaminated and are being washed prior to sterile gloving or working within a sterile field, *surgical asepsis handwashing* is performed. The hands are thoroughly washed, sometimes with a brush, and rinsed with the elbows low over the sink so that the fingers are rinsed first and the water flows off the elbows into the sink. This procedure makes the fingers the cleanest part of the hands. Sterile gloves may be worn to protect the patient even further. For specific techniques, refer to Module 3, "Medical Asepsis," Module 36, "Sterile Technique," and Module 37, "Surgical Asepsis."

## Care of Linens

Linens fresh from the laundry are relatively free of pathogens due to the strong detergents and bleaches used in the laundering process and to the hot automatic ironers. In order to prevent contam-

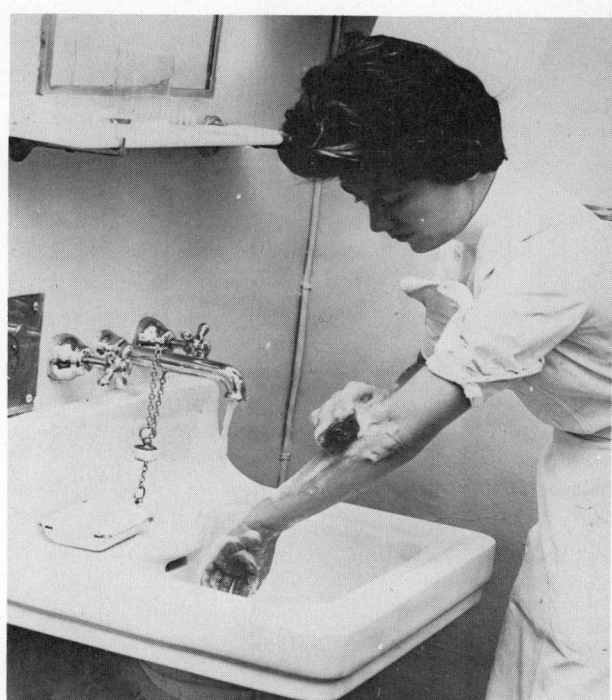

**Figure 11.3  Medical asepsis handwashing**
Lester V. Bergman & Assoc., Inc.

ination of linen, a clean place should be provided for them prior to use. Linen intended for one patient must not be put down at the bedside of another if the transfer of microorganisms from one patient to another is to be avoided. Neither clean nor dirty linen should be shaken; shaking spreads microorganisms by creating air currents. Linen dropped on the floor must be discarded, regardless of how wasteful this may seem, because the floor is usually heavily contaminated with dirt and the many organisms that settle out of the air. To prevent contamination of the nurse's uniform, used linen should be firmly bundled and carried away from the clothing. Hands are to be washed immediately after depositing soiled linens in the appropriate bag or hamper.

## Care of Equipment

In order to prevent cross-contamination, shared equipment must be appropriately cleaned before being moved from one patient to another. Thermometers, stethoscopes, and deep breathing machines fall into this category.

## Arrangement of the Patient's Unit

The physical arrangement of patients' units varies considerably. Some arrangements promote cleanliness better than others: the self-contained unit most effectively minimizes the likelihood of cross-contamination. Patients in these units have their own thermometers, bathing basins, emesis basins, bedpans, and urinals at their bedsides. These items are not shared with other patients. Even in self-contained units, however, nonhygienic practices that encourage the spread of pathogens can occur. Bedpans and urinals, for example, should never be placed on top of the bedside table or stand. They are kept, instead, in the compartments of the stand nearest the floor, where, because of gravity, the most microorganisms reside. The topmost drawers and compartments are reserved for the cleaner items used by the patient, such as toothbrushes, cosmetics, eyeglasses, and books. This arrangement allows microorganisms to settle downward from the cleanest to the dirtiest areas.

## Caring for More Than One Patient

When two or more patients request care simultaneously, it is best to determine which request is the most urgent and to respond to that patient first. After washing your hands, you may see to the needs of the second patient. This approach minimizes the spread of contamination from one patient to the other, which is very difficult to avoid if you are carrying objects to and from more than one patient.

## Methods of Killing or Reducing Infectious Agents

### Soap-and-Water Cleansing

Handwashing with soap and water is the single most effective measure against the spread of infection. Dishes and other objects that do not need to be sterile may be made medically aseptic by washing them with hot water and soap, using friction.

### Boiling

Boiling objects in water is rare now that more efficient methods are available. Boiling does eliminate many organisms, but sterility cannot be assured by boiling. If you ever practice abroad in a remote area where other methods are not available, you may have to resort to boiling as a method of cleansing.

### Ultraviolet Rays

Direct exposure to sunlight, of which less than 5 percent is ultraviolet rays (electromagnetic radiation), was once used in hospitals to promote antisepsis. Ultraviolet lamps were also used to reduce airborne pathogens, but because of the hazards of constant exposure to low-level radiation, this practice is now discouraged. Liquids cannot be sterilized by ultraviolet rays because the rays are neutralized when they are absorbed by the liquid. Extended exposure is necessary for nonliquid items to be made pathogen-free by this method.

### Antiseptics, Disinfectants, and Bactericidal Agents

Technically speaking, antiseptics, disinfectants, and bactericidal agents are distinguished by their differing effects on microorganisms. *Antiseptics* inhibit the growth of pathogens. These are usually mild enough to be used on the body. *Disinfectants* kill pathogenic microorganisms in addition to inhibiting their growth. Disinfectants are strong enough to be harmful to body tissue if applied directly. *Bactericidal agents* kill all microorganisms, pathogens and nonpathogens alike. In practice, the same agent may be used for all three purposes, depending on the strength of the solution. Clearly, all bactericidal agents are also disinfectants and antiseptics, and disinfectants are antiseptics as well. Thus, you may hear the terms used interchangeably.

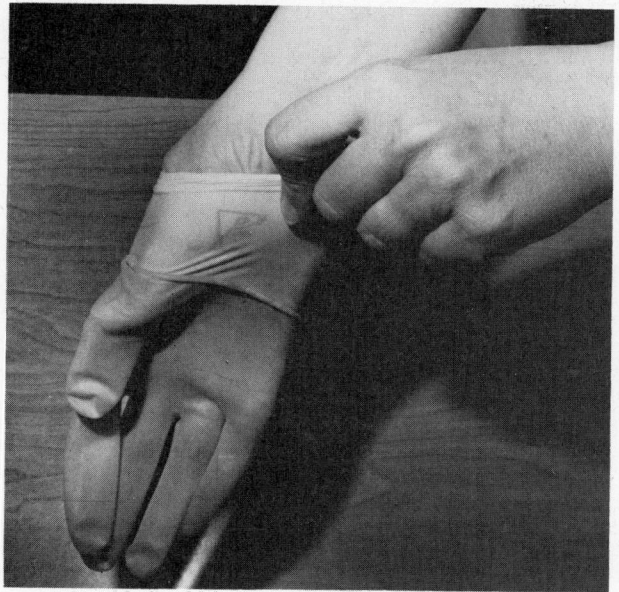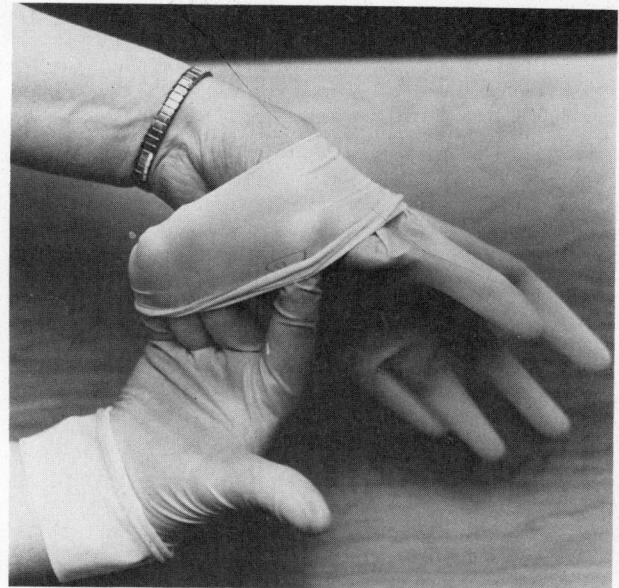

**Figure 11.4  Putting on sterile gloves**

*Left:* Pick up the right glove with your left hand, touching only the folded cuff, and put it on. *Right:* Grasp the left glove under the cuff and put it on. (Courtesy Ivan Ellis)

Alcohol- and iodine-based solutions are the antiseptics most commonly used on body tissue. Solutions containing phenol and formaldehyde are most commonly used in moderate strength for cleaning the hospital environment and in concentrated strength for soaking items used in direct patient care. Soaking times vary, depending on the agent and solution strength. You should become familiar with the solutions used in the facility in which you practice. Be sure that you understand the appropriate concentration as well as the type of solution to be used for a specific purpose.

## Autoclaving

*Autoclaving* is a process involving steaming under high pressure for a specific period of time. A special tape with which you should be familiar, is used on the wrappings. When the object being autoclaved has been exposed to the prescribed temperature and pressure long enough to render it sterile, the tape will show a particular marking, often but not always a black diagonal stripe. If a sterile packet is not designated sterile in some such way, it should be immediately returned for exchange. If autoclaved packets are not dry from the steam in the autoclave, they must be consid-

ered contaminated since dampness allows for the transfer of pathogens. Supplies and instruments for the operating room and delivery room and for use in sterile procedures are commonly autoclaved.

## Gas Sterilization

Gas sterilization as a method of destroying microorganisms is becoming increasingly widespread in hospitals. Exposure to the gas ethylene oxide kills all organisms. This method is particularly appropriate for delicate pieces of equipment that could be damaged by exposure to moisture or high temperatures.

## Aseptic Conscience

It is essential for you as a nurse to develop an *aseptic conscience,* or strict, rigid, and constant monitoring of your adherence to technique. Aseptic conscience can apply to both medical and surgical techniques. If, for example, you have begun to prepare a patient's tray for feeding and suddenly remember that you have not washed your hands since leaving the patient in the next bed, your aseptic conscience directs you to leave the tray and go directly to the nearest sink to wash, offering your patient at least partial protection from pathogens. If, while performing a catheterization, you inadvertently touch the surrounding unsterile drape with the tip of the catheter, your aseptic conscience tells you to secure another catheter and discard the first.

To remedy deviations from technique—and every nurse does at times fail to conform to technique—often takes time and is at best inconvenient. Though the patient will not always develop an infection as a result, the outcome cannot be predicted; the patient may be subjected to pain and further suffering due to infection resulting

from just such a lapse. A nurse who knows that medical or surgical technique has been broken and does not rectify it is a poor representative of the profession of nursing. If you observe a lapse in aseptic technique by someone else, you are equally obligated to see that the lapse is rectified to protect the patient. Simply commenting that contamination has taken place and offering to secure new equipment is usually sufficient. Sometimes the other person does not know such a lapse has occurred and will appreciate your intervention. Even if the nurse only *suspects* that technique has been deviated from, steps must be taken to correct the possible lapse. With regard to asepsis, nothing is assumed.

## Control of Infection With Drugs

Decreasing the number of pathogens within a host decreases the likelihood of a spread of infection. Although modern drugs are very effective in infection control, it is mistaken and often dangerous for nurses to believe that the need for precaution is lessened if a patient is on one of these medications.

There are several hundred such *antimicrobial* drugs, many simply variations of one another. Antimicrobials are subdivided into three large categories. The *sulfonamides*, low-cost synthetics usually given orally, have an antibacterial effect. The second group are the *antibiotics*, both natural and synthetic. Natural antibiotics are derived from yeasts and molds that have a destructive effect on the more virulent pathogens. The third group, the

*antifungals*, are agents used specifically against resistant fungal infections.

When you administer these preparations, it is your responsibility to know not only their actions but also their contraindications and side effects (see Chapter 10). Because these drugs have varied and potentially dangerous side effects, close observation is always in order. Besides watching for the allergic reactions that may occur in response to antimicrobials, you will be monitoring the effect of a particular drug on the patient and his or her progress. You might note, for example, a diminishing fever, lessening of the general malaise that frequently accompanies an infection, the improved appearance of an infected wound, or the patient's reported feeling of increased well-being.

## Nursing Care of Infection

Whether the patient has a generalized or a localized infection, the nurse can help fight the infection process. As we have noted, the ill person needs adequate rest, and an ill person with an infection needs additional sleep and rest. Providing for such rest sometimes requires ingenious

planning of nursing care. Because infection makes increased demands on the body, the diet must not be deficient. Intake of protein and carbohydrates is especially important: protein helps in healing damaged tissue and carbohydrates serve to meet the increased metabolic requirements caused by infection. High fluid intake prevents dehydration resulting from fever and aids in the excretion of toxins (poisonous protein substances produced by pathogens) from the body (see Chapter 21).

Meticulous hygiene should be observed when caring for a patient suffering from an infection. Such patients are often diaphoretic (perspiring) due to fever, which necessitates frequent bathing. General malaise may prevent the patient from performing adequate self-hygiene. Infection can also cause foul odors, unpleasant to the patient and the staff alike, which can be alleviated by good hygiene. For example, the patient with a *suppurating* (pus-discharging) wound needs frequent dressing changes and cleansing of the wound area (only, however, on the physician's order). The patient suffering a severe throat infection needs extra oral care.

Finally, the patient with an infection needs emotional support from the nurse. Infection is an assault on the body, psychologically as well as physically. It is often interpreted by the patient to mean that things are not going well or as planned. Infection is frequently called a *complication*, which understandably makes the patient anxious. An explanation of the vigorous efforts being made to treat and control the infection usually serves to reassure the patient.

## Isolation

When a patient is known to have an infection, or to be especially susceptible to infection, special precautions are taken to separate him or her from other patients. These precautions are called *isolation* technique.

In most settings the physician determines the type of isolation to be employed and the length of time it is to last. The presence of an infection is determined by examining the laboratory findings, which indicate the type of organism or pathogen present, its virulence, and, with knowledge of microbiology, its route of transmission. In such cases the goal of isolation is to protect others from infection. If the patient has a condition that lessens resistance to infection, such as severe burns or leukemia, the physician will choose protective isolation until the patient's own resistance becomes adequate.

If assessment leads you to conclude that a patient is either infectious or in need of special protection from infection, you may make a decision to isolate the patient appropriately and then consult the physician. Isolation procedure can always be discontinued if it proves unnecessary.

### Types of Isolation

Isolation has two possible purposes: to protect the environment from the pathogens infecting the patient or to prevent pathogens from infecting the patient. There are four types of isolation designed to protect others from the pathogens infecting the patient: *strict isolation, respiratory isolation, wound and skin precautions,* and *enteric isolation*. Protecting the patient is called *protective isolation* or *reverse isolation*. The requirements of the various types of isolation are listed in Table 11.2.

### Strict Isolation

*Strict isolation* is undertaken to restrict pathogens that may be transmitted through the air or by contact. The patient is placed in a private room free of all unnecessary equipment and furniture. The door is kept closed. Gowns and masks must be worn by all individuals, including visitors, entering the room. Hands are washed at a sink within the room on entering and leaving. Depending on the virulence of the organism, gloves may be required of all persons entering the room and discarded inside the room before leaving, or worn only for dressing changes and direct contact.

All linens and other articles used in the room must be *double-bagged* and clearly marked as contaminated, whether they are to be thrown away or returned to another department in the hospital. Double-bagging is performed by two people, the nurse who has been caring for the patient and a

Table 11.2
**Requirements of Isolation**

| | Strict isolation | Respiratory isolation | Wound and skin precautions | Enteric isolation | Protective isolation |
|---|---|---|---|---|---|
| **Route of transmission** | Air and contact | Air | Contact | Contact | Air and contact |
| **Room assignment** | Private with door closed | Private with door closed | Private is desirable | Private if a child | Private with door closed |
| **Gowns** | Worn by all | Unnecessary | Worn by all who have direct contact | Worn by all who have direct contact | Worn by all |
| **Masks** | Worn by all | Worn by all | Unnecessary except when changing dressings | Unnecessary | Worn by all |
| **Hands** | Washed by all on entering and leaving room | Washed by all on entering and leaving room | Washed by all on entering and leaving room | Washed by all on entering and leaving room | Washed by all on entering and leaving room |
| **Gloves** | Worn by all | Unnecessary | Worn by all who have direct contact with dressings | Worn by all who have direct contact | Worn by all who have direct contact |
| **Articles** | All articles must be wrapped or discarded with care | Precautions for those with secretions | Special handling of linens, dressings, and instruments | Special handling of articles contaminated with urine or feces | All articles entering room must be as clean as possible; sterile items often required |

"clean" partner, who stands outside the isolated unit with a bag of appropriate size for the object to be double-bagged (see Figure 11.5). By cuffing this bag and placing the hands safely under the cuffing, the partner prepares to receive the contaminated bag. The nurse closes the contaminated bag and drops it directly into the outer bag, making sure that it does not open. The partner then folds over the top of the outer bag, closes it securely, and disposes of the parcel. The linen outer bags are usually clearly marked with a wide red stripe of fabric; if not so marked, you can mark them yourself by pinning on a note or labeled tape. Trays or dishes, if not disposable, can also be double-bagged. In fact, double-bagging is a safe way of transporting many items. Specimens can be placed in small plastic bags for transport to the laboratory. It is the responsibility of health care workers to protect one another, as well as patients, from infection. Only an unsafe practitioner knowingly allows contaminated materials to be passed unmarked to others. Even trash is double-bagged for this reason.

## Respiratory Isolation

*Respiratory isolation* is designed to control pathogens that are exclusively airborne. Again, the patient is housed in a private room with a closed door. Gowns and gloves are not needed, but masks are a necessity and should be discarded on leaving the room. Hands are washed on entering and leaving. Any article contaminated with secretions must be carefully disinfected or double-bagged for disposition. Individuals with known respiratory ailments or predispositions should be discouraged from visiting, and all visitors should be educated appropriately.

## Enteric Isolation

*Enteric isolation* is undertaken when the pathogen is transmitted by direct contact and the mode of transmission is the gastrointestinal system. The physician writes such an order. A private room is desirable for adults and a necessity for children because of the difficulty of controlling children's desire to socialize. Gowns and gloves are worn by all those who have direct contact with the patient, but masks are not necessary. Hands are carefully washed when entering and leaving the room. Linen should be double-bagged, and any items contaminated with urine, feces, or vomitus must be carefully discarded or disinfected. The substances themselves should be disposed of in an adjoining private toilet facility. (Urine is considered contaminated because of its proximity to the intestinal tract and the rectum.)

## Wound and Skin Precautions

*Wound and skin precautions,* taken if there are microorganisms in a wound that may be spread by contact, do not require the patient to be isolated; however, a private room is desirable. This procedure is sometimes called *dressing isolation.* Gowns must be worn when in direct contact with the patient, and gloves are mandatory when in direct contact with the infected area. Hands are always washed on entering and leaving the room. Instruments, linen, and dressings are double-bagged to be sent to central supply or the laundry or discarded.

## Protective Isolation

*Protective isolation,* sometimes called *reverse isolation,* requires the practices outlined above and others as well. The nurse garbs to protect the patient from any pathogens that could be carried on the nurse's body or clothing. Cloth boots over the nurse's shoes may be required. Any object introduced into the room is considered a potential hazard to the patient. For example, a newspaper taken from inside the stack at the newsstand is likely to be freer of pathogens than the one on the top. In some facilities, food trays are prepared and handled by a single worker to prevent cross-contamination of food. Bottled or canned beverages are poured directly into paper containers held by the nurse just inside the door of the room or the containers themselves are sponged with hot water and soap or alcohol. Paperback books and magazines must be chosen with care from the newsstand to ensure that they are clean (hardback

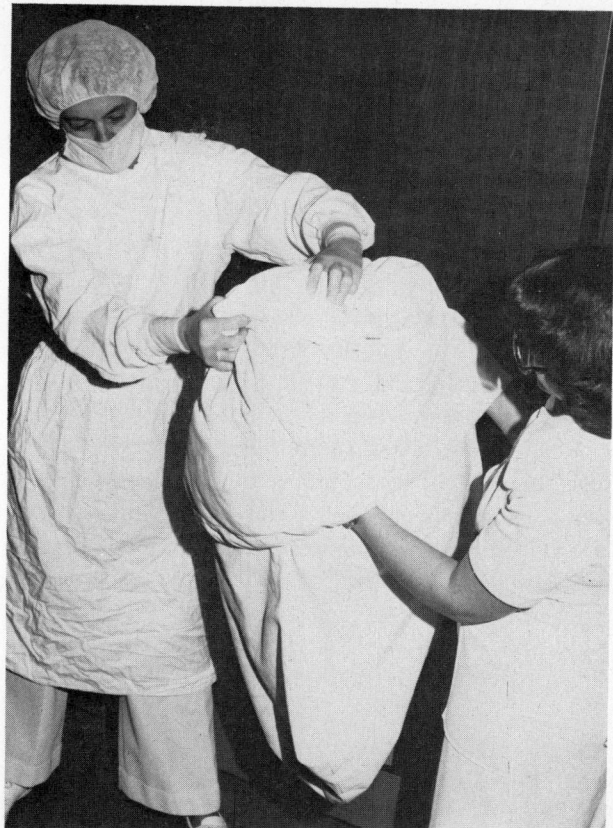

**Figure 11.5 Double-bagging**
Courtesy Ivan Ellis

books are discouraged because they are difficult to clean). The nurse's wristwatch is not considered clean, and should be removed, pinned under the gown, or carried in a clean plastic bag. Studies have shown that pathogen growth is minimal on metal watchbands, due to the properties of the metal, but extensive on plastic or cloth bands. Money and mail envelopes can also carry harmful pathogens: the patient's money should be kept at the nursing station to be spent on the patient's behalf when requested, and only the contents of envelopes should be given to the patient.

Because the room used for protective isolation is considered clean, all items and equipment used there can be safely removed and disposed of or cleaned in the usual manner. Double-bagging is not necessary.

Some of the practices described above will seem extreme, and not all will be employed in every case. Individual need determines how stringent isolation must be. It is important to keep in mind the purpose of these measures: the patient for whom an infection could prove fatal needs every protection.

Specialized medical centers that perform bone-marrow transplants and similar procedures have special laminar air-flow rooms to protect patients who are at extremely high risk of infection. Specially filtered air enters the closed room through one vent, flows through the room, and exits at another vent. Thus the air is constantly circulating and as free of contaminants as possible. Pharmacists often mix and process intravenous medications under laminar air-flow hoods in order to minimize contamination.

Research to evaluate the need for and effectiveness of protective isolation is underway. In all types of isolation, stringent and conscientious handwashing remains the single most effective measure.

## Psychological Isolation

Because communication is difficult through masks, and because of the inconvenience of garbing for isolation, the isolated patient rarely receives as much attention and interchange as nonisolated patients. Holding the hand of a severely ill or depressed patient through a glove is not a wholly satisfying experience for either nurse or patient. As a result, such patients can become irritable, restless, and depressed.

The nurse can help minimize the emotional and sensory deprivation the isolated patient experiences by spending extra time with the patient, in addition to the time devoted to physical care. Some ideas for creative intervention are offered in Module 22, "Isolation."

The patient's self-concept frequently suffers as a result of being considered infectious. Psychological support for the patient throughout this difficult experience is an essential part of total care. Care providers sometimes carelessly use the words "dirty" or "contaminated" when referring to areas of isolation. A patient who overhears such a remark may construe it to mean that he or she is also dirty and a danger to others. Comments of this kind should thus be studiously avoided.

# The Role of the Nurse in Isolation Technique

The nurse plays a definitive role in isolation technique. You must understand causes of infection as thoroughly as the physician so that you will know the rationale for specific practices and be able to explain it to visitors and other personnel. All isolation techniques are designed to create barriers that interrupt the transmission of disease.

*Isolation technique is only as effective as the least careful person.* Therefore, everyone having any contact whatsoever with the patient, including not only the health-care team but also the family, visitors, the chaplain, the newspaper deliverer, the housekeeper, the librarian, and others, must be fully instructed on the necessary routine and required to observe it.

It is essential that isolation rooms be unmistakably marked for all to see. In most hospitals, cards are affixed to the door of the room to identify the type of isolation in effect. Standardized cards are available from the National Center for Disease Control in Atlanta, Georgia. Alternatively, plain white cards, cards color-coded for various types of isolation, cards with complete instructions and cards simply labeled "Isolation" are used. It may be necessary for you to make your own sign; if so, it is wise to print in large letters the type of isolation being observed and, beneath it, the five or six steps for doing so. Sometimes an additional sign is posted asking all visitors to report to the nurses' station for instructions. This is a particularly good idea since it gives the nurse an opportunity to instruct visitors in isolation techniques as well as to make contact with the family and friends of the patient.

Regardless of the type of infection or isolation, a small stand containing all the items needed to carry out effective isolation technique is usually placed outside the room. It may contain gowns, masks, protective caps, gloves, or even cloth boots. Equipment needed by the patient, such as thermometers, blood-pressure cuffs, materials for hygiene, and other items can be kept in the room itself. A laundry hamper is kept in the room.

Watches and other jewelry should be removed when caring for a patient in isolation since path-ogens can be carried in crevices and even under tight-fitting wedding bands. For the same reason, fingernails should be closely trimmed and meticulously clean.

## Staff and Visitor Acceptance of Isolation

Patients do not enjoy being isolated. Nor do the staff and visitors derive pleasure from participating in isolation practices, which are inconvenient, bothersome, and at times uncomfortable. A visitor may, in frustration, pull the mask below the nose or remove a cap he or she construes as looking silly. It is then up to you to remind the visitor of the agreed-on precautions and to enforce them kindly but firmly.

## Community Efforts to Control Infection

### Hospitals

In addition to their efforts at infection control internally, hospitals also participate in control of infection in the surrounding community. In order to be accredited by the Joint Commission on Accreditation of Hospitals (JCAH), every hospital must have an active infection-control committee, usually chaired by a physician or an infection-control nurse. The infection-control nurse gathers data on all patients in the hospital who have infections, reports such data to other agencies (such as the public health department), conducts in-service education for hospital staff members, and serves as a resource person with regard to infection control. Infection control is a growing specialty area for nurses. The infection-control committee assists in the surveillance of infections within the hospital by reviewing data, and it makes policy and reviews and recommends procedures related to infection control.

### Counties

Counties compile statistics on infectious diseases occurring within their jurisdiction. Outbreaks of influenza, measles, and other infections are reported by counties to the state. If a particular infection is confined to a single county, the county infection-control physician may outline prevention and treatment for inhabitants of the county.

### States

Immunization programs, particularly for schoolchildren, are mandated by many states; some states prohibit children from attending school unless they have received prescribed immunizations. Measles has recently been added to the mandatory immunization laws of several states.

### The National Center for Disease Control

The National Center for Disease Control (CDC) in Atlanta, Georgia, funded by the federal government, acts in an advisory capacity to any individual or group requesting information. The CDC has just completed a computerized surveillance study of nosocomial infections, which will lead to further research. The CDC also distributes publications regarding infection control and treatment.

## The World Health Organization

The World Health Organization (WHO), a subsidiary of the United Nations, promotes the control of infection internationally. The recent massive increase in international travel has made the transfer of disease a problem with worldwide implications. The WHO has been studying the spread of influenza and other infectious diseases among nations. Smallpox, a devastating disease with no known treatment, was until recently widespread throughout the populated areas of the world. Through the cooperative efforts of the WHO and other international health-care organizations smallpox has been effectively eradicated.

# Conclusion

The patient with an infection has multiple problems, involving hygiene, threatened health status, and the burden of being a potential threat to others in the environment. The patient being protected from infection feels equally burdened. The nurse who knows both the theory and the skills of infection treatment and control can be extremely helpful to patients in both situations. It is rewarding to the nurse to grasp the relationship between the patient and the environment and to perform nursing actions that combat infection. Isolation is a unique situation in which care planning and nursing skills evolve directly from an understanding of the invisible world of microorganisms.

infectious agent
isolation
  enteric
  protective
  respiratory
  reverse
  strict
  wound and skin
    precautions
means of transmission
microorganisms
normal flora
nosocomial
orifice
parasitic worms
pathogen

portal of entry
portal of exit
precaution
prophylactic
protozoa
reservoir
spore
staph infection
sterile technique
sulfonamide
suppurating
susceptible host
vectors
vehicle
virulent
virus

## Study Terms

aerobic
airborne
anaerobic
antibiotic
antifungal
antimicrobial
antiseptic
asepsis
  medical asepsis
  surgical asepsis
aseptic conscience
autoclaving
bacteria
bactericidal
barrier

carrier
clean technique
complication
contact
direct contact
disinfectant
dressing isolation
droplet
double-bagging
fungus
handwashing
helminthic
host
indirect contact
infection

## Learning Activities

1. Examine each of the isolation cards used at your clinical facility.
2. Visit the laundry, kitchen, and medical laboratory of the facility to which you are assigned to observe treatment of contaminated articles.
3. Using the infection chain as a diagram, illustrate the transmission of each type of pathogen in respiratory, enteric, wound, and reverse isolation.
4. When caring for a patient with an infection, note on the nursing care plan special precautions and nursing actions that might be taken.
5. Role-play with another student: a nurse gives instructions on garbing for strict isolation to a visitor. Include the rationale for isolation garb.

## Relevant Sections in
## Modules for Basic Nursing Skills

| Volume 1 | Module |
|---|---|
| Medical Asepsis | 3 |
| Isolation | 22 |
| **Volume 2** | |
| Sterile Technique | 36 |
| Surgical Asepsis: Scrubbing, Gowning, and Gloving | 37 |
| Sterile Dressings | 40 |

## References

American Nurses Association, Division on Medical-Surgical Nursing. *Practice Draft: The Nurse and Infection Control.* Kansas City: ANA, 1976.

Aspinwall, Mary Jo. "Scoring Against Nosocomial Infections." *Nursing '78* 8 (October 1978): 1704–1707.

Birum, L. H., *et al.* "Catheter Plugs as a Source of Infection." *American Journal of Nursing* 71 (November 1971): 2150–2152.

Bullough, B. "When Should Isolation Stop?" *American Journal of Nursing* 72 (April 1972): 733.

Castle, M. "Isolation: Precise Procedures for Better Protection." *Nursing '75* 5 (May 1975): 50–57.

Chavigny, K. H. "Nurse Epidemiologist in the Hospital." *American Journal of Nursing* 75 (April 1975): 638–642.

DeGroot, J., and Kunin, C. M. "Indwelling Catheters." *American Journal of Nursing* 75 (March 1975): 448–449.

Donaldson, D. "Computer-Taught Epidemiology." *Nursing Outlook* 24 (December 1976): 749–751.

Fox, M. K.; Langner, S. B.; and Wells, R. W. "How Good Are Handwashing Practices?" *American Journal of Nursing* 74 (September 1974): 1676–1678.

Gallucci, Betty B., and Reheir, Christine E. "Infection, Nutrition and the Compromised Patient." *Clinical Nursing: Infection Control* 1 (July 1979): 23–33.

Hardy, C. S. "Infection Control: What Can One Nurse Do?" *Nursing '73* 3 (March 1973): 18–24.

"Historical Look at Infection." *Point of View/Ethicon* (1977): 8–9.

Jenny, J. "What You Should Be Doing About Infection Control." *Nursing '76* 6 (June 1976): 78–79.

Larson, Elaine. "Hands: the Healers and Killers." *Clinical Nursing: Infection Control* 1 (July 1979): 59–65.

Osborne, P. H. "Developing and Maintaining an Infection Control Program." *Supervisor Nurse* 8 (December 1977): 16–18.

Palakanetz, Sandra. "Nosocomial Infections: The Hidden Cost in Health Care." *Hospitals* 32 (16 August 1978): 101.

Turner, J. G. "The Nurse Epidemiologist: Selection and Preparation." *Supervisor Nurse* 9 (April 1978): 33–41.

U.S. Department of Health, Education and Welfare, National Center for Disease Control. *Isolation Techniques for Use in Hospitals.* Washington, D.C.: Government Printing Office, 1975.

U.S. Department of Health, Education and Welfare, National Center for Disease Control. *Outline for Surveillance and Control of Nosocomial Infections.* Washington, D.C.: Government Printing Office, 1974.

# Chapter 12
# Communication

To communicate is, according to the dictionary, "to make known." This is precisely what communication is all about: making oneself and one's ideas, thoughts, and feelings known to another individual. Effective communication requires both interest and skill. The skill can be learned; the interest must come from within you.

Communication is critical to every phase of the nursing process. Assessment requires effective communication in order to gather accurate and comprehensive information about a patient. Planning involves communicating with other members of the health-care team and with the patient and family. Explaining your actions to the patient is an ongoing component of direct care. It may also prove necessary to teach self-care skills or to help the patient cope with emotional problems accompanying illness. Finally, evaluating the effectiveness of nursing care involves communicating with all those who provide care as well as with the patient.

Thus communication has many different purposes for the nurse. The effectiveness of any given communication is enhanced by the use of skills and techniques appropriate to its purpose. Some skills are valuable in all situations; a few are valuable in one setting or for one purpose but not others. This chapter will examine how communication skills and techniques can be incorporated into your nursing care.

## The Nature of an Interaction

*Interaction* is communication between two individuals. The word is used in two senses, to describe both a particular episode of communication, such as a conversation, and an ongoing relationship. A single interaction may be seen as having three variables: the sender, the message, and the receiver.

### Variables in an Interaction

The *sender* is the person trying to communicate. Many factors about the sender affect the interaction. When you are the sender, your skill will facilitate the interaction. When the other person is the sender, awareness of his or her degree of verbal skill will help you bridge difficulties in communication.

The *message* is that which is being communicated by the interaction. The message may or may not be clear in the mind of the sender. If you are the sender, you should clearly define your message for yourself in order to communicate it effectively. If the other person is the sender, your awareness that the message may be unclear to him or her should prompt you to focus all your attention on understanding it. Sometimes a message is mixed, which means that conflicting ideas and/or feelings are being communicated simultaneously. A mixed message may make sound decisions impossible without more information.

The *receiver* is the person trying to understand the message. The receiver's skill also contributes to the effectiveness of the interaction. The receiver must *listen*. Though this sounds simple, it may not be. It is very easy for the receiver to think about what he or she will say next, rather than listening to the sender. The receiver must also *observe*: the message is conveyed not only in words but also in the behavior of the sender. The third component of skillful receiving is *attending*—that is, thinking about the words you hear and the behavior you observe. To understand the message fully, you need to attend closely to the interaction.

*Perception* is understanding of, and insight into, the message on the part of the receiver. Accurate perception of the message is the desired result of the interaction. In addition to the message itself, perception is influenced by the receiver's prior experience, relationship with the sender, and feelings about the interaction. When trust exists between sender and receiver and when previous efforts of communication have been successful, perception is enhanced.

Having perceived the message, the receiver responds to the communication. The interaction is not complete until the receiver responds. The roles

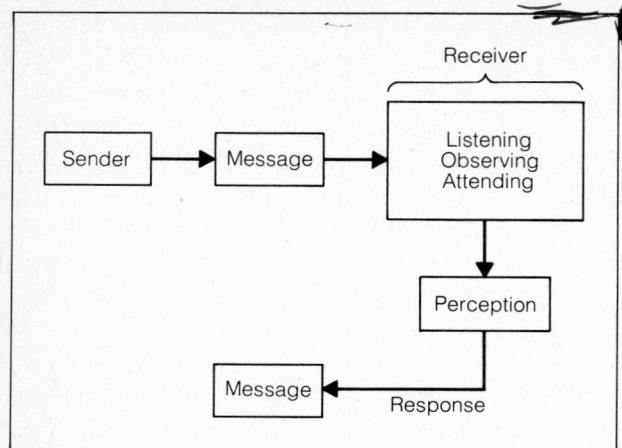

**Figure 12.1   The interaction**

of sender and receiver alternate within a single conversation.

The process of *validation* is crucial to all communication. Validation is verifying your perception of the message by telling the sender what you understand him or her to be saying and asking if you are correct. You may validate your perception by asking a specific question or by restating what you understood. Until you have validated a message, do not assume that you received it as the sender intended.

## Phases of an Interaction

A long-term interaction is not a static phenomenon but a changing, growing process that occurs between two people. Experts in the field of communication have subdivided interaction into three phases: the introductory phase, the working phase, and the termination phase (see Exhibit 12.1). The length of each phase depends on the interaction and its purpose.

### The Introductory Phase

The introductory phase of an interaction establishes the relationship between the participants. It may involve the exchange of factual information about both people and the purpose of the interaction. During this phase, the participants work out what the nature of their relationship will be and develop mutual trust. Until trust is well es-

**Exhibit 12.1**
**The Phases of an Interaction**

| Phase | Purpose |
|---|---|
| 1. Introductory | Establishing the relationship |
| 2. Working | Pursuing the relationship's goals |
| 3. Termination | Ending the relationship |

tablished, only superficial and factual communication can occur.

Trust is established by being *genuine*—that is, being authentically yourself and not adopting a facade. Focusing on the other person promotes trust, as does willingness to treat the other person's concerns as foremost. In nursing, a key to establishing trust is meeting the other person's immediate perceived needs before pursuing your own agenda. The maintenance of appropriate confidentiality is also critical to trust: if you will be sharing information you acquire from the interaction with others on the health-care team, you must make this clear to the other person at the outset so that he or she does not feel confidentiality was betrayed. Though the relationship is established during the introductory phase, it will continue to grow and change throughout the lifetime of the interaction.

### The Working Phase

The working phase of the interaction is the period during which its purposes are accomplished. This phase varies in length depending on those purposes, which might include teaching, therapy, or coordination of care.

### The Termination Phase

The termination phase is the end of the interaction. Ideally, the patient is prepared for termination from the beginning by knowing the purpose of the interaction and its expected goal. However, if the relationship is a meaningful one, termination can be difficult even when it is expected and prepared for. If it is not adequately prepared for, termination can be detrimental to the vulnerable patient and/or family. It is helpful to review the interaction's purpose and expected end throughout its duration, especially if it lasts a long time. The actual termination should be a summing-up: the purpose of the interaction is reviewed, and the work, accomplishments, and conclusions summarized. Leave-taking is formal recognition that the interaction or relationship is at an end. A short-term interaction may end with a brief farewell and acknowledgment that the interaction is over. If the relationship has been prolonged, bringing it to a smooth conclusion may require several sessions.

## Methods of Communicating Messages

Meaning is conveyed in a variety of ways, both verbal (using words) and nonverbal (using gestures and facial expressions). Understanding how these two aspects of communication can be varied to clarify the transmission of an intended message will help you be a more effective nurse.

### Using Verbal Communication

Verbal communication consists of all the words people exchange. Words can be a source of considerable confusion: you can probably recall becoming involved in an argument only to discover that you and your adversary differed only over the meanings of terms, not basic ideas. In addition to the words themselves, *pacing* and *voice tone* significantly affect the receiver's perception of verbal messages. Finally, it is important to choose communication techniques capable of accomplishing the purpose you have in mind.

### Language Usage

Words have different meanings to different people. The word "expensive," for example, means something very different to a welfare recipient than it does to a surgeon. Similarly, two people who both answer "fine" when asked how they feel may be in very different states of mind and health.

Furthermore, people's vocabularies vary a great deal. Technical words and abbreviations are like a foreign language to many patients. As a nursing student, you undoubtedly know how it feels not to understand all the technical terms being used around you.

It is important to take into account the patient's educational level, degree of sophistication, and fluency in English when choosing your words. Because it is crucial to communicate with patients, even if they speak little or no English, many facilities have developed resource lists of people on the hospital staff or in the community who are willing to serve as translators. If such a list does not exist in your facility, you might promote the development of one.

The use of volunteer translators can, however, create problems. The translator may not know technical terms in English or the other language, which can lead to incomplete or inaccurate communication. Thus health-care facilities that treat many patients who speak a particular language often employ a professional translator, who thus acquires familiarity with the health-care setting and with technical terminology.

In general, clarity, brevity, and simplicity are desirable. *Clarity* involves choosing words whose meaning is clear and unmistakable. *Brevity* means presenting your message briefly and without unnecessary digressions, so as to avoid confusion about what is important and what is less so. *Simplicity* involves choosing simple, commonly used words in preference to technical or seldom-encountered terms.

### Pacing

Pacing is the rate at which you speak. It is a common error to forget to pause between statements or questions to allow the receiver time to process the message and formulate a response.

## Voice Tone

Voice tone can change the meaning of words: something said in a loud voice can mean something entirely different than the same thing said softly. Voice tone also expresses urgency, impatience, sarcasm, condescension, anger, and many other attitudes and emotions; most people are quick to perceive such feelings, though they may not realize they are doing so.

When speaking to a person with a hearing impairment, it is important to speak not only loud enough but also slowly and clearly. Avoid mumbling. Using lower tones and speaking more slowly will assist the hearing impaired person to hear more clearly.

## Techniques of Verbal Communication

A large repertoire of communication techniques, and skill at using them, is extremely valuable in nursing. It is also important to recognize and work at avoiding responses that tend to interfere with communication.

## Asking Questions

It is appropriate to ask a patient questions only if you need the information to assess his or her problems and plan nursing care. You have an obligation to let the patient know the purpose of your questions and the uses that will be made of the answers. If you will be sharing the information you gain with others on the health-care team, you should say so before you ask any questions. If, for example, you will share the information you acquire from an interview with your instructor, you might say, "My instructor will review my interview with me to help me plan care." If you are recording the answers to your questions on the nursing record, the fact that you are doing so conveys the message that the information will be shared.

When specific information is needed in order to plan and provide care, you will need to ask specific questions. Such questions are of two types: open-ended and closed. *Open-ended* questions allow for the other person to respond in detail; an example is "What are your plans for managing your care after discharge?" The newspaper reporter's traditional litany—who, what, where, when, and how—may be of value to you in posing open-ended questions. Questions that can be answered with a brief yes or no are called *closed questions*; an example is "Will you have help when you go home?"

By deciding whether or not you want a detailed answer, you can determine when to use each kind of question. In general, open-ended questions are far more useful. Closed questions are essential when the person is unable to speak but capable of nodding or shaking the head. Such questions need to be planned very carefully in order to gain the necessary information without "putting words in the patient's mouth."

Plan your questions to proceed from the general to the specific in a branching manner. Doing so will help the patient concentrate and will demonstrate that your questions are purposeful. For example:

**Nurse:** What are your plans for care after you're discharged?
**Patient:** Well, I'm not sure. Guess I haven't thought much about it.
**Nurse:** Your physician said you should limit your activity. What is your understanding of what that means?
**Patient:** I believe he said something about not doing any housework or cooking.
**Nurse:** How will you arrange for meals?

If you have no specific questions in mind, but wish instead to explore the patient's feelings, worries, or uncertainties, direct questions may be of less value than facilitating responses.

## Facilitating Responses

Responses that encourage the other person to communicate with you are called *facilitating responses*. Though they are occasionally called "therapeutic techniques," we believe it is the entire interaction that is therapeutic, not merely a particular statement or response. Facilitating responses are tools whose purpose is to encourage and support the other person in communicating and personal problem-solving. Use of facilitating techniques is based on belief in the other person's integrity, worth, and ability to solve his or her own problems. Only if you believe in this concept will you be able to act as a facilitator and not try to be the patient's problem-solver.

Facilitating responses may be subdivided into three categories: nondirective comments, exploratory responses, and aids to decision making. Though each has a purpose, nondirective comments are generally the most useful.

*Nondirective comments* encourage the other person to continue talking in the same vein. Comments such as "yes . . .," "go on . . . ," and "mm-hmmm" indicate that you are attending to what is being said and demonstrate willingness to continue listening. Such comments are called *general leads*. Another type of nondirective response is *reflecting*, or simply repeating the patient's exact words in the form of a question. The patient says, for example, "I just can't stand staying in bed any longer!" and the nurse replies, "You can't stand staying in bed any longer?" This response allows the patient to hear what he or she is saying and to think about it. Overuse of this technique can, however, make the patient uncomfortable and self-conscious. A third type of nondirective response is *restating*, or repeating the other person's statement in different words. This technique helps the other person recognize the message that is being received. If, for example, the patient says, "I need a stronger sleeping pill," the nurse may reply, "Your present sleeping pill isn't effective?"

*Exploratory responses* help encourage the other person to examine a situation more completely. Placing events in *time sequence,* for example, might be promoted by asking, "Was that before or after . . . ?" or "What happened next?" *Focusing* the conversation involves identifying an important statement and pursuing it: "You said your brother is helpful. Could you explain more about that?" *Encouraging comparisons* may help the other person weigh and evaluate the significance of something: "Does this feel like . . . ?" *Seeking clarification* is asking for a clearer explanation of something that has been said: "I don't quite understand what you

mean. Could you explain more fully?" *Validating,* which we have already mentioned, involves identifying what you believe the other person is trying to say and asking whether you are correct: "Do you mean . . . ?"

*Aids to decision making* are responses that encourage the other person to make informed decisions. One way to do so is by serving as a *resource,* providing information or directing the patient to

---

Exhibit 12.2
**Responses That Facilitate Communication**

| Response | Example |
|---|---|
| **Nondirective comments** | |
| General leads | "Yes," "Go on," "mm-hmmm." |
| Reflecting | Patient: "I'm really scared." |
| | Nurse: "You're really scared?" |
| Restating | Patient: "I just can't seem to sit still." |
| | Nurse: "You're feeling nervous?" |
| **Exploratory responses** | |
| Placing events in time sequence | "When did that happen?" |
| | "Was this before or after . . . ?" |
| Encouraging comparisons | "Was this similar to . . . ?" |
| | "Are there differences this time?" |
| Focusing | "You said. . . . Could you explain that more fully?" "This seems to be an important point." |
| Seeking clarification | "What would you say is the main concern?" |
| Validating | "What I understand from what you said is. . . . Is that correct?" |
| **Aids to decision making** | |
| Serving as a resource | "Children under 14 can visit if special arrangements are made." |
| Pointing out information | "Have you considered . . . ?" |
| Reviewing | "Now you said the main concerns are. . . ." |
| Considering consequences | "If you do . . . , what might happen?" |
| Encouraging formulation of a plan | "What do you think you might do?" |

an appropriate source of information. Information-giving is appropriate only when the patient has indicated need for or interest in such information. If such a need is not apparent to the patient, information-giving might be construed as interfering or directive. In such a situation, *pointing out information* that might be of help lets the other person know that certain information is available, but allows him or her to decide whether to pursue it. *Reviewing* is helping to summarize what has been said, consider diverse approaches, and organize ideas. It is sometimes appropriate to encourage the patient to *consider the consequences* of proposed plans of action. When doing so, let the patient imagine and work out all the possible consequences; this process promotes independence and self-direction. The final step is encouraging *formulation of a plan*. This might involve constructing a time frame: "What do you think you might do first?" "What would come next?" You can encourage the patient to be specific in planning by saying, "Can you give me an example of what you plan to say?" or "Would you explain how you will go about that?" It is important to keep in mind that your role is to encourage the patient to formulate a plan; you must neither formulate a plan for the patient nor encourage him or her to adopt your plan.

## Blocking Responses

Responses that hinder communication, express lack of interest in what the patient has to say, or undermine his or her sense of adequacy are called *blocking responses*. A single blocking response will not usually destroy the effectiveness of an interaction, but many blocking responses will tend to make communication shallower, less sharing, and less effective at promoting problem-solving.

*Stereotyped comments*—overused, automatic phrases—are probably the commonest blocking responses. People tend to interpret the use of stereotyped comments as indicating lack of interest, condescension, or evasion. *Clichés* like "Things will be better tomorrow" and "Keep a stiff upper lip" are almost always perceived as unfelt and insincere. *Belittling* is the use of clichés to minimize the seriousness of the patient's problem: "Lots of patients here are much sicker than you are!" *False*

*reassurance* is the use of clichés to insist that all is well: "You'll be back on your feet again in no time!"

Introducing an *unrelated topic* into a conversation effectively communicates that you do not want to talk about the foregoing topic. For example, the patient brings up worries about discharge from the hospital and you reply, "Well, that's a long way off. I notice you have several new cards here." Usually the patient recognizes your discomfort and abandons the previous topic.

The various types of *opposing* responses are readily recognizable as blocking. *Rejecting* the patient's statement, such as by saying, "Don't think about that," indicates that you do not want to listen. *Denying* the truth of the patient's statement— "That's ridiculous!"—effectively discourages further sharing of feelings or ideas, as does *challenging* its validity: "How can you possibly know something like that?" *Defending* other staff members or the institution against the patient's complaints puts you in the position of opposing the patient. Responding defensively tells the patient, "I'm on the other team, not on your side." A more appropriate response takes such complaints seriously without necessarily agreeing with them.

*Pseudoprofessional comments*—remarks phrased in the language of psychology but not professional in context—are becoming more commonplace as people become more familiar with psychological concepts and terminology. They can be very detrimental to relationships with patients. *Probing*— asking for personal information unrelated to the patient's health care—is inappropriate if you are merely satisfying curiosity; doing so can undermine the patient's trust. The patient should be free to share only what he or she decides to share. When such information will be used to plan care, the patient ought to be informed of the purpose of the questions. Probing often grows out of a mistaken belief in the value of extensive information for its own sake, without regard to its usefulness in planning care. *Demanding an explanation* for the patient's expressed feelings or behavior can cause the patient extreme discomfort. Though sometimes intended to promote self-understanding, such a response rarely has that effect because the meaning is outside the patient's awareness. *Interpreting* the patient's comments can be perceived as demeaning or as an invasion of personal

Exhibit 12.3
**Responses That Block Communication**

| Response | Example | Response (*continued*) | Example (*continued*) |
|---|---|---|---|
| Stereotyped comments | | Defending | Patient: "I'm not sure that doctor knows what he's doing." |
| Clichés | "Chin up." "It's for your own good." | | Nurse: "Now you have a very good doctor. He certainly wouldn't do anything that wasn't in your best interest." |
| Belittling | Patient: "I don't want to live like this." Nurse: "You'll feel differently in the morning." | | |
| False reassurance. | "You'll be just fine!" "Nothing to worry about!" | Pseudoprofessional comments | |
| Introducing an unrelated topic | Patient: "Am I going to get better?" Nurse: "Well, the color of that robe sure makes you look better. Blue really is your color." | Probing | "Now you must tell me everything about your relationship with your son." |
| | | Demanding explanations | "*Why* do you feel that way?" |
| Opposing | | Interpreting | "Underneath you really feel anger at. . . ." |
| Rejecting | Patient: "I feel as if I'm never going to get well." Nurse: "Don't think like that, it's depressing." | Personal opinions | |
| | | Agreeing | "That's right. You do need to look at the bright side." |
| Denying | Patient: "I'm not worth bothering about." Nurse: "Of course you are. That's silly." | Disagreeing | "I don't think you understand." "No, you're wrong about that." |
| Challenging | Patient: "Just touching her hand made me well." Nurse: "It isn't possible for that to happen." | Approving | "I'm glad to see you're cheerful today." |
| | | Disapproving | "Now don't be so glum." |

rights. In general, only the person who makes the comment has the right to interpret it.

*Offering personal opinions* is a common blocking response. Whether you are *agreeing, disagreeing, approving,* or *disapproving* all indicate that you believe one viewpoint to be correct and others incorrect. Such a message can have several undesirable effects. A patient struggling uncertainly to make a personal decision may give up and defer to you. A patient who disagrees with your expressed belief or opinion may be reluctant to say so since "You are the professional." If you agree or approve of an expressed feeling, the patient may not share less positive feelings later in the belief that they will meet with your disapproval. Feelings should never be labeled correct or incorrect, good or bad; they simply are.

It is important to distinguish health teaching (see Chapter 13) from the less formal situations we have been discussing. It is appropriate in health teaching to approve of a given behavior you want to promote since the desirability of that behavior is demonstrable and not merely a matter of opinion.

## Understanding Nonverbal Communication

Nonverbal behavior may communicate feelings and attitudes more effectively than words. Nonverbal behavior can convey meaning independently or it may enhance or contradict verbal communication. Touch, tone of voice, and facial expressions communicate feelings to an infant before that infant is able to understand the meaning of any spoken word. At the other end of life, a warm touch communicates caring to a person so near death that words are no longer meaningful.

## Types of Nonverbal Behavior That Communicate

Almost any type of human behavior can communicate a message. The first step in understanding nonverbal communication is to learn to identify significant behavior. You will need to practice looking for such behavior in yourself as well as others: it is as important to be aware of the messages you are sending nonverbally as it is to understand those you receive from others.

The *position* of your body in relation to that of

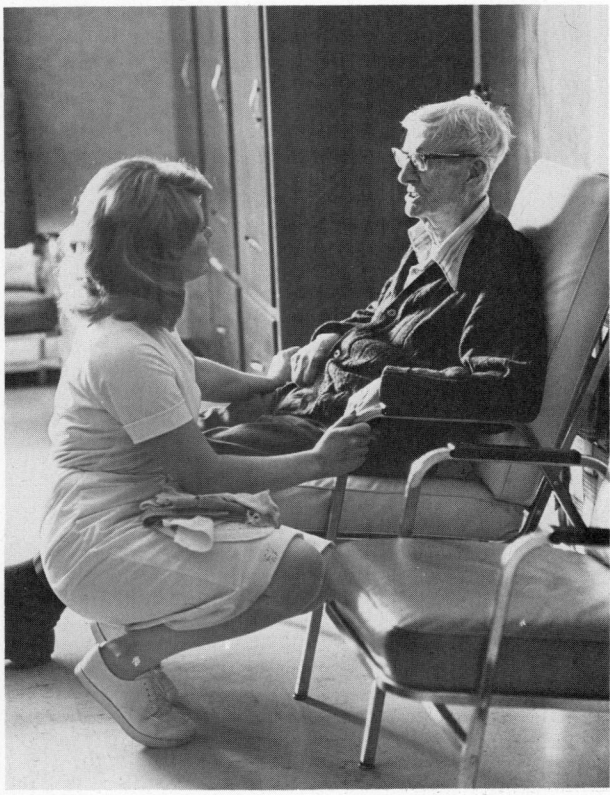

**Figure 12.2**
Sitting at eye level conveys a message of personal interest and equality of relationship. (Jim Harrison/Stock, Boston)

the patient expresses relative attentiveness and power. Directly facing a person usually indicates interest and attention. When the two people's faces are at the same level, communication is encouraged because they tend to feel of equal importance. If two people are positioned unequally, the lower person usually perceives the higher person as authoritarian.

*Gestures* are expressive movements of the hands and head. Common gestures include pointing and using the hands for emphasis, as well as nodding and shaking the head. Nodding is usually taken as indicating attention, agreement, or approval. Gestures can also express such spontaneous feelings as agitation, elation, despair, worry, and relief.

The *physical distance* between people communicates the degree of emotional intimacy existing or desired. Many studies have found distance to be related to people's perceptions of the space around their bodies, often termed *territory* or *personal space*. The area within which normal body odors can be detected, approximately twelve to eighteen inches, is perceived as one's *intimate space*. People often feel invaded and threatened when another person moves abruptly into their intimate space. Because nurses must often do so in the course of caring for patients, it is important to proceed slowly at first, explaining what you plan to do, and asking permission.

*Personal distance*, between approximately eighteen inches and four feet, is close enough to speak quietly and personally but allows for more independence and seems less threatening than intimate distance. It is a comfortable distance for most people. *Social distance*, from four to twelve feet, is more formal. Conversations conducted at this distance can be heard by casual passers-by, and people usually choose their words with this in mind. Most people are reluctant to talk about personal matters at this distance. *Public distance*, over twelve feet, is appropriate for speaking to groups rather than individuals. Communication at this distance is often formal, preplanned, and focused on ideas rather than feelings.

Culture deeply affects people's perceptions of appropriate physical distances. People of Hispanic, Southern European, and Middle Eastern background tend to be more comfortable at closer distances than people from Asian, Native American, and Northern European backgrounds.

*Facial expression* is the most accessible aspect of nonverbal communication. The position of the mouth, eyebrows, and eyes expresses feelings overtly. However, it is very easy to misinterpret familiar facial expressions. Although smiling usually indicates pleasure and frowning expresses displeasure or unhappiness, some people habitually smile when they are nervous or anxious and others frown when they are concentrating or lost in thought. Assumptions about the patient's mood on the basis of facial expressions are thus risky; always validate your perception.

*Eye contact* is also subject to different interpretations. In most Western cultures, eye contact is perceived as expressing honesty, straightforwardness, and attentiveness. In some Native American and Asian cultures, however, looking straight into the eyes of a person you do not know well may be considered rude. In situations that require you to wear a mask, such as isolation, eye contact can have a reassuring effect on the patient.

Most people associate *touch* with mothering, comfort, and caring. In fact, touch can express car-

Exhibit 12.4
**Aspects of Nonverbal Communication**

Position
Gestures
Distance
Facial expressions
Eye contact
Touch
Silence

ing when no other mode of communication can bridge a barrier between two people. Touch may be a way of expressing feeling, releasing tension, or simply making contact with another human being. Thus the nurse may touch the dying patient to express grief; the patient may grasp the nurse's hand for reassurance. But people's perceptions of touch depend on past experience, assumptions, and the nature of the situation. Some people associate touch with discipline, rejection, or pain. It is important to be alert to the meaning and value of touch for both the patient and yourself. When using touch with patients, evaluate primarily its value and meaning to the patient. Touch may be

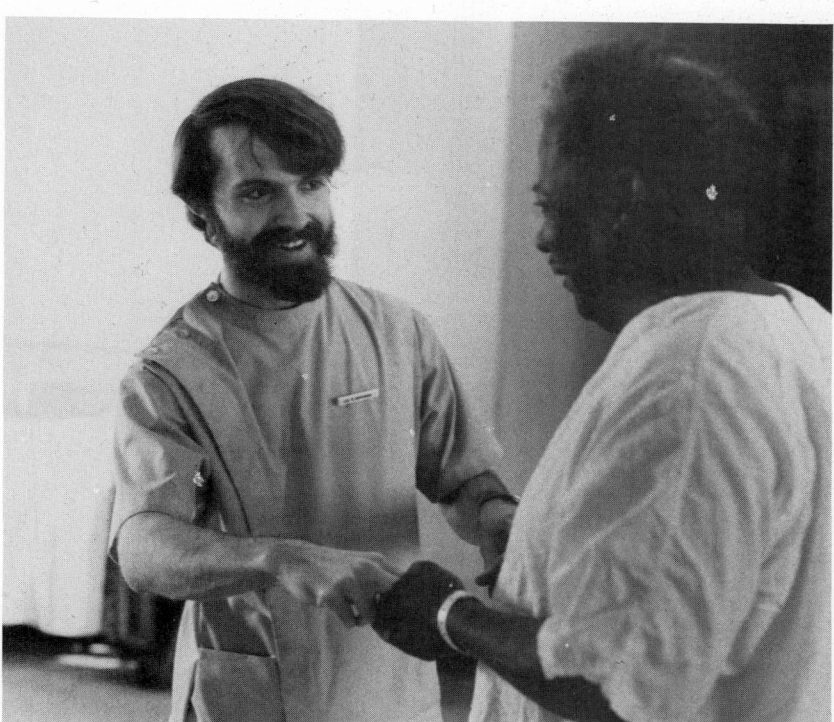

**Figure 12.3   Touch: a nonverbal expression of caring**
Elizabeth Wilcox

inappropriate, for example, if the patient misinterprets it as a sexual gesture. It may sometimes help to state what you are trying to convey with touch: "It's hard to be alone at a time like this. I'll stay with you during the test."

*Silence* also conveys meaning and can enhance communication. Silence at an appropriate moment in a conversation may communicate your willingness to let the other person think about a reply. Silence on the part of a patient may indicate that he or she is digesting information or marshaling personal resources. Sometimes sitting quietly with a patient communicates unconditional acceptance. However, silence makes many people anxious; such anxiety, conveyed by other nonverbal behavior, defeats the purpose of silence. You may be able to overcome anxiety by initially limiting silences to a few minutes and gradually increasing their duration as you become more comfortable. If five minutes is the most you can handle without becoming anxious, you might articulate this limit in advance by saying, "I'll stay another five minutes with you and then I'll leave."

## Interpreting Nonverbal Communication

Interpretation of nonverbal behavior ought to be approached systematically. You might begin by consciously noting the usual meanings of common types of nonverbal behavior.

The second step is to broaden your understanding and sharpen your ability to interpret nonverbal communication by familiarizing yourself with different cultures' typical nonverbal styles. Many (though not all) Southern European, Middle Eastern, Hispanic, and black people tend to use more vivid nonverbal language than Northern Europeans and Asians. It is easy to interpret behavior erroneously if you use your own background as a reference point for everyone you meet.

The third step is to read as much as you can about nonverbal cues. Many of the publications listed in the references at the end of this chapter make fascinating reading. You might also discuss them with other nurses to broaden your understanding.

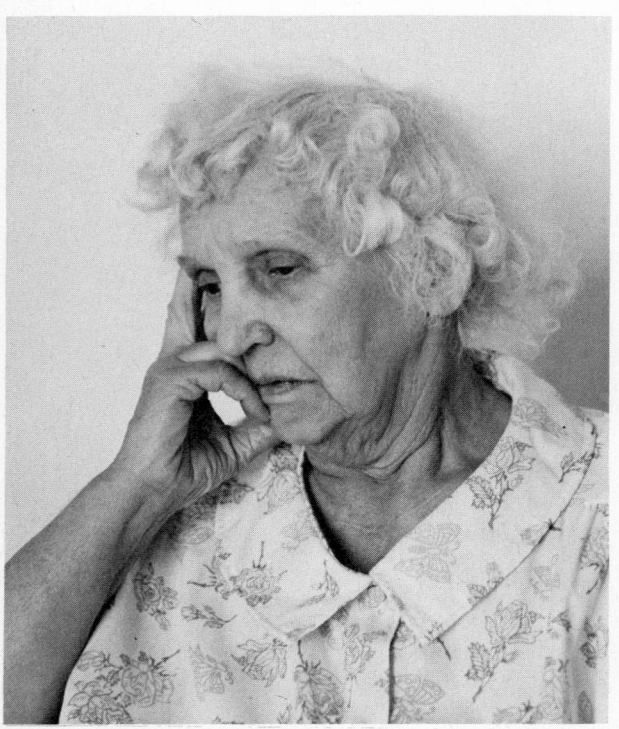 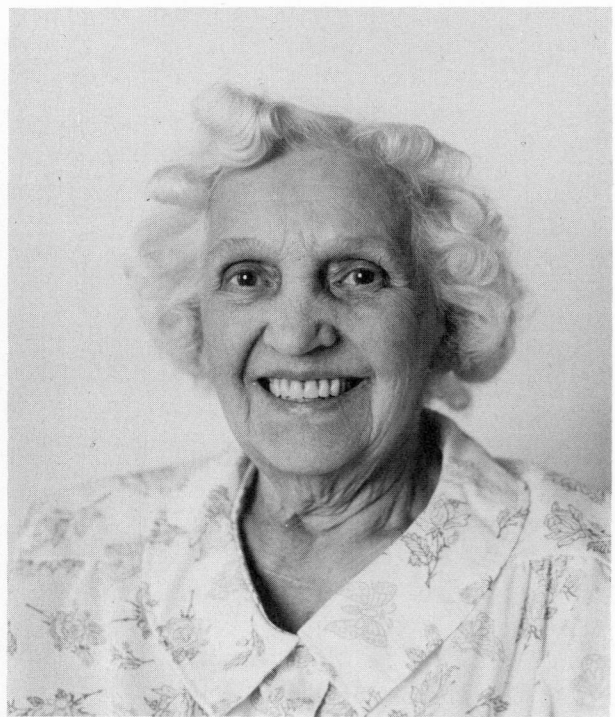

**Figure 12.4  Nonverbal communication and the patient**
What message is the patient communicating in each picture? (Russ Kinne/Danbury Hospital/Photo Researchers, Inc.)

The most definitive step, of course, is to validate your perception of a person's behavior by describing what you observed and asking him or her whether you interpreted it correctly.

## Intervention Based on Nonverbal Communication

Once you are sure you have interpreted a given behavior correctly, you can plan your nursing intervention. If the patient validates your interpretation, you may proceed accordingly. If he or she denies your interpretation, you should first consider the possibility that you might be in error. Interpreting nonverbal behavior is by no means simple, and such errors are common. But if further observation and objective data reinforce your interpretation, you might want to seek the opinion of another nurse. Then, if your interpretation is seconded, try responding to the nonverbal message you interpreted. For example, a patient admitted for diagnostic studies is tossing and turning, unable to sleep. Approaching the patient, the nurse says, "I notice you're having difficulty sleeping, and you look tense. Are you feeling worried?" The patient replies, "Oh, I'm O.K. I'm sure you have lots to do with so many sick patients." The nurse reconsiders the original observation and decides to respond to the nonverbal behavior rather than the patient's statement. The nurse sits down to talk to the patient and helps relieve the patient's worries. The patient finally falls asleep. In many instances, it helps significantly more to respond to the patient's nonverbal behavior rather than to a verbal denial of that behavior's message.

# Purposes of Communication

The appropriateness of the various techniques of verbal and nonverbal communication depends on the purpose of the interaction.

## Socializing

Socializing is engaging in ordinary social conversation; its content may include such impersonal topics as the weather and politics and such personal topics as children, family, and occupation.

A facility in which nurses rarely socialize with patients would be perceived as cold and unfriendly. Socializing is pleasant and relaxing and enhances our knowledge of one another. However, the nurse's social conversation with patients has been a cause of concern for many practitioners. The patient's physical well-being is a prime consideration—social conversation should not promote fatigue or interfere with needed rest. Another issue is the patient's privacy—social conversation should not pry into personal and family matters. A third concern is the patient's emotional well-being—it may be that the appropriate response to the concerns or feelings the patient expresses should be therapeutic, not social. Finally, social conversation should not become a forum for the nurse's problems and opinions.

As a nurse, you need to assess the situation and decide what the patient needs. If you decide that socializing is appropriate, it is your responsibility to make sure such conversation does not create a problem where none existed, by, for example, causing undue fatigue or probing into personal matters. Socializing is not an opportunity to talk about topics of personal interest to you but a time for patients to discuss topics that interest them.

What you reveal about yourself will vary considerably in different situations and with different patients. The crucial guideline is that socializing must not undermine the effectiveness of the professional relationship. A student nurse might feel comfortable sharing personal thoughts with a patient of the same sex. With a patient of the opposite sex, however, such talk might be misconstrued as romantic interest and interfere with future therapeutic interaction. Some nurses feel comfortable revealing their thoughts and feelings to other people, while others are more private even in their personal lives. Each nurse must decide how much and what to share in each situation. What is right for one may not be right for another.

There are those who question whether nurses should establish long-term friendships with patients that will persist outside of the care setting. Again, this is an individual matter. Sometimes such relationships are successful. In other instances, the two people find they have little in common once the professional connection ends. The nurse needs to be aware that a one-sided loss of interest can be painful for the other person. The ex-patient is apt to be more dependent emotionally and thus to be more hurt when the friendship ceases. Again, recognition of the various possible outcomes, critical self-evaluation, and a well thought-out decision constitute the best course of action.

## Interviewing

An interview is an interaction in which you gather information for purposes of assessment. The nursing care history is a *structured interview*—that is, an interview in which the questions are planned in advance. Other types of interview are *unstructured*—the questions are not planned in advance but arise in the course of the interview in response to previous answers.

When preparing for an interview, review pages 188–191 and plan your questions carefully. Sometimes facilitating responses prove very useful, as does your insight into nonverbal communication. Consider the physical setting of the interview carefully: comfort and privacy enhance the success of an interview.

## Therapeutic Interaction

When a patient experiences unpleasant feelings or has a decision to make or a problem to solve, the nurse can help him or her minimize anxiety, handle grief, clarify feelings, or work out the problem. Interaction for this purpose is called *therapeutic interaction.*

Therapeutic interaction proceeds systematically, in accordance with the four steps in the nursing process. First, the need for therapeutic interaction must be identified. In your nursing assessment, you will note and evaluate such things as nonverbal cues indicating anxiety, statements of feelings, and signs of grief. The problem confronting the patient should be identified, if it is known.

Second, you will plan your interaction. In order to do so effectively, you will first set a goal. What is your purpose in interacting with this particular patient? It may be for the patient to exhibit behavior less indicative of anxiety, to state that anxiety is less, or to plan action to solve a problem. In most cases, a nondirective approach using facilitating responses proves most helpful. When possible, plan for time to sit down and talk with the patient unhurriedly. This is a particularly appropriate time to review what you know about nonverbal messages in order to enhance communication.

Third, you will implement the planned interaction by talking with the patient, encouraging him or her to discuss concerns and feelings. Often this alone enables patients to manage their own feelings. You may also want to encourage a patient's problem-solving efforts. Remember that the patient benefits from the least possible directiveness on your part.

The last step, of course, is to evaluate the effectiveness of your interaction, examining the results in terms of the planned goal. If the goal was not met, consider the possible explanations. It is often helpful to review your interaction with particular attention to the facilitating responses and blocking responses you might have made. Try to determine whether such responses may have been responsible for failure to meet your goal. It is important to guard against unrealistic expectations, in terms both of the goal and the effort required to achieve it. Several interactions over a period of days may be more effective than a single interaction.

## Other Purposes of Communication

Health teaching and coordinating care with other members of the health-care team both require skillful communication. The importance and complexity of both processes warrant devoting a separate chapter to each. Chapter 13 is devoted to health teaching; Chapter 14 will examine coordination of care.

# Conclusion

Skillful communication is essential to effective functioning as a nurse. The skills you are developing now will continue to be broadened and honed throughout your nursing career. Fully as important as making yourself understood clearly and unmistakably are the related skills of eliciting needed information, interpreting feelings and behavior sensitively, and providing comfort and reassurance.

## Care Study  A therapeutic interaction

Mrs. Shadle is a seventy-five-year-old patient in an extended care facility for care following the repair of her fractured hip. Mrs. Langley is the registered nurse in charge of the unit. Entering Mrs. Shadle's room on her nursing rounds, Mrs. Langley notes that Mrs. Shadle is sitting in a wheelchair with her hands in her lap, hair uncombed, shoulders down, and head bowed. Mrs. Shadle emits a long sigh and does not look up as the nurse approaches.

**Nurse:** "Mrs. Shadle, you look like you're feeling down this morning."
**Patient:** "Who wouldn't? I'll never leave this awful place."
**Nurse:** "Never leave this awful place?"
**Patient:** "That's right—I can't ever go home because I can't walk, can't do a thing." Tears start to flow down her cheeks.
**Nurse:** (She sits down beside Mrs. Shadle and takes her hands.) "Mrs. Shadle, do you mean that you believe you won't be able to walk again?"
**Patient:** "That's right—and I can't be home in this thing." (She points at the wheelchair.)
**Nurse:** You are going to Physical Therapy. Can you tell me what you did there yesterday?"
**Patient:** "I stood up between those bars and tried to walk—but I could only go halfway and I got so tired."
**Nurse:** "Yesterday you went halfway. Do you remember what you were doing in Physical Therapy last week?"

**Patient:** "That was when I first started going. It took two of them to hold me up."
**Nurse:** "So last week it took two people to hold you up and this week you walked halfway down the bars."
**Patient:** "I guess that is better, isn't it? But it goes so slowly."
**Nurse:** "It's a slow process but it has been steady. What do you suppose you might be doing next week at this time?"
**Patient:** "Maybe I'll be able to walk the whole way." (Her face brightens.)
**Nurse:** "You may even be using a walker so you can walk around the room." (Mrs. Langley has communicated with the Physical Therapy Department and knows that this is the plan.)
**Patient:** "Really? I might be able to go home if I could use a walker."
**Nurse:** "Mm-hmm."
**Patient:** "I guess this isn't such a bad place for a while."
**Nurse:** (She gives Mrs. Shadle's hand a squeeze and stands up.) "I'll have Miss Johnson, the aide, help you comb your hair and clean up to go to Physical Therapy. I'll be back to check on how you're getting along. If you get to feeling down again, call me. O.K.?"
**Patient:** "Thank you, Mrs. Langley."

## Study Terms

agreeing-disagreeing
aids to decision
  making
approving-
  disapproving
belittling
blocking responses
challenging
clichés
communication
considering
  consequences
defending
demanding
  explanations
denying

distance
encouraging
  comparisons
exploratory responses
eye contact
facial expressions
facilitating responses
false reassurance
focusing
formulation of a plan
general leads
gestures
interaction
interpreting
interviewing
introductory phase

leave-taking
message
nondirective comments
nonverbal
opposing
pacing
perception
personal opinions
pointing out
  information
position
probing
pseudoprofessional
  comments
receiver
reflecting
rejecting
resource

restating
reviewing
seeking clarification
sender
silence
socializing
stereotyped comments
structured interview
termination phase
time sequence
touch
unrelated topic
unstructured interview
validating
verbal
voice tone
working phase

## Learning Activities

1. Complete a nursing history on a patient in the clinical facility.

2. Plan a five-minute conversation with a given patient. After leaving the patient, write down the entire conversation. Note nonverbal as well as verbal interaction. Identify the type of interaction: socializing, teaching, or other.

3. Plan a conversation in which you will encourage the patient to explore his or her feelings about hospitalization or illness.

4. Review the section on facilitating techniques as you plan. Carry out the planned interaction. Record the interaction, noting nonverbal as well as verbal interaction. Review your interaction.

## References

Barnett, Kathryn. "A Theoretical Construct of the Concepts of Touch as They Relate to Nursing." *Nursing Research* 21 (March–April 1972): 102–110.

Brammer, Lawrence M. *The Helping Relationship: Process and Skills.* Englewood Cliffs, N.J.: Prentice-Hall, 1973.

Burnside, I. M. "Caring for the Aged: Part 5, Touching Is Talking." *American Journal of Nursing* 73 (December 1973): 2060–2063.

Chappelle, M. L. "The Language of Food." *American Journal of Nursing* 72 (July 1972): 1294–1295.

Egolf, D. B., and Chester, S. L. "Speechless Messages." *Nursing Digest* 4 (February 1976): 26–29.

Epstein, C. "Breaking the Barriers to Communication in the Health Care Team." *Nursing '74* 4 (December 1974): 63–68.

Fast, Julius. *Body Language.* New York: Simon and Schuster, 1970.

Field, W. E., Jr. "Watch Your Message." *American Journal of Nursing* 72 (July 1972): 1278–1280.

Goldsborough, Judith. "On Being Non-Judgmental." *American Journal of Nursing* 70 (November 1970): 2340.

Gordon, T. *Parent Effectiveness Training.* New York: Wyden, 1970.

Hall, Edward. *The Silent Language.* New York: Doubleday, 1973.

Hein, Eleanor. "Listening." *Nursing '75* 5 (March 1975): 93–102.

Kreiger, Doris. "Therapeutic Touch: The Imprimatur of Nursing." *American Journal of Nursing* 75 (May 1975): 784–787.

Loesch, L. D., and Loesch, N. A. "What Do You Say After You Say Mm-hmmm?" *American Journal of Nursing* 75 (May 1975): 807–809.

Lynch, J. J. "The Simple Act of Touching." *Nursing '78* 8 (June 1978): 32–36.

Radulovic, P. O. "Under the Cover of His Charm." *American Journal of Nursing* 73 (October 1973): 1731–1737.

Robinson, L. "The Crying Patient." *Nursing '72* 2 (February 1972): 16–20.

Sathre, Freda S., et al. *Let's Talk: An Introduction to Interpersonal Communication,* 2nd ed. Glenview, Ill.: Scott, Foresman, 1977.

"Touch: A Symposium." *Nursing Forum* 18, no. 1 (1979).

Veninga, R. "Communications: A Patient's Eye View." *American Journal of Nursing* 73 (February 1973): 320–322.

# Chapter 13
# Health Teaching

## Objectives

After completing this chapter you should be able to:
1. Define learning.
2. Compare and contrast the three types of learning.
3. List internal and external influences on learning.
4. Specify assessment data needed to identify learning needs.
5. Outline the essential components of a teaching plan.
6. Explain how evaluation relates to the type of learning desired.

## Outline

Health teaching is helping people learn what they need to know in order to maintain or regain health. As life expectancy increases, more and more people must learn to live with complex regimens for managing chronic illnesses. At the same time, healthy people are increasingly eager for information about how best to maintain their own and their families' health. Thus both the opportunities and the responsibilities of the nurse continue to grow. Nurses' knowledge of health and illness, as well as their constant interaction with patients, makes them particularly well suited to do health teaching. In turn, health teaching provides for a unique and fruitful application of the nursing process. In your role as a health teacher, you will (1) assess the patient and the situation to determine his or her learning needs and readiness to learn, (2) select goals and devise a teaching plan to meet them, (3) implement the plan, and (4) evaluate the effectiveness of your teaching.

Most health teaching is pursued with one learner at a time. However, nurses also teach groups of people, which requires skill and experience in working with groups (see Chapter 6) as well as mastery of the material to be taught and familiarity with the teaching/learning process. Clearly, this chapter can be no more than a foundation for the teaching skills you will develop over time. Let us first examine the teaching/learning process.

## Understanding the Teaching/Learning Process

Learning may be defined as a change in behavior not due to growth or fatigue. In this context, *behavior* means both observable activities (such as taking medications and eating special foods) and those that cannot be seen (such as thinking and planning). A *learning need* is thus a need for a change in behavior. Assessing a patient's learning needs involves consideration of a wide variety of health-related factors.

### Types of Learning

There are three types of learning: psychomotor learning (acquiring physical skills); cognitive learning (gaining knowledge); and affective learning (changing attitudes). All three types of learning occur continually throughout the life cycle as aspects of normal development, as well as in planned learning situations.

### Psychomotor Learning

Patients often need to learn new physical skills, such as giving themselves injections or changing colostomy bags. Plenty of opportunity to practice

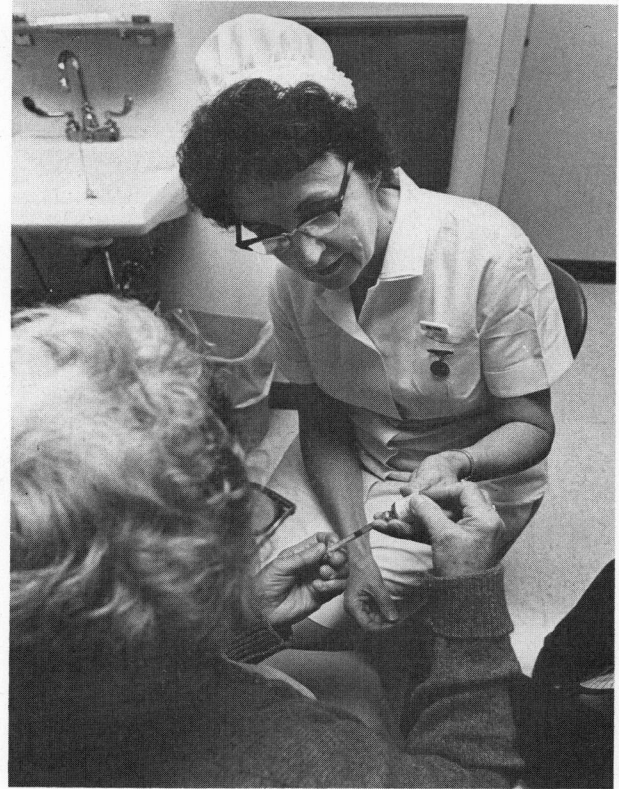

**Figure 13.1**
Psychomotor learning is acquiring new physical skills.
(Dan Bernstein)

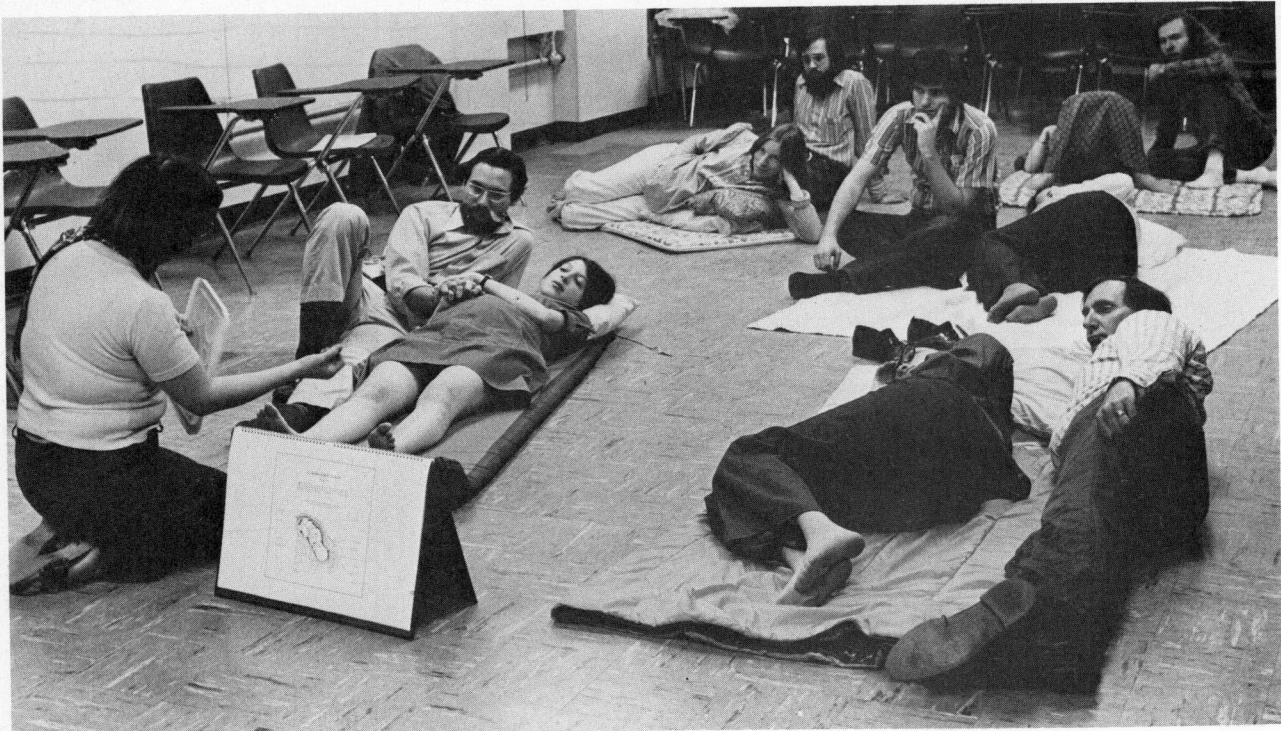

**Figure 13.2**
Cognitive learning is absorbing new knowledge. (Elizabeth Hamlin/Stock, Boston)

such skills is crucial. Evaluation is based on the patient's ability to perform the skill adeptly.

## Cognitive Learning

People need repeated exposure to new information in order to absorb it thoroughly. Some people learn best by receiving information visually; others prefer it presented verbally. Most people learn best through a combined verbal and visual approach.

## Affective Learning

Acquisition of new attitudes and values is usually the most gradual type of learning as well as the most difficult to measure. A patient learning to cope with a particular health problem may master new psychomotor skills and knowledge well before new attitudes are firmly established. Affective learning involves working through one's feelings about presently held attitudes and beliefs as well

as the new values being considered. Learning has occurred when new beliefs are accepted. Participation in therapeutic interaction and/or group discussion is helpful to the process of affective learning.

## Internal Influences on Patient Learning

The first considerations in planning patient teaching are the *internal characteristics* of the learner: (1) previous education and experience, (2) physiologic status, (3) vocabulary level, (4) anxiety level, and (5) motivation (see Exhibit 13.1).

## Previous Education and Experience

*Previous education and experience* make a great deal of difference in the patient's approach to learning. An individual who has enjoyed school and other types of learning may enjoy this new challenge. A person who associates education with shame

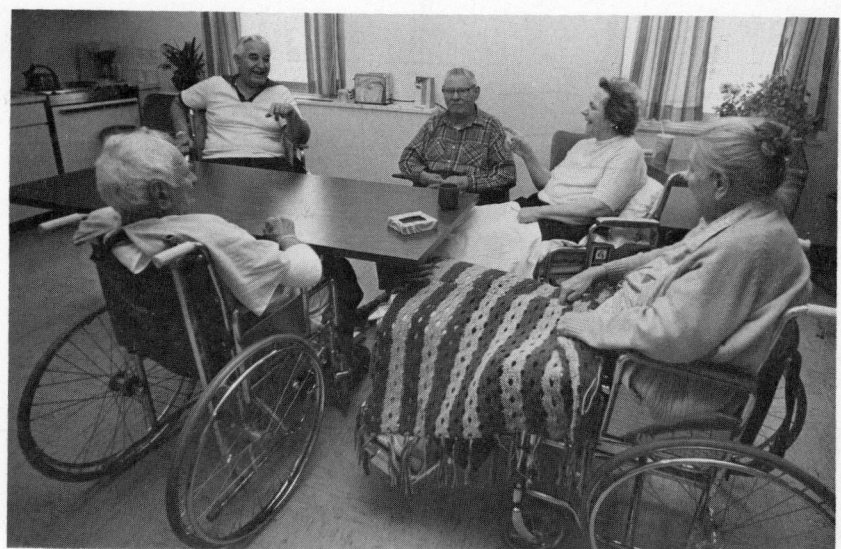

**Figure 13.3**
Affective learning is adopting new beliefs and attitudes. (Russ Kinne/Danbury Hospital/Photo Researchers, Inc.)

and failure will, however, be hesitant to embark on new learning. A patient whose college work included extensive study of the biological sciences will respond to learning how illness is affecting the body's functioning very differently than a person who has avoided anything scientific and knows little about normal functioning of the human body. A parent of three small children has very different preparation for learning to care for a handicapped baby than a person who has never cared for an infant. Sometimes the desired learning will occur only if you provide basic background information, such as teaching normal nutrition in order to teach about a special diet.

## Physiologic Status

*Physiologic status*—fatigue, hunger, lack of oxygen, altered blood components, drugs, and the like—significantly affects learning. Needless to say, this is a matter of particular concern to nurses since many patients have physiologic problems. Adaptations may have to be made in teaching to accommodate such problems. In order not to tire the patient, teaching may have to be pursued in small segments. You may need to reassure the patient that slow learning is a result of illness and fatigue, not an indication of lack of ability or effort. If the pace is so slow as to frustrate both the patient and the nurse, teaching may have to be postponed un-

til the patient's condition improves. Immediate needs must be met before secondary needs: a patient whose mind is absorbed with the effort of breathing is not likely to be interested in learning about a new diet. By planning for rest, providing medication for pain relief, and promoting comfort, you may be able to minimize the effects of physiologic factors.

## Vocabulary

The extent and level of the learner's *vocabulary* affects his or her ability to understand written material and oral explanations. The individual may interpret some words differently than you do. As a beginning nursing student encountering a new vocabulary, you ought to have a heightened sensitivity to the patient's unfamiliarity with medical language. Sometimes the desired learning will occur only if you first explain the terms you are using.

## Anxiety

Mild *anxiety* may facilitate learning by focusing the learner's full attention on the task. Higher levels of anxiety interfere with learning by diffusing attention or focusing it on only a part of the situation. An individual who is very anxious may leap from one thought to another, unable to concentrate on a single idea. High anxiety also tends to orient the individual to the present rather than the future. A therapeutic interaction may help to lower the patient's anxiety. Sometimes anxiety-relieving medications are given to make learning more effective. If, on the other hand, the patient demonstrates total lack of anxiety and concern, pointing out potential problems that could be solved by the proposed learning may elicit enough anxiety to facilitate learning.

## Motivation

*Motivation* is an internal tendency or desire to learn. Motivation is greatest when the individual feels a need and recognizes that the proposed learning would satisfy it. For example, a person living in a foreign country needs to learn its language in order to relate to others. Because the need to learn is great, effort and attention will be correspondingly great. But needs for new knowledge are often less readily obvious. A male patient who is to eat a special diet at home but expects his wife to plan and cook all his meals may not perceive a need to know about the diet. As a result, he would be likely to devote minimal effort and attention to learning about it. Trying to motivate an individual to learn is a challenging task. Merely pointing out a person's needs does not guarantee that they will be perceived as needs. The most effective strategy is usually to help the person think through the situation and arrive at an independent decision that a need exists.

The teacher, as facilitator of the learning process, is responsible for assessing the internal influences described above and determining the patient's degree of *readiness to learn*. Readiness to learn is determined by the combined effect of in-

---

Exhibit 13.1
**Internal Influences on Learning**

Previous education and experience
Physiologic status
Vocabulary
Anxiety
Motivation

---

ternal factors. If readiness is at a very low level, it may be necessary to postpone teaching. In other instances, the teacher can alter or affect internal factors sufficiently to enable the person to learn.

## External Influences on Patient Learning

The teacher can also facilitate learning by changing or adapting factors *external* to the learner: (1) physical environment, (2) privacy, (3) timing, (4) the teacher's vocabulary, and (5) teaching strategies (see Exhibit 13.2).

### Physical Environment

The *physical environment* may need to be modified to ensure that temperature, light, noise, and the like are at levels compatible with optimum functioning. It may be necessary to find another setting for teaching or to consult with those responsible for the physical plant. Simply opening windows or doors to provide ventilation may help. If the learner will need to read or to examine a fine scale, such as on a syringe, the lighting should be appropriate.

### Privacy

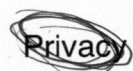

The nature of the task or material to be taught will determine the degree of privacy required. It may be necessary to wait until the patient's roommate is absent or visitors have left in order to provide privacy. In other cases, however, it might be helpful for a family member to be present. Sometimes closing the curtains or shutting the door ensures adequate privacy. A task such as colostomy irrigation may be taught in a bathroom whose door can be locked to protect privacy.

### Timing

The *timing* of teaching is too often determined by the nurse's convenience rather than its appropriateness to learning. For example, the arthritic who is stiff and sore on first arising may need to learn

Exhibit 13.2
**External Influences on Learning**

Physical environment
Privacy
Timing
The teacher's vocabulary
Teaching strategies

___

manual skills later in the day. The elderly diabetic who typically arises very early, while other patients are still asleep, may learn best then, when he or she is freshest and most alert. Scheduled diagnostic tests and other procedures should also be taken into account. Of course, if your teaching concerns the test itself, it should be scheduled prior to the test. If it concerns something else, the patient's preoccupation with the test may make the period preceding it inappropriate for teaching. Teaching scheduled too far in advance of the patient's need for the information may seem unimportant or provoke anxiety. If, on the other hand, the teaching is scheduled immediately before the knowledge is needed, there may not be sufficient time for learning.

## The Teacher's Vocabulary

The teacher should suit the *vocabulary level* used in explanations to the understanding of the learner. Consider the patient's education and socioeconomic background, as well as cultural factors, when determining what vocabulary to use. However, many otherwise well-educated people are not familiar with such medical terms as "void" or "stool specimen." Rather than asking whether the patient understands the words you are using, you might ask him or her to restate what you have said. This approach reveals whether you are conveying your message satisfactorily and provides you with a sample of the patient's vocabulary.

The following situation, in which a student nurse once found herself, exemplifies communication breakdown due to vocabulary differences. An elderly man hospitalized for diagnostic tests was very friendly and anxious to please, but his English was broken and difficult to understand. His physician ordered a stool specimen, which the nurses repeatedly explained to the patient. Over

and over he smiled, nodded, and later walked to the bathroom, had a bowel movement, and flushed it down the toilet. The staff was becoming upset. The student nurse reviewed her information on the patient and found that he had worked at manual labor all his life and had very little education. Concluding that he probably did not understand what was wanted, she tried a variety of terms—to no avail. Finally, in desperation, she said, "Shit in the pan," and pointed at the bedpan. The patient's face lit up. "Sure!" he said, and the problem was solved. This was not the student's customary vocabulary—but it *was* the patient's.

## Teaching Strategies

The following teaching strategies have been shown to promote learning. Keep them in mind as you plan your teaching and select methods and materials (see Exhibit 13.3).

*Reinforcement*—rewarding the learner for making the desired response—is considered by many theorists to be the primary basis for learning. Anything the learner perceives as rewarding can be a reinforcement. Praise is the most common reinforcement, since most people have learned to value it. For some individuals, more tangible rewards—such as reading a story to a child or allowing a teenager extra time to talk on the telephone—may be more appropriate. The most effective reinforcement follows immediately after the desired response, without delay. Punishment for inappropriate responses has less effect on behavior than does reward for appropriate responses. In fact, many theorists believe that ignoring inappropriate responses eliminates them more effectively than punishment.

Frequent opportunities to *practice* new skills increase the rate of learning. Practice spaced out over time is generally more effective than a single long session, since fatigue can undermine performance. Practice immediately following instruction is more helpful than delayed practice because less is forgotten. *Feedback*—comparison of the individual's performance during practice to the desired objective—promotes rapid learning.

*Active participation* appears to facilitate learning. The learner can exercise several modes of input—touch, motor action, hearing, sight, and so on—

by practicing each segment of the skill as it is explained. Writing down important points is another means of active participation; some learners benefit considerably from doing so.

*Audiovisual aids* are an alternative mode of communication that can enhance direct verbal interaction, particularly if they relate to the learner's previous knowledge or experience. Many audiovisual aids for health teaching, including slide/tape presentations, films, and posters, are produced commercially and by voluntary associations. Anatomical models may help the person visualize the parts of the body being discussed. Some hospitals stock many such aids and a number of pamphlets and books appropriate for health teaching. It is a nursing responsibility to determine what audiovisual aids are needed and to communicate these needs to the administration of the health-care facility. One may do so individually or by serving on special patient-care committees.

The *sequence* in which material is presented can have a direct effect on the rate and extent of learn-ing. Proceeding from familiar to unfamiliar material helps the learner put new information in perspective. In order to do so, you must first find out what the learner already knows. Never make assumptions about a person's level of knowledge: whether the patient is a doctor or a laborer, an individualized assessment is needed. A dermatologist, for example, may be totally unfamiliar with routine preparations for kidney x rays in a particular hospital, while a laborer may have undergone such x rays on a number of previous occasions. Be sure to validate your impressions of the patient's knowledge before proceeding.

In general, proceeding from simple ideas to complex ones, from what is known to what is unknown, from an understanding of the normal to understanding of the abnormal, and from concepts involving wellness to concepts pertaining to illness, helps the learner absorb new information in an orderly way.

## Behavior Modification and Nursing Practice

*Behavior modification* is a method of teaching characterized by an explicitly stated behavioral goal, systematic reinforcement of the desired behavior, and ignoring (or other negative treatment) of undesired responses. The objective is to increase the incidence of desired behavior and decrease that of undesired behavior.

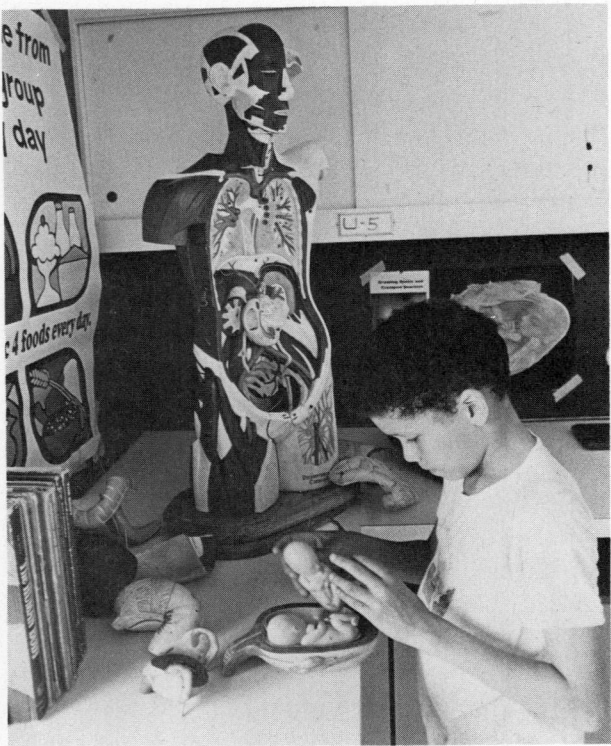

**Figure 13.4**
Audiovisual aids can facilitate learning. (Patricia Gross/Stock, Boston)

---

Exhibit 13.3
**Basic Principles of Learning**

**1.** Reinforcement enhances learning.
**2.** Frequent opportunities to practice new skills will increase the rate of learning.
**3.** Feedback facilitates learning.
**4.** Active participation promotes learning by providing for several modes of input: touch, motor action, hearing, and observation.
**5.** Audiovisual aids are an alternative mode of communicating that can supplement direct verbal interaction.
**6.** Appropriate sequencing facilitates learning. Information should proceed from
    **a.** simple to complex.
    **b.** known to unknown.
    **c.** well to ill.
    **d.** normal to abnormal.

---

Behavior modification is extremely clear-cut methodologically. There are techniques to evoke the desired behavior at the outset, to identify an appropriate means of reinforcement, and to respond to undesired behavior. There are a number of good texts on behavior modification.

Behavior modification is widely used in health care and has proven particularly successful in helping the mentally retarded, the disabled, and people in chronic pain. Success appears to be greatest when behavior modification is part of a total team approach to care. For a fuller discussion of behavior modification in health care, see the text by Berni and Fordyce listed in the end-of-chapter references.

Some nursing writers view behavior modification as mechanistic and thus fundamentally at odds with the humanistic mission of nursing. Questions have also been raised about the ethics of undertaking behavior modification without the knowledge and consent of the patient. Unconsented-to behavior modification might be considered manipulative and an infringement on individual human rights. Since the success of such techniques is in no way compromised by informing the patient fully, most facilities that employ behavior modification have policies of full disclosure, allowing the patient to decide whether or not to participate.

## Assessment in Health Teaching

The first step in health teaching, like other nursing responsibilities, is thorough assessment. Assessment in turn has several components.

### Assessing the Patient's Learning Needs

First you must verify that a learning need exists. As we have said, a learning need is a need for a change in behavior, new knowledge, or new attitudes. You will need to decide whether the patient might benefit from acquiring skills, knowledge, or attitudes he or she cannot be expected to develop without help. The following questions will help you identify learning needs.

Must the patient perform a new task or use a new skill? For example, a person on crutches must walk in an unfamiliar way. Stairs, ramps, and doorways all require new movements and means of balance. Instruction in these skills is needed. Similarly, the mother of a first baby will be expected to bathe, change, and feed the infant when she goes home. Does she know how? Has she ever done it before? Situations such as these abound in a hospital.

Will the patient's pattern of daily living have to change? A woman with a serious heart problem may need to rest during the day and avoid strenuous activities. What is she allowed to do? What specific exertions should be avoided? The diabetic needs to adopt a stable pattern of meals and activity. Does this mean that each day must be exactly the same? How are necessary variations provided for? Of course, teaching the patient to adopt a new life style is not your only responsibility. You can also help the person deal with the feelings aroused by such a change, as outlined in Chapter 12.

Does the patient need information on which to base judgments? The diabetic may be instructed to carry candy or sugar for use in an emergency. What constitutes an emergency? How much candy is enough? When must a physician be called? Many similar, if less dramatic, judgments need to be prepared for. A mother must decide when a child is ill enough to require a visit to the physician. She must decide when to increase an infant's food intake. The health-related decisions we make throughout our lives need to be based on sound information.

Will the current problem be of continuing concern? Short-term problems call for very different teaching than do long-term problems. Joint disability due to a sprain requires different adaptations and planning than does joint disability due to rheumatoid arthritis, which is a lifetime health problem.

Is the immediate situation unfamiliar to the patient? A person who is about to undergo a diagnostic test needs to know what is to be done, how it will feel, what he or she is expected to do, how long it will take, and so forth. The person scheduled for surgery needs to know about preparation for surgery, recuperation, and expectations for his or her behavior. It has been documented that patients who have had thorough preoperative teaching have fewer postoperative complications.

Other common learning needs involve medications to be taken after discharge, special diets or activities that must be continued at home, symptoms that ought to be reported to the physician, and continued management of a chronic illness.

## Assessing Current Level of Knowledge or Ability

The second step in assessing learning needs is determining the patient's current knowledge, degree of skill, and/or attitudes. If you assume no prior knowledge of sound dietary habits or the components of a special diet the patient may have been adhering to for years, he or she may feel justifiably insulted or patronized. Sometimes nurses fail to recognize that the patient's learning need is not for information (such as about a special diet) but for a change in attitude (such as learning to value adherence to the diet).

## The Patient's View of the Learning Need

Once you have determined that a learning need exists, it is necessary to find out whether the patient also recognizes the need. If the patient does not perceive a learning need, your best efforts at teaching may be unsuccessful. You will find the techniques of therapeutic interaction helpful in this aspect of assessment. By means of therapeutic interaction, you may be able to help the patient consider the situation and acknowledge learning needs. For example, a patient might recognize a need for affective learning by being willing to discuss feelings and concerns.

## Identifying Internal Influences on Patient Learning

Finally, internal factors that affect learning—fatigue, vocabulary, anxiety, and the like, discussed on pages 202–204—must be assessed before embarking on your teaching plan. Otherwise your planning may prove to be unrealistic or inappropriate for the patient in question.

# Planning Patient Teaching

When a learning need has been mutually acknowledged, specific goals (often termed learning objectives) and a plan for achieving them must be established in cooperation with the patient.

## Relating Goals to the Type of Learning

The goals or objectives you select ought to correspond to the type of learning in question. For a psychomotor skill, the goal should be something the patient will *do*. If the proposed learning is to be cognitive, the goal will be for the patient to state or explain something. For affective learning, it is difficult to specify goals. Merely professing a new belief or attitude may or may not indicate genuine change. A more reliable indication is the patient's subsequent behavior. Thus the goals of affective learning are often stated as desired changes in behavior that would imply the adoption of a new attitude. If, for example, the affective change desired is that the patient believe in the importance of adhering to a special diet, the goal might be for the patient to stay on the diet voluntarily.

## Individualizing Goals

Nurses commonly err by trying to impart to the patient all the information on a given subject they themselves possess. An effective way to correct this tendency is to be alert for nonverbal cues from the patient as to the information he or she will use and can absorb at the time. For example, a patient who is very worried about giving himself an injection may be uninterested in considering any other aspect of his care until he has mastered that skill. Immediate needs must be addressed first.

In some cases it may be advisable to outline a series of objectives, recognizing that you are only beginning the teaching process. The patient may then continue learning at a later time, either independently or with another teacher. For example, the patient who has a complicated medication regime to understand may spend an hour discussing her learning needs and formulating objectives with you. The next day she might initiate further discussion with the nurse who administers her morning medication. The nurse working in the evening might help her devise a means of keeping track of when medications are due. Thus the entire team might become involved.

Such team involvement may be planned in advance and facilitated by a health-teaching flow sheet on the patient's record. The objectives are listed on the flow sheet, and each nurse involved in teaching records what has been accomplished. The more specifically the goals and objectives are

stated, the easier it will be for the patient to plan and pursue learning and to measure and evaluate progress. A goal as general as "to learn about the prescribed medications," while accurate, provides too little direction for someone who does not know what is important to know about medications. More specific objectives might be "(1) to know the name and dosage schedule for each medication, (2) to know the purpose of each medication, and (3) to know what untoward signs and symptoms should be reported to the physician." This kind of objective enables the patient to ask appropriate questions and to evaluate his or her learning: the patient can review the medications and determine whether or not more learning is needed. A patient who is discharged from the hospital before completing the objectives will also be able to continue learning with a nurse in the physician's office, a public health nurse, or someone else involved in his or her care.

## Planning the Teaching Process

In planning the actual teaching process, you will need to reflect in turn on each aspect of the teaching/learning process. Your assessment will indicate what *environmental factors* you must modify to accommodate the patient's needs, as well as the *language level* and *timing* and *duration* of teaching most likely to facilitate learning. Appropriate *reinforcement* for the particular patient in question

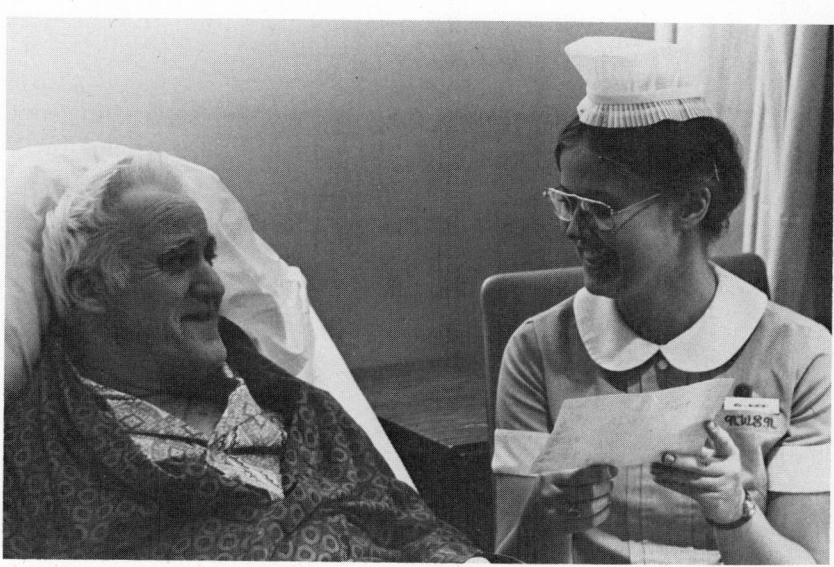

**Figure 13.5**
A warm relationship facilitates the teaching/learning process. (Lynn McLaren, courtesy of Newton-Wellesley Hospital)

deserves attention. Your plan should include opportunities for *active participation*, if possible, and *feedback* on the patient's progress. You may wish to track down or make some appropriate *audiovisual aids*. Finally, you must plan the *sequence* in which the material will be presented.

When learning needs are short-term, simple, and capable of being met by a single individual (such as teaching the patient how to operate the call system), a written plan may not be necessary. This emphatically does not mean *no* plan is necessary; it means that, having formulated it, you can carry it in your mind.

Long-term learning needs necessitate a written plan. The more specific the plan, the more easily it will be implemented by the members of the team. The plan should specify the material to be taught, the objectives or goals to be reached, the methods to be used, the individuals who will do the teaching, and the duration of time in which it is to be accomplished. The more detailed your attention to external factors that are subject to modification, the greater will be the continuity of the teaching/learning process.

## Implementing Your Teaching Plan

When you carry out your teaching plan, remain alert to the patient's needs and responses. It may be necessary to modify the pace or some other aspect of your teaching in light of the patient's progress. For example, if the patient is more fatigued than you expected, you will have to shorten your teaching time. Similarly, if you find that a skill is much more difficult for a patient than you had anticipated, you will have to plan additional time for practice.

## Evaluating Learning

Evaluation involves comparing the learner's achievement to the goals initially specified. It may be necessary to devise tests or trials in order to evaluate learning adequately. In the case of psychomotor learning, such a test might consist of demonstration of a skill; cognitive learning might be tested by recitation; and affective learning by, for example, the successful assumption of certain responsibilities.

To be most helpful, progress in learning should be evaluated during the teaching process as well as at its completion. Ongoing evaluation allows you to modify your teaching plan if necessary and gives the learner helpful feedback regarding his or her progress. If an opportunity for feedback is not provided at each step, the person may learn misinformation or practice incorrectly.

Success should be praised freely, since praise tends to motivate further achievement. Praise should focus on specific accomplishments and learning, not personality traits. To a child learning to give an injection, you might say, "You did a good job of measuring the medicine. You showed real skill!" *Not* "Good girl!" Make a conscious effort to enlarge your vocabulary of praise.

Be cautious with regard to failure. After pointing out errors, encourage renewed efforts in a nonthreatening way; failure can lead to depression and withdrawal. Criticism can easily be interpreted as personal rejection if it is not phrased with care.

The learner should be encouraged to evaluate his or her own learning, which necessitates familiarity with the objectives. The learner may need your assistance in comparing his or her performance with the desired objectives.

If learning fails to occur or if the rate of learning is too slow, reassess the internal and external factors affecting the teaching/learning situation and replan your teaching.

# Teaching Groups

We have thus far focused exclusively on teaching individuals. Though most health teaching is one-to-one, nurses also teach groups of people, such as families and groups of patients with the same health problem.

## Advantages of Group Teaching

Teaching groups offers some significant benefits in addition to simple time-saving. Mutual sharing of feelings and problems within the group helps meet the individual group members' psychosocial needs for support, self-esteem, and belongingness. The wide-ranging discussion of issues possible in a group is particularly valuable in promoting affective learning.

As members of the group raise questions, pertinent information is introduced and cognitive learning is fostered. Members who have coped successfully with a given problem in the past may have helpful and concrete suggestions to offer. For example, a group of people with diabetes may share hints about how to stick to a special diet when eating at a restaurant, as well as their feelings about being set apart by their special diet.

In practicing new skills, some patients may be encouraged by the company of other beginners; for others, self-consciousness and fear of failure makes practice in a group setting very threatening.

## Disadvantages of Group Teaching

Teaching a group requires greater interpersonal skill on the part of the teacher than does individual teaching. Maintaining interaction with five, ten, or more people at once poses a complex and constantly varying challenge.

Group size is a major factor in the effectiveness of teaching. Ten to fifteen people is probably the largest group that allows for a free interchange of feelings and an opportunity for all to participate. A larger group may need to be subdivided. A group of five or six people may be optimal for establishing the necessary trust to share feelings as well as thoughts.

When you teach a group of people, the possibility always exists that the material presented will be irrelevant to some members. By definition, group teaching cannot be as individualized or personal as one-to-one teaching can be.

Evaluation may be more difficult in a group. It is also difficult to prevent feelings of failure on the part of those individuals who perform less well. If one person is consistently less able than others in the group, his or her self-esteem may be impaired.

## Planning Group Teaching

The basic principles that guide individual health teaching apply equally to group teaching.

Group teaching always requires a formal written plan. The characteristics of the group should be spelled out, and goals and objectives specified with that particular group in mind. Sharing the written goals and objectives with prospective class members will enable them to decide for themselves whether the group will meet a personal learning need.

Your plan for teaching should allot sufficient time for every member of the group to participate at every stage in the teaching process. Ordinarily, therefore, group teaching requires a longer time span than individual teaching.

The setting for group meetings merits thought. Keep in mind the number of people in the group and the learning activities you have planned. Too large a space may inhibit discussion and participation, while too small a space will constrict activity and comfort. Sometimes the space available dictates the maximum size of the class.

Group meetings should be scheduled for a time of day when most of the individuals you hope to reach will be able to participate. If you are planning to teach a family, the evening is likely to be best. For a group of inpatients, an afternoon after all routine daily care is finished might be optimal.

The interpersonal relationships that develop within the group will be crucial to its success. You will need to assume leadership in fostering positive relationships and controlling members who would otherwise monopolize discussion or undermine others' self-esteem through criticism.

Referring to the material on group interaction in Chapter 6 will help you plan effective group teaching.

## Evaluating Learning in a Group

Evaluation of a group requires ample time—considerably more time than evaluation of individual learning. More formal techniques may also be called for, such as a written quiz instead of an informal discussion. If psychomotor skills are to be evaluated, each person in the group will need an opportunity to demonstrate accomplishment.

## Conclusion

As you progress in nursing, your opportunities for involvement in health teaching will grow. It is a mistake to undertake very large projects independently until you have had a chance to teach on a limited scale or with someone else. As patients in your care become increasingly self-directed as a result of skills and information you have taught them, you will begin to understand why some writers consider health teaching the most important function of the nursing practitioner.

## Care Study  Teaching about an upper G.I. x ray

Mr. Stokes has been admitted to the medical unit for diagnostic tests. His admitting problem is "recurrent epigastric pain." His orders specify "Upper G.I. series in a.m., routine preparation."

Mr. Kyle, a registered nurse, is assigned to care for Mr. Stokes. In the process of taking a nursing history, Mr. Kyle notes that this is Mr. Stokes's first hospitalization, that he is quite upset, and that he has a high school education and is currently employed as a salesman. The nurse asks what Mr. Stokes knows about the planned tests and decides on the basis of his answers that Mr. Stokes has a learning need. He thus formulates a tentative goal and plan and discusses it with the patient.

**Nurse:** "Mr. Stokes, it seems that you would like to know a little more about what is going to be happening."
**Mr. Stokes:** "Sure would!"
**Nurse:** "Right now I must pass four o'clock medications.

I'll come back at five, and we'll discuss the preparation you will have this evening, what will be done here before you go to x ray, and exactly what will happen in x ray. While I'm gone, you can think of any specific questions you'd like to ask. I'll leave a pencil and paper so you can jot things down if you'd like."

When Mr. Kyle returns, he gives Mr. Stokes a printed form outlining the preparation for an upper G.I. x ray and goes over it with him point by point. He answers all Mr. Stokes's questions about his test and makes simple anatomical drawings to clarify information.

Later that evening, Mr. Kyle approaches Mr. Stokes to review what they discussed earlier. Mr. Kyle clarifies a few points that were not clear to Mr. Stokes.

Mr. Kyle then records his assessment of the learning need, the teaching he performed, and the patient's learning.

## Study Terms

active participation
affective
audiovisual aids
behavior
behavior modification
cognitive
environment
external influences on
   learning
feedback
goal
internal influences on
   learning
learning
learning need

motivation
objective
physiologic status
practice
psychomotor
readiness to learn
reinforcement
sequence
   known to unknown
   normal to abnormal
   simple to complex
   wellness to illness
teaching/learning
   process
vocabulary level

## Learning Activities

1. For a patient in the clinical area,
   a. identify a learning need.
   b. set a goal or objective.
   c. plan the teaching.
   d. carry out the teaching.
   e. evaluate its effectiveness.

The learning need chosen should be simple. It may be written up or reported verbally.

2. Review the card index (Kardex) in the clinical area to identify at least three patients who might be expected to have learning needs. Be prepared to describe these patients, their learning needs, and your rationale for choosing them in a discussion group.

3. If your clinical facility has a health teaching record or flow sheet, make a copy and demonstrate its use to record a teaching plan.

4. Design a health teaching flow sheet for use in your clinical facility.

## References

Aiken, L. H. "Patients' Problems Are Problems in Learning." *American Journal of Nursing* 70 (September 1970): 1916.

Ballantyne, D. J. "Closed Circuit T.V. for Patients." *American Journal of Nursing* 74 (February 1974): 263–264.

Berni, R., and Fordyce, W. *Behavior Modification and the Nursing Process,* 2nd ed. St. Louis: C. V. Mosby, 1978.

Brylski, E., and Gillin, J. "Audio-visuals Made to Order." *Nursing Outlook* 20 (June 1972): 385–387.

Collins, R. D. "Problem-Solving: A Tool for Patients, Too." *American Journal of Nursing* 68 (July 1968): 1483–1485.

Dziurbejko, M. M., *et al.* "Including the Family in Preoperative Teaching." *American Journal of Nursing* 78 (November 1978): 1892–1894.

Haferkorn, V. "Assessing Individual Learning Needs as a Basis for Patient Teaching." *Nursing Clinics of North America* 6, no. 1 (1971): 199–209.

Lee, E. A., *et al.* "How Is Inpatient Education Being Managed?" *Nursing Digest* 6 (Spring 1978): 12–16.

Murray, R., and Zentner, J. "Guidelines for More Effective Health Teaching." *Nursing '76* 6 (June 1976): 44–53.

Palm, M. L. "Recognizing Opportunities for Informal Patient Teaching." *Nursing Clinics of North America* 6 (December 1971): 669–678.

Piepgras, R. "All Nurses Are Teachers." *Nursing Outlook* 17 (October 1969): 49–51.

Redman, B. K. "Patient Education as a Function of Nursing Practice." *Nursing Clinics of North America* 6 (December 1971): 573–580.

———. *The Process of Patient Teaching in Practice,* 3rd ed. St. Louis: C. V. Mosby, 1978.

Sharp, A. E. "Four Steps to Better Patient Teaching." *RN* 37 (May 1974): 62–63.

Shuler, C. "Documenting Patient Teaching." *Supervisor Nurse* 10 (June 1979): 43–45.

Smith, D. "Writing Objectives as a Nursing Practice Skill." *American Journal of Nursing* 71 (February 1971): 319–320.

Steagall, B. "How to Prepare Your Patient for Discharge." *Nursing '77* 7 (November 1977): 14–16.

Walters, J. "Four Practical Questions to Ask When Organizing Preoperative Classes." *American Journal of Nursing* 79 (June 1979): 1090–1091.

Wood, M. M. "300 Valuable Booklets to Give to Patients and Their Families: A Source Guide." *Nursing '74* 4 (April 1974): 43–50.

# Chapter 14

# Coordination of Care

## Objectives

After completing this chapter, you should be able to:

1. Explain the nurse's role in coordination of care.
2. Outline the responsibilities of the student nurse with regard to reporting on and off.
3. List items that should be included in an intershift report.
4. Discuss the purposes of team conferences.
5. Outline the responsibilities of the nurse for maintaining nursing-care plans.
6. Discuss the strengths and weaknesses of traditional narrative charting and problem-oriented records.
7. Explain the purpose of an incident report.
8. List information that should be included in a referral.
9. Discuss ways you can facilitate the functioning of the nursing team.
10. Explain the audit approach to formal evaluation of nursing care.

## Outline

Verbal Reports
    Reporting On and Off
    Intershift Report
    Team Conferences
Nursing Care Plans
Charting
    Traditional Narrative Charting
    Problem-Oriented Records
    Abbreviations and Charting Style
Incident Reports
Planning for Continuity of Care
    The Discharge Planner

Writing a Referral
Working With a Team
    In-Service Education
    Directing Others in Care
        The Nursing-Process Approach
        Styles of Leadership and Supervision
    Consideration of Feelings
    Encouraging Growth
Evaluating Care
    Audit of Records
    Direct-Care Audit

Beginning nurses often mistakenly think that co-ordination is a function only of nurses in super-visory or administrative positions. On the con-trary, it is characteristic of the professional nurse to be concerned from the outset with the total con-text of the health-care situation and its impact on the patient. In all daily activities then, the nurse can help the system function more effectively for the patient's benefit.

Coordination of care is basically a matter of communication within the health-care team. Everything you know and will learn about com-munication will be pertinent to this aspect of your practice. Some communication with other person-nel will be oral and some written. Though it is common—and understandable—for nurses to complain about paperwork, written records are absolutely essential to quality care. Time spent on these records is by no means wasted; it is part of patient care. As a practicing nurse, you will of course want to facilitate any effort to make record-keeping more efficient and less time-consuming so that it does not detract from direct care.

The understanding of people you have acquired to prepare you for patient care will also be of value as you work with other health-care team mem-bers. Insight into the feelings and motivations that influence people's behavior, familiarity with the functioning of groups, and well-developed com-munications skills are all extremely valuable in the coordination of care.

## Verbal Reports

Your first experiences in coordinating care are likely to be verbal reports to another nurse. These may occur when reporting on and off, in giving and receiving intershift reports, and in team con-ferences.

### Reporting On and Off

As a student, when you arrive on a unit to care for patients, you are in a unique position because you are not part of the ongoing staff of that unit. You may be unfamiliar with such things as the routines of the facility and the location of equip-ment, and the regular staff will not know you or your abilities. Although your instructor will com-municate with the staff on your behalf, this cannot take the place of your own communication with staff members.

If you will be on the unit for less than a full shift, it is important to find out who will be re-sponsible for care of the patient after you leave. Even if you will be present for the full shift, many facilities assign a staff person to each patient cared for by a student in order to serve as a resource for the student. Find out who this staff person is and meet with him or her. Communicate clearly what your abilities and responsibilities are. It is impor-tant to state straightforwardly the limits of your own abilities and what you expect to accomplish with the patient. If the patient has needs you are not yet prepared to fulfill (such as a procedure you have not yet learned), clarify this with the other care giver.

When you leave the unit, whether for a break or at the end of your assigned stay, you must again contact the staff person to outline what has been accomplished and the patient's status. You may also be expected to report off to a team leader or charge nurse, in addition to the person assigned for care.

Tension sometimes develops between regular staff members and student nurses. Conscien-tiously maintaining clear communication with the staff can prevent or alleviate such tension.

### Intershift Report

Most health-care facilities require an oral report between one shift and the next (such as the night shift and the day shift). The purpose of the *inter-shift report* is to provide essential information and current assessment data about each patient.

When you are receiving a report, the extent of

| Room | Name | Diagnosis, Surg. & Date | Physician | Activity | Diet | I & O | Drsg. | Tubes Drains | I.V. | Other |
|------|------|------------------------|-----------|----------|------|-------|-------|--------------|------|-------|
| | | | | | | Pertinent Assessment Data | | | | |
| 208 | John James | Diabetic Ing. hernia Rep 12/5 | Evans | up ad lib | Reg. | — | Clean + Dry | — | — | no pain |
| 209A | Stella Washington | Chole 12/6 | Jefferson | Chair t.i.d. | NPO | V, O.K., 250/ 1175 | Clean + dry | N.G. to suction | D₅W | |
| 209B | Vacant | | | | | | | | | |
| 210A | Judy Brown | abd. hyst. 12/5 | Cole | up | soft | 950⁻820 (low) | mod. sero. sang. | | out ©10 | Gas |
| | | | | | | | | | | |
| | | | | | | | | | | |

**Figure 14.1  Intershift report form**

the notes you take will be determined by the nature of your responsibilities. If your responsibility is clearly limited to one or two patients, you will want to note carefully all information about those patients. If your responsibilities include answering lights and serving meals to other patients, you will need to take notes on the diagnosis, activity level, and diet of each patient. Figure 14.1 illustrates a form on which you might record information received at an intershift report.

If you are responsible for giving a report, you must prepare very carefully. Some facilities specify the information to be included; others rely on the individual nurse to decide what to include. The intershift report form might also be used to record information you wish to include when giving a report.

After reviewing or deciding what to include, make careful notes so as to have all the facts at hand. A report is usually given using a card index or notebook containing basic care information on all the patients. Proceed through the card index (Kardex) carefully, checking your notes periodically so you do not forget any important information. Go slowly enough to allow those to whom you are reporting to take notes and ask questions. Though time should not be wasted, hurrying can make for incomplete communication.

## Team Conferences

In facilities that employ the team method of patient care, whereby a group of staff members work together to care for a group of patients, team conferences are held regularly. The purpose of such conferences may vary. Some team conferences are devoted to discussing the care of a patient who presents particularly difficult nursing problems.

Another purpose of the team conference is to explore a given aspect of care that may affect many patients, such as the admission nursing interview. Such a conference is more educational in intent.

A team conference is an occasion for sharing. The better prepared each individual is to contribute, the more valuable the conference will be. In order to prepare, consider the topic or patient to be discussed. Review the patient's chart. Then think about what you might contribute or questions the team might discuss. If the conference has no predetermined subject, you might bring up problems or topics you would like to have discussed.

When you participate in team conferences, keep in mind what you have learned about effective functioning in groups. Review Chapter 6, and consider how you can be supportive of the group's purpose.

## Nursing Care Plans

The primary purpose of a written nursing care plan is to communicate to the entire nursing care team what is to be done for the patient. Its secondary purpose is to serve as evidence that the patient is receiving ongoing and appropriate nursing care. Written documentation is increasingly being required by the federal government (through Medicare and Medicaid) and insurance carriers for purposes of evaluating health care. Nurses also use written records—both the care plan and the chart—to assess and improve patient care; care reviews are routinely undertaken by nursing committees within the employing institution. Finally, accrediting bodies require written nursing care plans for each patient.

The initial nursing care plan, usually written by the nurse responsible for admitting the patient, is based on the initial nursing history and examination. Figure 14.2 illustrates how a standard nursing care plan may be adapted for use with an individual patient.

The nursing care plan must be updated and reviewed on an ongoing basis. This responsibility may be assigned to the primary nurse who is responsible and accountable for the patient's care or it may be shared by all the nurses who care for the patient. In general, the nursing care plan is more likely to be kept up-to-date if one nurse is responsible.

Whether or not one person is responsible, others can contribute ideas and information to the nursing care plan. As a student nurse, it is your responsibility to find out the appropriate procedure for updating a care plan. Then, when you feel you have something to contribute, you can follow through by consulting with the appropriate nurse.

Since the nursing care plan is the nurse's responsibility, it is important to appraise both content and form critically to ascertain whether it is fulfilling its purposes adequately. In evaluating any written nursing care plan, the following questions may be used as guidelines:

**1.** Can the patient's current problems be quickly discerned?
**2.** Are the goals or objectives of care, both immediate and long-term, identified and clearly stated and measurable?
**3.** Are the prescribed nursing actions paired with the problems they are intended to alleviate, so their effectiveness can be evaluated?
**4.** Are the prescribed nursing actions stated clearly enough that anyone responsible for care can follow them accurately?

The written nursing care plan may be in a card index, on a separate sheet on the chart, or in a variety of other locations. The only requirement is that it be available to those who care for the patient. In some settings, nursing care plans are erased, changed, and eventually discarded when the patient is discharged. Though this approach makes it easier to change the care plan as the patient's needs change, it greatly hampers ongoing review of the situation and subsequent evaluation.

## Charting

The patient's chart is a tool for communication among health-care team members about the patient's illness, therapies, tests, and response to care. It is the legal record of care and as such may be used in a court proceeding. The chart is also used for monitoring quality of care and for conducting research.

All members of the health-care team have responsibilities for the patient's official record, but nursing is usually charged with primary responsibility for seeing that the record is properly set up, that all pertinent forms and records are added when they become available, and that the chart accompanies a patient who moves within the health-care system for treatments and tests. After the patient has been discharged, the medical-records department assumes responsibility for the record, reviews it for completeness, obtains missing information, and stores the record for use in various evaluation, statistical, and research pro-

BASIC CARE PLAN

DIAGNOSIS: KNEE SURGERY

ANTICIPATED OUTCOMES:

DISCHARGE PLANNING:

*Tomlin, Arthur*
*542-40-572*
*Age 22*
*Dr. A. Bradshaw*

| DATE | USUAL PROBLEMS | EXPECTED OUTCOMES | DEADLINES | NURSING ORDERS |
|---|---|---|---|---|
| 12/8 | poss. anxiety due to fear of surg. and unknown | lessened anxiety | 12/8 | 1. Pre-op teaching by T.L. on adm<br>2. Reinforce teaching by T.L. morn of sug. Include Quad sets & SLL<br>3. Allow pt. to voice fears<br>*J. Reynolds RN* |
| 12/9 | poss. pain due to surg. | verbalize reasonable comfort | ✓ q 4° | 1. Offer pain med q 4° 1st 24 then prn.<br>2. ✓ alignment & reposition as nec<br>3. Give pain med prior to P. & ambulation as needed.<br>*J. Reynolds RN.* |
| 12/9 | poss. impaired circ. due to edema, tissue trauma or constricting dressing | Pedal pulses present Warm pink foot | *at discharge* | 1. ✓ circ. q 2° on even hr. 1st 24°<br>2. Position leg as ordered.<br>3. Notify M.D. for severe pain on passive stretch<br>*J. Reynolds, R.N.* |
| 12/9 | poss. inability to SLL due to fear of pain or poor muscle tone | Quad sets at will | *By discharge* | 1. Instruct to do quad sets 10X hr. while awake 1st 24°<br>2. Obtain order for crutch-walking p̄ SLL - ½ wt.<br>*J. Reynolds, R.N.* |
| 12/9 | poss. constipation due to immobility & pain meds | BM q.o.d. | ✓ *daily* | 1. Offer juice @ 10ᵃ and 8ᵖ<br>2. Min. fluids - 2000/24 hr<br>3. Offer lax q.o.d. @ HS<br>*J. Reynolds. R.N.* |
| 12/10 | *Anxiety over job disruption* | *verbalizes resolution of problems related to job.* | *discharge* | *1. Encourage him to express concerns and formulate a specific plan of action*<br>*J. Reynolds R.N.* |

**Figure 14.2  Nursing care plan**
Courtesy Ballard Community Hospital (Seattle, Washington)

grams. The record is available for reference if the patient is readmitted.

In addition to overall responsibility for the chart, the nurse must also record data related to the nursing process: assessment data, including subjective and objective information and problems; nursing actions; and evaluation of the effectiveness of those actions. Keep in mind that you need to record enough information to communicate adequately with other members of the health-care team and to demonstrate the level of care provided. Many evaluation systems operate on the assumption that actions not recorded have not been performed. Adequate recording is also a legal safeguard for you personally. If questions arise about the appropriateness or adequacy of care, the chart is accepted as proof of the care given. See Module 2, "Charting," for detailed directions on charting techniques.

## Traditional Narrative Charting

Traditional patient records provide separate forms for each discipline caring for the patient: doctor's progress notes, nurse's notes, a physical therapy record, and the like. Each discipline records information gathered and actions taken on the appropriate form. Routine information is also recorded on a variety of graphs and checklists.

The nurse's notes are usually organized chronologically. For each shift, the nurse notes assessment data (both subjective and objective), problems identified, actions taken, and evaluation of those actions (see Figure 14.3). The narrative may be modified to organize information around body systems, human needs, or in any other manner agreed upon by the facility.

Most people find traditional narrative notes easy to write, which increases willingness to make appropriate entries in the chart. New types of information can be included in the narration without difficulty. For precisely the same reasons, however, a narrative record may be disorganized; it may be difficult to find needed information without reading through paragraphs of irrelevant narration. Module 2, "Charting," includes examples of adaptations of narrative charting.

## Problem-Oriented Records

The problem-oriented record (POR), or problem-oriented medical record (POMR) as it is sometimes called, is designed to encourage all members of the health-care team to use a problem-solving approach to patient care and to organize the record so that information is readily available (Weed, 1970).

The basic components of the POR are (1) the data base, (2) the problem list, (3) the initial plan, (4) progress notes, and (5) flow sheets. The *data base* consists of all initial information on the patient, the physician's history and physical, the nursing admission interview and examination, and the admitting laboratory work. The patient's admitting problems are identified from the data base and are stated with as much specificity as possible. If later information provides more insight or allows for more accurate labeling of a problem, the statement of that problem will be revised. Each problem is then numbered and titled, and the resulting *problem list* serves as a combined table of contents and index to the record. If further problems are identified, they are added to the list; when problems are resolved, their resolution is noted on the problem list (see Figure 14.4).

The *initial plan* outlines what will be initially done for the patient, including any further diagnostic studies, specific treatment, plans for patient education, and/or plans for eventual discharge. The physician usually writes the initial problem list and plan.

*Progress notes* are written by all members of the health-care team and are organized in a specific manner commonly referred to as *SOAPing*—an acronym for the order in which information is entered in the progress note (see Figure 14.5). First, the problem under discussion is identified by number and title. Then *subjective* information (symptoms) is recorded, followed by *objective* information. Next comes an *analysis* of the data (Weed calls this step "assessment," a slightly different use of the term than is common in nursing). Finally, a *plan* of action is specified. Progress notes need not always contain all these elements. For example, if the patient is unable to respond, there would be no subjective data. Similarly, if you have

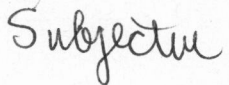

Subjective

## PATIENT RECORD

| DATE | HOUR | ASSESSMENT |
|------|------|------------|
| 12/6/80 | 4:00 p. | ADMITTED PER _walking_ GLASSES _yes_ CONTACTS — |
| | | DR. _Burton_ NOTIFIED TIME _4:15 p._ DENTURES (NATURAL) — |
| | | T.P.R. 98⁴-88-22 B.P. 138/86 (ARTIFICIAL) ↑ and ↓ |
| | | WEIGHT 185 # ADMISSION BATH — HEARING AID — |
| | | LAB WORK DONE: BLOOD ✓ URINE ✓ TRANSFUSIONS (YES) (NO) ✗ |
| | | MEDICINES (BRING TO DESK) _None_ (WHERE) (WHEN) |
| | | ALLERGIES _Sulfa_ PREGNANCIES — |

_See Admission Hx + P.E. for all systems review._
_Psych-Soc. Expresses high level of anxiety._
_Constantly jiggling keys or pacing the floor._
_Time spent listening to concerns and explaining_
_routines resulted in some ↓ in level of anxiety._
_Integ. Routine abdominal prep. done for colon resection._
_G.I. Enema prep. begun. See Flow sheet for details_

_L. Donahue R.N._

| Patient Assessment | Circulatory (Circ.) | Central Nervous System (C.N.S.) | Dermatology (Derm.) | Gastrointestional (G.I.) |
|---|---|---|---|---|
| | Genitourinary (G.U.) | Musculoskeletal (Musc.-Skel.) | Psycho-Social (Psy.-Soc.) | Respiratory (Resp.) |

Cormand, Thomas
827-06-572
Age: 62
Dr. A. Burton

**BALLARD COMMUNITY HOSPITAL**
SEATTLE, WASHINGTON

P-194 Rev. 5/73

**Figure 14.3 Traditional narrative charting**
Courtesy Ballard Community Hospital (Seattle, Washington)

GROUP HEALTH COOPERATIVE OF PUGET SOUND

MASTER PROBLEM LIST

Mitchell, Carl A
m - 58
420 - 473 - 1129
11/5/80 - Dr. M. Reynolds

| PROBLEM NUMBER | DATE PROB. ACTIVE | PROBLEM – ACTIVE | PROBLEM – RESOLVED | DATE RE-SOLVED |
|---|---|---|---|---|
| 1 | 11/5/80 | Chest pain / M. Reynolds M.D. | | |
| 2 | 11/5/80 | Anxiety rē hospitalization/ J. Kirkland R.N. | | |
| 3 | 11/5/80 | Constipation due to inactivity / J. Kirkland R.N. | | |
| | | | | |
| | | | | |
| | | | | |
| | | | | |
| | | | | |
| | | | | |
| | | | | |

**Figure 14.4 The problem list**

Courtesy Group Health Cooperative of Puget Sound (Seattle, Washington)

EVERGREEN GENERAL HOSPITAL — KIRKLAND WASHINGTON

7/77

STD. FORM C5

| DATE AND HR. | PROBLEM ORIENTED PROGRESS NOTES |
|---|---|
| | **INSTRUCTIONS:** Problem oriented progress notes should have: Date; Time; Name of Problem; and S.O.A.P.: (Subjective, Objective, Assessment, Plan) format. |
| 1/15/81 | 7:30 p.m. #1 Preoperative Anxiety |
| S | - "I've never had surgery before. My stomach is twisted in Knots. Maybe I'll die!" |
| O | - Face drawn. Paces the floor when left alone. Asks the same question over and over. |
| A | - Moderate to severe anxiety interfering with ability to comprehend preoperative teaching and potential adverse response to surgery. |
| P | - R.N. to spend one-to-one time with patient using interaction to decrease anxiety. Omit group preoperative session. Notify surgeon. Martha Reynolds R.N. |

NOTE PROGRESS OF CASE - COMPLICATIONS - CONSULTATIONS - CHANGE IN DIAGNOSIS - CONDITIONS ON DISCHARGE - INSTRUCTIONS TO PATIENT - AND FINAL SUMMARY.

STAMP HERE

MILLS, JEFFREY R.
DR. WILSON NO. 723-081
B.D. 10/18/59 AGE 21 SEX M

PROGRESS REPORT

PROBLEM ORIENTED PROGRESS REPORT 5

**Figure 14.5 POMR progress notes**
Courtesy Evergreen General Hospital (Kirkland, Washington)

nothing new to add to the analysis of data, you would not include that section in your progress note. Module 2, "Charting," includes examples and directions for writing SOAP progress notes.

The last part of the problem-oriented record consists of *flow sheets*—graphs and charts used to record simple data most easily absorbed in that form. Flow sheets reduce the volume of narration and the bulk of the chart while providing a record of important information (see Figure 14.6). They are commonly used for vital signs, neurological checks, a bowel training program, and so forth.

The advantages of the POR are that it encourages a problem-solving approach, all team members record on the same form and thus see one another's comments, redundancy is reduced, and the chart is less voluminous. Another advantage is the ease with which the course of a specific problem may be followed through the record.

A disadvantage is that POR charting is new to many members of the health-care team and extensive in-service education may be needed to implement it. Another potential drawback is that people occasionally have information they feel should be recorded but cannot find a place for it within the structure of the chart, and thus will omit it. The solution to this dilemma is to consult with others to decide where the information can be added, even if it means beginning a new flow sheet or checklist. Recording one-time actions may also prove problematic, since they do not fit easily into the progress note or merit a flow sheet. This problem may be solved by recording on the progress note that the action is planned and then adding a date, time, signature, and the word "done" when it is completed. Perhaps the biggest problem arises when a particular item of data is pertinent to a number of problems such as in the case of a critically ill patient. In this situation, data might be organized by body systems and all relevant problems charted together. The POR is most successful when such difficulties are approached creatively and not treated as stumbling blocks.

## Abbreviations and Charting Style

The typically extensive use of abbreviations and incomplete statements in patients' charts often makes them hard to read. Module 2, "Charting," illustrates how to simplify statements when charting. Appendix A consists of a list of common abbreviations; you may also wish to ask whether your facility has a list of approved abbreviations. Appendix B provides a list of abbreviations of common medical diagnoses. You may need to look up an abbreviated diagnosis in this list before consulting your other reference books for information on nursing care. Appendix C lists prefixes and suffixes combined to form medical terms. Familiarity with these terms will make it much easier to understand patients' charts.

## Incident Reports

When an untoward incident or accident—such as a fall, cut, or medication error—occurs in a health facility, an *incident report* is filed in the record department. Incidents involving staff and visitors, as well as patients, are reported. If a patient is involved, the incident is also noted on the patient's chart. The purposes of incident reports are to highlight recurrent problems, to serve as a record for insurance and legal reference, and to indicate a need to modify procedures and/or plan in-service education.

The staff member who discovers or witnesses the incident is usually responsible for filing the incident report. Doing so does not constitute responsibility for the problem.

In the event of an incident, assess the situation to determine whether injury has occurred. If there is any possibility of injury, a physician is notified or the injured person is sent to the emergency department of the hospital. Make out the report as soon as possible after seeing to immediate needs so that the details will be fresh in your mind.

EVERGREEN GENERAL HOSPITAL — KIRKLAND, WASHINGTON
## GENERAL PURPOSE FLOW SHEET

2-72

**INSTRUCTIONS:** Label problems at top and enter parameters to be followed: H&P; Measurements: Lab data; Blood pressures, etc.

PROBLEM: #3  Decubitus ulcer on coccyx

| PARAMETERS | DATES/TIME | | | | | | |
|---|---|---|---|---|---|---|---|
| | 1/5/80 8 a.m. | 1/5/80 8 p.m. | | | | | |
| Size of open area | 2" x 3" | 2 x 3 | | | | | |
| Color of tissue | Pale Pink | Pink | | | | | |
| Drainage – Am't | Lg. | Mod. | | | | | |
| Drainage – Color | Yellow | Yellow | | | | | |
| Cleaned c̄ N.S. | ✓ | ✓ | | | | | |
| Heat Lamp 20 min. | ✓ | ✓ | | | | | |
| | | | | | | | |
| Initials | R.J. | M.O. | | | | | |

↓STAMP HERE↓

EDISON, ROBERT K.          8-009-021
LAST NAME        FIRST        INITIAL    HOSPITAL No.

KELLEY                          476
PHYSICIAN                      CODE

11/19/05        75            M
BIRTH DATE      AGE          SEX

GENERAL PURPOSE FLOW SHEET                    4

**Figure 14.6  POMR flow sheet**
Courtesy Evergreen General Hospital (Kirkland, Washington)

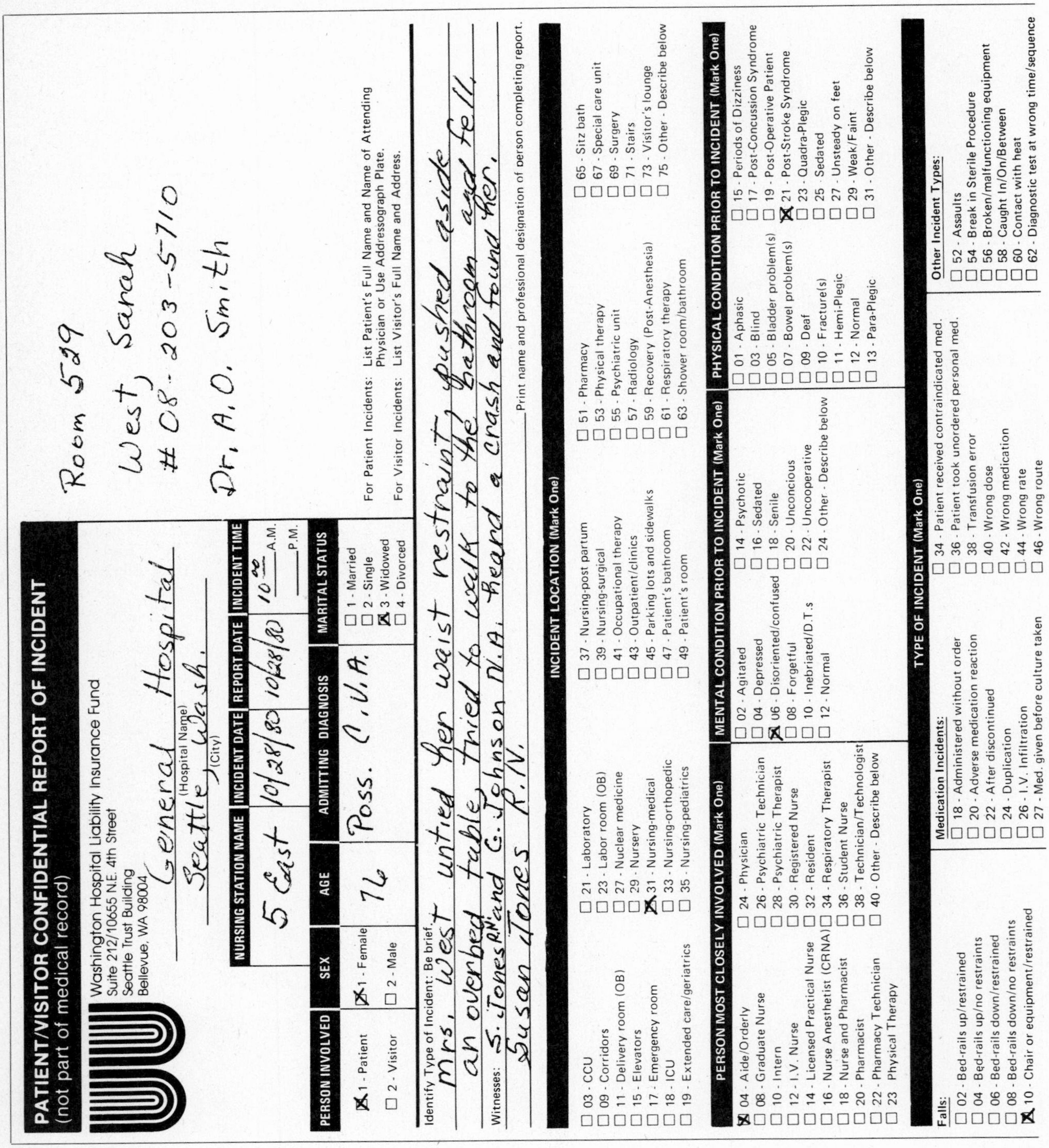

**PATIENT/VISITOR CONFIDENTIAL REPORT OF INCIDENT**
(not part of medical record)

Washington Hospital Liability Insurance Fund
Suite 212/10655 N.E. 4th Street
Seattle Trust Building
Bellevue, WA 98004

General Hospital (Hospital Name)
Seattle, Wash. (City)

Room 529
West, Sarah
# 08-203-5710
Dr. A.O. Smith

| NURSING STATION NAME | INCIDENT DATE | REPORT DATE | INCIDENT TIME |
|---|---|---|---|
| 5 East | 10/28/80 | 10/28/80 | 10:00 A.M. / ___ P.M. |

| PERSON INVOLVED | SEX | AGE | ADMITTING DIAGNOSIS | MARITAL STATUS |
|---|---|---|---|---|
| ☒ 1 - Patient<br>☐ 2 - Visitor | ☒ 1 - Female<br>☐ 2 - Male | 76 | Poss. C.V.A. | ☐ 1 - Married<br>☐ 2 - Single<br>☒ 3 - Widowed<br>☐ 4 - Divorced |

For Patient Incidents: List Patient's Full Name and Name of Attending Physician or Use Addressograph Plate.
For Visitor Incidents: List Visitor's Full Name and Address.

Identify Type of Incident: Be brief. Mrs. West untied her waist restraint, pushed aside an overbed table, tried to walk to the bathroom and fell.
Witnesses: S. Jones RN and G. Johnson N.A. heard a crash and found her.
Susan Jones R.N. — Print name and professional designation of person completing report.

**INCIDENT LOCATION (Mark One)**

☐ 03 - CCU
☐ 09 - Corridors
☐ 11 - Delivery room (OB)
☐ 15 - Elevators
☐ 17 - Emergency room
☐ 18 - ICU
☐ 19 - Extended care/geriatrics
☐ 21 - Laboratory
☐ 23 - Labor room (OB)
☐ 27 - Nuclear medicine
☐ 29 - Nursery
☒ 31 - Nursing-medical
☐ 33 - Nursing-orthopedic
☐ 35 - Nursing-pediatrics
☐ 37 - Nursing-post partum
☐ 39 - Nursing-surgical
☐ 41 - Occupational therapy
☐ 43 - Outpatient/clinics
☐ 45 - Parking lots and sidewalks
☐ 47 - Patient's bathroom
☐ 49 - Patient's room
☐ 51 - Pharmacy
☐ 53 - Physical therapy
☐ 55 - Psychiatric unit
☐ 57 - Radiology
☐ 59 - Recovery (Post-Anesthesia)
☐ 61 - Respiratory therapy
☐ 63 - Shower room/bathroom
☐ 65 - Sitz bath
☐ 67 - Special care unit
☐ 69 - Surgery
☐ 71 - Stairs
☐ 73 - Visitor's lounge
☐ 75 - Other - Describe below

**PERSON MOST CLOSELY INVOLVED (Mark One)**

☒ 04 - Aide/Orderly
☐ 08 - Graduate Nurse
☐ 10 - Intern
☐ 12 - I.V. Nurse
☐ 14 - Licensed Practical Nurse
☐ 16 - Nurse Anesthetist (CRNA)
☐ 18 - Nurse and Pharmacist
☐ 20 - Pharmacist
☐ 22 - Pharmacy Technician
☐ 23 Physical Therapy
☐ 24 - Physician
☐ 26 - Psychiatric Technician
☐ 28 - Psychiatric Therapist
☐ 30 - Registered Nurse
☐ 32 - Resident
☐ 34 - Respiratory Therapist
☐ 36 - Student Nurse
☐ 38 - Technician/Technologist
☐ 40 - Other - Describe below

**MENTAL CONDITION PRIOR TO INCIDENT (Mark One)**

☐ 02 - Agitated
☐ 04 - Depressed
☒ 06 - Disoriented/confused
☐ 08 - Forgetful
☐ 10 - Inebriated/D.T.s
☐ 12 - Normal
☐ 14 - Psychotic
☐ 16 - Sedated
☐ 18 - Senile
☐ 20 - Unconcious
☐ 22 - Uncooperative
☐ 24 - Other - Describe below

**PHYSICAL CONDITION PRIOR TO INCIDENT (Mark One)**

☐ 01 - Aphasic
☐ 03 - Blind
☐ 05 - Bladder problem(s)
☐ 07 - Bowel problem(s)
☐ 09 - Deaf
☐ 10 - Fracture(s)
☐ 11 - Hemi-Plegic
☐ 12 - Normal
☐ 13 - Para-Plegic
☐ 15 - Periods of Dizziness
☐ 17 - Post-Concussion Syndrome
☐ 19 - Post-Operative Patient
☒ 21 - Post-Stroke Syndrome
☐ 23 - Quadra-Plegic
☐ 25 Sedated
☐ 27 - Unsteady on feet
☐ 29 - Weak/Faint
☐ 31 - Other - Describe below

**TYPE OF INCIDENT (Mark One)**

Falls:
☐ 02 - Bed-rails up/restrained
☐ 04 - Bed-rails up/no restraints
☐ 06 - Bed-rails down/restrained
☐ 08 - Bed-rails down/no restraints
☒ 10 - Chair or equipment/restrained

Medication Incidents:
☐ 18 - Administered without order
☐ 20 - Adverse medication reaction
☐ 22 - After discontinued
☐ 24 - Duplication
☐ 26 - I.V. Infiltration
☐ 27 - Med. given before culture taken
☐ 34 - Patient received contraindicated med.
☐ 36 - Patient took unordered personal med.
☐ 38 - Transfusion error
☐ 40 - Wrong dose
☐ 42 - Wrong medication
☐ 44 - Wrong rate
☐ 46 - Wrong route

Other Incident Types:
☐ 52 - Assaults
☐ 54 - Break in Sterile Procedure
☐ 56 - Broken/malfunctioning equipment
☐ 58 - Caught In/On/Between
☐ 60 - Contact with heat
☐ 62 - Diagnostic test at wrong time/sequence

**Figure 14.7 Incident report**
Courtesy Washington Hospital Liability Insurance Fund (Seattle, Washington)

## CAUSE OF FALL - PATIENT (Mark One)

- 05 - Call light not used
- 07 - Improper footwear
- 09 - Pt. Confused/disoriented
- 11 - Pt. Fainted
- 13 - Pt. Incontinent
- [X] 15 - Pt. Inebriated/D.T.s
- 17 - Pt. Lost Balance
- 19 - Pt. Lowered side rail(s)
- 21 - Pt./family refused restraints
- [X] 23 - Pt. removed restraint(s)
- 25 - Pt. Sedated
- 27 - Pt. Senile
- 29 - Pt. Unable to follow instructions
- 31 - Pt. Uncooperative
- 33 - Pt. Violated activity order
- 35 - Other - Describe below

- 12 - Chair or equipment/no restraints
- 14 - While ambulating/with permission
- 16 - Other - Describe below

## CAUSE OF FALL—HOSPITAL (Mark One)

- 01 - Call light not answered promptly
- 03 - Call light unavailable
- 04 - Failure to assist Pt. adequately
- 05 - Inappropriate activity order
- 07 - Lack of Pt. care staff
- 09 - Lack of Pt. safety assessment/care planning
- [X] 11 - Lack of Pt. supervision
- 13 - Poor maintenance of beds, Pt. transport equipment, etc.
- 15 - Poor maintenance of floors, handrails, etc.
- 17 - Poor technique in lifting/moving patient
- 19 - Restraints inadequate/unavailable
- 21 - Restraints not applied
- 25 - Side rail(s) left down
- 27 - Transfer belt not used
- 29 - Other - Describe below

- 28 - Medication on hold
- 30 - Medication theft/missing medication
- 32 - Omission
- 47 - Wrong site
- 48 - Wrong time
- 50 - Other - Describe below

- 64 - Electrocution
- 66 - Fire
- 70 - Hospital acquired infection
- 72 - Lost/damaged Pt./Visitor property
- 74 - Lost specimens
- 76 - Missing instrument(s)
- 78 - Missing needle(s)
- 80 - Missing Sponge(s)
- 82 - Omitted diagnostic test
- 84 - Omitted treatment
- 86 - Patient escape
- 88 - Struck against
- 90 - Struck by
- 92 - Surgery check list not completed
- 94 - Wrong diet
- 95 - Wrong treatment/diagnostic test
- 96 - Other - Describe below

## ACTIVITY ORDERS (Mark One)

- 02 - Ambulate with Assistance
- 04 - Ambulate without Assistance
- 06 - Bathroom Privileges with Assistance
- 08 - Bathroom Privileges without Assistance
- 10 - Dangle with Assistance
- 12 - Dangle without Assistance
- [X] 14 - Up in Chair
- 16 - Up with Assistance
- 18 - Up without Assistance
- 20 - Other - Describe below

## MEDICATION INVOLVED (Mark All Appropriate)

- 02 - Analgesic
- 04 - Antiarrythmic
- 06 - Antibiotic
- 08 - Anticoagulant
- 10 - Anticonvulsant
- 12 - Antidepressant
- 14 - Antihistamine
- 16 - Antineoplastic
- 18 - Diuretic
- 20 - Insulin
- 22 - Narcotic
- 24 - Sedative/Tranquilizer
- 26 - Steroid
- 30 - Vasodilator
- 32 - Vasopressor
- 34 - Other - Describe below

## CAUSE OF MEDICATION INCIDENT (Mark One)

- 02 - Container contents not checked
- 04 - Container improperly labeled
- 06 - Container label not checked
- 08 - Copy of order not sent to pharmacy
- 10 - Direct copy of physician's order not checked
- 12 - Discharge cancelled
- 14 - Error in blood crossmatching
- 16 - Error in blood typing
- [X] 18 - Failure to chart correctly/promptly
- 19 - Failure to have second nurse double check dosage of potent drug
- 20 - Faulty IV equipment
- 22 - Incorrect calculation of dosage
- 24 - Injection technique
- 26 - IV not monitored
- 27 - Med. card lost or misfiled

- 28 - Med. card not compared with unit med. profile/Kardex
- 30 - Med. cup not compared with med. card
- 32 - Med./IV not received from pharmacy
- 34 - Med./IV placed in wrong location (shelf, unit dose tray, etc.)
- 36 - Med./IV received late from pharmacy
- 38 - Patient drug profile not kept up-to-date and accurate in pharmacy
- 40 - Patient drug profile/Kardex/med. card not kept up-to-date and accurate on unit
- 42 - Patient not counseled on hazards of unordered pers. meds.
- 44 - Patient not observed until medication (oral) was taken
- 46 - Patient out of room
- 48 - Patient's allergies not checked
- 50 - Patient's I.D. band not checked
- 52 - Patient's personal medication(s) not confiscated
- 54 - Patient transferred
- 55 - PDR or package insert not checked

- 56 - Physician's order misread
- 57 - PRN medication given early without physician approval
- 58 - Questionable med. order not questioned or challenged
- 60 - Time lapse since last dosage not verified
- 64 - Unclear order not reviewed with physician
- 65 - Unit med. profile/Kardex/med. card misread
- 66 - Unit med. profile/Kardex/med. cards not checked frequently as reminder
- 68 - Unit med. profile/Kardex/med. cards not compared with direct copy of physician's order
- 72 - Wrong dosage or strength from pharmacy
- 74 - Wrong IV equipment used
- 76 - Wrong med. from pharmacy
- 78 - Other - Describe below

## NATURE OF INJURY (Mark One)

- 01 - Abrasion
- 03 - Aggravation of pre-existing condition
- 05 - Allergic Reaction
- 07 - Amputation
- 09 - Asphyxia/Anoxia
- 11 - Back or Disc injury
- 13 - Blindness
- 15 - Broken tooth/teeth
- 17 - Burns
- 19 - Comatose
- [X] 21 - Contusion
- 23 - Deceased
- 25 - Fracture-Dislocation
- 27 - Head/Brain injuries
- 29 - Hip fracture
- 31 - Incontinence
- 33 - Infection/contag. disease
- 35 - Internal injury
- 37 - Laceration
- 39 - Loss of hearing
- 41 - No apparent injury
- 43 - Paralysis
- 45 - Puncture
- 47 - Sprain/strain
- 49 - Other - Describe below

WAS PHYSICIAN NOTIFIED? [X] YES  [ ] NO  TIME NOTIFIED 10:30 [X] A.M. [ ] P.M.

WAS PERSON SEEN BY A PHYSICIAN [X] YES  [ ] NO  TIME SEEN 10:30 [X] A.M. [ ] P.M.

CLINICAL INFORMATION/FOLLOW-UP OR OTHER SENSITIVE FACTS OR EXPLANATIONS (FOR MORE SPACE USE REVERSE SIDE):

IF ANSWER IS OTHER, LIST ITEM NO. AND DESCRIBE BELOW

*Bruise on left shoulder. No other injuries apparent.* — A. B. Smith, M.D.

**WASHINGTON HOSPITAL LIABILITY INSURANCE FUND COPY**

WHLIF - 2/79

**Figure 14.7** (continued)

Your report should include all pertinent facts, including exact times and the sequence of events. The language should be objective; remember that the incident report is a legal document. Any corrective action taken to remedy the problem should also be noted. Figure 14.7 illustrates a type of incident report structured to elicit maximum factual data and to minimize the time spent writing the report.

# Planning for Continuity of Care

It is the nurse's responsibility to assure that needed nursing care continues when a patient is discharged or transferred to another health-care facility. Patients are often discharged from acute-care facilities while still in need of nursing care and rehabilitative support that cannot be provided by their family and friends or managed in their own homes. There are various alternative approaches to continuing care for such patients. Though most require a physician's referral, it is often the nurse who points out the most appropriate source of help and makes out the referral.

## The Discharge Planner

Many hospitals give responsibility for discharge planning to a nurse known as the *discharge planner*. This nurse may follow patients' progress throughout hospitalization or may depend on the referrals of staff nurses to identify patients in need of discharge-planning services.

The discharge planner meets with the patient and family to explore alternatives for continuing care. Such alternatives include home health aides, who assist with routine personal care and household tasks for a limited time; visiting nurses, who can provide skilled care; and residential skilled-nursing facilities. Once a decision is made, the discharge planner makes the arrangements for post-hospital care and transfer of care to the agency selected.

In a facility without a discharge planner, responsibility for planning discharge is typically diffused among the staff members responsible for the patient's care. The physician may meet with the patient and family to plan appropriate post-discharge care. A social worker may arrange the placement if a residential facility is needed; the nurse may arrange for visiting nurse services. The referral form is usually made out by the staff nurse. In some localities, the community health nurse visits the patient before discharge to facilitate continuity of care.

## Writing a Referral

When a patient is ready for discharge, it is the staff nurse's responsibility to complete a *referral form*. At this time it is both appropriate and legally permissible to share information about the patient with individuals outside the facility; the agency that will be responsible for the patient's care needs such information to provide sound care. By accepting a referral, the patient gives implied consent for appropriate information to be shared with the agency. Appropriate information is defined as that which is pertinent to sound care.

The patient's condition at the time of discharge is summarized, often in the form of a brief system review of all data pertaining to each body system. Current nursing care problems and planned interventions are then outlined. Information on special needs, such as a technique for transfer, a means of communication, or food habits, should be included. The form also provides for the physician to write discharge orders. In some settings, the nurse fills out the form, after clarifying with the physician which current medications and orders are to be continued. The physician then simply signs the form.

# PATIENT DISCHARGE RESUMÉ

**DIET**

2 Gm. Na Low Cholesterol; Low Saturated Fat Diet reviewed with patient and wife before discharge

**ACTIVITY**

Increase activity gradually as directed by M.D. Begin with self care, frequent rest periods; no stairs.

**PROCEDURES**

None

**COMMENTS**

Pt. Has discussed need for stress reduction with various individuals. Plans to enroll in course on stress management next month. M.D. has given tentative approval. Understands need to avoid aspirin and aspirin containing products.

Awareness of Diagnosis (Patient aware of reason for hospitalization): Pt. can verbalize what happened during his heart attack. Can outline possible contributing factors in his life style.

Reportable signs & symptoms: Any chest pain not relieved by nitroglycerin. Shortness of breath on exertion. Fluid retention as seen by puffy ankles or weight gain. Any bleeding problems—gums, urine

Medication instruction & schedule (Home bound medications only)

| | MEDICATION | DOSAGE | TIMES |
|---|---|---|---|
| 1 | Coumadin | 2.5 mg. (1 tablet) | Each a.m. — To have blood test weekly — every Wednesday. |
| | 2. Nitroglycerin | 0.3 mg. (1 tablet) | As needed for chest pain. Under the tongue. May be repeated in 5 min. x 2. Still no relief call M.D. |

Patient and/or family verbalizes awareness of above instruction ☒ YES ☐ NO

**DISCHARGE DATA**

Date 12/5/80  Time 2:15  T.P.R. 98⁸-78-18  B.P. 132/84  DESTINATION Home
Personal belongings returned? ☒ YES ☐ NO ☐ N/A  Returned to: patient
Medications returned ☐ YES ☐ NO ☒ N/A
Discharged: Person escorted by _____  Wheel Chair ☐ Ambulatory ☐ Ambulance ☐

Special Instruction Sheets (specify type): Diet Instructions

Office visit on: 12/20/80  ☒ call office on arrival home for appointment _____

Konold, Dwayne
870-50-682
Age 58
Dr. M.F. Woodey

CHART COPY

Referral made to Home Health ☐ YES ☒ NO
PATIENT SIGNATURE D. Konold
EMPLOYEE SIGNATURE C. Kling R.N.
TITLE

BALLARD COMMUNITY HOSPITAL
5409 BARNES AVENUE NORTHWEST • SEATTLE, WASHINGTON 98107 • 782-2700

**Figure 14.8 Patient Discharge Resume**
Courtesy Ballard Community Hospital (Seattle, Washington)

# Working With a Team

Even when "team nursing" is not the primary mode of care, the various nurses who care for a given patient constitute a team. Working effectively with this team is an important aspect of nursing. When you take part in team conferences (see pages 216–217) and committees on nursing policies and procedures, reviewing the information on groups in Chapter 6 will help you participate most effectively.

## In-Service Education

On occasion you may be asked to lead an in-service teaching session for other nursing personnel. If, for example, a patient on your unit has a new type of colostomy irrigation and all staff members need to learn how it is to be done, you may be asked to research the literature on the subject, plan a presentation, and lead the class. This is an opportunity to put into practice the principles of teaching outlined in Chapter 13. You will need to plan appropriate goals and objectives, select teaching methods suitable to the type of learning in question, and develop a means of evaluating learning. It is usually best to evaluate progress in such a way that only the person being evaluated knows his or her own evaluation results; this approach serves to preserve the self-esteem of those having difficulties. You should also devise a method of evaluating your effectiveness as a teacher.

## Directing Others in Care

Even if you are not a team leader, charge nurse, or head nurse, it sometimes becomes necessary to direct others in care. For example, you may find yourself directing a single aide with whom you are working or several students less experienced than yourself. A nursing-process approach is suitable to such situations.

## The Nursing-Process Approach

The first step in the nursing-process approach is to carefully assess the abilities of those with whom

you are working: spend a few minutes talking with each individual about his or her past experience or consulting with other nurses. You will also need to know what the facility expects of an individual with a given job title. Is there a job description for aides or nursing assistants? What kind of in-service preparation are nursing assistants given in your facility?

The next step is to analyze the level of difficulty of each component of the task or assignment and decide what you will ask someone else to do and what you will need to do yourself. You should also plan a method of self-evaluation so that, after implementing your plan, you can evaluate the effectiveness of your decisions and actions.

## Styles of Leadership and Supervision

Authoritarian relationships—simply telling other people what to do and checking to see that they have done it—tend to be effective in accomplishing many tasks in a short time. They are notably less effective, however, in terms of long-term job satisfaction. A more democratic and cooperative relationship thus has important benefits for the patient as well. When people are satisfied with their jobs, they are more likely to manifest a positive attitude in their work and to apply their own problem-solving and creative abilities, which results in better patient care. Chapter 6 describes the functioning of a democratic group.

## Consideration of Feelings

Occasionally some of your colleagues will experience problems related to working with patients. Many stressful events occur in health-care facilities, and the demands on the emotional stability of care givers can be extreme. Be sensitive to the feelings of those around you. People often need a genuinely concerned listener to help them sort out their feelings. Nurses can be very helpful to one another by offering a therapeutic ear when the occasion requires. For example, when a patient is very difficult to care for or criticizes the nursing staff, some members of the nursing staff may become discouraged or self-doubting. By active listening you can help them identify effective ways of responding and reinforce their feelings of self-esteem by pointing out what they do well.

In settings where nurses provide this kind of support to one another and to other care givers, staff turnover is minimized and better working relationships ensue.

## Encouraging Growth

Nursing is a highly demanding profession, and all nurses need to grow continually in knowledge and ability to care for patients. We can encourage one another in such growth by praising those who do well, acknowledging those who pursue continuing education, and refraining from personal criticism. When you notice that someone is not functioning appropriately, make an effort to point out better methods without appearing unduly critical. When your work is criticized constructively, try to keep in mind that the criticism is not directed at you as a person; it is an effort to help you move toward better practice.

Nurses are often guilty of expecting excellence from one another but failing to acknowledge it. Learn to be free with praise. Receiving praise for your nursing care enhances self-esteem, and the result is usually renewed effort to maintain high-quality care.

# Evaluating Care

Formal evaluation of nursing care is becoming increasingly commonplace. Though evaluation of nursing is not yet required by law anywhere, some accrediting agencies do insist on it.

## Audit of Records

The usual means of evaluating nursing care is an *audit* of records. First, a committee of nurses identifies a commonly occurring patient-care situation, such as care of the patient with a cholecystectomy (gall-bladder surgery). The committee then outlines criteria that would indicate good nursing care had been delivered. Such criteria may be of two kinds: outcome and process. *Outcome criteria* specify documentable end results, such as that the patient's temperature is normal for 24 hours prior to discharge and that the patient is able to repeat discharge instructions. *Process criteria* specify actions that should have been taken by the nurses, such as preoperative teaching before surgery and regular inspection of dressings after surgery. It is common for both types of criteria to be established.

The next step is to ask medical-records personnel to retrieve pertinent charts, such as the charts of all patients who have undergone cholecystectomies in the last six months. These charts are systematically reviewed for conformity to the criteria. The results of the review are collated and documented on an easily reviewed form to facilitate study.

A nursing committee then reviews the information collected and decides on the next step. If all charts meet the criteria, letters of congratulation to the nurses are in order. If deficiencies are found, the committee must try to determine whether they are deficiencies in charting or deficiencies in care. In-service education is then planned to correct such deficiencies.

## Direct-Care Audit

A less common method of evaluating care is the *direct-care audit.* The criteria for a direct-care audit are set by nurses. A nurse auditor—a supervisor, a nurse from another unit, or an outside nurse hired as an auditor—visits the patient care unit and reviews the patients, the records, and the activities of the nurse in light of the criteria. The results of this kind of audit are used in the same manner as those of the record audit. Because it is very time-consuming, the direct-care audit is less common.

## Conclusion

Coordinating patients' care is a complex task that will draw fully on and enhance your knowledge of groups and individuals and your communication skills. Though intricate and demanding, coordination of care can be profoundly rewarding in terms of sound patient care and job satisfaction.

### Study Terms

| | |
|---|---|
| audit | nursing care plans |
| coordination | outcome criteria |
| data base | problem list |
| direct-care audit | problem-oriented |
| discharge planner | record (POR) |
| flow sheets | process criteria |
| incident report | progress notes |
| initial plan | referral form |
| intershift report | report |
| narrative charting | SOAPing |

### Learning Activities

1. Attend a team conference.
2. Draw an organizational chart of the nursing staff in the facility to which you are assigned.
3. Go to an intershift report. Take notes. In a discussion in your clinical group, review the information you received. Identify any information you needed but did not receive.
4. Accompany a patient to another department for a procedure (such as x ray or physical therapy). Identify any nursing actions that could be taken

before and after to assist the staff in the other department and/or the patient. Share your information and ideas with your clinical group.

### Relevant Sections in
### Modules for Basic Nursing Skills

| Volume 1 | Module |
|---|---|
| Charting | 2 |

### References

Atwood, J., et al. "Symposium on the Problem-Oriented Record." *Nursing Clinics of North America* 9, no. 2 (June 1974).

Blount, M., et al. "Documenting With the Problem-Oriented Record System." *American Journal of Nursing* 79 (September 1979): 1539–1542.

Burba, M., et al. "The Evaluation of Patient Care Through the American Nurses' Association Standards of Nursing Practice." *Supervisor Nurse* 9 (May 1978): 58–59.

Epstein, C. "Breaking the Barriers to Communication in the Health Care Team." *Nursing '74* 12 (December 1974): 63–68.

Forman, M. "Building a Better Nursing Care Plan." *American Journal of Nursing* 79 (June 1979): 1086–1087.

Hover, J., et al. "Nursing Quality Assurance: The Wisconsin System." *Nursing Outlook* 26 (April 1978): 242–248.

Kerr, A. H. "Nurses' Notes: Making Them More Meaningful." *Nursing '72* 9 (September 1972): 6–11.

Moore, K. R. "What Nurses Learn From Nursing Audit." *Nursing Outlook* 27 (April 1979): 254–258.

Nerland, E. "Patient Transfer Form Provides Continuity of Care." *Hospitals* 52 (October 1978): 151–152.

Schell, P. L. "POMR—Not Just Another Way to Chart." *Nursing Outlook* 20 (April 1972): 510–514.

Vasey, E. K. "Writing Your Patient's Care Plans Efficiently." *Nursing '79* 9 (April 1979): 67–71.

Weed, L. L. *Medical Records, Medical Education and Patient Care.* Cleveland: Case Western Reserve University Press, 1970.

Wiley, L. "The Nursing Care Plan: A Communication Plan That Really Works." *Nursing '78* 8 (March 1978): 28–33.

# Part Five

## Psychosocial Needs of the Person

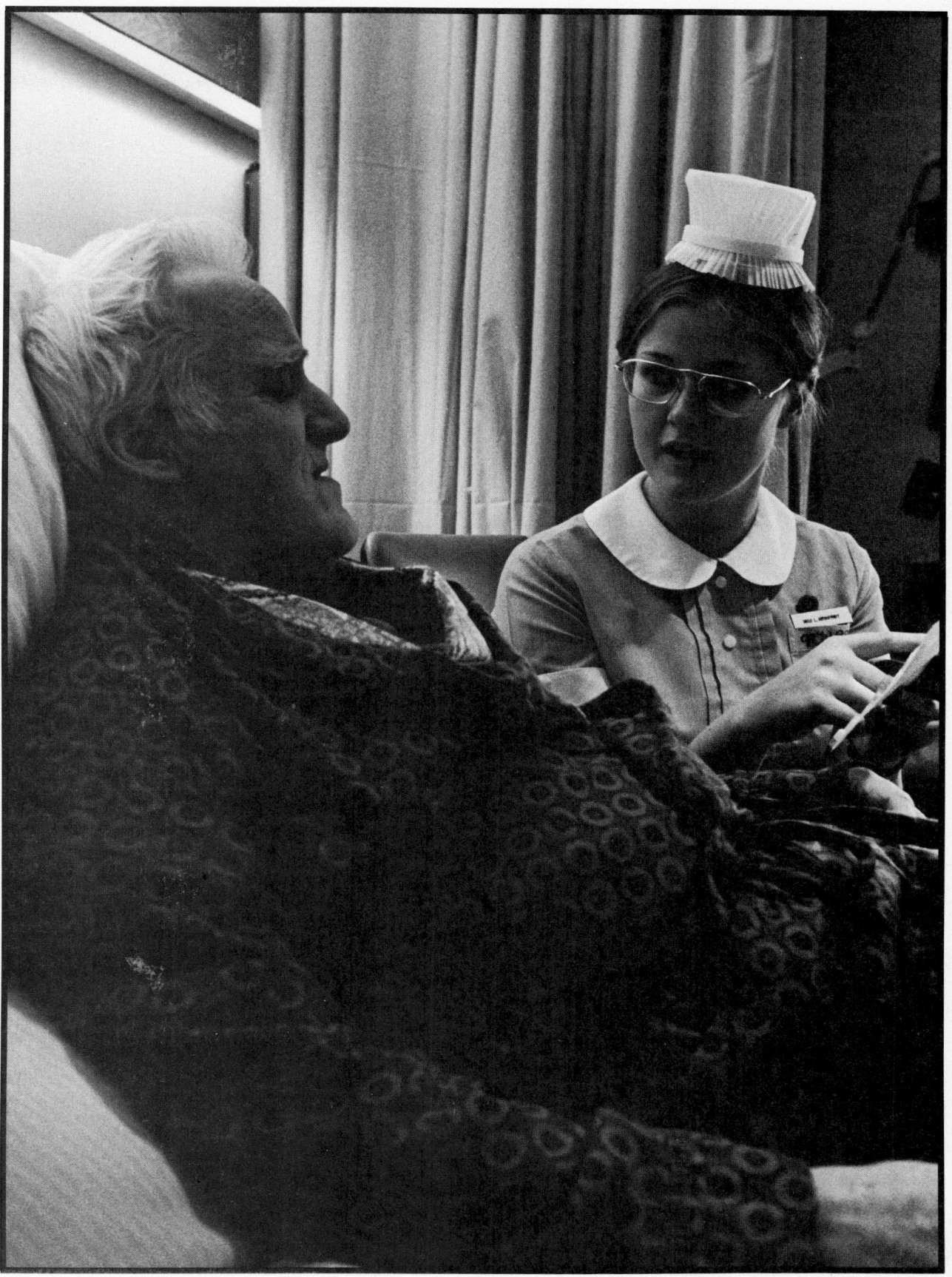

# Chapter 15
# Mental Health

Mental health can be defined as a set of emotional and cognitive patterns conducive to effective functioning in one's own particular life situation. These patterns are positive for the individual in that they facilitate coping with life. Mental health encompasses thoughts, feelings, and responses to life and is closely related to physical health. Although many components of mental health have been identified, most can be seen as aspects of the human needs Maslow identified. When the needs for love, belongingness, and self-esteem are met, positive patterns can develop.

The exact nature of positive patterns of thought and behavior varies from culture to culture. What is useful and constructive in order to function in one society might not be useful in another. For example, if submissiveness and deliberate submergence of one's personal views are a cultural norm, the person who deviates in the direction of personal assertiveness is likely to be considered abnormal; the result may be isolation from others and loss of self-esteem. In a culture that values aggressiveness, however, the individual who would be out of place in a submissive culture might be highly respected.

Mental health is also a very individual matter. Whereas one person might derive satisfaction and a sense of belongingness from dependence on someone else, dependence might arouse major inner conflicts in a person who views it as evidence of a personal deficiency.

The level of a person's mental health at any given time is usually ascertained by examining his or her ability to function in relationship to the self and the environment. The models used to describe health and illness in Chapters 3 and 7 also apply to mental health. Mental illness is a state characterized by inability to function in daily life due to psychological problems. This chapter will focus on the person who is basically healthy but who may need assistance and support to function more effectively due to a troubling life situation.

## Basic Concepts in Mental Health

Let us consider some basic mental health concepts that are central to nursing in terms of human needs (see Exhibit 15.1).

### The Whole Person

Mental health cannot be considered in isolation from physical health. *A human being is made up of interrelated components—physical, mental, emotional, and spiritual—and must be viewed as a whole person.* Problems that are basically emotional also affect physical health. Thus it is never appropriate for a nurse to focus on one aspect of a person at the expense of another aspect. Because of this interrelationship, actions aimed at relieving mental health problems may also help alleviate physical problems. The reverse is also true: when physical problems are under control, mental health is likely to improve. Thus mental health, like physical health, is a dynamic phenomenon, affected by events and always in flux.

### Self-Esteem

*Self-esteem*, according to Maslow, is valuing oneself positively. We speak of those who attribute negative values to the self as having low self-esteem. *Self-esteem is an important factor in coping with daily life*, and many aspects of life that affect self-esteem have pertinence for you as a nurse.

### Self-Concept

One's *self-concept* is one's total view of the self—the psychosocial-spiritual-intellectual self as well as the physical self. Though the term is often used interchangeably with *self-esteem*, they are not identical. Self-esteem refers only to the value one places on the self, while one's self-concept encompasses other feelings and ideas about the self in addition to one's sense of value. Self-concept is the basis of self-esteem.

One's view of oneself directly affects one's ability to function. If you see yourself as competent and resourceful, you will tend to behave in ways that reinforce this perception. Seeing yourself as incompetent, on the other hand, may make you reluctant to attempt tasks or even destine you to failure before you begin.

Your self-concept derives from many factors, among the most potent of which is *feedback,* or information about other people's impressions, responses, and opinions. When others respond to you in ways that indicate acceptance, you tend to see yourself as acceptable; if they reject you, you are likely to regard yourself as unacceptable.

## Body Image

One's concept of one's physical self is called one's *body image.* In addition to feelings and attitudes about one's physical self, body image is based on sight, sound, touch, and proprioceptive input (stimuli from within the body). How one sees one's physical self is central to self-esteem.

*Any mutilation or change in body structure or function will affect an individual's self-concept and relationships with others and must be understood in terms of the individual's feelings about the change.* If a person undergoes a perceptible change in the body, such as the removal of a body part, he or she must be reoriented toward the body, reappraise others' responses, and adjust his or her self-concept. Body image changes may affect feelings about oneself as a sexual partner (see Chapter 17), as a worker, and as a family member. A minor change, such as a small appendectomy scar, may not cause difficulty. The loss of a leg, however, represents a major problem in adjustment. In assessing the seriousness of the difficulty and deciding whether or not the individual needs assistance in dealing with the change, the most significant factor is the meaning of the change for the individual (see Chapter 29).

## Human Dignity

*The concept of human dignity rests on faith in the individual's worth, regardless of race, sex, creed, culture, or behavior* (Dunn, 1962). Recognition of the intrinsic worth of each individual is the basis of all supportive, helpful human relationships and is central to effective nursing. Belief in this principle underlies efforts that go unnoticed and supports work toward goals that are not realized. When acted upon, the concept of human dignity promotes in others a belief in their own dignity and worth.

## Self-Understanding

Another critical factor in self-esteem is the degree of self-understanding an individual possesses. Seeking self-knowledge tends to promote self-esteem in that it brings about recognition of one's positive features.

Self-understanding is particularly important for the nurse. *Understanding oneself promotes an understanding of others.* As a nurse your capacity to understand others will be called on in many situations, and the basis for doing so lies in an understanding of yourself. Self-understanding is not a static state but a dynamic process of striving to know yourself in relation to each new experience and each new person you encounter. Consider the applicability of all you learn about mental health to your own life and think about the ways such concepts can enhance your self-understanding. Then seek an understanding of their applicability to your relationships with family, friends, patients, and co-workers.

## Love and Belongingness

Every individual, according to Maslow, needs to feel loved and cared about. From infancy on, the feeling of being cared about is essential if one is to thrive. Although the nurse cannot permanently fill the role of a provider of love and belongingness in a patient's life, the nurse can certainly help meet this need.

## Individuality and Group Identification

*People respond and function both as individuals and as members of social groups.* It is important to see others as individuals whose responses grow out of their own experiences and to abandon expectations of behavior based on stereotyped views of "the good patient," racial and ethnic groups, or males and females. On the other hand, we must not ignore the group to which an individual belongs. A person's family and ethnic group inevitably affect the way he or she responds and functions. Finding an appropriate middle ground between stereotyping and inattention to individual backgrounds is a difficult task, as is distinguishing between behavior based on individual differences and behavior characteristic of the group to which the person belongs. However, a continuing effort to do so will help you deal more effectively with others. For example, some family groups respond to the illness of a member by gathering together and becoming intensely involved in the person's care. An understanding of this practice and its meaning to those involved is necessary if the patient is placed in a unit where the number of visitors and length of visits are very restricted. On the other hand, the patient may prefer that the family not be so intimately involved. As a nurse, your first responsibility in such a situation is to the patient.

Many people derive a necessary sense of belongingness from identification with a group. If we undermine this group identification in the care setting in order to "treat everyone alike," we are failing to recognize the importance of belongingness for mental health. Our attitude toward the group of which the patient is a member will also affect the patient's self-esteem, since people typically interpret the value placed on their social group as the value placed on them as individuals.

## The Need to Communicate

*Mental health requires that the individual have adequate means for communication with others and/or self-expression.* Some consider communication the most important single factor in mental health. Undeniably, anything that hampers communication with others—whether laryngitis, a language barrier, or a mental attitude—poses a threat to mental health. Inability to communicate significantly affects recovery from any illness, as is most dramatically apparent in the case of the stroke patient. If two patients have equal motor function but differ in speech capacity, the patient who can communicate will invariably be rehabilitated to self-care more easily and rapidly.

Communication reflects one's belongingness to the human community. Only communication can pierce an individual's isolation, by allowing for him or her to feel close to another person. It is the nurse's responsibility to help provide the patient with a means of communication. Doing so might require seeking the help of another person, such as the speech therapist, or using sign language, pictures, or gestures. For the patient in isolation, it could mean setting aside time to talk together; for the deaf patient, you might provide a "magic slate" for writing messages. With patients whose mental attitudes block communication, the nurse must work skillfully and patiently at using the nursing process to establish some form of communication.

## Feelings and Behavior

*Feelings* are subjective experiences of emotion, such as happiness, fear, or anxiety. Feelings are often verbally expressed, but they may also be indicated by behavior. It is generally much more difficult to identify others' feelings accurately on the basis of behavior alone than when the person can express feelings verbally.

## The Validity of Feelings

*Feelings and sentiments are real and must be treated as such whether or not they appear to be based on fact.* If we accept a person's feelings and sentiments without judging them to be right or wrong, we strengthen the interpersonal relationship and build mutual trust. It is usually easy to accept feelings—our own or others'—for which we can discern reasons; if we doubt the validity of the reasons, however, we may tend to label the feelings inappropriate.

## The Meaningfulness of All Behavior

*All behavior has meaning and purpose for the individual.* Behavior can solve problems, relieve anxiety, and/or help people cope with stress. Though you may not understand certain behavior, or be able to discern its purpose, recognition that behavior has meaning to the individual can help you be more accepting even when your understanding is only partial. Because behavior is not always understood by the individual who engages in it, your efforts to understand may serve to guide him or her to greater self-awareness. If you are attempting to help someone change his or her behavior, it may be essential to search for and understand the meaning and purpose of the behavior you hope to modify.

## Self-Actualization and Capacity for Growth

Self-actualization is, according to Maslow, becoming what one is capable of becoming. Although self-actualization is often thought of as a remote end-point, it is more helpful to see it as a process of growth.

*Each individual has the basic capacity for growth.* As a person's immediate goals and needs are met, new ones arise to take their place. We are expecting growth when we ask individuals to adopt new ways of functioning, learn new skills, and/or deal with a variety of complex feelings and problems. If an individual does not appear to be striving for growth, the prevailing conditions need to be examined. Are his or her immediate needs going unmet? Is energy available for growth or is all the patient's available energy being devoted to maintenance? Are you providing a climate suitable for growth?

# Threats to the Hospitalized Patient's Mental Health

We all assume a number of different roles in our daily lives. For example, a woman may be a daughter in one setting, an employee in another, and a mother in still another. Each of these roles is characterized by a set of expected behaviors. The term *mother* evokes widely shared expectations, within whose general outlines each person develops a particular way of responding on the basis of life experience and background.

Becoming a patient requires a person to adopt a new role. The nature of this role may vary, depending on whether the setting is an outpatient clinic, the home, or an acute-care hospital. People's responses to the role of patient also depend on their families and cultural backgrounds, which teach them various interpretations of appropriate behavior for the sick person, and on their previous experiences with the patient role.

Individuals differ in their views of health and illness. A person with multiple handicaps who needs ongoing supervision by a health-care team may consider himself healthy as long as he does not have an acute illness. His response to the patient role will be quite different from that of the person who perceives a sprained ankle as a serious threat to health and assumes a totally dependent role. When the patient's concept of health differs from that of the health-care team members, conflict may result. This situation calls for the skillful use of interpersonal communication techniques to resolve the conflict. If it is not possible or desirable to alter the patient's perception, the health-care providers may have to alter their expectations and approaches.

## Threat to the Self-Concept

Whatever the setting, certain common problems confront the person who must take on the patient role. The first such problem is the threat to the person's self-concept posed by illness and the patient role. "I'm not a whole person anymore." "I can't fulfill my usual role in life." "What will other people think of me? How will they treat me now?" The answers to these and other questions may require a change in the view of the self. During a temporary illness, such changes may be very minor and easily dealt with by the patient. A major illness, on the other hand, frequently requires profound changes, and the patient may need assistance and support in dealing with his or her feelings.

## Loss of Privacy

A second problem is the loss of privacy. The patient may be asked personal questions by a number of different people. There may be physical examinations that offend modesty. In the hospital, personal belongings are often carefully inspected, inventoried, and stored elsewhere for safekeeping. Elimination may have to take place while other people are present or separated only by a curtain. In brief, the hospital setting requires the patient to suppress a set of feelings and behaviors related to maintaining personal privacy and modesty.

Belief in human dignity and worth mandates protecting the privacy of the individual in every way possible. It requires that you be sensitive to the patient's feelings and recognize that they may differ from your own. With this principle as your guide, you will also provide a full measure of privacy to the individual who is not able to claim it independently: the comatose individual, the child, or the person without speech. Concretely, providing privacy means using blankets for draping, pulling curtains, and being discreet when you talk with the patient about personal matters.

## Loss of Control

Adults in Western society are used to the sense of controlling their own lives. In the health-care setting, tests may be ordered, forms filled out, and plans for care made by others; the person may feel as if swept along on the tide. Giving consent does not necessarily mean that the patient thoroughly understands all that is happening.

Loss of control may also be a threat to the self-image and thus may create anxiety. This outcome can be prevented or alleviated by allowing patients to retain control over as much of their lives as possible. Whenever feasible, you can give the patient choices regarding care. For example, does he prefer a bath now or in an hour? In what order does she prefer the tasks of care? Too often such decisions are made arbitrarily by nursing personnel even when a choice is feasible. To help the patient feel more control over the situation, you ought to introduce unfamiliar members of the health-care team, describe their functions, and carefully explain all that is going to happen, including time schedules. You must also explain how beds and call lights work, where the bathroom is, and how the telephone operates. Fear of loss of control over elimination is very prevalent, especially in the elderly. Calm acceptance of such problems and shared planning to solve them can restore dignity and some control to the patient, even when physical control is lost. As for control over broader matters, review the Health Consumer Bill of Rights in Chapter 1 and consider how you can support the patient in the exercise of these rights.

## Uncertainty About Expected Behavior

Patients also experience uncertainty as to the behavior expected of them. "How is a patient supposed to act?" "Is it permissible to ask questions?" "Do I have to ask for pain relief or can I expect it

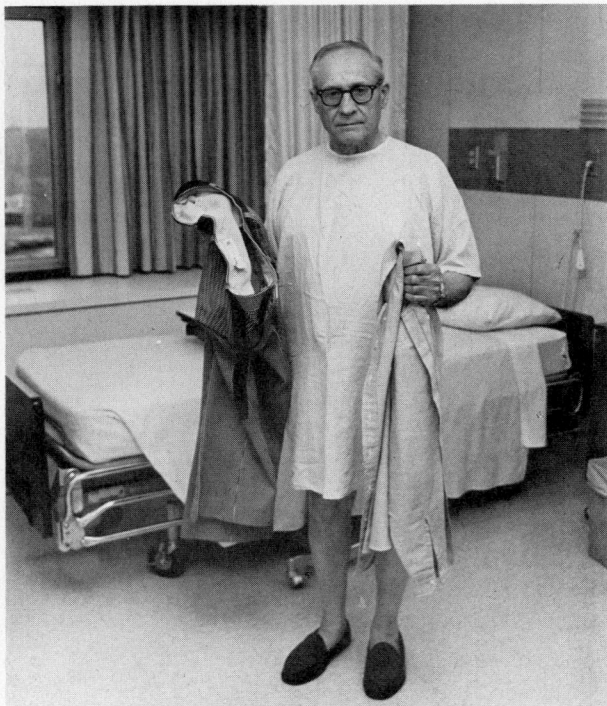

**Figure 15.1**
Uncertainty about the behavior expected in the health-care setting creates stress. (Russ Kinne/Danbury Hospital/Photo Researchers, Inc.)

to be provided without asking?" You have faced such uncertainty yourself if you have ever sat in a doctor's examining room wondering what you should do next. "Am I expected to wait in the examining room until the doctor returns or should I get dressed and go to the desk?" Such uncertainty may be multiplied many times over when the entire environment is unfamiliar and one's contact with the health-care system has been limited. Anxiety may be especially pronounced among individuals from cultural backgrounds other than those of the health-care workers.

You can assist the patient by describing the behavior you expect. The most routine admission to the hospital may be a completely new experience for the patient. "Am I expected to take all my clothes off under that gown?" "Can I leave my underwear on?" "Am I expected to go right to bed?" "Do I ring the buzzer or will you automatically come back?" Explanations of all such matters are necessary, as are any orders regarding activity, the policy on leaving the area, and the patient's

responsibilities for his or her own care. Be sure to elicit the patient's questions and concerns as well. Hospital admission is not the only time when expected behavior needs to be explained. Explanations are also needed when a new procedure or treatment is to be performed, when the patient is to go to another department for a test, and when changes occur in care. The need for clear statements of expected behavior continues throughout the patient's contact with the health-care system.

## Unfamiliar Routines

In the hospital the patient must adopt an entirely new pattern of living. The schedule may be drastically at odds with his or her own. In spite of attempts to individualize care, most institutions find that certain routines and schedules are necessary to function smoothly. As a nurse, you might consider which of the patterns prescribed by the institution are really essential and whether it is possible to adapt them in any way to the needs and desires of the patient. Certain aspects of our routines are indeed based on necessity, but others are unquestionably the result of long-standing traditions that have no rationale and have never been questioned.

## Worry Over Expenses

A major problem facing the consumer of health care in the United States is its cost. For most people, an extensive illness or hospitalization costs more than insurance pays. Health-care costs have been rising much more rapidly than most other sectors of the economy. Even those whose health-care plans pay all the costs of illness may be subject to loss of income, expenses for child care, and/or the cost of homemaking services. The nurse is not usually in a position to alleviate a patient's financial concerns directly. However, the nurse can refer the patient to others with the ability and knowledge to do so, such as the social worker. Some hospitals employ individuals to help patients with their financial problems. Sometimes the patient can deal with such problems independently if he or she has access to the business office or insurance carrier. Developing a sound knowledge of available community resources can equip you to make appropriate referrals.

## Uncertainty About the Outcome

Though some people enter the health-care environment with relatively simple problems whose favorable outcome is a virtual certainty, a great many patients carry a heavy burden of undisclosed fears. Sometimes such fears arise from realistic knowledge of the seriousness of the illness. A person who enters the hospital for treatment of kidney failure, for instance, may clearly recognize that the outcome cannot be predicted with certainty and that there is a possibility of prolonged treatment or death. Another patient may feel very threatened by surgery the hospital staff regards as routine. For example, he or she may fear never waking up from the anesthesia. Such fears are often exacerbated by physicians' caution about making absolute predictions. Full disclosure of the possible adverse effects of treatment may intro-

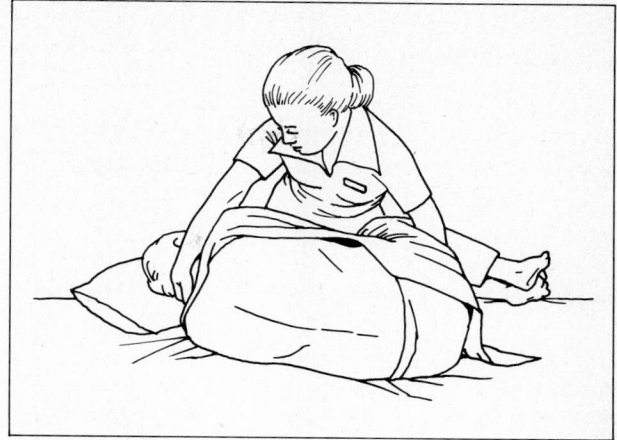

**Figure 15.2**
It is especially important for the nurse to assess the psychological response of the patient during a potentially upsetting procedure. Here, the nurse watches the patient's face during a lumbar puncture.

duce or exaggerate fears. Uncertainty of this kind is very threatening to most individuals. People are usually more successful at handling their anxieties when the nature of the problem is clear-cut.

# Feelings Created by Threats to Mental Health

People respond in varying ways to threats to mental health, though their responses typically exhibit patterns that you will gradually learn to recognize. Feelings of anxiety, depression, anger, and hostility are common. Behavior may change in an effort to cope with the situation and the feelings being aroused. If the situation seems overwhelming, a crisis may occur.

## Anxiety

Anxiety is a subjective experience of apprehension initiated by a threat to oneself, whether physical, mental, emotional, or spiritual (Peplau, 1963). Since becoming a patient involves so many potential threats, you can expect most people to experience some degree of anxiety during their interaction with the health-care system. Because of the interrelationship between physical and psycholog-

ical well-being, this will hold true whether the initial problem is physical or psychological. Helping the patient to reduce anxiety to a manageable level is an integral part of nursing practice.

Table 15.1 provides an overview of anxiety. As you will note, mild anxiety is not harmful. It helps one focus on the problem at hand, motivates one to solve that problem, and provides energy or drive. In fact, mild anxiety characterizes much of life. As anxiety increases, however, it becomes increasingly dysfunctional. With the advent of moderate anxiety, one begins to suffer deficits in ability to function. As anxiety becomes progressively more severe, ability to function diminishes until the person reaches a state of panic.

In addition to subjective feelings and effects on ability to function, there are also physiological signs of anxiety; these too become progressively more abnormal as anxiety increases. In order to identify anxiety then, you will need to note phys-

Table 15.1
**Characteristics of Anxiety**

| | No anxiety (−) | Mild anxiety (+) | Moderate anxiety (+ +) | Severe anxiety (+ + +) | Panic (+ + + +) |
|---|---|---|---|---|---|
| **Pulse** | Resting rate | Slightly faster | Noticeably faster | Rapid, possibly irregular | Very rapid and irregular |
| **Respiration** | Resting rate | Slightly faster | Noticeably faster | Rapid and irregular | Very rapid, possible hyperventilation |
| **Blood pressure** | Resting level | Slightly elevated | Noticeably elevated | High | High; if profound, may suddenly drop and cause fainting |
| **Muscle tone and effect on activity** | Flaccid, not ready to act; lethargic | Slight tension, ready to act; acts with purpose | Increased tension; may have headaches and other aches; may engage in repetitive mannerisms to release tension; may pace | Extreme tension— may be almost unable to move; no purposeful action; repetitive actions increased in speed and intensity | Extreme tension; either immobilization or eruption into erratic behavior; almost uncontrollable |
| **Mood** | Calm; may feel lethargic | Alert; feels ambitious and ready to act | Nervous, somewhat upset | Very upset, feels loss of control | Out of control, panicky |
| **Effect on perception** | Not alert, easily distracted | Alert, sees details well; extraneous material excluded from attention | Focuses more narrowly; may not perceive whole situation | Focuses on random detail; misses whole situation | Perception distorted |
| **Effect on learning** | Slow | Enhanced, optimal | Slow or limited | Greatly diminished or absent | No learning possible |

ical signs, behavior, and expressions of feeling by the patient.

# Depression

*Depression* is a mental state in which one feels in low spirits, dejected, and even without hope. Mild depression is a component of normal life. When it is a response to real circumstances or events, it is usually short-lived and begins to recede when the person is able to respond to the situation effectively or when the situation itself changes.

Depression may also be pathological—that is, related to abnormal functioning. Pathological depression is by definition much more extreme than would be expected in view of the prevailing circumstances, or it may occur in the absence of any visible life problem. Pathological depression renders the person unable to act effectively, and self-esteem is very low. Pathological depression requires professional help.

Let us consider the signs and symptoms that characterize all depression (see Table 15.2).

## Cognitive Signs

A person who is depressed is less able than usual to concentrate on the tasks at hand and exhibits a lack of interest in life. Learning is usually slowed. The entire thinking process may be slow, requiring more energy than is available.

## Behavioral Signs

A person who is depressed tends to move very slowly and may sit for long periods of time doing nothing at all. Sleep is often disturbed; early wak-

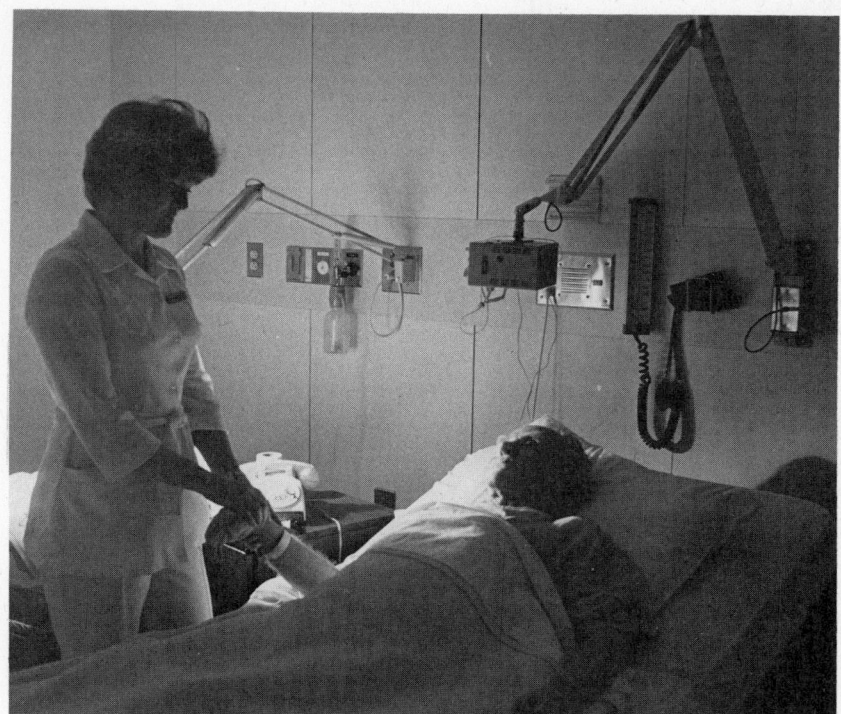

**Figure 15.3**
The person who is depressed exhibits characteristic physical signs. (Russ Kinne/Danbury Hospital/Photo Researchers, Inc.)

ing is common. The person may cry or sigh frequently, and appetite is typically poor.

## Physical Signs

Body function may slow down, resulting in slow pulse, lowered blood pressure, and slowed respirations. Constipation is common. When depression persists for a long period of time, the skin often becomes dry and the hair lifeless. The posture of the depressed person is characterized by slumped shoulders and a tendency for the head to be bent. The person may appear to be carrying a great weight. The face seems to droop and the expression is typically sad.

## Anger and Hostility

*Anger* is a feeling of extreme displeasure with someone else, often stemming from the feeling that he or she is "against" you or preventing you from acting as you wish. *Hostility* is viewing the other person as an opponent or enemy. Anger and hostility often go hand-in-hand.

Patients in health-care settings may express anger toward their families, friends, and care givers. Often anger is an appropriate response to events or circumstances. For example, a person who has been left lying on a stretcher in a hallway for forty-five minutes while waiting for a test may be justified in feeling extreme displeasure toward the

Table 15.2
**Signs of Depression**

| Cognitive signs | Behavioral signs | Physical signs |
|---|---|---|
| Decreased concentration | Slow movement | Slow pulse |
| Lack of interest | Inactivity | Slow respiration |
| Slowed learning | Sleep disturbance | Low blood pressure |
| | Early waking | Constipation |
| | Crying | Dry skin and hair |
| | Sighing | Slumped posture |
| | Poor appetite | Bowed head |
| | | Sad expression |

people responsible for the resulting discomfort and fatigue. If a file is misplaced, necessitating that a test be repeated, the patient's anger is appropriate—though it is inappropriate to direct such anger at the person who performs the repeated test if he or she was not responsible for the original error.

When a patient expresses anger, your first response should be to examine the situation and determine whether the anger appears to be appropriate. When it is, it is the responsibility of the health-care team to try to correct or remedy the situation. When it proves impossible to do so, you should at least acknowledge to the patient that his or her anger is justified and say that you will try to see to it that the situation is not repeated. This kind of response may prevent hostility and preserve a relationship in which the patient and the health-care workers are "on the same team" rather than opponents.

When you cannot identify an objective provocation for a patient's anger, you might consider whether it is serving as a defense mechanism, such as projection or displacement (see pages 247–250). Anger that seems inappropriate is often a means of coping with anxiety. Could the patient's anger be an attempt to relieve anxiety?

## Crisis

A *crisis* is "a situation which threatens to overwhelm the individual" (Aguilera, 1978). Specifically, it is a situation in which the coping patterns that proved successful in the past are no longer adequate. Such a situation can be considered a major stressor.

## Types of Crises

There are two types of crises. The first is the *maturational* or *developmental crisis*, which arises out of changes that occur in the context of the life cycle. You will recall from Chapter 4 that Erikson identifies each stage of the life cycle with a characteristic developmental crisis. Developmental crises are thus relatively predictable in the life of the individual. For example, the adolescent can be ex-

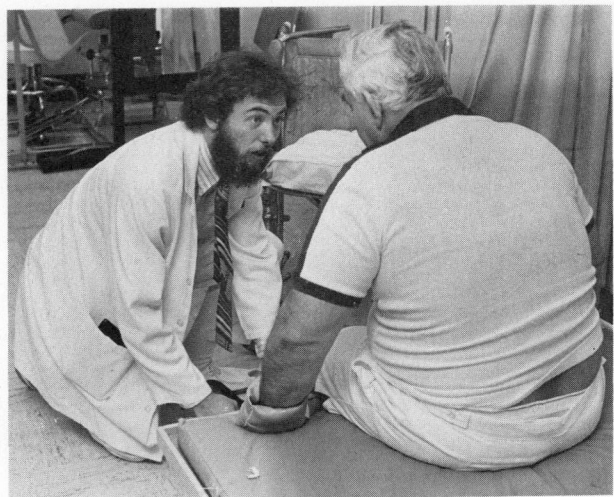

**Figure 15.4**
It is important to acknowledge when a patient's anger is justified. (Russ Kinne/Danbury Hospital/Photo Researchers, Inc.)

pected to undergo a crisis involving the process of developing an identity as an independent individual. Conflicts and difficulties surrounding this process are not unexpected. By recognizing normal developmental crises, you will be better able to help an individual successfully resolve such a crisis.

The other type of crisis is a *situational crisis*. Situational crises are those that involve specific occurrences in a person's life. The occurrence might be a single incident, such as an assault, or a particular stage in a relationship. In some cases, the precipitating incident itself may not appear overwhelming; the crisis occurs because of accumulated stress, which allowed for the incident to precipitate the person beyond his or her ability to cope successfully.

## Identifying Crises

In a crisis, a person becomes unable to function effectively in most areas of life. He or she might be unable to go to work or, if there, unable to do the job. Decision making becomes almost impossible. Anxiety is typically very high, approaching the panic state.

# Coping Behavior

Whenever a person experiences unpleasant emotions, he or she tries to alleviate them by means of some type of behavior. Thoughts or actions directed toward alleviating unpleasant feelings are called coping behaviors, or *coping mechanisms*. Not all coping mechanisms are successful, and some create additional problems for the person.

## Problem Solving

The most effective coping usually involves efforts to eliminate the unpleasant feelings by remedying the situation from which they arose. This problem-solving approach is the most positive and provides the longest-lasting remedy. In many situations, however, the individual is not capable of problem solving. This is particularly true in crises, when we typically see other behaviors.

## Defense Mechanisms

*Defense mechanisms* are largely unconscious mental processes that serve to relieve feelings of anxiety and tension. Though they do not solve the initial problems, defense mechanisms help to alleviate feelings of anxiety temporarily. Freud, who originated the concept of defense mechanisms, defined them narrowly as totally unconscious behaviors. Subsequently a variety of writers have expanded the list of defense mechanisms to include some that are not totally unconscious. The defense mechanisms discussed below are those most commonly encountered (see Exhibit 15.2).

Most people begin to use defense mechanisms in childhood to handle anxieties. A given individual will usually use only a few of the many mechanisms that have been identified. People typically continue to use those that have proven successful for them in the past.

It is usually inappropriate to try to stop an individual from using defense mechanisms since the loss of defense mechanisms can arouse overwhelming anxiety. If defense mechanisms become dysfunctional—that is, create more problems than they solve—they must be overcome in order for progress to be made. Professional counseling is often needed in such instances. If consistent emotional support is available, a person will often abandon a defense mechanism independently when he or she is able to cope effectively without it.

## Regression

A person who regresses behaves in a way more appropriate to an earlier stage of development. Thus an adult may become dependent and a three-year-old child may revert to drinking from a bottle. Regression is a very common response to illness. Though the person will need to re-establish age-appropriate behavior in the process of recovery, an episode of regression is not harmful to ongoing development.

## Rationalization

To rationalize is to find intellectual reasons to justify behavior and feelings that are in reality based on unconscious thoughts and feelings. For example, a person who works slowly and fails to finish a project on time may rationalize that it was done more thoroughly. Similarly, things that are desirable but unattainable may be characterized as unwanted or not valuable: a person who cannot afford a private room in the hospital may state that private rooms are undesirable because "you never get any attention there."

## Repression

Repression is the process of putting stress-provoking thoughts and/or feelings completely out of one's awareness. Repression is not deliberate but unconscious, and the ideas repressed cannot be voluntarily recalled to awareness. If confronted

Exhibit 15.2
**Common Defense Mechanisms**

| Defense mechanism | Definition | Defense mechanism | Definition |
| --- | --- | --- | --- |
| Regression | Exhibiting behavior characteristic of an earlier stage of development. | Substitution | Consciously redirecting energy from a blocked goal to another endeavor. |
| Rationalization | Offering intellectual justifications for behavior and/or feelings that are in reality based on unconscious thoughts and feelings. | Projection | Attributing one's own feelings, ideas, or characteristics to another person. |
| Repression | Unconsciously putting stress-provoking thoughts and/or feelings completely out of one's awareness to the extent that they cannot be voluntarily recalled. | Displacement | Transferring feelings aroused by one person or situation onto another person or situation. |
| | | Identification | Adopting attitudes and behaviors characteristic of an admired individual. |
| Suppression | Consciously putting troubling thoughts and/or feelings out of one's awareness on a temporary basis. | Reaction formation | Adopting attitudes or behaviors diametrically opposed to those of a person or group with whom one is in conflict. |
| Denial | Unconsciously refusing to acknowledge a painful truth or situation. | Conversion | Developing a physical illness or disability to substitute for a painful emotional or mental conflict. |
| Compensation | Emphasizing some personal trait to make up for perceived lacks in the self. | Restitution | Relieving guilt by "making up" in some way for the actions that aroused the guilt. |
| Sublimation | Unconsciously redirecting energy from a blocked goal to another endeavor. | Fantasy | Using one's imagination to create alternatives to reality. |

with the repressed material, the person will truthfully declare that he or she has absolutely no recollection of it. An example is a student who was told that his clinical performance was unsatisfactory and later insisted that this was never said; the information was so threatening that the student repressed it.

## Suppression

Suppression is similar to repression in that the troubling material is withdrawn from conscious thought; the difference is that the withdrawal is a conscious or semiconscious act and that the material can be recalled if needed. The person simply chooses to be impervious or not to remember. For example, a nurse with a serious personal prob-

lem might go to work, concentrate on performing well, and effectively exclude all thoughts of the personal problem until something recalls it to consciousness.

## Denial

Denial is an unconscious mechanism whereby a person simply refuses to acknowledge a threatening reality. The event, situation, or feeling is treated as nonexistent. Denial is a common response to a very severe shock or crisis. For example, the initial reaction to being informed of impending death is often to say, in effect, "No, there must be some mistake. It could not be true." Denial may be indicated by behavior as well as by words: a person who has been told that his or her illness is life threatening but continues to plan for the future, ignores directions for treatment, and acts happy and content may be denying the reality of the illness. Denial serves to protect the person from an overwhelming reality.

Denial is often abandoned gradually. That is, the person may appear to acknowledge the reality of the situation in one instance and in another to behave as if it were not true. Denial is usually abandoned when it no longer serves to protect the self from awareness of the situation. In some instances, however, denial may persist. If it interferes with recovery and rehabilitation, professional intervention may be called for. Persistent denial may not be harmful, however, if there are no alternatives and the situation cannot be changed.

## Compensation

Compensation is emphasis on some trait or traits to make up for perceived lacks in the self. A member of a musical family who has little musical ability may strive to demonstrate athletic proficiency. When the lack is real, compensation may be of value in redirecting the person's energies toward a sphere where success is possible.

## Sublimation

Unconscious redirection of energy from an unattainable goal to another endeavor is called sublimation. A person who wanted to have children but was unable to do so, for example, might sublimate by focusing all his or her energies on a job. This process would be unconscious, not deliberate.

## Substitution

Substitution is a consciously planned redirection of energies from a blocked goal to an accessible one. For example, a nurse who had planned to go to graduate school but was unable to do so because of family responsibilities might redirect his or her energies into a course in coronary-care nursing.

## Projection

Projection is the attribution of one's own feelings, ideas, or characteristics to another person. It is usually undesirable feelings and traits that are projected. For example, a man who is angry at others might perceive others as angry at him.

## Displacement

Displacement is the transfer of feelings aroused by one person or situation onto another person or situation. It typically occurs when it would be too distressing to admit the real object of such feelings. If a patient's anger is aroused by the perceived lack of support of close family members, expressing such anger toward them might further erode their support. The patient's anger may therefore be displaced onto the nursing personnel.

## Identification

Admiration and affection for another person may prompt one to adopt attitudes and behaviors characteristic of that person. For example, a new graduate nurse who admires an experienced head nurse might begin to use similar expressions and gestures. Valuable behaviors might also be adopted in the process of identification. An important aspect of child development, identification originates unconsciously but sometimes affects conscious behavior.

## Reaction Formation

Almost the exact opposite of identification, reaction formation is rejection in oneself of any characteristics one shares with a person or group one fears or despises and adoption of the diametrically opposed behavior and attitudes. Reaction formation also occurs when an individual is trying to establish independence or autonomy: in rejecting dependence, a teenager may also reject the person on whom he or she was formerly dependent, adopting behavior patterns highly antagonistic to those of the parent.

## Conversion

Conversion is the process by which a person experiencing painful emotions and mental conflict develops a physical illness or disability that then substitutes for the psychological problems. A psychological problem is thus "converted" into a physical one. A dramatic example is paralysis in a young army recruit ordered to participate in a military operation. Concern about his own survival, beliefs about duty and courage, and fear of what others will think of him may create an intolerable conflict, which the paralysis resolves by taking decision making out of his hands. A person experiencing a conversion reaction is often amazingly calm and accepting of what most people would view as a major life crisis because, rather than representing crisis, it represents relief from crisis. Conversion is an unconscious mechanism.

## Restitution

Restitution is an effort to relieve guilt by means of behavior that "makes up" for the cause of the guilt. A woman who was very angry at her husband just before he was injured in an accident may feel guilt over her anger; she may spend long hours at the hospital in an effort to compensate for her previous antagonistic feelings. Restitution is unconscious in origin.

## Fantasy

Fantasy is the use of one's imagination to construct alternatives to reality. Children use fantasy a great deal, daydreaming about the present and the future and constructing elaborate scenes in which they star. Fantasies of the self as competent, resourceful, and capable can be very productive for several reasons. First, the fantasy serves as a problem-solving forum in which alternative behaviors can be explored, allowing the individual to choose the best course of action. Second, fantasy can be self-fulfilling. Imagining oneself as a certain type of person makes one more likely to act in ways that will make the fantasy a reality. Seeing ourselves as strong and capable may result in our becoming exactly that. The converse is also true: fantasy that focuses on oneself as the victim of outside forces may have a negative effect on self-confidence and self-esteem.

# Helping the Patient Maintain Mental Health

## Assessment

Assessment of mental health is complex, subtle, and requires close and sustained attention. Train yourself to listen carefully to what the patient says, being especially alert to expressions of *feelings*. Encourage the patient to discuss feelings in order to learn how he or she is responding to what is happening.

Second, observe the patient's *behavior*. Look at his or her body posture, facial expressions, gestures, and responses to ordinary tasks and events. Does the patient's behavior indicate anxiety, depression, or anger?

Third, consider *physical signs* in light of the patient's behavior and expressed feelings. Pulse, blood pressure, and respiration are valuable guidelines in assessing mental as well as physical health.

Another aspect of assessing mental health is taking into account the person's *current situation* and *stage of psychosocial development*, which can hold important clues to his or her mental health status.

Finally, you will need to put all these data together in order to identify any problems that you as a nurse may be able to assist in resolving.

## Planning Intervention

Intervention in most mental health problems approximates the following general model, which you will need to modify and adapt to the specific situation and the individual in question (see Exhibit 15.3). Communication skills are the major tools for resolving mental health problems. Therapeutic interaction is used in the following way.

## Ventilating Feelings

Perhaps the most helpful thing you can do for a patient is to be a concerned listener and encourage the free expression of feelings. An opportunity to express feelings and to be assured that someone else is concerned about those feelings may be all that is needed or possible. In any situation, ventilation of feelings is always the first step. General leads, such as reflecting, restating, and nondirective comments, are the most effective techniques for encouraging expression of feelings. When feelings are expressed, it is important to maintain an accepting attitude. Remember that the validity of feelings is a central mental health concept.

## Gaining Intellectual Understanding or Insight

This is a more demanding step. In order for the patient to gain insight into the stress-producing situation, he or she must think through and explore the situation independently. For you to explain the situation is often of no value at all. Instead, the use of facilitating techniques can help the person to consider all aspects of the situation. At this point you may wish to use the exploratory responses, which help the person to consolidate information. If the patient is occasionally unwilling to work at this task, it is best simply to express concern and willingness to listen and plan to talk further when the patient is more ready to proceed.

## Exploring Ways of Coping

When the patient has gained some insight into the situation, it is appropriate to encourage him or her to recall successful methods of coping with stressful situations in the past. This approach encourages the person to see himself or herself as a capable person able to cope with stressful situations. It also helps the person to focus on specific actions

---

**Exhibit 15.3**
**Intervention for Mental Health Problems**

1. Ventilating feelings
2. Gaining intellectual understanding or insight
3. Exploring ways of coping
4. Decision making
5. Referral
6. Providing skilled care

---

rather than generalized concerns. It is sometimes appropriate to point out information in a nondirective manner. For example, you might say, "Some people find that talking directly to the person they are angry with is helpful. Have you considered that approach?" Giving directions or direct suggestions ("You should . . ." or "You ought . . .") undermines autonomy.

## Decision Making

Finally, you can help the person choose a course of action that might alleviate stress. In most instances, making such a decision is in itself anxiety-relieving. Again, the use of facilitating techniques is appropriate in encouraging someone to move toward a decision. When a decision has been made, it is helpul to summarize the process by which the person has arrived at a decision, reinforce the idea that he or she is capable and able to cope, and offer assistance if it is needed to implement the decision. Such assistance might include providing the name and telephone number of somebody to contact, obtaining appropriate booklets or pamphlets, or accompanying the person when he or she talks with someone else.

## Referral

Occasionally you will conclude that the problem a patient is experiencing is beyond the scope of your own ability and understanding. In such a case, the appropriate step is referral to someone with the particular skills needed. For example, a mental health nursing clinician on the staff of the hospital may work directly with the patient or with the staff to develop appropriate nursing ap-

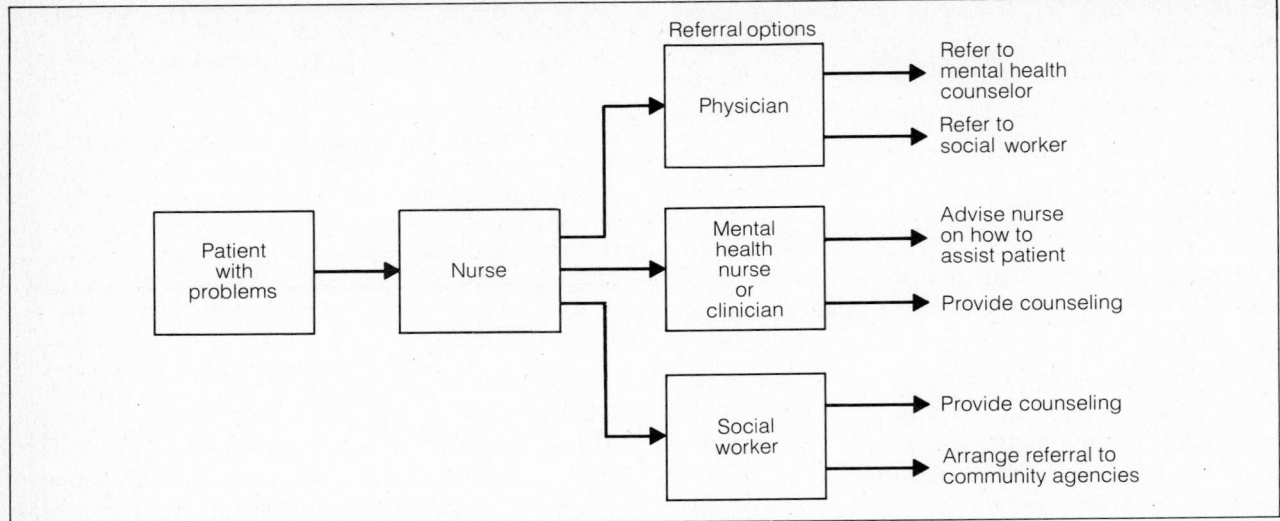

**Figure 15.5**
Referral is one avenue of intervention for patients with mental health problems.

proaches to the patient. Alternatively, referral to a social worker or mental health therapist may be indicated. If a physician's order is needed for such a referral to be made, you will want to consult with the physician, presenting the data you have gathered and explaining your rationale for wishing to make such a referral.

## Providing Skilled Care

An important method of supporting the patient's mental health, often overlooked, is providing for his or her physical needs with a high degree of skill. When physical needs are met by a skillful care giver, many anxieties are relieved and the person feels safe and able to relax. His or her energies can thus be directed toward the effort of coping with the illness and with recovery. When you experience uncertainties and doubts, they should be discussed with your instructor or an experienced nurse out of earshot of the patient. When you are in the patient's presence, strive for a calm and confident attitude toward the tasks you are carrying out. This does not mean that you should be untruthful with your patients, but merely that your worries and uncertainties should not become problems for them.

## Conclusion

Concern for the patient's mental health is a primary concern of the nurse and will be the impetus for your continuing efforts to deepen your understanding of mental health. As you progress in nursing, your increasing technical skill and skill in communication will both contribute to support the mental health of the patient.

## Care Study  A patient with anxiety

Betty Westman was pacing the floor of her hospital room when Mary Cedino, the team leader, walked in. Ms. Cedino noted that Ms. Westman was breathing rapidly and had a tight, pinched expression on her face. Ms. Cedino knew that Ms. Westman had been told by her physician that she was to be discharged that afternoon. Ms. Cedino was also aware that Ms. Westman was a single parent with several preschool children at home. All these factors suggested to Ms. Cedino that Ms. Westman was anxious about going home. She validated this hypothesis by saying, "You look upset. Can you tell me how you're feeling?" Ms. Westman replied, "I just don't know what to do!"

"Could we sit down together and talk?" suggested Ms. Cedino. Ms. Westman nodded affirmatively. Ms. Cedino then pulled up a chair and said, "Please explain to me what is worrying you." After listening for a short while as Ms. Westman talked about how apprehensive she was about managing at home, Ms. Cedino decided to move from using general leads to trying to help Ms. Westman explore the situation and understand it more thoroughly.

She encouraged Ms. Westman to discuss all the responsibilities at home that concerned her and to acknowledge that she was feeling anxious because she was worried about performing all the tasks of caring for her family.

Ms. Cedino then tried to help Ms. Westman think about previous occasions when she had been ill or away from home for a while and how she had managed then. Ms. Westman ventured that some jobs could be left undone and that once when she had been ill a neighbor had helped her with shopping. As the conversation progressed, Ms. Cedino encouraged Ms. Westman to identify actions she could take to make the home situation easier to manage. Ms. Westman decided that she would ask her neighbor to help with shopping again, hire a neighborhood teenager to take the children to the playground daily, and nap while the children were napping.

In conclusion, Ms. Cedino summarized the discussion and commented, "You have made some very constructive plans as we talked." Ms. Westman looked visibly more relaxed and replied, "Well, I've handled a lot of problems in my life and I guess I can handle this."

## Study Terms

| | |
|---|---|
| anger | human dignity |
| anxiety | identification |
| behavior | maturational crisis |
| belongingness | panic |
| body image | projection |
| cognitive | psychological |
| compensation | equilibrium |
| conversion | rationalization |
| coping mechanism | reaction formation |
| crisis | regression |
| defense mechanism | repression |
| denial | restitution |
| depression | self-actualization |
| developmental crisis | self-concept |
| displacement | self-esteem |
| emotional | self-understanding |
| fantasy | situational crisis |
| feedback | sublimation |
| feelings | substitution |
| hostility | suppression |

## Learning Activities

1. Write out goals for yourself aimed at increasing self-understanding. Try to achieve these goals during this term.
2. Participate in a discussion of mental health as it relates to you as a student and as a nurse.
3. Select a specific patient in the clinical area and identify a mental-health concept that appears to be of primary importance in your relationship with this patient.
4. Recall the last time you were particularly anxious. Consider how you responded in terms of ability to focus on detail and to learn.
5. Identify defense mechanisms that you have used in the past. Consider whether or not they were helpful.

# References

Aguilera, Donna, and Messick, Janice. *Crisis Intervention: Theory and Methodology,* 3rd ed. St. Louis: C. V. Mosby, 1978.

Belaief, L. "Self-Esteem and Human Equality." *Nursing Digest* 6 (Fall 1978): 59–67.

Carstairs, G. M. "Mental Health: What Is It?" *World Health* 26 (1973): 4–9.

Carter, F. M. *Psychosocial Nursing,* 2nd ed. New York: Macmillan, 1976.

Dobson, J. "Man and His Spirit: A Matter of Self-Esteem," Part 2. *Life and Health* 92 (February 1977): 28–29.

Dunn, H. L. *High-Level Wellness.* Arlington, Va.: R. W. Beatty, 1962.

Elliott, S. "The Day the Students Came." *American Journal of Nursing* 69 (April 1969): 551–552.

Farnsworth, D. L. "Mental Health: A Point of View." *American Journal of Nursing* 60 (May 1960): 688–691.

Grace, M. J. "The Psychiatric Nurse Specialist and Medical Surgical Patients." *American Journal of Nursing* 74 (March 1974): 481–483.

Issner, N. "The Family of the Hospitalized Child." *Nursing Clinics of North America* 7 (January 1972): 5–12.

Maynard, C. K., *et al.* "Guidelines for Dealing with Anger." *Journal of Psychiatric Nursing* 17 (June 1979): 36–41.

Meyer, V. R. "The Psychology of the Young Adult." *Nursing Clinics of North America* 8 (January 1973): 5–14.

Peplau, Hildegarde. "A Working Definition of Anxiety." In *Some Clinical Approaches to Psychiatric Nursing,* edited by S. Burd, *et al.* New York: Macmillan, 1963.

Porter, A. "Patient Needs on Admission." *American Journal of Nursing* 77 (January 1977): 112–113.

Rickles, Wathan, and Finkle, B. C. "Anxiety: Yours and Your Patients'." *Nursing '73* 3 (March 1973): 23–26.

Robinson, Lisa. *Psychiatric Nursing as a Human Experience,* 2nd ed. Philadelphia: W. B. Saunders, 1977.

Seeger, P. A. "Self-Awareness and Nursing." *Journal of Psychiatric Nursing* 15 (August 1977): 24–25.

Sloboda, S. "Understanding Patient Behavior." *Nursing '77* 7 (September 1977): 74–77.

Snyder, *et al.* "Elements of a Psychosocial Assessment." *American Journal of Nursing* 77 (February 1977): 235–239.

Stuart, G. W., and Sundeen, S. J. *Principles and Practice of Psychiatric Nursing.* St. Louis: C. V. Mosby, 1979.

Volicer, B. J. "Patients' Perceptions of Stressful Events Associated With Hospitalization." *Nursing Research* 23 (1974): 235–238.

White, C. M. "The Nurse-Patient Encounter: Attitudes and Behavior in Action." *Journal of Gerontological Nursing* 3 (May/June 1977): 16–20.

# Chapter 16

# Spiritual Needs

## Objectives

After completing this chapter, you should be able to:

1. Discuss the role of spiritual needs in illness.
2. Explain ways of assessing an individual's spiritual needs.
3. Discuss the role of the clergy in the care of a hospitalized person.
4. List actions the nurse might take to help meet a patient's spiritual needs.
5. Outline the major features of the following religions that directly affect health care: Roman Catholicism, Protestantism, Eastern Orthodoxy, Judaism, Islam, and Buddhism.

## Outline

Religious Development
    Infants and Toddlers
    Preschoolers
    School-Age Children
    Adolescents
    Adults
The Role of Spiritual Needs in Illness
Beliefs That Interfere With Health Care
    Illness as Punishment
    Illness as Self-Caused
    Prohibition Against Blood Use
    Trust in Miraculous Cures
Religions and Beliefs That Affect Health Care
    Roman Catholicism
      Baptism
      Holy Communion
      Anointing of the Sick
      Religious Objects

    Protestantism
      Diet
      Baptism
      Communion
      Anointing of the Sick
    Eastern Orthodoxy
    Judaism
    Islam
    Buddhism
    Philosophical Systems
Assessing the Patient's Spiritual Needs
Meeting the Patient's Spiritual Needs
    The Role of the Clergy
    Quiet Rooms
    Worship Services
    Additional Nursing Actions
Care Study: A Patient Manifesting Spiritual Needs

Those in scientific disciplines often overlook the spiritual or religious sphere of life: our wish to know life's ultimate meaning and purpose. Our efforts to care for the whole person, however, involve recognizing the role of spiritual needs.

# Religious Development

Religious development is difficult to characterize since it is so variable. Much depends on what the individual is taught in childhood and the importance of religion in the life of the family. Nevertheless, a general pattern can be discerned and correlated with the stages of cognitive and moral development.

## Infants and Toddlers

Infants and toddlers are not yet able to think abstractly. Young toddlers can be taught to imitate adult actions, such as bowing the head and folding the hands in prayer. Toddlers are acutely responsive to the feeling associated with religious practices. If the family's attitude toward their religion is one of contentment and happiness, the toddler will usually exhibit a relaxed and happy attitude toward religious observance. If an attitude of fear and restriction surrounds religious practices, the toddler is likely to carry these feelings into later life.

## Preschoolers

Preschoolers voluntarily imitate adult behavior when it is reinforced and thus may happily participate in religious rituals that are not too long or arduous. For example, a preschooler may enjoy saying a prayer before a meal or at bedtime, singing religious songs, or reciting short verses.

The preschooler thinks concretely and does not conceptualize. God may be likened to a person he or she knows, and religious thought typically centers on the self. Literal interpretation of the statement that prayers are answered, for example, may cause the toddler to think that he or she can cause events by praying.

Preschoolers have developed a sense of right and wrong, heavily influenced by any religious teaching the family has offered. Firm beliefs about the consequences of wrongdoing are typical.

According to Murray and Zentner (1979), the preschooler is never spiritually neutral. He or she perceives the beliefs of the family and accepts them totally even when they are not explicitly stated. This wholehearted acceptance is an outgrowth of the preschooler's belief in the omnipotence of his or her parents.

It is important for care givers to know what religious beliefs and observances are important to a hospitalized preschooler. If the child has religious rituals, such as a bedtime prayer, they should be continued in a hospital, since they serve to provide security and continuity.

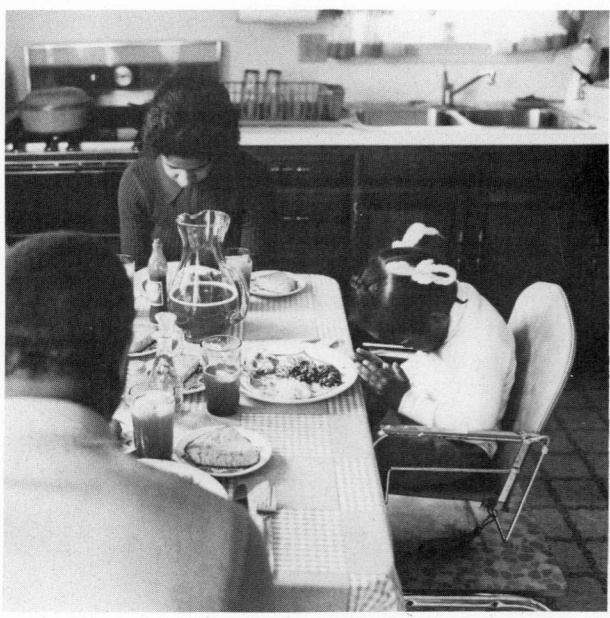

**Figure 16.1**
Preschoolers may be happy participating in religious rituals. (Owen Franken/Stock, Boston)

## School-Age Children

The school-age child is more likely to have had formal religious instruction. Belief is still largely concrete in nature, but the child may be gradually moving toward an understanding of the abstractions associated with religious belief. The school-age child may hold conflicting beliefs simultaneously without questioning them or expressing concern. Care givers ought not challenge or point out inconsistencies in belief. Although inconsistencies may be of concern to an adult, the child will only be confused by trying to sort them out. The family and religious teachers are the appropriate people to help the child do so as his or her religious instruction proceeds.

Certain religious rituals may be especially important to school-age children, who often believe in the magical value of ritual. Whenever possible, such rituals should be allowed the hospitalized child.

## Adolescents

The adolescent is acquiring the ability to deal with intellectual abstractions and may be preoccupied with puzzling philosophical and moral questions. In general, the adolescent is trying to figure out the world and his or her place in it. It is typical for adolescents to examine and challenge the beliefs with which they have been raised. It is also possible at this age to make an independent decision to embrace a particular religious belief system. Many religions recognize this capacity in a formal way. In the Jewish faith the ceremony of Bar Mitzvah confers on the adolescent the role of adult member of the congregation. In some Protestant churches, adolescence is the age when baptism as an adult is performed; in others, the capacity for independent decision making is formally acknowledged by confirmation. Young people who make an emotional and intellectual commitment to a faith are likely to draw on their belief to answer the questions of identity and purpose that arise during adolescence. The other extreme is a deliberate rejection of the family religion, which may be motivated by any number of factors, including reaction formation, rebelliousness, the urge to be independent, and loss of belief. Thus the adolescent in a family with firm religious beliefs may refuse to attend church, declare that religion stifles independence, and profess atheism. Adolescents want to be treated as adults in religious matters. They want to make independent decisions and to be taken seriously when they express beliefs.

## Adults

Spiritual life is not stagnant in adulthood. Throughout life, especially when confronting major crises, adults may re-examine their religious beliefs and practices. It is thus important that, as care givers, we never make assumptions about a person's wishes with regard to religious needs. Membership in a particular religious group does not automatically mean that a patient will welcome a visit from clergy of that faith. Similarly, a hospitalized member of the clergy may not want to attend religious services in the hospital. Patients who have no formal religious affiliation may wish to talk to religious counselors. Do not make assumptions about another person's spiritual needs; instead, validate your perceptions through facilitating interaction.

The adult who has made decisions regarding spiritual needs with which he or she is comfortable and which provide support to the self will usually have a broad outlook on life and will have confidence in its value and purpose.

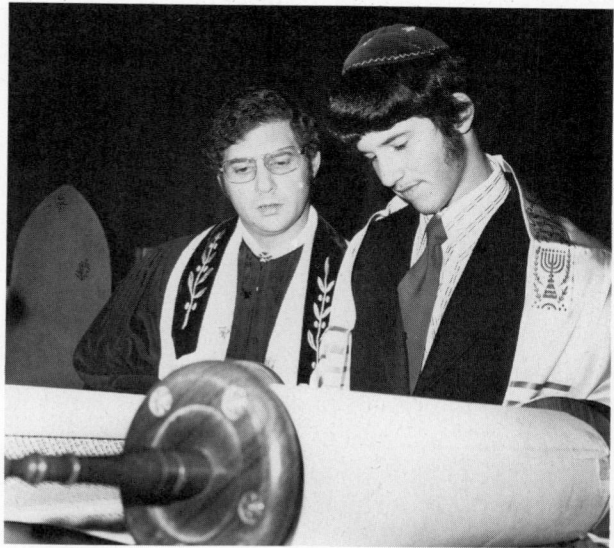

**Figure 16.2**
The adolescent may make a formal religious commitment. (Joe Ofria/Global Focus)

## The Role of Spiritual Needs in Illness

Folk cultures believe that spiritual forces are responsible for illness and for recovery or nonrecovery. In such cultures, the role of healer is combined with that of spiritual or religious adviser. Only in modern society have these two spheres of life been separated—a separation that involves losses and hazards for the ill person.

The modern study of illness focuses on multiple causation and individual susceptibility to the processes of illness. The more we understand the implications of this knowledge, the better able we are to understand the importance of people's spiritual needs.

Many people derive a comfort and inner strength from their religious beliefs that help them meet illness. When illness is overwhelming, religious beliefs sustain a person who is facing death. The force and value of personal faith should not be underestimated.

Spiritual belief is by no means limited to members of formal religions. There are many people who believe in the existence of God without necessarily subscribing to any particular faith's view of the nature of God. There are also those who do not believe in God but have a guiding philosophy of life. Many such people have highly developed personal beliefs about the meaning of life and ethical behavior.

## Beliefs That Interfere With Health Care

Some religious beliefs may prevent people from seeking health care or consenting to treatment.

### Illness as Punishment

The view of illness as punishment can be a barrier to effective health care. When ill, the psychological status of a person who adheres to such a belief is likely to be at a low ebb; self-esteem is greatly diminished by guilt. Lowered self-esteem may in turn discourage the person from seeking health care or complying with the medical regimen. The individual may view the outcome of illness as dependent on his or her ability to identify and remedy wrongdoing.

This belief system represents a difficult dilemma for the health-care worker. How can you interact with individuals to enhance their self-esteem and willingness to participate in care without interfering with personal religious beliefs? A member of the clergy may be able to offer valuable guidance in such a situation.

Preschool and school-age children are prone to view illness as punishment, due less to religious teaching than to the concrete interpretation of right and wrong typical of this age group. If you encounter this belief in a child, it is appropriate to consult the child's parents to learn whether the belief has a religious component. You might say to the child, "From what I know about being sick, I don't believe it happens because you are bad," and then provide for the kind of open interaction that allows for discussion of the child's belief.

### Illness as Self-Caused

There are those who believe that wellness is man's natural state and that illness results from incorrect living and lack of religious faith. Christian Scientists, for example, do not seek health care. When illness strikes, they seek instead to strengthen their religious faith and purify their way of living.

When such a person does enter the health-care system, it is often with feelings of failure and continuing reluctance to accept health-care technology. Staff often have difficulty accepting a patient who does not willingly comply with treatment, but a supportive and accepting attitude on the part of staff is essential to the self-esteem of these patients.

## Prohibition Against Blood Use

One of the most widely known restrictions on health care is the Jehovah's Witnesses' prohibition on the use of any blood or blood product as a part of care. This prohibition is based on their interpretation of the Bible. In the belief that violating this prohibition will result in God's punishment, Jehovah's Witnesses choose to die rather than accept a blood transfusion. When the patient is an adult, health-care workers may be distressed but must work diligently to be accepting of the patient's belief. When a child is involved, society—that is, the law—takes a different position. When a blood transfusion is considered essential to the survival of the child, a physician and hospital may take the case to the court. The court may then assume custody of the child for purposes of medical care and order the transfusion. The reasoning behind this approach is that the child's life should not be jeopardized when he or she is too young to make an independent commitment to a particular religious faith. In the case of an adolescent, however, the courts may be reluctant to intervene.

## Trust in Miraculous Cures

As professionals trained in the sciences, we must be careful not to dismiss without thought the possibility that spontaneous remissions and cures can

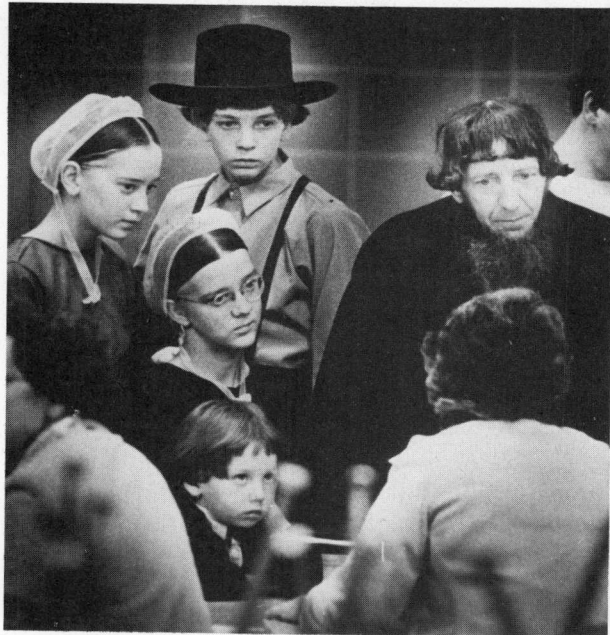

**Figure 16.3**
Sometimes members of a religion will permit medical treatment that is contrary to their beliefs. These Amish parents allowed their children to receive polio vaccine, a practice forbidden by their religion. (Wide World Photos)

occur even when objective evidence indicates a condition is irreversible. Belief in the possibility of such an occurrence is supportive and sustaining for many people.

At times, however, this belief prompts patients to abandon medical care. When health-care workers become adversaries of a patient's belief system, trust may break down. If, however, they demonstrate respect for the patient and acceptance of his or her beliefs, it may be possible to encourage the patient to continue medical care while hoping for a religious cure.

## Religions and Beliefs That Affect Health Care

Although individual members of the same faith differ in adherence to its tenets, it is helpful for the nurse to have a general familiarity with specific religious beliefs as they relate to health care. An understanding of theology is not expected of the nurse. Most of the following discussion will center on the major religious groups in the United States, with which many Americans maintain at least nominal affiliation; we will also briefly discuss other belief systems.

## Roman Catholicism

The Roman Catholic Church is a religious body characterized by uniform beliefs and fairly formalized ways of dealing with health-care problems. The specificity and uniformity of its guidelines facilitate appropriate action on the part of health-care workers. Three Catholic sacraments—Baptism, Holy Communion, and Anointing of the Sick—are of special significance to the ill Catholic.

### Baptism

Baptism is considered essential and is usually performed on the young infant. If an unbaptized person wishes to be baptized, a priest will be willing to come to perform the rite. If the patient is in danger of dying, the priest will come immediately, for it is the Church's wish that no one die without Baptism. If Baptism is truly desired and it appears that the person will die before a priest arrives, *any* person may perform this rite. Baptism has three essential components: (1) the sincere intent to baptize on the part of the person performing the rite; (2) sprinkling or pouring of any clear water over the head; and (3) recital of the words "I baptize you in the name of the Father, the Son, and the Holy Spirit" while the water is being sprinkled. The Baptism is then recorded on the chart, and a priest is notified immediately. It is appropriate but not necessary for a Roman Catholic staff member to perform the rite. Crises requiring such action occur most commonly in obstetrics, when a newborn child dies or a fetus is aborted. If the family is Catholic, the product of conception is baptized if there is any possibility that life is present. If it is known that the family is Catholic, Baptism might be performed even if the parent cannot be consulted first (if, for example, the mother is under anesthesia and the father is not present). The fetus is buried by the family, and special arrangements must thus be made.

### Holy Communion

The second sacrament of significance to the Roman Catholic patient is Holy Communion. When Communion is planned, the patient should be made presentable, the unit straightened, and a clean cleared table provided for the patient's use. The table may be covered with a linen hand towel if one is available. The patient may eat before Communion. Privacy is necessary during the priest's visit because the patient may wish to make a confession in conjunction with Communion. Communion is not commonly administered to the patient who is not allowed food because the communicant eats a bread wafer. An exception to the prohibition on food may be made in some circumstances.

### Anointing of the Sick

The third important sacrament is the Anointing of the Sick, administered by a priest to a Catholic who is ill. If a dying patient is known to be Catholic, a priest is always called even if the patient is unable to authorize such a call. The Anointing of the Sick may be administered to an individual more than once, but it is usually performed only once in a particular episode of illness. In the past this sacrament was called "Extreme Unction" or "Last Rites" and was commonly administered only to those about to die. Many patients still become very frightened when this sacrament is suggested, viewing it as evidence of impending death. The nurse should be prepared for such a response, especially from the older patient. A note should be made in the patient's record after this rite has been administered.

### Religious Objects

The Roman Catholic patient may use a rosary, which is a specially constructed chain of beads used as a guide to prayer, and may have various religious medals. These items are important to the patient, and special care is needed to guard against their loss in the hospital.

## Protestantism

Protestant religious groups account for the largest number of individuals in the United States. It is difficult to be specific about Protestant religious beliefs because there are many denominations, each with its own beliefs and practices. Even within a single denomination, individual beliefs and practices differ; thus it is especially important to consult the individual patient about his or her wishes.

## Diet

Few Protestant denominations have dietary restrictions. The Seventh-Day Adventists strongly advocate an ovo-lacto-vegetarian diet (see Chapter 21). The Church of Jesus Christ of Latter-day Saints, commonly called Mormon, does not approve of drinking coffee, tea, chocolate, or cola beverages because they all contain stimulants. Many Protestant groups disapprove of alcoholic beverages.

## Baptism

Baptism is a sacrament in most Christian churches. Some Protestants believe in infant baptism, and might wish to have a gravely ill infant or child baptized. Others, notably the Baptist churches, believe baptism should be deferred until the child reaches the age of responsible decision making, usually considered to be about twelve or thirteen years old. Thus infant baptism is not undertaken without explicit directions from the family. Protestant baptism is performed by ordained clergy.

## Communion

Communion, a sacrament in the majority of Protestant denominations, is conducted at a church with the congregation present. Although rarely performed for an individual patient in the hospital, communion may usually be provided if the person desires it.

## Anointing of the Sick

Most Protestant groups do not routinely anoint the sick, but some may do so in special instances. Many Protestants take great comfort in reading the Bible. It is common practice to visit a sick member of the congregation in the hospital.

## Eastern Orthodoxy

There are several Eastern Orthodox churches, each with a specific national origin, such as Russian Orthodox and Greek Orthodox. Because these churches are governed and function independently, the Eastern Orthodox patient will prefer a priest from his or her own church if a spiritual counselor is needed. If the community has no religious body of the individual's national background, the patient can be asked whether another Orthodox priest should be called. These churches do constitute a single faith, and in an emergency any Orthodox priest will serve the needs of an Orthodox patient.

The priest may perform confession and communion (or Holy Eucharist, as it is frequently called in the Orthodox Church) at the patient's bedside. There is also an ordinance for anointing of the sick, which is called Holy Unction. Preparation for these observances is the same as for the Roman Catholic sacraments.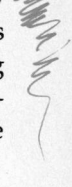

## Judaism

There are several Jewish groups, which differ in the strictness of their adherence to the laws of Judaism. The Orthodox Jew is the most strict and will usually wish to observe the *kosher* laws concerning food (see Chapter 21). Reform and Conservative Jews are less strict. The only Jewish ritual that might be performed in the hospital is circumcision of the male infant. Because a number of Jewish men, in addition to the rabbi, are present during the circumcision, special arrangements must be made. In areas where ritual circumcision is commonplace, a routine has usually been established. If not, planning in consultation with the rabbi is appropriate. Such a plan must also be approved by the physician in charge of the infant's care.

The death of an Orthodox Jew presents a unique challenge: burial should take place before the Sabbath, which begins at sundown on Friday. If the death occurs early in the week, this is not difficult, but a death on Friday requires prompt action. Orthodox Jews usually do not permit autopsies to be performed.

## Islam

Islam—the Muslim faith, based on the teachings of the prophet Mohammed—is the major religion in the Near East and North Africa. Islam emphasizes very precise individual rituals and prayers, and the Islamic patient will wish to carry out these devotions in private. The only Islamic dietary restrictions are disapproval of alcoholic beverages and of pork. There is a fasting period in the Muslim calendar, but the ill are exempt from this requirement.

A large group of Muslims in the United States originated as an independent black religious movement known as the Nation of Islam. This group has subsequently affiliated with the worldwide Islamic community and expanded its membership beyond the black community. Nevertheless, black pride, autonomy, and independence are still basic tenets of the faith.

Conservative Muslims retain the traditional restrictions on the freedom of women, who are not allowed to be seen unveiled by men other than members of the family. Health care for such women should be provided by female health-care workers.

## Buddhism

The number of Buddhists in the United States is growing. Many are of Asian background; others are young people who have converted to Buddhism. Like Christianity, Buddhism has many sects. Many Buddhists are vegetarian. In the belief that one's current actions affect one's later life and rebirth, Buddhists generally attempt to be peaceful and cooperative in their daily living. This system of belief encourages calm acceptance of whatever life has to offer, and as a consequence the patient may not express needs or ask for care. The nurse must be especially alert to nonverbal indications of needs and problems.

## Philosophical Systems

Some philosophical systems view life as completely predetermined: "That's fate" and "What will be will be" are common expressions that reflect this viewpoint. Adherents of such systems may not be willing to change their diets or life styles to improve their health in the belief that the future cannot be altered. Although concentrating on the present may enable you to assist such a person, you may not be able to change this attitude. Respect for one's philosophical beliefs is one of the rights of the patient.

An *agnostic* is a person who believes that human beings cannot know whether or not God exists. An *atheist* does not believe in the existence of God. A person who adheres to either of these beliefs bases ethical decisions on his or her philosophy of life. Such an individual will usually not wish to consult a member of the clergy but may wish to share his or her feelings and thoughts with an interested, caring friend.

## Assessing the Patient's Spiritual Needs

Nurses are often reluctant to ask about patients' religious needs or concerns, believing their questions may either be interpreted as prying or lead patients to erroneous assumptions about the seriousness of their illness. If you believe that it is a function of nursing to support the whole person, concern for the patient's spiritual needs will be a part of your nursing plan.

When you take a nursing history on admission to the hospital, you might ask if the patient has a religious preference and wishes a religious adviser, pastor, or church notified of his or her illness. The response will provide some information about the patient's spiritual concerns.

Observation of the patient's behavior provides additional information. Does the patient read the Bible or a prayer book? Does he or she wear religious medals or insignia or use religious objects, such as a rosary?

In conversation, does the patient discuss God or God's will? Does the patient talk about the meaning and purpose of his or her existence?

Expressions of guilt or a troubled conscience may be dealt with by the individual recognizing them as religious problems.

Many hospital admission forms provide a space in which to indicate religion. If the religious affiliation noted there would in some way affect health care, it should be taken into consideration when planning care. The family can usually give you specific information about the patient's religious practices if he or she is unable to communicate.

## Meeting the Patient's Spiritual Needs

### The Role of the Clergy

Many large hospitals have a chaplain, who serves as a member of the health-care team to identify and, if possible, meet patients' spiritual and religious needs. The modern chaplain has usually had special education in dealing with the spiritual needs of those who are ill. Familiar with a wide variety of religious beliefs, the chaplain is prepared to contact other clergy when patients have specific needs. Furthermore, the chaplain's understanding of health care makes him or her a valuable participant on the health-care team. Some very large hospitals may have more than one chaplain, representing various religions.

Chaplains' methods of operation vary, depending largely on the philosophy of the hospital. Often the chaplain visits each newly admitted patient. Although an ordained member of the clergy of a particular faith, the chaplain does not restrict his or her attention to members of the same faith. During the initial visit, the chaplain greets the patient and explains the role of the chaplain. A patient who has religious needs will often indicate them to the chaplain at this time. The chaplain is also available for referrals by the nurse or consultations with the staff about problems related to patients' religious needs. The chaplain may spend time with the patient simply visiting, reading scripture, or ministering in a variety of ways. A skilled chaplain assesses the patient's needs and relates in the way that is most helpful to the patient. In some settings the chaplain also helps the staff cope with the stresses of caring for patients who are critically ill.

When there is no hospital chaplain, the clergy in the community usually undertake to meet this need. Since they are often unfamiliar with hospital routine, they may need special assistance from the nurse in planning what they will do. If the patient wishes to see a member of the clergy, the patient, the family, or the nurse (with the patient's permission) may call one. If the patient is affiliated with a specific congregation, it is best for its clergy to be called. If the patient is far from his or her own congregation or does not belong to one, you may ask a few questions to ascertain the patient's general beliefs and then suggest several churches with similar beliefs whose clergy have expressed willingness to serve the needs of the sick.

Not all those with strong religious affiliations wish a member of the clergy to visit. For example, Jewish clergy are basically teachers of their congregations and have few special religious powers exceeding those of other Jews. Thus a Jewish patient may wish to see his or her own rabbi but be uninterested in seeing any other rabbi.

Some religious groups, including the Latter-day Saints and Christian Scientists, do not have ordained clergy. Instead, these denominations appoint lay people to minister to the sick, and their religious function should be recognized by the health-care worker. In Christian Science, this role is undertaken by the *reader*.

Occasionally, a member of the clergy may lack skill in dealing with the sick and may upset rather

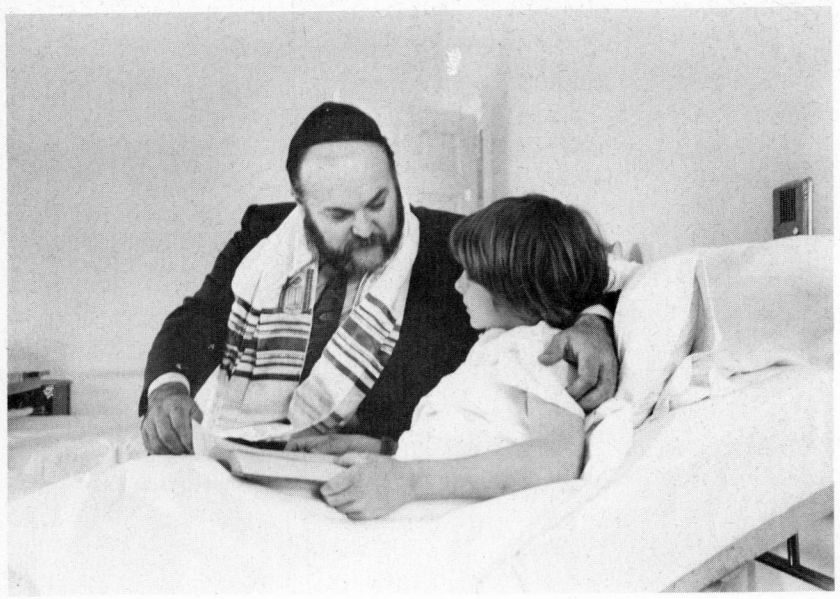

**Figure 16.4**
Members of the clergy may comfort and support the patient and the family.
(Chris Maynard)

than support the patient. In such a case, the nurse must explain this tactfully to the clergy member and suggest that he or she limit or abandon visits.

Well-intentioned but misguided members of some religious groups sometimes wish to visit many patients without regard for individual patients' wishes. Patients who would deny strangers entry into their homes often feel unable to control access to their hospital bedsides. Thus it is the nurse's responsibility to protect the patient's privacy.

## Quiet Rooms

Many hospitals have a chapel or quiet meditation room for use by patients, families, and staff. This room is usually nondenominational so that a wide variety of people will feel comfortable using it, though this may not be the case if the hospital is sponsored or affiliated with a specific religious group. Such a room can be of value to those who need a few moments of quiet thought, as well as those who wish to worship. It may be the only place where privacy and refuge from the hectic pace of the hospital are available to a family that has just lost a loved one. Wise use of this peaceful environment will be supportive to many people. Staff members, too, may need a few moments' refuge to gather strength for difficult situations.

## Worship Services

Worship services are held in some large hospitals and nursing homes. These services may be non-denominational, or separate services may be held for different religious groups. If such services are held, the nurse should offer information about them to the patient and the family. It is also the nurse's responsibility to plan the patient's care so that attendance is possible. A desire to attend religious services should be treated as a special need when determining priorities for care.

## Additional Nursing Actions

Sometimes a patient requests that a nurse read scripture to him or her. Most people would not consider doing so to be participation in a religious observance, but the individual nurse must decide how to respond in light of the specific situation. Often a volunteer will read scripture, or the patient's congregation will locate a member willing to do so.

If the patient has religious symbols or medals, their loss can, as we have said, be seriously upsetting. Every effort should be made to keep track of these items and to ensure that they are not inadvertently lost. Occasionally, a patient will request permission to take a religious object to the operating room. Although not common practice, arrangements to do so can usually be made with the surgeon, operating-room staff, and recovery-room staff. This alone may make a significant difference in the patient's ability to tolerate severe stress.

Patients may ask you to pray for or with them. If your religious beliefs coincide, you might join the patient in prayer. If your beliefs differ greatly, you might simply offer to stay while the patient prays. If you also find this difficult, you can seek another staff member who would be more comfortable in this role. If the patient asks you to pray on his or her behalf and you do not feel that it is appropriate for you to do so, you might say that you will continue to keep the patient in your thoughts and offer to contact a member of the clergy or other person who could meet this need.

If a patient feels guilt, with regard either to illness or to some other aspect of life, a member of the clergy is often best able to assist in its resolution. Some religions have prescribed means of absolving guilt; in others the process is less formalized. All major religions address issues of guilt and conscience and attempt to assist the individual in confronting them. The serious anxiety that guilt can arouse can be a barrier to healing. Thus resolution of guilt, which is a religious problem, contributes to recovery from physical illness.

Occasionally patients behave in ways related to their religious beliefs that create problems for the nurse. If a patient attempts to convert the nurse to his or her own religious beliefs, the nurse faces the difficult task of maintaining simultaneously a helpful nurse-patient relationship and personal religious or philosophical integrity. Acknowledging the importance of the patient's beliefs and redirecting the conversation to focus on the patient's needs is an effective way to deal with this problem.

When a member of the clergy or other person with a religious vocation, such as a nun, becomes a patient, health-care workers may have unrealistic expectations of their behavior. Such an individual is sometimes expected to continue to act in a supportive way toward others and to be exemplary in behavior and free from anxiety. This expectation is far from realistic. Clergy are people, with varying degrees of ability to tolerate and deal with the stresses of illness. Natural feelings of anxiety will be present, and the support and aid of others will be needed. Reducing staff expectations of exceptional behavior and carefully assessing the individual will ensure realistic care.

## Conclusion

The spiritual dimensions of patient care may easily be overlooked. Patients often feel that their spiritual lives and beliefs must be kept separate from their health care. This feeling often originates with health-care workers who feel that spiritual matters are not their concern. Recognizing and meeting spiritual needs, or making referrals to those who can meet them, is an aspect of caring for the whole patient and may significantly enhance the patient's ability to deal successfully with the stress of illness.

## Care Study A patient manifesting spiritual needs

Ms. Jennifer Nakima, a student nurse on the medical unit, was assigned to care for Mr. Stephen MacDougal. In the course of her assessment, she noted that Mr. MacDougal kept a well-worn Bible at his bedside. His admitting information sheet gave his religious preference as Protestant. She also noted that when she entered his room he would often put his Bible away and fold his hands expectantly.

**Ms. Nakima:** "Mr. MacDougal, I notice that you read your Bible a lot. It seems to be an important part of your life."

**Mr. MacDougal:** "Yes, it is. I was raised as a Christian and have been one all my life. Other people may be wishy-washy, but not me! I was an elder in my church for many years, but lately I've been sick too much to be able to take any responsibility."

**Ms. Nakima:** "Are you used to attending church on Sundays?"

**Mr. MacDougal:** "Never miss! Except now, of course."

**Ms. Nakima:** "Did you know that there is a nondenominational church service here in the hospital every Sunday?"

**Mr. MacDougal:** "No—who goes?"

**Ms. Nakima:** "Well, it's for patients mainly, but visitors and staff are welcome to attend too. Ministers from different churches conduct the service."

**Mr. MacDougal:** "When do they have it?"

**Ms. Nakima:** "It's at 1:30 in the afternoon. That's because most people are done with treatments and things and the staff can help them get there. Would you like to go? I could arrange it."

**Mr. MacDougal:** "Well . . . do you have to get dressed up to go?"

**Ms. Nakima:** "A robe and slippers are what most people wear."

**Mr. MacDougal:** "I'd like to go, then, if it isn't too much trouble."

**Ms. Nakima:** "I'll make the arrangements with the team leader who will be here Sunday and mark it on your care plan. Maybe you could remind the person who is taking care of you on Sunday, too. That would make a double-check."

**Mr. MacDougal:** "Sure. I won't forget, that's for sure."

In this instance, the student nurse assessed the patient's spiritual needs and identified an appropriate way to meet them. Her actions were carefully planned and made use of the unit's communication system to facilitate implementation. The patient was included at all points in the process: Ms. Nakima validated her assessment with him, he participated in making the plan, and he had a role in carrying out the plan.

## Study Terms

| | |
|---|---|
| agnostic | kosher |
| Anointing of the Sick | Muslim |
| atheist | Protestantism |
| Baptism | quiet room |
| Buddhism | rabbi |
| chaplain | reader |
| clergy | religious medals |
| Eastern Orthodoxy | Roman Catholic |
| Holy Communion | rosary |
| Islam | sacrament |
| Judaism | scripture |

## Learning Activities

**1.** Choose a religious group to contact for information about its response to illness and special help for those who are ill. This information can be submitted in writing or presented for class discussion.

**2.** Interview a nurse to determine what he or she sees as the most significant actions nurses can undertake with regard to spiritual needs.

## References

Berkowitz, P., and Berkowitz, N. "The Jewish Patient in the Hospital." *American Journal of Nursing* 67 (November 1967): 2335.

Damsteegt, D. "Pastoral Roles in Pre-Surgical Visits." *American Journal of Nursing* 75 (August 1975): 1336–1337.

Dickinson, Sr. C. "The Search for Spiritual Meaning." *American Journal of Nursing* 75 (October 1975): 1789–1793.

Dillenberger, J., and Welch, C. *Protestant Christi-*

anity. New York: Charles Scribner and Sons, 1955.

Morris, K. L., *et al.* "Team Work: Nurse and Chaplain." *American Journal of Nursing* 72 (December 1972): 2197–2199.

Murray, R., and Zenther, J. *Nursing Assessment and Health Promotion Through the Life Span,* 2nd ed. Englewood Cliffs, N.J.: Prentice-Hall, 1979.

Naiman, H. L. "Nursing in Jewish Law." *American Journal of Nursing* 70 (September 1970): 2378–2379.

"Patients' Religious Beliefs—Nurses' Responsibility." *Regan Reports on Nursing Law* 14 (April 1974): 2.

Pederson, W. D. "The Broadening Role of the Hospital Chaplain." *Hospitals* 42 (September 1968): 58.

Piepgras, B. "The Other Dimension: Spiritual Help." *American Journal of Nursing* 68 (December 1968): 2610–2613.

Pumphrey, J. B. "Recognizing Your Patient's Spiritual Needs." *Nursing '77* 12 (December 1977): 64–69.

Raciappa, J. D. "A Total Ministry." *American Journal of Nursing* 73 (April 1973): 645.

"Recognizing Your Patient's Spiritual Needs." *Nursing Update* 6 (July 1975): 1–2.

"Taking Patient's Spiritual History Is Called Important by the Surgeon." *O.R. Reporter* 8 (December 1973): 11.

Ware, T. *The Orthodox Church.* Baltimore: Penguin Books, 1972.

Westberg, G. E. *Nurse, Pastor and Patient.* Rock Island, Ill.: Augustana Press, 1955.

# Chapter 17
# Sexuality

## Objectives

After completing this chapter, you should be able to:

1. Differentiate between sexuality and sexual behavior.
2. Think about your own feelings on sexual variations and sexual behavior on the part of patients.
3. Name and define the most common types of sexual dysfunction.
4. List three major classes of drugs that may affect sexuality.
5. List the ways in which illness can increase or decrease libido.
6. Name and define the surgical procedures most likely to precipitate sexual problems.
7. Discuss the four aspects of sexuality likely to pose problems for the disabled.
8. Discuss the importance of sexual counseling as it relates to the care of the patient.

## Outline

Over the past several years, a new awareness of individual and group needs has emerged. Certain groups of people—the elderly, handicapped, and those who are disadvantaged by other circumstances—have gained recognition of their special needs, thereby securing greater control over their lives. Individual needs also have been re-examined, and as a result sexual attitudes are changing. A new openness with regard to sexuality is allowing people to explore their sexual feelings honestly. Such matters as abortion, family planning, and alternative sexual life styles, until very recently considered unmentionable in polite society, are now discussed frankly and openly. Women are claiming sexual freedom enjoyed in the past only by men.

It is important to keep in mind the distinction between sexuality and sexual behavior. *Sexuality*, regardless of how it is expressed, is an integral aspect of every person. Its components are awareness of one's body as a source of pleasure, perception of oneself as feminine or masculine, and a sense of oneself as an inherently sexual being. Although this chapter will focus on *sexual behavior*—the expression of sexuality—let us keep in mind the nature and universality of sexuality.

## Variations in Sexual Behavior

Sexual behavior is the expression of sexuality. *Heterosexuality*—sexual preference for the opposite sex—is the norm in American society. After collecting a massive volume of data, Alfred Kinsey and his colleagues published two books (1948, 1953) on the sexual behavior of the American male and female. These books reported the sexual practices of heterosexual men and women to be far more varied than had previously been acknowledged. They also documented a higher-than-expected incidence of two variations from the norm: *homosexuality*, or sexual preference for members of the same sex; and *bisexuality*, or sexual interest in members of both sexes. It is unclear whether more people are homosexual and bisexual now than at the time of Kinsey's research or whether greater public acceptance has simply made sexual variations more apparent. Until very recently, both homosexuality and bisexuality were considered "deviant" behavior, often punishable by law. In the last few years, homosexuals, most of whom prefer to be called *gay* (either sex) or *lesbians* (women), have formed groups for mutual support and to protest discriminatory practices against them. In 1973 and again in 1974, the American Psychiatric Association (APA) at its annual convention affirmed the position that homosexuality, in and of itself, does not constitute mental illness.

Just as a certain proportion of the general population is homosexual, so may be some members of the health-care team, including nurses. It is impossible, of course, to suppress our emotional and sexual lives entirely when practicing nursing. Our attitudes unavoidably influence our interactions with patients and with our peers. It must be understood, however, that nurses never impose their sexual views on their patients. Though remaining objective and nonjudgmental is not always easy, nurses should regard patients as people with problems who need care, regardless of their sexual life styles. Similarly, nurses should evaluate one another in terms only of nursing proficiency, not of sexual preference.

*Stereotyping*, unwise in any situation, is particularly futile when one tries to "guess" another person's sexual preference. The notion that males who are "limp-wristed" and females who are "mannish" are gay is simply false. Studies of gay people reveal no overwhelming preponderance of particular traits. These findings underline the wisdom of accepting people as they are, without preconceptions.

Although homosexuals have become much more vocal and many are speaking out honestly in defense of their sexual orientation, gay patients rarely divulge their homosexuality. In light of generally negative staff attitudes toward homosexual patients, such reticence is understandable. The overtly homosexual patient is still often socially ostracized, even to the point of being placed in a single room or alone in a multiple-occupancy room. The staff may avoid the usual light conversation and inquiries about the patient's job and family. The patient's visitors may be scrutinized by the staff, and attempts may be made to limit their visits. Some degree of relief is often evident when such a patient is discharged.

Attitudes are also changing regarding what is considered acceptable sexual behavior between two consenting adults. Alternative, creative techniques are being explored by couples as a means to more fully experience sexual satisfaction. This will be discussed in more detail later.

## Sexuality and Nursing Practice

It has been said that many nurses appear *asexual*, or *sexless*, and prefer to regard patients in the same light. Perhaps some nurses exaggerate their professional demeanor as an emotional defense to facilitate performing intimate tasks for patients.

If we consider nurses sociologically, we can better understand the sources of the judgmental attitudes nurses sometimes exhibit toward people whose sexual life styles differ from that of the majority. Nursing's roots are in religion; many schools of nursing were originally religious in nature. Even with the current prevalence of nonsectarian settings, nursing continues to be subject to dictates on moral and sexual conduct. Also, nurses are largely drawn from the middle class; few are very wealthy or very poor. The characteristic values of the middle class have tended to be conservative, particularly in the realm of sexuality. Social changes are usually initiated at the fringes of society and make their way into the mainstream gradually. Nurses, as representatives of the mainstream, may accept social change somewhat reluctantly.

It is incumbent on nurses to recognize that individuals have the right to fulfill their sexual needs however they desire, as long as others are not coerced or harmed in any way. It is important, furthermore, to respond objectively and professionally to gay patients and others whose life styles are unconventional.

### Data Gathering

Because sexuality is a delicate and emotion-laden subject, sexual information about patients is rarely solicited by means of direct questions. Many patients would consider such questions an invasion of privacy. Thus you may have no more than a "feeling" that a patient is confronting sexual problems. If this is the case, the best way to help may be to build a trusting relationship with the patient and signal your availability to explore any problems the patient may have. Other patients, or their sexual partners, may talk to you about such problems without prompting. A male patient may be more comfortable talking to a male nurse; female patients might also prefer to speak with a nurse of their own sex, though this is not always the case.

With medical or surgical conditions involving the reproductive or sexual organs, and possibly alterations in body image (see Chapter 29), the nurse can intervene more directly with a leading remark such as "Some patients who have this surgery are concerned about how their sexual performance might be affected. Have you and your physician talked about this, or is there anything I can help clarify for you?" Often the nurse's role is to facilitate communication about sexual matters between the physician, the patient, and perhaps the patient's sexual partner. At other times it may be to offer information and emotional support, particularly if sexual adaptations are necessary.

### Inappropriate Sexual Behavior

One sensitive problem you may occasionally encounter is a suggestive or seductive advance by a patient. Pretending such an incident did not occur

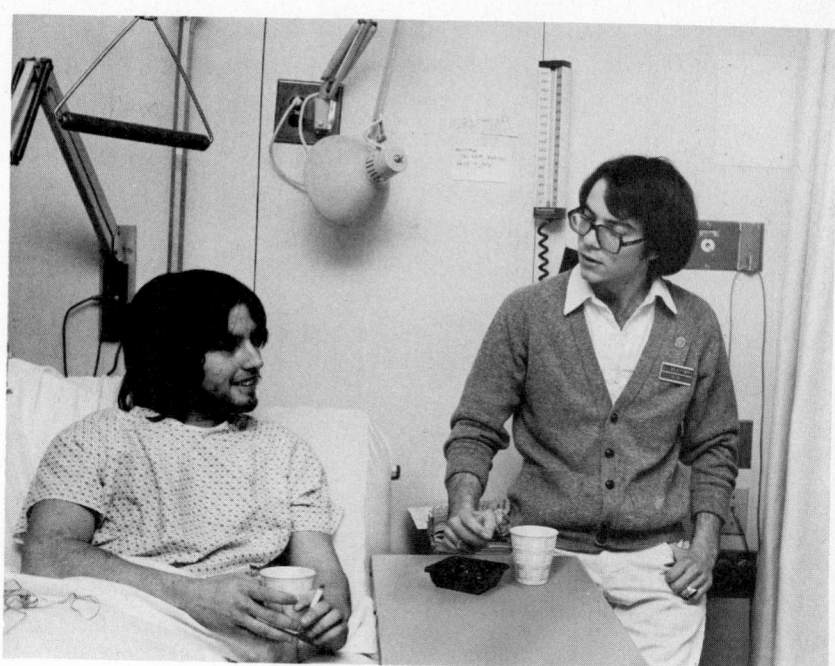

**Figure 17.1**
Sexual concerns are shared by patient and nurse. (Russ Kinne/Danbury Hospital/ Photo Researchers, Inc.)

is usually not helpful, since it allows for the same behavior to be repeated. It is usually more effective to confront the situation, saying calmly but briefly that you care about the patient professionally but that personal advances are inappropriate and may even interfere with care. If you express your concern for the patient as a person and do not respond to such an incident with rejection, a working relationship and a friendly professional atmosphere can usually be reinstated.

You must closely examine your own dress and behavior to discern whether, even unconsciously, you are "sending messages" that could be construed as sexually provocative. In general, women express sexuality more visually than do men; men do so more verbally. For example, a female nurse in a very short, form-fitting uniform may convey a highly sexual image to the patient. A male nurse may exhibit his sexuality by making a lighthearted but sexually suggestive remark to a patient. Neither is behaving professionally. Patients, who are typically bored and unable to pursue their usual forms of sexual release, are especially vulnerable to both visual and verbal nuances. Any frank sexual remark or overture to any patient by any nurse, regardless of the sex of either, is extremely inappropriate and unprofessional.

## Dealing With Erection and Masturbation

Such nursing tasks as cleansing the areas of elimination and the genitals can make both the nurse and the patient uncomfortable. It is not uncommon for a male patient to experience an *erection* of the penis during such care. This reflex should not be construed as a sexual overture. The erection mechanism is both voluntary, arising from the cerebral cortex, and involuntary, originating in the lumbar portion of the spinal cord. Even very young infants have erections, and adult males may experience them during the REM sleep stage. The adult male commonly awakens with an erection due to a distended bladder. An erection during care is usually simply a reaction to the stimulus of touch and not an expression of erotic feelings. If the patient shows signs of embarrassment or makes an apologetic remark, you might say that you hope he will not feel uncomfortable, since such an occurrence is not uncommon and is due to a reflex that is not under his control.

*Masturbation* is self-stimulation for the purpose of sexual pleasure, possibly terminating in sexual climax. Once thought harmful, masturbation is now increasingly accepted as a natural component of psychosexual development and a useful outlet for sexual tension for some individuals. Nevertheless, cultural taboos still surround masturbation, and it remains an emotionally charged subject. It may happen that you observe patients masturbating. Mental patients to whom cultural values are not for the moment important may masturbate openly. Only if such behavior becomes excessive and is preferred to normal relationships does it pose a problem. When the patient improves and re-establishes a sexual relationship, masturbation usually diminishes.

Retarded and brain-damaged people sometimes masturbate openly, as do many children. The family and the staff may become upset, viewing such behavior as indelicate. Understanding that such a person's emotional and intellectual life may be comparable to a child's helps make sense of this behavior. An example is a nineteen-year-old boy with considerable brain damage due to a motorcycle accident. As his state of awareness improved, he engaged in masturbation. His mother, embarrassed and upset, asked the nurse to do something to stop him. When the nurse explained that such behavior is not unusual in brain-injured patients, and could be a sign that the patient was becoming aware of himself and progressing toward fuller consciousness, the mother became more accepting.

What if the nurse happens in on an adult patient in the act of masturbating? Leaving the patient in privacy is an appropriate response. Such behavior should be regarded as satisfying an immediate need, and no response should be made that might cause the patient to feel guilty or ashamed. The same principles apply in the case of the elderly patient, male or female, who engages in masturbation. We now know that sexual interest persists late in life, and some elderly people have no outlet for it other than masturbation. Because the elderly who are institutionalized may suffer sensory deprivation, sexual self-stimulation can be therapeutic. Although encounters with masturbating patients will probably be very infrequent, you should prepare yourself to deal with the situation in the most knowledgeable and understanding manner possible.

## Age and Sexuality

The recent massive increase in pregnancy and venereal disease among teenagers is a matter of deep concern to health-care professionals, public policymakers, parents, and teenagers alike. Not to mention the problems unplanned pregnancy can cause young people themselves, research shows that infants of teenage parents have a high rate of developmental health problems (Marlow, 1977). As a student nurse or practicing nurse, you may be consulted by teenagers or their parents with regard to sexual matters. The best response is to encourage them to seek the help of a trained professional counselor.

Young adulthood and the middle years may also be characterized by a variety of sexual crises. Many couples experience sexual incompatibility or differing desires with regard to frequency, though more divorcing couples cite money and children rather than sexual problems as causes of estrangement.

Sex between people past childbearing age was once thought to be "not nice" and not necessary, but such attitudes no longer prevail. Sexual activity enjoyable for both partners may continue into one's eighties and beyond. Thus it is unjustifiable to assume that an elderly patient is no longer interested in sex and has no active sexual life. Some elderly couples have, for health-related or psychological reasons, mutually decided to conclude their sexual activity. In other cases, such a decision is made unilaterally, causing friction between the partners. Physiologically, the aging process causes structural and hormonal changes in the sexual organs that may bring about a decline in libido and sexual frequency. However, this circumstance should not have a disruptive effect on sexual interest and performance. Aging people need to know that sex in the later years is perfectly acceptable, enjoyable, and natural; nurses need to abolish any preconceptions they might have to the contrary.

# Common Types of Sexual Dysfunction

Nurses should be familiar with common sexual problems. Both men and women may experience low *libido,* or desire for sexual activity. The need for sexual activity varies greatly from one individual to another and becomes a problem only if it is perceived as such by the people involved. Sometimes decreased libido is a consequence of lack of a partner; this is particularly true of older widowed adults.

No realm of human activity is more clearly a blend of mind and body than sexuality. Few sexual problems are exclusively psychological or exclusively physical in nature. Psychological arousal promotes sexual performance; in turn, sexual performance draws on the emotions.

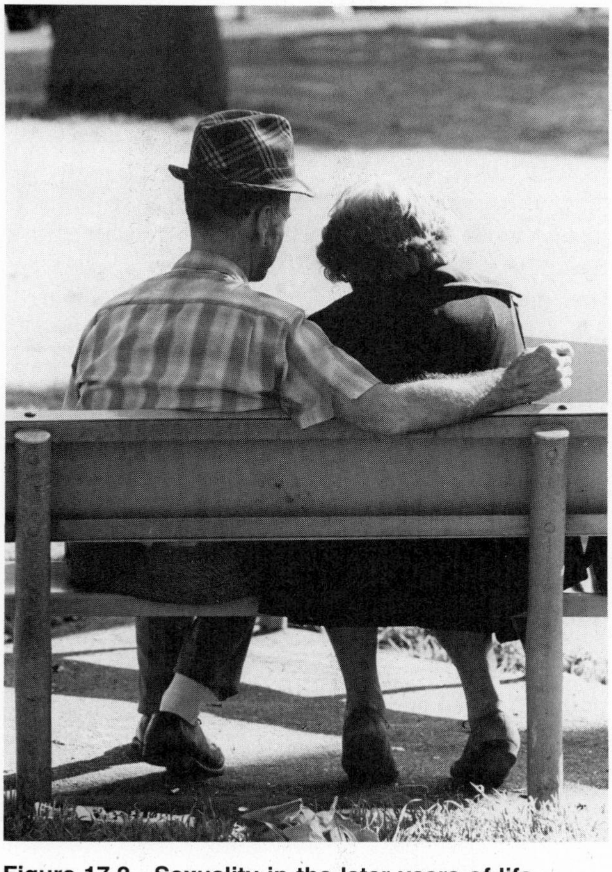

## Common Sexual Problems of Males

By far the most common sexual problem for males is *impotence,* the inability to produce or maintain a penile erection. Though it is commonly believed that impotence is usually psychological rather than physical in origin, a recent study found that 35 percent of the participants had previously overlooked disorders of the endocrine system, such as too little testosterone or overactive thyroids (Spark, 1980). Impotence can also be caused by motor nerve disruption, such as in cases of spinal-cord injury.

The second most common problem for males is *premature ejaculation,* usually defined as ejaculation of semen within thirty to sixty seconds of *intromission* or penetration of the vagina. Problematic because it interferes with the satisfaction of one or both partners, premature ejaculation may be caused by anxiety or other psychological mechanisms.

Less common is *inhibitory ejaculation,* which can take the form either of delayed ejaculation or inability to ejaculate. This problem may interfere with mutual satisfaction and is often psychological in origin.

**Figure 17.2  Sexuality in the later years of life**
Eric Kroll/Taurus Photos

## Common Sexual Problems of Females

*Frigidity* is a condition of the female characterized by low or absent libido. Frigidity may have a variety of underlying causes, including unpleasant sexual experiences in childhood, repressive attitudes imposed early in life, fear, and, often, an inept sexual partner.

*Nonorgasmic* women differ in that some have never had an orgasm while others can achieve orgasm only with difficulty. Some women who do not achieve orgasm through intercourse alone can do so with other forms of sexual play and may prefer such alternatives to intercourse. A woman may also feel satisfied occasionally without attaining an orgasm. Being nonorgasmic becomes a problem, in a large part, only if the woman perceives it as one or if it disturbs her partner.

*Vaginismus*—severe and painful spasm of the vaginal orifice brought on by attempts at intercourse—is a less common sexual problem and usually psychological in origin.

Painful intercourse, or *dyspareunia*, is often due to inadequate lubrication of the vagina, which in older women may be a consequence of estrogen deficiency. Occasionally, dyspareunia is caused by structural defects. Psychological causes have been reported as well.

## Drugs and Sexuality

Few, if any, drugs have no side effects. Such side effects are at best distressing to the patient and at worst dangerous. Physicians often choose to prescribe a certain drug, regardless of its side effects, because it is the best agent for a specific condition. Drugs commonly cause skin rashes, blood disorders, nausea, respiratory depression, and a host of other reactions and can cause changes and problems in every system of the body. Over 118 drugs may cause changes in libido or sexual performance (*Journal of Drug Research*, 1974). The three main classes of such drugs—*anorexic* (appetite-reducing), *antihypertensive* (blood-pressure–lowering), and *antidepressive*—generally cause a decrease in libido.

There are many other drugs that may affect sexuality. Some hormones and the dopamine derivatives can greatly increase libido, which can frighten the family, the staff, and the patient by dramatically altering the patient's self-image.

To retard malignant or abnormal cell growth, a hormone of the opposite sex may be prescribed in rather large dosage. Some masculinizing effect on the female and feminizing effect on the male undergoing such therapy is almost unavoidable, and a supportive, empathic attitude is essential on the part of the nurse.

Although many of the potential side effects of drugs are mentioned to the patient so that he or she will be sure to inform the physician if they occur, there is disagreement about whether information on possible sexual alterations should be provided in all cases. The issue is whether such information might be suggestive enough to trigger problems not otherwise caused by the medication. On the other hand, patients on some of these drugs have been known to become very upset over decreased libido and difficulty in sexual performance, not realizing that such changes are drug-induced.

The drug information circulated by pharmaceutical companies citing sexual difficulties due to certain drugs usually focuses on the male response: lack of sexual desire, failure to attain or maintain an erection, and ejaculation of semen too early or not at all. Such deficiencies in males appear to be more readily measurable than are deficiencies of response in females, but lack of sexual desire and inability to attain climax may occur in the female to an equally distressing degree. A trusted nurse is often the one person to whom the patient confides sexual problems. He or she may express great relief when you explain that it is *possible* such problems may be drug-related. When the physician is consulted, the drug may or may not be discontinued, depending on its importance in the treatment of the underlying condition. If the drug is not withdrawn, the patient and his or her partner may need continuing support and counsel with regard to the resultant sexual problem.

You can do patients a service by keeping in mind the drugs each is taking and by keeping an eye out for side effects. It is a strong argument for ongoing assessment that problems of a sexual nature are thus detected before causing the patient undue emotional distress and anxiety.

## Illness and Sexuality

Illness causes both general and specific sexual problems. The major changes in the patterns of daily living that illness brings about are exaggerated by the unfamiliar environment of the hospital. Not only sexual activity is postponed; work, hobbies, and family and community responsibilities are also interrupted.

Interest in sex is enhanced by rest and a state of well-being. Among the most common components of illness are fatigue and general malaise or listlessness, neither conducive to sexual activity. The body's resources are all engaged in combating the illness; the patient's mind is focused on his or her health and possibly also on missing work and the burden the illness represents for the family. Illness is also typically accompanied by some degree of mental depression, which is known to reduce libido.

Certain specific illnesses can affect sexuality. Diabetic men, for example, experience more sterility and impotence than the general population, while diabetic women tend to give birth to larger-than-normal infants. Sex provokes anxiety in some epileptics who equate sexual excitement with the advent of a seizure. However, there is no evidence to substantiate the notion that seizures are brought on by sexual activity. Living as normally as possible is desirable for the epileptic.

A rather special case is the patient recovering from a heart attack. Heart attacks occasionally occur during sexual intercourse, due to the increased expenditure of energy, so fears about resuming sex on recovery are not entirely unrealistic. Only the physician can determine what instructions are appropriate for a given patient, but sexual activity need never be entirely eliminated. Depending on their cardiac status, some people resume sexual relations almost immediately and others must delay doing so. If there is risk for a male patient, his partner can be encouraged and instructed to assume the more active role in intercourse. Audiovisual materials are available to teach the patient and his partner sexual adaptations that may be indicated.

We have noted the decrease in libido caused by illness, fatigue, and hospitalization. It is not uncommon for this circumstance to be followed by its opposite. For example, a recovering heart patient, under orders for bedrest, who feels refreshed and no longer extremely anxious, may begin to joke or talk about sex. The nurse should realize that persistent talk about sex may indicate accumulated sexual tension or worries and problems the patient wants to address. This is a situation calling for assessment and evaluation. First, you should acknowledge the patient's behavior by saying something like "You certainly have quite a repertoire of jokes" or "You must be improving to be showing so much interest in sex." You might go on to say that it is not unusual for patients who are beginning to feel like their old selves again to experience renewed interest in sex. This opening can lead to discussion if the patient wishes to talk.

Sex therapists agree that sexual interaction be-

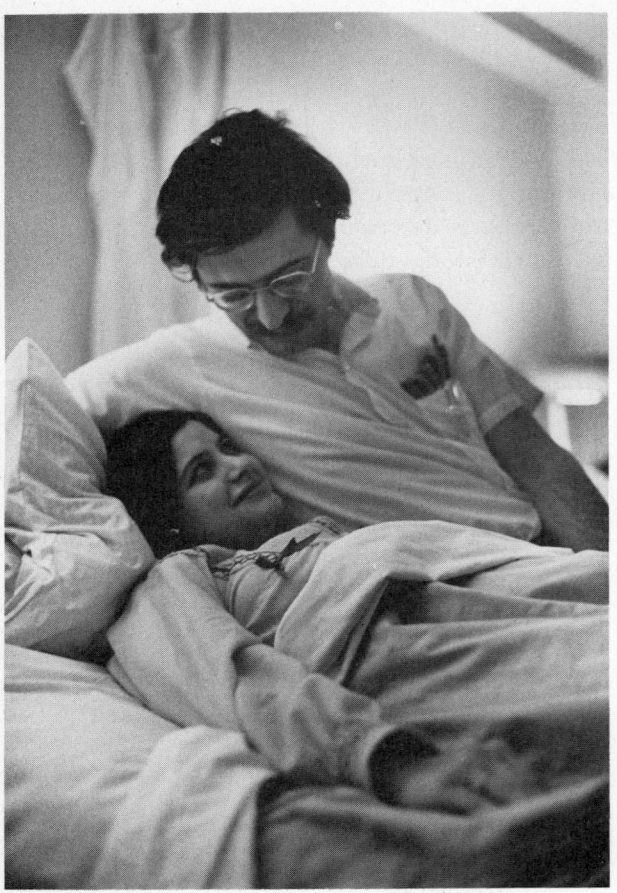

tween a chronically ill patient and the sexual partner should not be discouraged by health-care providers. For the sexually active patient, long-term interruption of sexual activity can be a stressor that intensifies illness. However, a hospital is not an appropriate setting for sexual interaction because it lacks privacy. Many hospitalized patients could safely be allowed to go out on a "pass"—that is, to remain registered as a patient but make a home visit. This option would be particularly valuable for patients undergoing intermittent treatment or lengthy rehabilitation.

**Figure 17.3**
The hospitalized patient faces temporary disruption of his or her sex life. (Chris Maynard)

## Surgery and Sexuality

Some surgical procedures that involve the genitourinary system have an undeniable effect on sexuality. Moreover, *any* surgical procedure that alters body image can alter the patient's feelings about his or her sexuality.

The male patient who undergoes a bilateral *orchidectomy* (removal of both testicles) suffers almost total loss of libido due to cessation of androgens. He may or may not receive hormonal supplements, depending on the characteristics of his illness. The female who undergoes "surgical menopause" (removal of the uterus, fallopian tubes, and ovaries) may experience a decline but not a

total loss of libido, depending on her particular hormonal system. Again, hormonal supplements may or may not be administered. Whenever libido is lost partly or completely, sexual counseling is in order to minimize feelings of failure, guilt, or inadequacy. You can be very helpful in encouraging the patient and the patient's sexual partner to undertake sexual counseling.

Other sexually related conditions requiring surgery, though they have no direct physiological effect on libido or performance, have vivid psychological implications that can bring about sexual problems even in medically sophisticated patients.

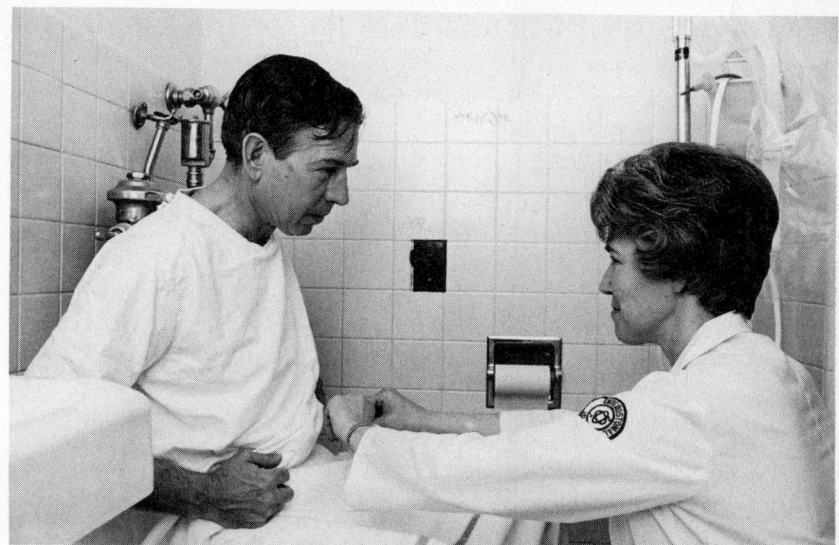

**Figure 17.4**
The manner in which the care provider responds to the colostomy affects the patient's self-concept. (Courtesy American Cancer Society)

The impact of such psychological factors must never be minimized. For example, a man who chooses to have a *vasectomy*—an interruption of the tubes that deliver sperm—for purposes of contraception may encounter unexpected problems with sexual performance following the procedure. In fact, this consequence is so common that physicians now recommend counseling before the procedure is performed.

Women sometimes experience decreased libido after a *hysterectomy*, or removal of the uterus, which does not physiologically affect sexual interest. Particularly in a society that equates ample breasts with womanliness, the woman who must undergo a *mastectomy*, or removal of a breast, experiences sexual trauma. She may feel that she is no longer the woman she once was, and is therefore diminished sexually. The emotional support of her sexual partner is essential. The nurse can often talk honestly and openly with both partners, together or separately, in order to help reinstate the patient's feelings of femininity.

The patient, male or female, who has had a *colostomy* needs very special attention from the nurse with regard to sexuality. A colostomy, which is performed for many medical conditions, is the surgical interruption of the intestines, a portion of which is brought through the lower abdominal wall to form a new opening for the excretion of feces. The intestinal opening or *stoma* appears moist and of normal pink hue and varies in size from individual to individual. Your responsibility for helping the colostomy patient maintain sexual integrity begins when you perform the first dressing change. If your face reflects acceptance, without a flicker of aversion, a significant step has been taken toward acceptance on the part of the patient. The displacement of the intestine is no minor matter for the patient psychologically, and the patient's emotional status should be treated as a priority in the process of assessment. After discharge from the hospital, unexpected excretions, the wearing of ostomy bags, and possible odor may affect sexual desire on the part of both participants. Ideally, such problems are short-lived. A light dressing and/or attractive underclothing to cover the stoma can minimize feelings of repugnance. Pamphlets on daily living after colostomies, including information on sexual activity, are available from several organizations.

In all cases of amputation, scarring, and incisions that violate the body's integrity, the nurse ought to be aware of possible problems of body image and, consequently, sexuality. Each surgical patient warrants a realistic assessment for potential sexual problems.

# Sexuality and the Disabled

Many people suffer from chronic conditions and diseases of the muscular, skeletal, cardiovascular, and nervous systems that render them medically handicapped. Of necessity, their lives consist of numerous adaptations and adjustments in order to function as normally as possible. Health-care personnel have traditionally focused primarily on helping handicapped patients ambulate, dress and feed themselves, and perform basic hygiene. Only recently have those caring for the handicapped begun to consider their sexual needs. It must be remembered that the patient's sexual needs usually involve another person equally and fully.

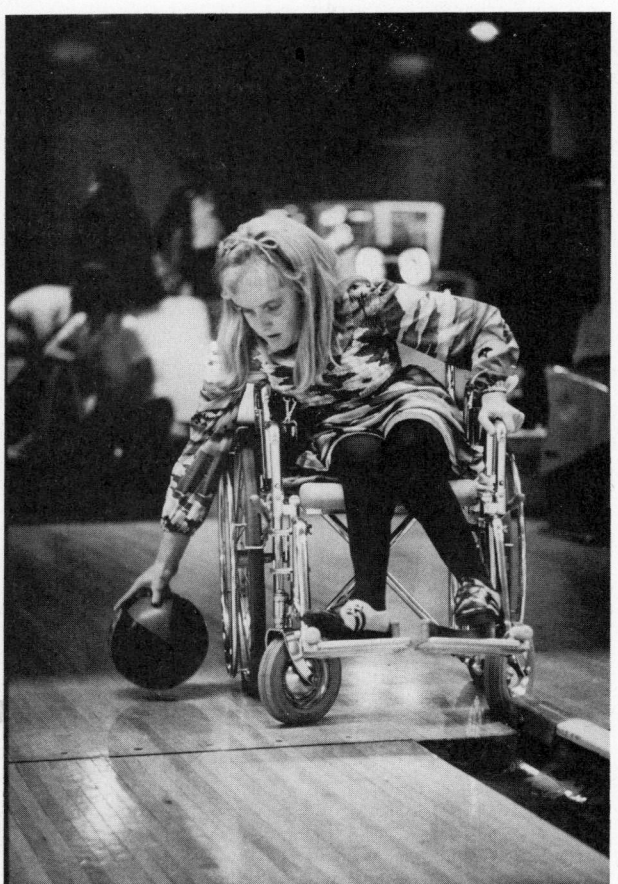

**Figure 17.5 Wheelchair athletes**
Anestis Diakopoulos/Stock, Boston

With therapy and walking devices, the patient may learn to walk again. But this could be only a hollow triumph in the wake of a broken marriage or the loss of a meaningful relationship.

In one study, a group of young men confined to wheelchairs because of spinal-cord injury were asked which they would choose if they had a choice between being able to walk or to function sexually; by far the majority chose sexual function ("Sex and the Paraplegic," 1972).

There are certain preconditions for the development of a friendship that leads to a caring sexual relationship. The disabled face some unique problems establishing such a relationship—problems involving body image, conveying sexuality, finding a partner, and sexual performance.

## Body Image

Body image is one's concept of one's physical self. Achievement of a body image that is both favorable and realistic is one of the central tasks of development, particularly in adolescence. Such a body image in turn contributes to a strong self-concept. For the disabled, as for everyone else, body image is deeply influenced by the reactions of others. Furthermore, a sense of control over one's body is central to one's self-concept (Bogle, 1979). People disabled since birth or early childhood may be less prone to body-image distortion that those disabled in adulthood. To come to terms with disability in a realistic and accepting way frees a person to reach out for friendship that can grow into a sexual relationship.

## Conveying Sexuality

Visible disability can be a barrier to attracting another person into an intimate relationship. Inability to stand may hinder the initial sexual phase. To make eye-to-eye contact with someone in a wheelchair or bed, the nondisabled person must sit. If the upper limbs are affected, embracing is left to the nondisabled partner. The disabled can, however, learn to use expressive body language.

Appliances such as braces convey a feeling of being cold, hard, and angular, characteristics that do not convey sexuality. (More often, sexuality is thought of in terms of warmth, softness, and roundness.) Appliances and body distortion, such as limb atrophy, can be frightening to people unaccustomed to physical disabilities.

## Finding a Partner

It is a delicate process to transform a friendship into an intimate sexual relationship. The process usually begins with subtle probing to find out whether the desire to do so is mutual. There may follow a covert testing period, which can be anxiety-provoking. If the relationship does not become sexual, thus disappointing one of the people involved, he or she may suffer feelings of rejection and unworthiness. In addition to these universal problems, the disabled have the added disadvantage that many nondisabled people consider them incapable of sexual arousal.

## Sexual Performance

A disabled person with a willing, accepting partner can find sexual variations that will prove mutually satisfying. Though each case is entirely individual, recent studies are optimistic about sexual activity for the handicapped. New sexual techniques must often be learned, and adaptations made, but the joy of relating sexually need not end. Such adaptations may be as simple as trying a new position or as delicate as accommodating to the presence of a catheter or stoma. Some disabled people have succeeded in enhancing the *erogenous* potential of parts of the body other than the genitals, even to the point of experiencing orgasmic equivalents in such areas as the abdomen, buttocks, and ears. This experience is called a *paraorgasm* (Bogle and Shaul, 1979).

## Counseling for Sexual Problems

The guidance of a trained counselor in sexuality can often help troubled couples reaffirm their relationship and achieve mutual sexual satisfaction. Some facilities require that the patient's attending physician agree to a referral for sexual counseling. Sex counselors use many techniques. With newly paralyzed or incapacitated patients, the first step after separate interviews with the partners is usually to create a climate in which each can share with the other fears about their sexual status. The male patient might be thinking, "Am I really still a man at all?" "Will my partner leave me if I can no longer satisfy her sexually?" or even "Is it fair to her to remain together?" His partner may be thinking, "Can he ever be the man to me he once was?" or "I feel it's wrong for me to have sexual longings when he cannot participate in sex," or even "There is no way I can leave him now without unbearable guilt," or "I'm locked into a relationship no longer sexually alive." The airing of these guilt-provoking thoughts allows the couple to begin to come to grips with the problem they share. Constructive therapy can then begin. The problem is often less severe if it is the woman who is handicapped, since she may still be capable of participating in sex receptively, though not actively. When it is the man who is handicapped, the wife may be encouraged to assume a more active role and to take the superior position during intercourse. Social stereotypes sometimes make it very difficult for the man to be sexually receptive and the woman active without feelings of humiliation on both parts. Several excellent films are available illustrating sexual intercourse in the female-dominant position. The long-term guidance of a trained counselor can often lead couples to reaffirmation of their relationship and mutual sexual satisfaction.

Until quite recently, little had been written for the health professional on the treatment of sexual dysfunction. The current plenitude of articles on the subject in the health literature is welcome, since sexual dissatisfaction has played a prominent role in the dissolution of many marriages and caused unhappiness for many single people as well. Patients are increasingly likely to discuss sexual problems with nurses or physicians in an effort to seek help.

*Conjoint therapy,* which is now in favor, is the treatment of a couple by a male and a female therapist, one or both of whom is a physician. Often the nonphysician is a nurse with special training. Each sees the patient of the same sex alone, after which the four interact to resolve problems.

You should know how to guide couples or individuals looking for a competent, reputable therapist or counselor. Most large hospitals and university medical centers now have sexual dysfunction clinics, and there are many private clinics that treat sexual dysfunction and other mental health problems. In all probability, smaller communities too will have such resources in the not-too-distant future. A telephone call to the nearest university, large hospital, or medical society will usually elicit the names of one or more practitioners or groups trained in treatment of sexual dysfunction.

It is important to warn patients to avoid or carefully check up on sexual dysfunction clinics that advertise. Regulations establishing guidelines for sex therapy have not yet been implemented, and there are disreputable therapists who use questionable techniques. Sound counseling, however, has enabled large numbers of people to find new satisfaction in their sexual lives.

## Sexual Assault

Sexual assault—the imposition of any sexual behavior on an unwilling person—includes acts ranging in severity from simple exposure to rape. It is important to understand that these acts of sexual assault are more hostile and violent than sexual in motivation. Statistics on the incidence of sexual assault are difficult to gather; the majority of cases are not reported because the victim feels fear, guilt, or humiliation.

As a nurse, you may be consulted by a patient or a friend seeking counseling or support for a victim. Sexual assault violates the dignity and bodily integrity of the victim and can be highly damaging emotionally. Subsequent sexual problems may arise between the victim and the usual sexual partner. The person may develop socially incapacitating fears. For these and other reasons, the victim should be strongly encouraged to seek professional help. A physical examination should be performed to rule out venereal disease and pregnancy, and psychological help is highly desirable to offset emotional trauma. Nurses can provide support and caring for victims of sexual assault.

Most large urban areas have sexual assault clinics or rape relief agencies whose purpose is to aid victims medically, psychologically, socially, and legally. Privacy is respected. You should encourage the victim and/or the family to draw on such community resources, which can do a great deal to minimize the trauma of sexual assault.

## Conclusion

It is time for us as nurses to broaden our vision and acknowledge sexuality as an integral aspect of patients' personalities. Sexual attitudes are changing massively, and nurses must adapt or lose opportunities to respond fully to patients' needs.

Buffeted by the physiological and psychological

strains of illness, patients face a multitude of problems. Dealing sensitively with sexual problems requires a high degree of trust between patient and nurse. Though we must not overtly express our own sexuality in nursing practice, professionalism does not require us to appear so forbiddingly asexual as to be unapproachable by patients with problems. Many patients, no matter how trustful of the nurse, are reticent about divulging their sexual worries and problems openly. It falls to the nurse to assess for problems and provide opportunities for the expression of concerns and the offering of appropriate referrals.

## Care Study  A patient in need of sexual counseling

Ed Jefferson, a twenty-seven-year-old *quadriplegic* (a person with paralysis of all four extremities), is in a rehabilitation unit. He has an attractive wife, who visits regularly, and a young daughter. During the seven weeks since his injury, he has been highly motivated in his sessions with the physiotherapist and has talked about regaining all function. A minimal degree of shoulder movement has returned, but the physician has told Mr. Jefferson that he will probably never regain the use of his legs.

Ms. Stevens, a registered nurse, has been caring for Mr. Jefferson. She perceives a potential problem in the physician's statement and the patient's subsequent depression. Ms. Stevens knows that, although many quadriplegics can maintain a penile erection, Mr. Jefferson's sexual function may be compromised.

Ms. Stevens notices that Mr. Jefferson is becoming increasingly quiet. He develops a headache or nausea just before the physiotherapist's visits and pleads not to have therapy. He no longer initiates conversation, simply answering direct questions and making his immediate needs known. He watches less television than he once did and spends long periods of time awake but with his eyes closed. Just before his wife's daily visit, he complains about all sorts of minor matters. He appears edgy and apprehensive at these times, and his wife also appears unusually quiet and at times uncomfortable. They talk together primarily about their child.

The possibility that the patient's sexual function may be compromised appears to be affecting the psychological status of both husband and wife and the relationship between the two. Ms. Stevens decides that nursing intervention is needed. She recognizes that she cannot provide sexual counseling but knows that a sexual counselor is available in the community.

While bathing Mr. Jefferson one day, Ms. Stevens says, "You know, many people who are paralyzed worry a great deal about whether or not they'll be able to function sexually. It's certainly normal to have this concern, and if you have had some feelings about this, would you like to talk to someone trained in this area who can guide both you and your wife toward some solutions?" In the process of validating her conjecture, she has formulated an appropriate plan to refer the couple to someone equipped to offer counseling.

A look of relief comes over Mr. Jefferson's face as he admits that sexual functioning has been one of his primary concerns. After consulting with the physician, the nurse makes a referral to a therapist trained in sexual counseling.

Ms. Stevens feels satisfaction as she realizes that her goal has been reached: Mr. Jefferson and his wife will receive help. Evaluation of her nursing action is positive.

## Study Terms

androgens
anorexic
antidepressive
antihypertensive
asexual
bisexual
body image
climax
colostomy
conjoint therapy
contraceptive
disabled
dyspareunia
ejaculation
erection
erogenous
fallopian tubes

frigidity
gay
heterosexual
homosexual
hysterectomy
impotence
inhibitory ejaculation
intromission
lesbian
libido
mastectomy
masturbation
menopause
nonorgasmic
orchidectomy
orgasm
ovaries

paraorgasm
premature ejaculation
quadriplegic
semen
sexual assault
sexual behavior
sexuality
sexual variations

sperm
stereotyping
stoma
testicles
uterus
vaginismus
vasectomy

## Learning Activities

1. Visit a sexual dysfunction clinic in your area and/or talk with a sexual dysfunction counselor.
2. Write a paper assessing the sexual development and awareness of three of your patients. (Do not use their real names.)

# References

Blanchard, Mabel G. "Sex Education for Spinal Cord Injury Patients and Their Nurses." *Supervisor Nurse* (February 1976): 20–28.

Bogle, Jane, and Shaul, Susan. *Seminar on Sexuality and Family Planning for the Disabled.* Seattle, Washington. May 25, 1979.

Comarr, A. E., and Gunderson, B. B. "Sexual Function in Traumatic Paraplegia and Quadriplegia." *American Journal of Nursing* 75 (February 1975): 250–255.

Costello, Marilyn K. "Sex, Intimacy and Aging." *American Journal of Nursing* 75 (August 1975): 1330–1332.

Dlin, Barney, and Perlman, Abraham. "Sex After Ileostomy or Colostomy." *Medical Aspects of Human Sexuality* (July 1972): 32–43.

Fine, Herbert L. "Sexual Problems of Chronically Ill Patients." *Medical Aspects of Human Sexuality* (October 1974): 137–138.

Hanlon, K. "Maintaining Sexuality After Spinal Cord Injury." *Nursing '75* 5 (May 1975): 58–62.

*Journal of Drug Research,* 10 (May 1974). Published by the Society for the Study of Sex.

Keaveny, M. E.; Hader, L.; Massoni, M.; and Wade, G. "Hysterectomy: Helping Patients Adjust." *Nursing '73* 3 (February 1973): 8–12.

Kinsey, A. C.; Pomeroy, W. B.; and Martin, C. E. *Sexual Behavior in the Human Male.* Philadelphia: W. B. Saunders, 1948.

———. *Sexual Behavior in the Human Female.* Philadelphia: W. B. Saunders, 1953.

Krizinofski, M. T. "Human Sexuality and Nursing Practice." *Nursing Clinics of North America* 8 (December 1973): 673–681.

Kroah, J. "How to Deal With Patients Who Act Out Sexually." *Nursing '73* 3 (December 1973): 38–39.

Lief, Harold I., and Payne, Tyana. "Sexuality: Knowledge and Attitudes." *American Journal of Nursing* 75 (November 1975): 2026–2029.

Lindl, K., and Rickerson, G. "Spinal Cord Injury: You Can Make a Difference." *Nursing '74* 74 (February 1974): 41–45.

Marlow, Dorothy R. *Textbook of Pediatric Nursing.* Philadelphia: W. B. Saunders, 1977.

Moore, Karen; Folk-Lighty, Marie; and Nolen, Mary Jane. "The Joy of Sex After Heart Attack." *Nursing '77* (June 1977).

Pengelley, E. T. *Sex and Human Life.* Reading, Mass.: Addison-Wesley, 1974.

Pogoncheff, Elaine, and Brossart, Jean. "The Gay Patient." *RN* 42 (April 1979): 46–52.

Puksta, Nancy Sallese. "All About Sex—After a Coronary." *American Journal of Nursing* 77 (April 1977): 602–605.

"Sex and the Paraplegic." *Medical World News* (14 January 1972).

Smith, J., and Bullough, B. "Sexuality and the Severely Disabled Person." *American Journal of Nursing* 75 (December 1975): 2194–2197.

Spark, Richard, *et al.* "Impotence Is Not Always Psychogenic." *Journal of the American Medical Association* (22–29 February 1980): 750–755.

Stanford, Dennyse. "All About Sex—After Middle Life." *American Journal of Nursing* 77 (April 1977): 608–611.

U.S. Department of Health, Education and Welfare, National Center for Health Statistics. "Advance Report: Final Natality Statistics, 1976." *Monthly Vital Statistics Report* 26 (29 March 1978). Supplement.

Watts, Rosalyn Jones. "Dimensions of Sexual Health." *American Journal of Nursing* 79 (September 1979): 1568–1572.

Wilson, R. "Counseling Patients About Sex Problems." *Nursing '73* 73 (November 1973): 44–46.

Woods, Nancy Fugate. *Human Sexuality in Health and Illness.* St. Louis: C. V. Mosby, 1975.

# Part Six

## Physiological Needs of the Person

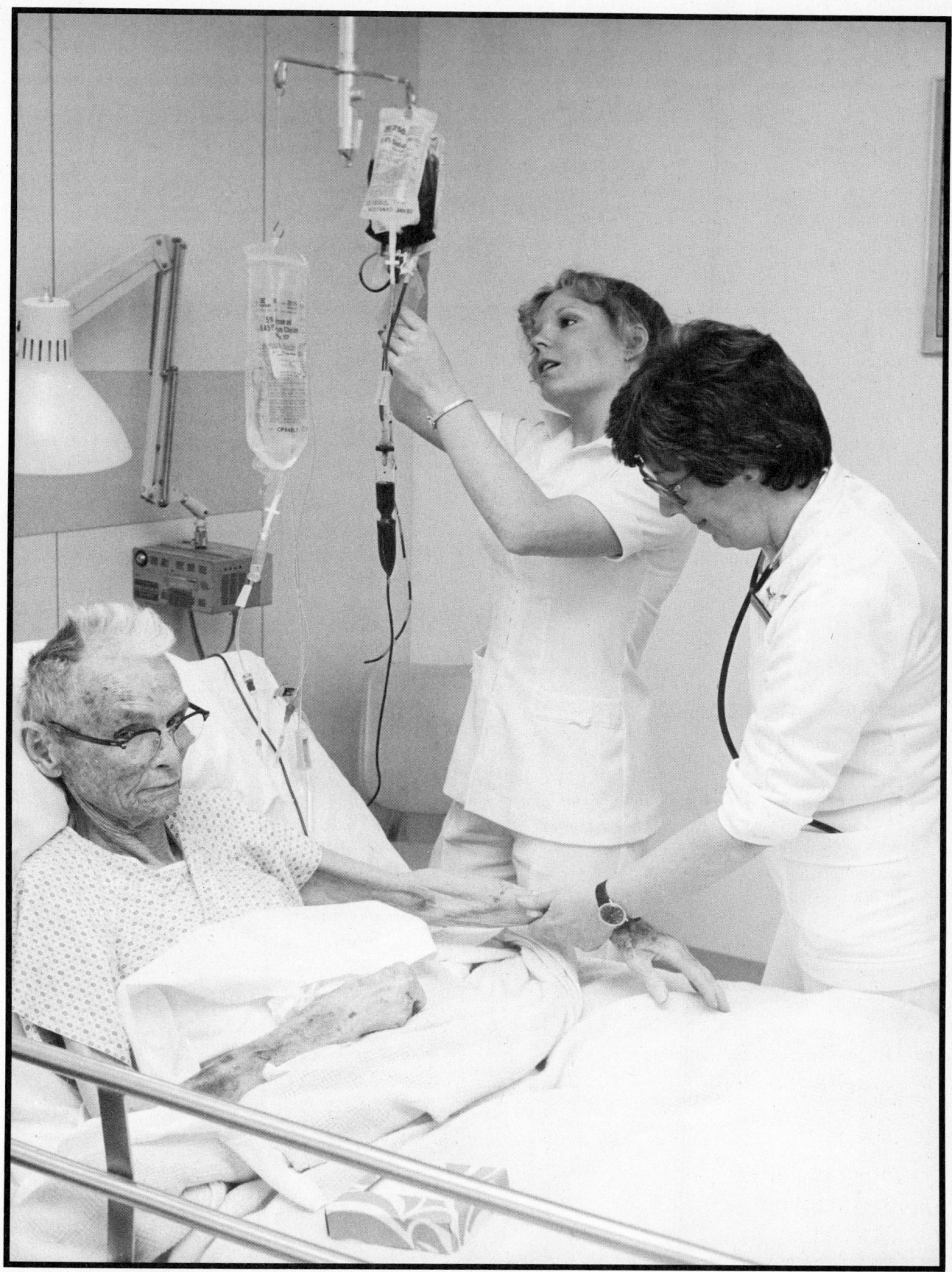

# Chapter 18

# Hygiene

## Objectives

After completing this chapter, you should be able to:
1. Describe the appearance of a nurse who practices good hygiene and looks well groomed.
2. Specify when during the hospital day hygiene may be administered to the patient.
3. List factors important in assessing the patient's hygienic needs.
4. Compare normal and abnormal skin findings.
5. Describe five methods of bathing a patient.
6. Briefly discuss procedures other than bathing that contribute to total hygienic care.
7. Describe variations in care appropriate for black and other dark-skinned patients, including skin assessment and hair care.

## Outline

Hygiene may be defined as those practices that bring about personal cleanliness, comfort, and feelings of well-being. Because such practices vary greatly from one setting to another, it is important to be cognizant of prevailing hygiene habits and general life style. In the hospital setting, being clean, tasteful, and neat conveys to the patient that you know the importance of good personal hygiene. In urban and rural outpatient settings, where standards of hygiene and general appearance differ from those of hospitals, nurses' wearing apparel and hair styles may conform to those of the facility's clients. If you administer skillful and knowledgeable hygiene, the patient's confidence in your ability to perform other tasks will be enhanced. Helping patients maintain hygiene tells them that you care about their comfort.

## Culture and Hygiene

One has only to walk through European palaces and castles to realize that cold and dampness kept their early occupants from bathing frequently. Burning herbs and fragrances was a common practice, both to ward off disease and to disguise unpleasant odors resulting from poor hygiene. As late as the beginning of this century, bathing was infrequent; in fact, many people believed that frequent bathing was injurious to health.

People have become much more hygiene-conscious over the last few years. The development and sale of hygiene products is an enormous national business. Central heating and ample supplies of hot water have made daily bathing more feasible than in the past, and the traditional Saturday-night bath is no longer a way of life. Showers have come to supplement or replace bathtubs in many homes. Deodorants, shampoos, oils, powders, lotions, and a wide variety of soaps, some antibacterial in nature, enhance individual hygienic practices.

Among the many patients who do not regard a daily bath as healthful or necessary may be the economically disadvantaged persons whose dwelling does not provide proper bathing facilities or privacy and the older person who chills easily and perspires very little. Dry skin is a chronic problem for many people, young and old, partly because of the warmth and dryness typical of American homes. Unless oils are used, daily bathing can aggravate dry skin. Finally, people who were not taught as children to bathe daily do not make it a practice as adults.

## The Nature of Hygiene

The administration of hygiene has three main goals, the first of which is maintenance of healthy skin. Massaging and cleansing increases cellular nutrition and circulation, thus keeping the skin intact as a defense against infection. Second, hygiene provides for the removal of transient microorganisms from the body, decreasing the chances of infection. Third, hygiene contributes to the patient's comfort. Feeling refreshed and clean contributes to subjective well-being and thus to self-esteem. Encouraging women to continue using makeup and prompting men to shave or trim their beards regularly also enhance self-worth.

In addition to bathing, oral care, and hair care, hygiene includes maintenance of a clean, neat unit and proper handling of linens. Each component of hygiene will be discussed in detail in the remainder of this chapter. For specific information about equipment and steps in each procedure, see Module 6, "Bedmaking"; Module 7, "Assisting

With Elimination and Perineal Care"; and Module 8, "Hygiene." In order to use your time as efficiently as possible while providing hygiene to the patients in your care, it is important to make a careful assessment of their needs.

## The Nurse's Personal Hygiene and Appearance

Many of the functions nurses perform are physical in nature, and thus stimulate more perspiration than do sedentary tasks. And synthetic uniforms, which do not "breathe" as do cotton fabrics, allow perspiration to remain on the skin and deteriorate, which can sometimes cause unpleasant odors. Personal cleanliness is essential for nurses, regardless of their work setting. Many nurses bathe immediately after arriving home from work, to remove any pathogens that might have been transmitted to them. This is a prudent practice.

### Uniforms

It is advisable to wear a uniform only once before laundering it and to remove it immediately on arriving home. This practice prevents pathogens from being spread to the home environment. Concern for the welfare of others also suggests that a uniform worn in the hospital should not be worn in other settings, such as stores and offices. Your uniform should also be clean when you enter the clinical area so as not to bring microorganisms to the susceptible patient. Some hospitals provide locker facilities where nurses may change clothes. Pediatric units have pioneered in the use of large apronlike smocks, which are worn over the uniform and can be changed during the day as needed. They are usually provided and laundered by the hospital.

### Oral Care

The nurse should practice good oral care. Brushing the teeth regularly makes the mouth clean and odor-free. *Caries* (cavities) can be prevented; if they do occur, they ought to be repaired promptly: carious teeth create a persistent mouth odor that is not relieved by brushing or mouthwash. Smokers should brush even more frequently than non-smokers. The use of chewing gum to mask mouth odor is discouraged, since it is distracting to patients and other workers; breath mints and mouthwashes are preferable.

### Hair

Hair should be worn short or secured close to the head to prevent it from falling forward and ob-

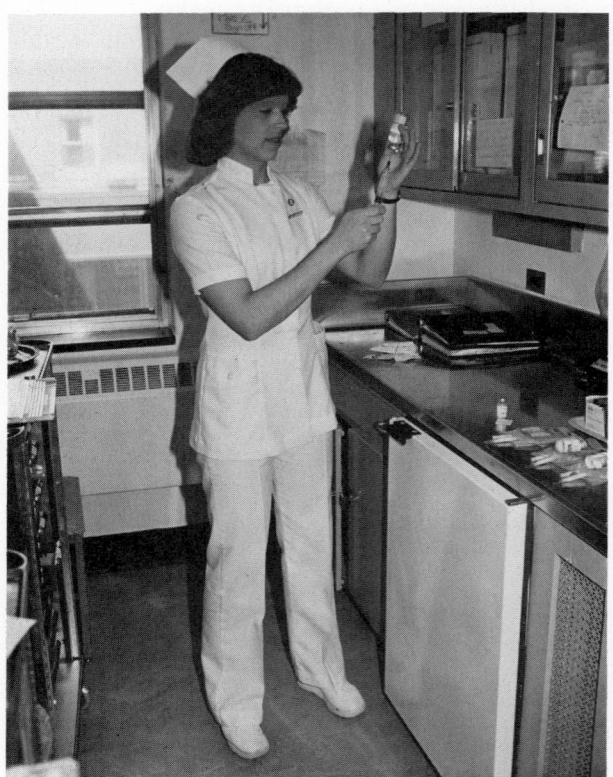

**Figure 18.1   The well-groomed nurse in the hospital**
Russ Kinne/Danbury Hospital/Photo Researchers, Inc.

scuring your vision. In addition to convenience and neatness, such styling makes it unnecessary to use your hands to rearrange your hair; this practice is unhygienic since it transmits microorganisms from hands to hair and vice-versa and can scatter organisms about the immediate surroundings. Long, loose hair can also hang over patients' food trays and over open wounds whose dressings are being changed, creating a general hazard of transmittal of microorganisms. Beards should be short and well-groomed for the same reasons. Regular shampooing gives all hair a shiny, healthy look.

## Fingernails

Fingernails that are well-trimmed and filed are easy to keep clean and unlikely to scratch a patient. Because nail polish can chip and fall into a patient's bed or, worse, into a sterile field, its use is generally discouraged. If worn, it must be in good repair and of an undistracting pale shade.

## Jewelry

The nurse should wear little personal jewelry in the hospital setting. Acceptable items are a wedding band, watch, and posts or studs in pierced ears. Jewelry not only looks unprofessional, but it can be damaged or lost in the practice of nursing. More serious is the danger of scratching a patient's skin or catching rings or bracelets in a patient's hair. Loop earrings that accidentally catch in hanging equipment or are grasped by an agitated patient could lacerate the nurse's earlobes. Thus jewelry should be reserved for a social setting.

## Name Pins

Proper identification of health-care personnel is crucial, since there are so many different providers. A name pin that designates the wearer's role is an official part of the nurse's uniform and should always be worn. Patients greatly appreciate knowing the name and function of those caring for them, and the name pin serves as a reinforcement to the oral introduction.

## Caps

The wearing of nursing caps by female nurses has become controversial. While some facilities' dress codes dictate the wearing of caps by all female nursing personnel as a matter of policy, caps are worn infrequently or not at all in other facilities. Female nurses may question the need for a cap inasmuch as their male counterparts are never required to wear them. If worn, a cap should always be clean and neat.

## Dress Code for Nonhospital Settings

The uniform traditionally worn by hospital-based nurses is not appropriate in many schools, community health clinics, and other agencies that employ nurses. Nurses in such facilities often wear street clothes, sometimes covered by a lab coat for asepsis and appearance. If you wear street clothes, they should be appropriately tailored and your name pin should be clearly displayed. Regardless of the setting, personal hygiene and appearance are important for nurses in their professional roles.

# Skin, Mucous Membrane, Nails, and Hair

Most nursing-care hygiene procedures involve the *integument*, or skin, mucous membrane, nails, and hair. The cleanliness of these parts of the body is essential to prevent the colonization or growth of microorganisms. Before considering specific procedures, let us look at the composition of healthy skin, mucous membranes, nails, and hair.

The skin is composed of two main layers, a thin

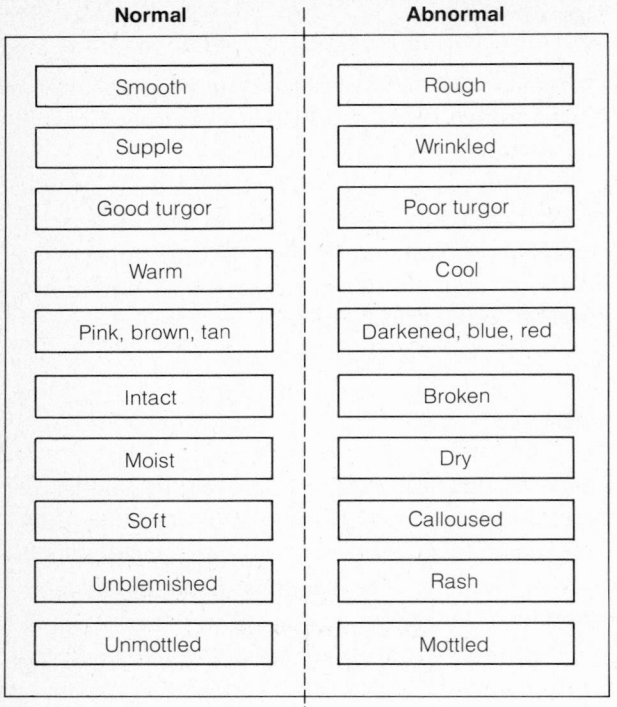

| Normal | Abnormal |
|---|---|
| Smooth | Rough |
| Supple | Wrinkled |
| Good turgor | Poor turgor |
| Warm | Cool |
| Pink, brown, tan | Darkened, blue, red |
| Intact | Broken |
| Moist | Dry |
| Soft | Calloused |
| Unblemished | Rash |
| Unmottled | Mottled |

**Figure 18.2  Characteristics of normal and abnormal skin**

outer layer called the *epidermis* and a thicker inner layer called the *dermis*. The skin has three functions. It serves as a protection for underlying tissue and a barrier to pathogens. By excreting moisture and salts, the skin helps maintain water and electrolyte balance. Lastly, the skin is a system for sensation. That is, the brain receives information about environmental changes through the receptors in the skin and can thus respond appropriately to maintain homeostasis. Healthy skin is warm, moist, supple, and of a color consistent with the person's ethnic heritage (see Figure 18.2).

The passageways that open to the surface of the body, such as the mouth and digestive tract, the nose and respiratory tract, and the genitourinary tract, are lined with *mucous membrane*, which consists of a thin layer of *epithelial cells* supported by underlying connective tissue. Mucous membrane protects these passages from the invasion of microorganisms, secretes the substance *mucus,* which is a lubricant, and is able to absorb water and various salts. Healthy mucous membrane is pink in color, moist, and intact.

The nails are made up of epidermal cells containing a hard protein substance called *keratin*. We can only suppose that the nails served to protect the fingers when our early ancestors used their hands for agricultural labor. Healthy nails are hard but not brittle, smooth, and oval in contour. The color of the nail beds should be pink above a white crescent (the lunula). The color of the nailbeds is a good indicator of the status of oxygenation, pallor indicating a deficit.

Except for the soles of the feet and the palms of the hands, the entire human body is covered with hair. Like the nails, the hair is composed of keratin, in shafts extending upward from the roots, which are embedded in the dermis of the skin. The shaft and root, containing an outer layer of connective tissue and an inner layer of epithelial cells, make up what we call a *hair follicle. Sebaceous glands* at the base of each hair follicle secrete oil that lubricates the follicle. Hair in the nose and around the ears and eyes serves the protective purpose of keeping out dust and foreign bodies. Body hair, including that on the head, may have been more abundant in early man and provided warmth to the body. Healthy hair is strong, not brittle, and appears shiny and lustrous.

## Hospital Routines for Hygiene

In most hospitals it has long been the policy to bathe each patient completely every day. In nursing homes, where staff-patient ratios are lower, patients are necessarily bathed less frequently. Some hospitals are beginning to modify the rigid policy of daily bathing.

*Complete morning care* usually consists of a bath or shower, special perineal care, a backrub, and care of the mouth, hair, and nails. All bed linens are changed. The unit is tidied, and unused items are discarded or put aside with the patient's permission.

*Partial care* involves washing of particularly soiled areas of the body, usually the face, neck, hands, *axillae* (armpits), and perineum. Oral care and hair care are also provided, and a backrub may be included. The unit is made neat, and soiled linens are changed. It is a thoughtful practice to change the pillowcase so as to give the patient a sense of freshness.

Both complete care and partial care are sometimes referred to as "a.m. care." The practice of bathing patients in the morning disregards the wishes of the individual who prefers to bathe in the evening or just before bedtime, and a few facilities are beginning to offer baths at times other than the morning. This practice helps relieve the strain on staff time during the busy morning hours and accommodates the patient who sleeps well after an evening bath.

*Early a.m. care,* often provided by the night staff before the nurses' report in the morning, is preparation for the morning meal. Toilet facilities are offered and the face and hands are washed. The stand is straightened and cleared to make room for the food tray. Oral hygiene may accompany the cleaning of teeth or dentures. It is also appropriate to clean eyeglasses before giving them to the patient.

*H.s. care* (evening or bedtime care) is given in the evening just before sleep. If you think of the things you like done before sleep, you will recognize their importance to the patient. A clean gown or pajamas are often appropriate. The face, hands, and back are washed and a relaxing backrub is given. Glasses and dentures are carefully put away for the night and soiled dressings or linens are replaced. Oral care is given.

There are also other times when hygiene is appropriate. After using a bedpan, urinal, or toilet, the patient should be given an opportunity to wash his or her hands in order to remove microorganisms. If the nurse has assisted, the nurse's hands should also be washed. Handwashing before eating should also be encouraged.

# Assessment

## Assessing the Patient's Hygienic Needs

An admissions bath is usually given to a patient new to the facility. To assess the patient for this initial procedure, you will need to know several things. What is the patient's diagnosis? If the patient is in pain, has difficulty breathing, or appears fatigued, you should not further tire him or her with extensive hygiene. If the patient has come directly from home and is clean, comfortable, and rested, you may choose to delay or omit the bath. If, on the other hand, the patient was admitted in a soiled condition—such as a person involved in a pedestrian accident who has dust or dirt on the skin—immediate special hygiene may be indicated.

What does the patient see as his or her hygiene needs, and how can these needs be incorporated into hospital routine most easily and comfortably for the patient? Does the patient prefer a shower or is a bed bath more appropriate due to fatigue? Would the patient like a shampoo? If possible, let the patient help you plan care for hygiene. Patients have far too few decisions to make in the hospital and should be given some control over their care whenever possible.

With regard to an established inpatient, evaluate the hygiene the patient has been receiving. Read the record to determine whether there have been problems and identify them clearly. How might you modify care? For example, if the patient has been given tub baths but since yesterday has developed a fever from a bladder infection and has an indwelling catheter, a bed bath with cool but comfortable water is appropriate. Another patient who has been showering may have reported fatigue after the shower yesterday and slept through most of the lunch hour. You may decide to give a partial bath instead to allow the patient to rest. (A partial bath involves cleansing the face, axillae, hands, back, and perineal area.)

The tasks of hygiene provide the nurse an opportunity to assess the patient. Physical assessment can focus on the patient's general appearance or on such specifics as relative strength and the presence or absence of stiff joints. Muscles may be observed for turgor and skin for color, dryness, and the presence of lesions. The condition of the hair, nails, teeth, and gums may also become apparent in the course of care. The time spent with the patient can also be an occasion for psychological assessment and interaction, allowing you tactfully to explore the patient's feelings and concerns. States of confusion, depression, contentment, and elation can all become obvious to the nurse who is sensitive to others' feelings.

## Assessing the Hygienic Needs of More Than One Patient

You should realistically and carefully assess the hygienic needs of each of the patients assigned to you on any given day. If, for example, you are to administer a.m. care, you should determine which patients need a complete bath and which might appropriately be given a partial bath (assuming, of course, that your facility allows you to make such decisions and does not require daily morning baths for all patients). In fact, if you are to administer morning care to as many as five or six patients, it would be difficult to give each a complete bed bath. Often patients can perform part of their own care. Allowing patients to participate in their own care helps promote and maintain a sense of independence and can be beneficial psychologically. Some patients who are free of drainage and body odor do not need a complete bath daily. Others may need to bathe more than once a day. In addition to the patient's needs, the nurse's time must also be considered. The two factors must be weighed together in order to use your time as advantageously as possible for the patients under your care.

In practice, you may choose to strip the bed of top linen, replacing it with the bath blanket, and bring the bath water and other items needed for one patient to perform self-care while you administer a bed bath to another. Communicating this procedure clearly to the patients involved allows such scheduling to run smoothly.

## Bathing

Bathing affords generalized physiological benefits to the patient. The activity and movement it elicits stimulate the respiratory system and improve circulation. The movement of muscles and joints maintains and promotes mobility. Since the muscles are relaxed by exposure to warm water, it is appropriate for the patient to perform range-of-motion exercises in the bathtub. Cellular nutrition and circulation are enhanced by the application of friction to the skin, and some microorganisms and dead epithelial cells are thereby removed from the skin.

Bathing is an excellent occasion to assess the skin of the patient. Observe whether the skin is dry or moist, warm or cool. Are some areas of the skin different in appearance from others? Particular attention must be given to beginning skin breakdown. If reddened areas do not blanch upon massage, there may be poor circulation in the area that could lead to a pressure sore and interruption of skin integument. This happens more often over bony prominences. Very dry skin may lead to cracking and *decubitus ulcers*, or bedsores (see Chapter 19).

Assessing skin color in a patient with dark skin is easier if you know the patient and are familiar with his or her normal skin tone. Flushing is manifested as a red tinge on dark skin. Pallor gives the skin an ashen look. As with white-skinned patients, you may look for pallor of the nail beds, mucous membranes, and conjunctiva of the eyes. *Cyanosis*—a bluish discoloration of the skin due to inadequate oxygen in the blood—may be more difficult to identify (Roach, 1977) but can often be detected by examining the soles of the feet and the palms of the hands for a blue color.

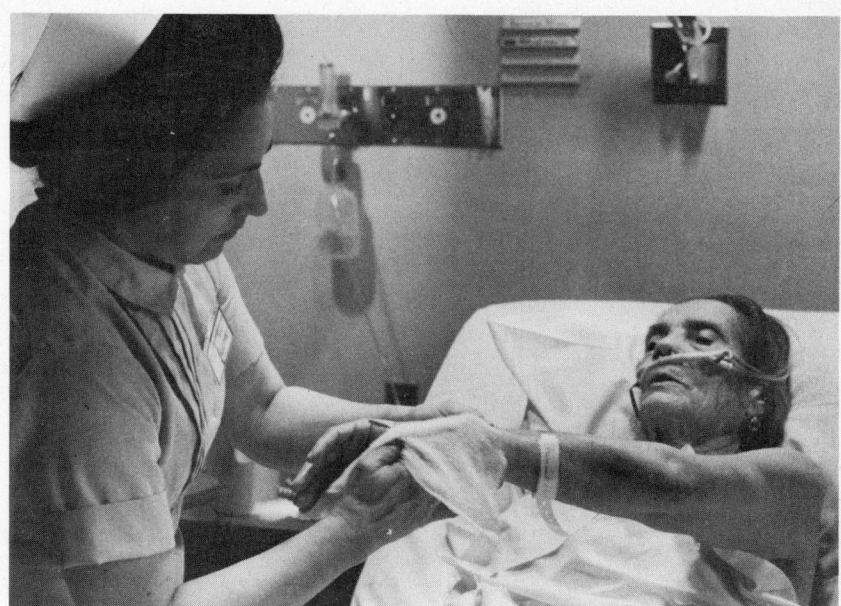

**Figure 18.3 Giving a bed bath to a hospitalized patient**
Elizabeth Wilcox

*Jaundice* is the presence of bile salts in the skin, which gives the patient a yellowish appearance. Jaundice may be detected at an early stage by examining the sclera, or white portion of the eyeball, for a yellowish cast. A patient with jaundice may also have clay-colored stools and/or dark urine.

Whatever type of bath is chosen for the patient, safety is a prime consideration. Water temperature always poses a hazard and must be carefully checked. Tubs are filled and showers run *before* the patient enters, and water for the bed bath is checked before being applied to the patient. A bath thermometer is sometimes difficult to find, but if you are unsure of the temperature, an ordinary thermometer can be used. With practice, most nurses become quite adept at recognizing safe temperatures by testing the water on their wrists; until you become skilled at doing so, always test the water with a thermometer. It is advisable to ask patients whether or not they use soap on their faces: soap can be irritating, and dangerous to the eyes, if not used with care. Many soaps are drying, and oil might be added to the bath water for patients with obviously dry skin. The patient who showers could apply a small amount of oil after the shower. Safety is a major factor in a patient's bath or shower. Most facilities have installed handrails in the tub or shower area, and the patient should be encouraged to use them.

## Types of Baths

Methods of bathing patients consist of the bed bath, the tub bath, the Century tub, the standing shower, and the chair shower. Module 8, "Hygiene," and Module 9, "Basic Infant Care," provide specific directions for bathing. The types of baths are discussed here.

## The Bed Bath

A bed bath is performed by a nurse, who bathes the patient in bed using basins of warm water. Special draping prevents the patient from being chilled or unduly exposed. Washing is accomplished in long, smooth strokes, moving from the cleaner parts of the body to the more soiled parts. A variation of the bed bath is the *towel bath*, performed with very large towels or flannel bath blankets. The folded towels are placed in a large plastic bag containing hot water and a small amount of a special antiseptic solution that need not be rinsed from the skin. Wringing out the towels and placing them on the patient, the nurse lightly massages the patient from the feet upward, advancing the clean top sheet as the bath progresses. The back is then washed in the same fashion. Because the massage is beneficial to patients incapable of

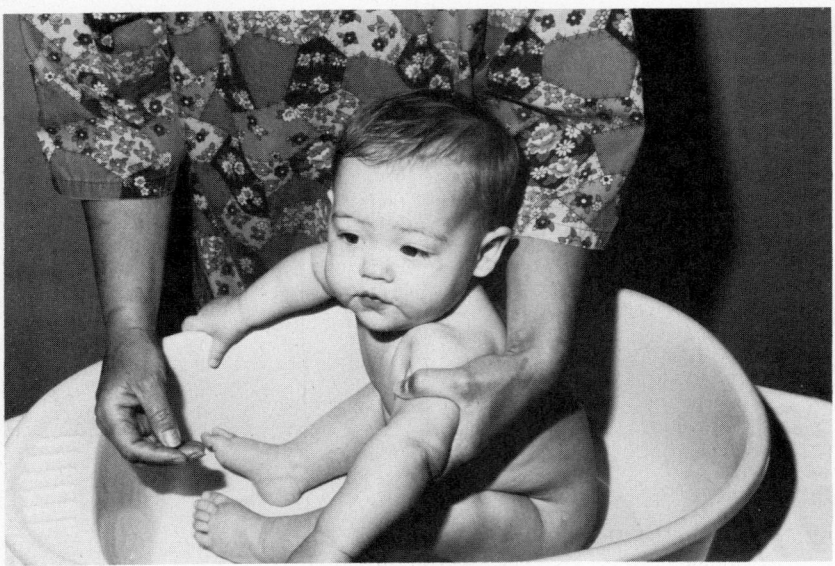

**Figure 18.4 Bathing an infant in a basin**
Courtesy Ivan Ellis

much exercise, this type of bath might be alternated with a complete bed bath. Its advantages are that the patient is not likely to be chilled if the bath is properly performed and that the skin is rendered moist and soft.

## The Tub Bath

A tub bath is virtually the same as a bath the patient would take at home. The water temperature should be carefully monitored: very cool water may chill the patient since most body surfaces are in contact with the water, and water that is very warm or hot can be dangerous to the circulatory system, particularly in the elderly. A bath towel on the bottom of the tub prevents slipping. Transferring a patient to the tub from a wheelchair is facilitated by positioning the wheelchair at the back of the tub or facing its side. The patient's legs can easily be lifted over the lip of the tub and a two-person assist used to lift him or her into the water. Module 15, "Transfer," describes and illustrates techniques for transferring a patient.

## The Century Tub

The Century tub (a brand name), frequently used in chronic-care settings, consists of a plastic chair in which the patient sits. Straps are fastened to secure the patient, and the entire chair then locks

to a hydraulic lift, which raises, turns, and lowers it into a high tub that can accommodate the sitting patient. A special oil soap is added to the water, and the patient can be bathed or whirlpool outlets can be activated to stimulate and further clean the body surfaces.

## The Standing Shower

Showers are the most thorough method of cleansing since the water is rinsed from the body, carrying off microorganisms. Before arranging a shower, be sure the patient feels strong enough to undertake it. You may wish to place a chair nearby in case the patient feels sudden fatigue. Use a bathmat to prevent slipping and place the call signal in an accessible spot, explaining its presence and use to the patient.

## The Chair Shower

A chair shower is administered in a cabinet that allows the patient to remain seated in a shower chair. A waist-high partition may enclose the shower area, permitting the nurse to assist while remaining dry. It is questionable, however, whether the nurse can give an effective shower from such a position. A newly available device consists of a horizontal shower cabinet that allows a bedridden patient to be showered on a special stretcher.

# Implementing Other Hygienic Measures

Other than bathing, complete hygiene also includes the use of deodorants, bath powders, and soaps; perineal care; the backrub; shaving; oral, eye, nail, and hair care; and care of the patient's bed.

## Using Deodorants, Bath Powders, and Soaps

Individuals respond differently to products like deodorants and bath powders. If a person habitually uses a certain product, there is probably no danger of toxicity. But if such a product is new to the patient, it is prudent to use it sparingly until its safety has been established.

The active ingredient in many antibacterial soaps and hygiene products is *hexachlorophene*. In the early 1970s a study revealed that use of this chemical in high concentration caused brain lesions in newborn monkeys. Though such serious effects have not been demonstrated in humans, the U.S. Food and Drug Administration issued a warning that hexachlorophene in concentrations of more than 3 percent should not be used on newborn infants. This policy has since been extended to most over-the-counter hygiene products today, making them safe to use.

Growing preoccupation with meticulous hygiene has created a market for what advertisements call "feminine hygiene sprays." These products are, in fact, perineal deodorant sprays whose value is questionable. They are quite irritating to many women and have been proven to cause severe reactions in some.

## Perineal Care

The perineal area requires meticulous care. It is characterized by a heavy concentration of bacteria, because the excretion of feces and urine and the deep creases of the groin provide moisture and warmth in which bacteria can grow. A thick, cheesy secretion called *smegma*, largely composed of dead epithelial cells in the area of the perineum, can act as a reservoir for bacteria. Good perineal care is thus a matter of careful cleansing. Cleansing ought always to be performed from front to back, or from the urinary orifice to the intestinal orifice, to prevent contamination of the urinary tract with intestinal organisms. It is important to emphasize the necessity of frequent perineal care for the patient who has an indwelling catheter in place. The region around the catheter should be cleaned well before cleansing the remainder of the area.

Patients who are able should be given the opportunity to perform their own perineal care. While providing the patient with clean water, soap, a cloth, and a towel, you might ask, "Would you like to finish your own bath now?" or ". . . wash between your legs," ". . . wash your genitals," or ". . . wash the crotch area." Use words the patient is likely to understand and allow sufficient time and privacy. If the patient is unable to perform this task unaided, undertaking it in a professional, efficient manner will help relieve anxiety and embarrassment on either side. This aspect of care may discomfit the inexperienced student, but practice makes it a more routine matter; patients will become more relaxed as you do. Module 7, "Assisting with Elimination and Perineal Care," provides more detailed directions on giving perineal care.

A *douche* is an irrigation of the vagina. The fluid used may be any of a variety of commercial products, a mild vinegar solution, or tap water. Because douches can destroy the normal *flora*, or residing organisms, in the vagina, leading to infection, douching is regarded as unnecessary for the normal healthy woman.

## The Backrub

The backrub is a cherished nursing art. It is thus disconcerting when a nurse pours a bit of lotion on his or her hand, briskly rubs up and down the patient's back, and considers the patient to have had a backrub. A backrub or massage is given for two purposes: stimulation and relaxation. A rub after a morning bath may be given to stimulate the skin and muscles; before sleep, a soothing backrub

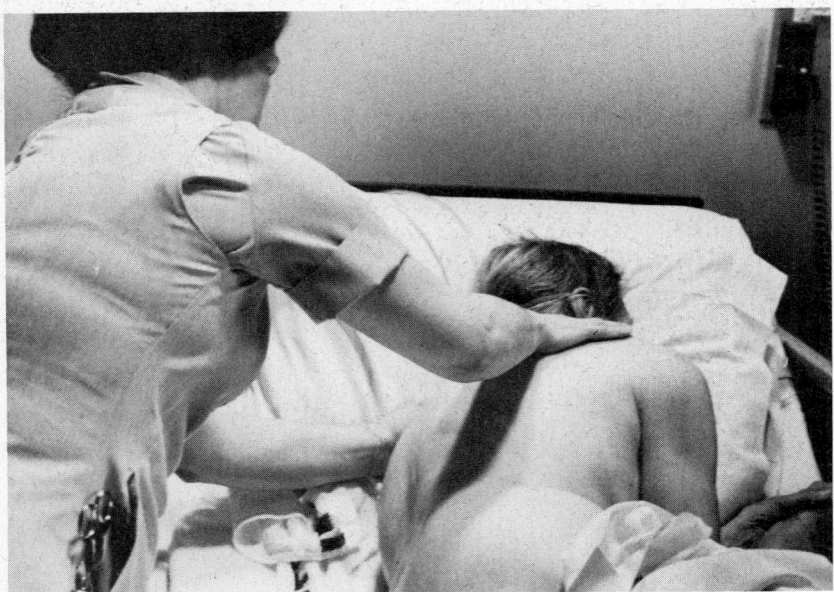

**Figure 18.5 The backrub**
At least one hand should remain in contact with the patient's back at all times, even when you are pouring lotion. (Let the back of your hand rest on the patient's back.) (Elizabeth Wilcox)

encourages rest. If the patient falls asleep during a backrub of the latter type, the nurse should feel a sense of success. Both the extent of the backrub and the type of stroke used, including the amount of pressure, will determine the effect on the patient.

It is good practice to keep the hands in constant contact with the patient's skin, using long smooth strokes. There are various correct methods of massage, all of which focus on the *coccyx* and buttocks and the full length of the spinal column. The nurse's hands radiate upward and over the shoulders, giving extra treatment to the muscles of the neck, which typically become quite taut when the patient spends a lengthy time in bed. Lotions are the most popular lubricants to use for massage: they replace the moisture lost in the skin, have a pleasant odor, and allow the hands to move smoothly. Powder also makes for a smooth rub, but it is both drying to the skin and potentially dangerous if inhaled. If powder is used, care must be taken to prevent inhalation by the patient or nurse. If the patient has a fever, alcohol is occasionally used; it evaporates quickly and cools the patient. On cooling, however, it becomes sticky in consistency and makes for jerky strokes unless more alcohol is added. Alcohol also has a drying effect on the skin.

The backrub is a part of the administration of the bath, and should be considered as such. When a backrub is offered, the patient may decline on the basis that "it's too much trouble" for the nurse. The nurse should explain that it is no trouble because the patient's skin, which is in contact with the bed, needs such care. Most patients very much enjoy backrubs and many ask for such attention. Because it brings pleasure to the patient, the nurse may also enjoy it. It is often an opportune occasion to talk quietly with the patient and convey a caring attitude.

## Shaving the Patient

You may prefer to shave the male patient before beginning a bed bath. Alternatively, placing warm, moist hand towels over the patient's face while you are administering a bed bath feels good to the patient and softens the hair follicles for easier shaving. Bed patients should always be shaved before the bottom linen is changed since small hairs that fall into the bed can cause discomfort.

Daily shaving is necessary for many men to appear and feel well-groomed. Some men with beards shave the edges to give it the shape they desire. Furthermore, some patients develop skin irritations if they do not shave; the hairs hold perspiration on the skin, causing a fine rash. Male patients quite often bring their own razors to the hospital, but some hospital units have electric ra-

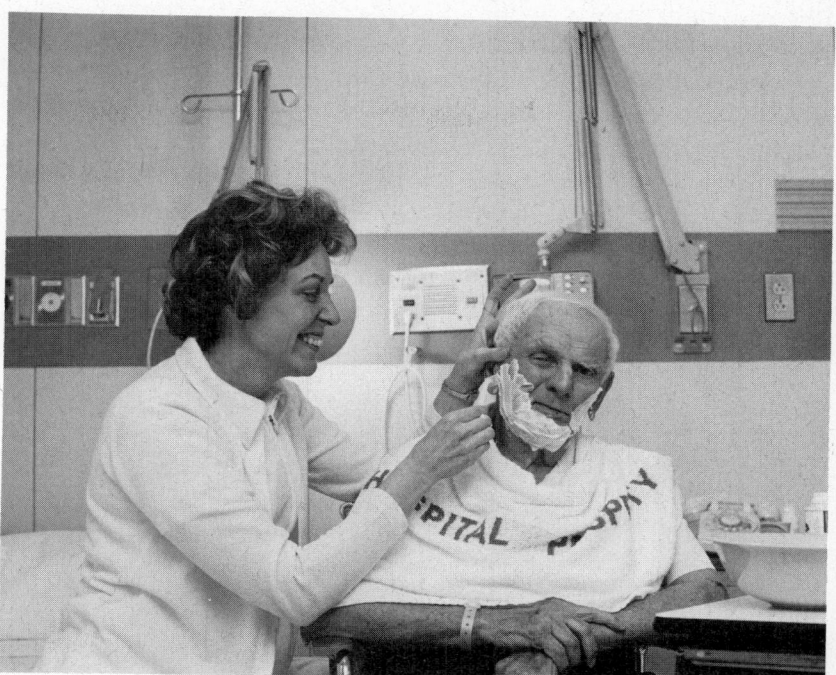

**Figure 18.6  Shaving a patient**
Russ Kinne/Danbury Hospital/Photo Researchers, Inc.

zors available for patients' use. The blades of such communal razors must be soaked in disinfectant solution between patients. Alternatively, disposable safety razors designed for one-time use are very efficient. If you stretch the skin slightly taut, shaving a patient is not a difficult task. The shaving soap the patient customarily uses is the best choice.

## Oral Care

Oral care consists of assessment, treatment, and care of the teeth, mouth, and gums. Illness and contingent problems involving diet and fluids cause the patient's mouth to need almost constant attention. The patient becomes uncomfortable if the mouth becomes dry and unpleasant-tasting due to the accumulation of sordes. *Sordes* are composed of mucus, epithelial cells, and bacteria that adhere to the teeth and inside the mouth. The lips or tongue may develop painful cracks or fissures, and a foul odor may be present.

Patients who are in relatively good health can perform oral care as they would at home. For those who must be given oral care, the nurse should assess what is needed. In general, the teeth are brushed and the inside of the mouth and the lips cleaned and moistened. Dentures can be brushed with a special denture brush or an ordinary toothbrush. Commercial powders and creams are sold for this purpose, but if the patient does not have these items, toothpaste or even plain water can be used. Dentures may be stored overnight in a safe container, immersed in a solution or dry, depending on their composition. *Mouthwashes*, though pleasant and refreshing, do not kill microorganisms. Dental hygienists tell us that the use of *dental floss* is as effective or more so than brushing and removes sordes that cannot be removed with a brush. Another recently developed aid to oral hygiene is the high-pressure water appliance known as an oral irrigator or water spray unit. Though improper use can cause gum damage, its effectiveness has now been proven.

For patients unable to perform their own oral care, a number of techniques are needed. If the patient can hold water in the mouth and spit it back out without choking, the nurse may perform regular oral care with a toothbrush and dental floss. If the patient is unconscious, oral care becomes both more difficult and more necessary, since sordes accumulate rapidly when a person mouth-breathes and cannot swallow saliva. Because conventional flushing techniques may cause the patient to aspirate fluid, the teeth are cleaned

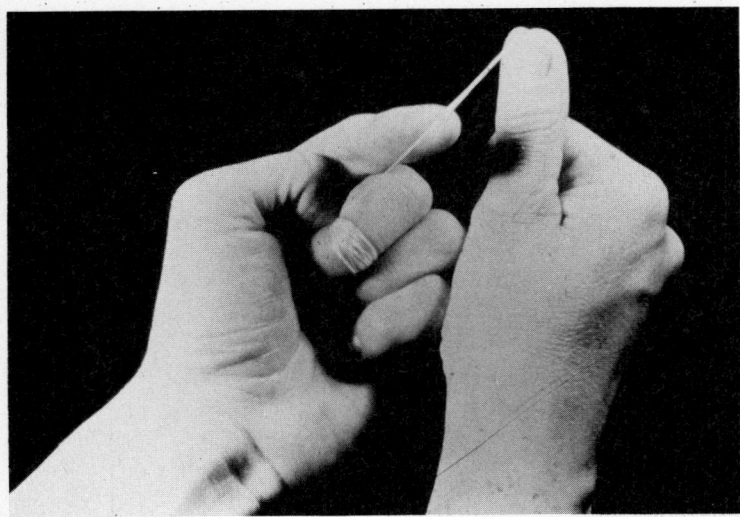

**Figure 18.7 Flossing the teeth**
Courtesy Ivan Ellis

with cotton swabs dipped in a solution. You may wish to make up an oral hygiene tray containing various solutions, all clearly labeled, and cotton swabs. Whether you use commercially made swabs or make your own, care must be taken that the gauze or cotton is secure and cannot be inhaled or ingested. Nurses have different preferences on solutions to use for oral care. A diluted solution of hydrogen peroxide, with a small amount of mouthwash added for esthetic purposes, has good cleaning properties. Buttermilk was popular until it was proven to promote the formation of caries. A mixture of glycerine and lemon is still widely used, but lemon can damage tooth enamel if used for a long time. Glycerine, rather than moistening the mouth, can absorb moisture from mouth tissues, contributing to damage of the mucous membranes.

If the patient's lips are dry, a light coating of a *water-soluble* jelly, A&D ointment (containing the vitamins A and D, which promote healing of irritations), or petroleum jelly may be applied. These should always be applied sparingly since inhalation of non–water-soluble products can obstruct lung tissue and cause pneumonia. Patients who are receiving oxygen or have a tube inserted through the nose need more frequent oral care. Oxygen is very drying, and patients with oxygen hunger tend to mouth-breathe, which dries the tissues of the mouth, increases the accumulation of sordes, and causes cracking of the mucous membranes.

## Eye Care

Most patients' eyes do not need special care since the tears produced by the lacrimal glands constantly wash over the surfaces of the eyes, freeing them of dust or other contaminants. There are times, however, when eye care is needed. If there is a discharge, the eye can be irrigated with sterile water or normal saline. This procedure is described in Module 38, "Irrigations." Crust on the lashes or lids composed of dried discharge material can be removed with moistened gauze.

The eyes of an unconscious patient should be frequently inspected and irrigated during hygiene if necessary. The physician may order that a solution of *artificial tears*—a neutral, sterile lubricating agent—be instilled if natural tearing is deficient. If one or both eyes of an unconscious patient remain open and unblinking, they are taped closed with gauze and paper tape in order to prevent drying of the surfaces and injury. The tape must be removed frequently and the eyes inspected for irritation or infection.

Occasionally a patient will have a prosthetic (artificial) eye. If the patient is unable to care for the prosthesis, the nurse can open the eye and place a clean finger under the lower edge to break the suction and remove the glass or plastic eyeball. The eye can then be washed in normal saline and replaced by opening the lid and placing the prosthesis firmly under the upper lid. It will fall into place and reseal.

Contact lenses are worn by many patients. Lenses may be hard, semisoft, or soft, and the cleansing and storage procedures vary. If you are unsure of the type, consult with the patient or family. A pharmacist would also be able to tell you how to care for a particular type of lens. A sterile, cotton-tipped applicator moistened with normal saline can be used to remove hard or semisoft contacts. With the tip, gently push downward on the lower edge of the lens. This will raise the top edge of the lens so you can remove it. The larger soft lenses are removed by bending them between the fingers and lifting outward. Lenses should be stored according to directions. To replace a lens, wet the surface with a commercial wetting solution. Hold the eyelid open with the fingers of one hand and, with the lens on the tip of a finger of the other hand, place it directly onto the *cornea* (the middle of the convex surface of the eye).

## Nail Care

Complete hygiene also involves attention to the nails. Pointed nail cleaners are often kept on hospital units for the purpose of cleaning under patients' nails where secretions, loose skin, and pathogens can collect. Many institutions allow only a registered nurse or a *podiatrist* (specialist in care of the feet) to trim the nails of diabetic pa-tients, in view of the fact that diabetics are very prone to difficult-to-heal infections. The very slightest nick may have such a consequence. Filing the nails of diabetic patients is thus often safer than cutting. Filing is also preferable in the case of the older patient with extremely hard and thick toenails, which can be almost impossible to cut with scissors or clippers. Soaking the nails before cutting is usually beneficial. It is important to examine the patient closely for rough nails, which can cause abrasions of the skin if the patient should scratch.

## Hair Care

Hair can become a significant problem in the hospital, for both the patient and the staff. Long hair quickly becomes matted from rubbing against bedding. A small amount of alcohol or vinegar applied to the hair, followed by brushing, will usually remove such tangles, but alcohol dries the hair and should be used only occasionally. To avoid problems, it is advisable to arrange the hair in an attractive and convenient manner of the patient's choosing soon after admission. (Braids are a popular way of arranging long hair.) You can usually assess the frequency of the patient's need for shampooing. Most hair need not be washed every day. Dry shampoos may be used with bed pa-

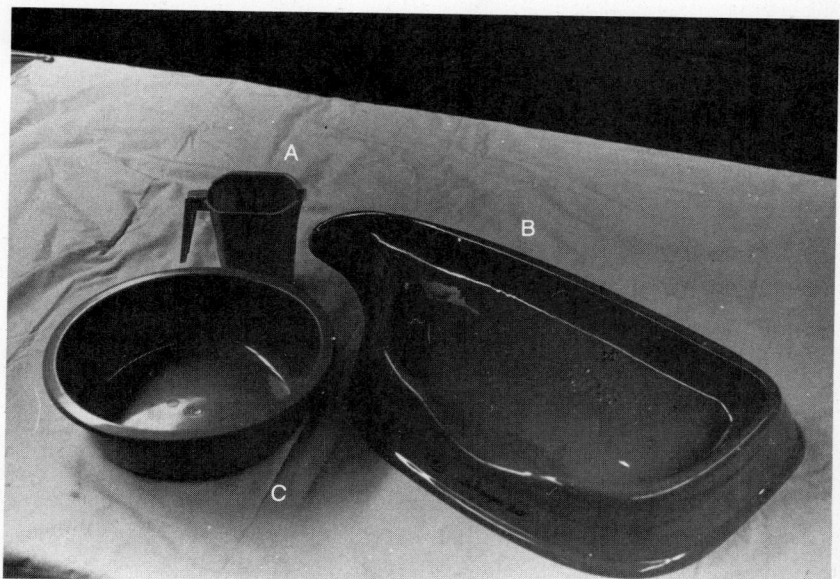

**Figure 18.8  Equipment for shampooing patient's hair in bed**
Water is poured from the pitcher (*A*) over the patient's hair, drains down through the trough (*B*) beneath the patient's head, and falls into the basin (*C*) below. (Courtesy Ivan Ellis)

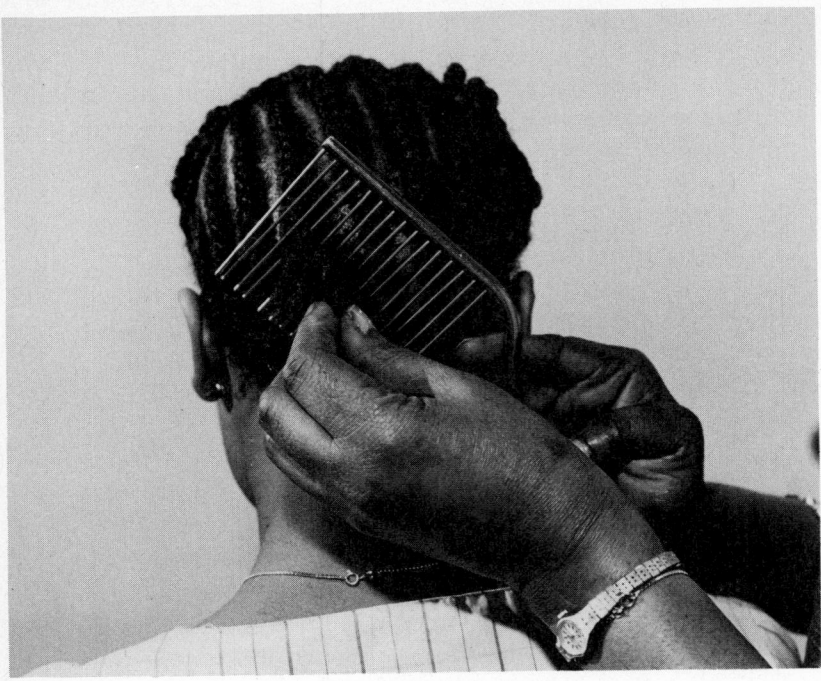

**Figure 18.9  Caring for the hair of a black patient**
Lawrence Cherkas

tients, but they can cause itching of the scalp and discomfort; some patients can be placed on a stretcher and taken to a basin where, with padding under the head, the scalp and hair are washed. Using a device that combines a funnel with a plastic or rubber sheet, you can wash the hair of a patient unable to be moved from bed (see Figure 18.8). The desire for clean hair can become preoccupying for patients, especially women with long hair.

A nonblack nurse may feel uncertain about caring for the hair of a black patient due to unfamiliarity with its texture and style. If the patient's hair is elaborately styled, such as in "cornrows" (intricate tiny head braids) be sure to ask for permission before dismantling the style. The patient and family may object, because such styles are very time-consuming to arrange. If you shampoo very curly black hair, style it before it is completely dry. It becomes very curly when dry. Comb small sections of the hair away from the scalp, taking care not to put undue tension on the hair roots. The smooth hair of Native Americans and Asians is easier to arrange. Consult the patient, if possible, when caring for the hair of a person from an ethnic group other than your own.

## Care of the Patient's Bed

The patient's bed is his or her environment. Because patients spend long periods of time in bed, nurses must pay careful attention to making the bed a place of comfort and safety.

Proper placing of linens, such as draw sheets, incontinent pads, and turn sheets, allows the bed's cleanliness to be easily maintained and saves the nurse and the patient the inconvenience of having to change the entire bed. For the patient who cannot turn without help, a *turn sheet* can be made from a bath blanket folded in quarters or a draw sheet folded in half and placed under the heavier portion of the patient's body. It is much easier for nurses to turn a patient by grasping the sides of this device than by grasping the patient's extremities, and this method is also more comfortable and safer for the patient.

When making a bed, whether the patient is in the bed at the time or not, four goals should be kept in mind. First, the surface under the patient should be smooth and free of wrinkles. The patient with sensitive skin can develop pressure sores, or decubitus ulcers, because of the slightest wrinkle. Even wrinkles in the underbedding—

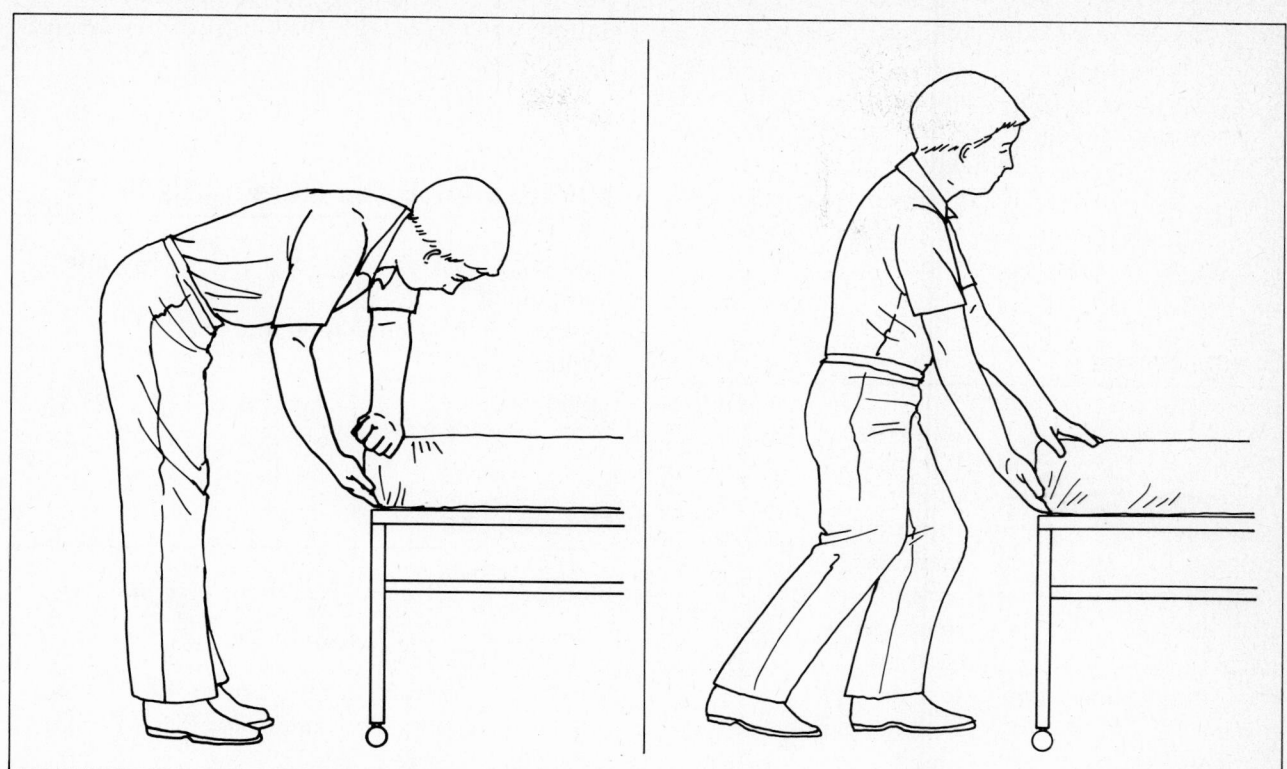

**Figure 18.10  Posture for bedmaking**
*Left:* Back bent over to reach bed (incorrect). *Right:* Back straight, knees bent (correct).

such as the mattress pad, bottom sheet, or plastic sheet—must be smoothed to prevent such occurrences. Second, all surfaces that touch the patient must be meticulously clean. To protect the patient from microorganisms, the linens nearest to the body must be changed as needed. Third, enough bedding should be used to keep the patient warm. The physical work you do may make you feel quite warm, but you should not assume that the patient resting quietly in bed is equally so. A good index is to ask patients how many blankets they want. A single blanket is usually enough, since hospitals are kept quite warm. Finally, the well-made bed must give the patient room for adequate movement. An overly neat bed that constricts movement is not a service to the patient. Loosening the bedding over the feet is especially important so that, when the patient is lying on his or her back, the feet are not in constant extension but remain in anatomical position, the toes pointing upward.

Comfort and safety are more important considerations, but a neat appearance should be strived for in making a bed. It is possible to make a neat bed without ignoring the more important factors.

## Conclusion

In providing hygiene, you are performing tasks the patient would undertake if able. To the patient, conscious or unconscious, this is a valuable service. In learning the skills that comprise good hygiene, you, as a beginning student, will gain needed confidence in your own abilities. The performance of these skills combines theory and practice in many aspects of nursing, such as asepsis, control of infection, maintenance of mobility, and physical and psychological assessment. Hygiene is total patient care and never an isolated task. To leave a formerly soiled, disheveled, and uncomfortable patient in a state of cleanliness, comfort, and repose is a reward in itself.

## Study Terms

| | |
|---|---|
| artificial tears | hexachlorophene |
| axilla | h.s. care |
| backrub | hygiene |
| bed bath | integument |
| caries | jaundice |
| Century tub | keratin |
| chair shower | massage |
| coccyx | mottled |
| complete morning care | mouthwash |
| cornea | mucous membrane |
| cyanosis | mucus |
| decubitus ulcer | oral care |
| dental floss | oral irrigator |
| dentures | partial care |
| deodorant | perineum |
| dermis | podiatrist |
| deterioration | sebaceous glands |
| douche | shower |
| early a.m. care | smegma |
| epidermis | sordes |
| epithelial cells | towel bath |
| eye care | tub bath |
| flora | turn sheet |
| genitals | water-soluble |
| hair follicle | |

## Learning Activities

**1.** When bathing yourself, pay close attention to the pressure and strokes used. Decide what is most comfortable.
**2.** Visit a large drugstore and take note of the hundreds of hygienic products offered for sale.
**3.** Practice giving a backrub to a classmate or family member.
**4.** Plan general hygiene for a patient in the clinical area.

**5.** Identify the factors that guided your plan in Activity 4.

## Relevant Sections in
## Modules for Basic Nursing Skills

| Volume 1 | Module |
|---|---|
| Bedmaking | 6 |
| Assisting With Elimination and Perineal Care | 7 |
| Hygiene | 8 |
| Basic Infant Care | 9 |

## References

Block, P. L. "Dental Health in Hospitalized Patients." *American Journal of Nursing* 76 (July 1976): 1162–1164.

Davis, M. "Getting to the Root of the Problem— Hair Grooming Techniques for Black Patients." *Nursing '77* 7 (April 1977): 60–65.

Derbes, Vincent J. "Rashes: Recognition." *Nursing '73* 3 (March 1973): 44–49.

Dyer, E. D.; Monson, M. A.; and Cope, M. J. "Dental Health in Adults." *American Journal of Nursing* 76 (July 1976): 1156–1159.

"Four Proven Steps for Preventing Decubitus Ulcers." *Nursing '77* 7 (September 1977): 58–61.

Greenleaf, J.; Staley, R.; and Payne, P. A. "Portable Shower for Bed Patients." *American Journal of Nursing* 74 (November 1974): 2021.

Grier, M. E. "Hair Care for the Black Patient." *American Journal of Nursing* 76 (November 1976): 1781.

Gruis, Marcia L., and Innes, Barbara. "Assessment: Essential to Prevent Pressure Sores." *American Journal of Nursing* 76 (November 1976): 1762–1764.

Hogan, R. "Mr. O'Brien's Beard." *American Journal of Nursing* 77 (January 1977): 61.

Johnson, B. "The Meaning of Touch in Nursing." *Nursing Outlook* 13 (1965): 59.

Maurer, J. "Providing Optimal Oral Health." *Nursing Clinics of North America* 12 (December 1977): 671.

Michelsen, D. "How to Give a Good Back Rub." *America Journal of Nursing* 76 (November 1976): 1762–1764.

Price, J. H. "Oral Health Care for the Geriatric Patient." *Journal of Gerontological Nursing* 5 (March/April 1979): 25–29.

Reitz, M., *et al.* "Mouth Care." *American Journal of Nursing* 73 (October 1973): 1728–1730.

Roach, L. B. "Color Changes in Dark Skin." *Nursing '77* 7 (January 1977): 48–51.

Rubin, B. A. "Black Skin: Here's How to Adjust Your Assessment and Care." *RN* (March 1979): 31–35.

Sykes, Julie; Kelly, A. Paul; and Kenney, John A., Jr. "Black Skin Problems." *American Journal of Nursing* 79 (June 1979): 1092–1094.

Zucnick, Martha. "Care of an Artificial Eye." *American Journal of Nursing* 75 (May 1975): 835.

# Chapter 19

# Activity and Rest

## Objectives

After completing this chapter, you should be able to:

1. Define and describe the different types of musculoskeletal activity.
2. Discuss the role of rest in maintaining health.
3. Describe the effects of immobility on the body's systems.
4. Outline the use of the nursing process to meet activity and rest needs.
5. List measures other than activity that can be used to combat the effects of immobility.
6. Define rehabilitation.
7. Discuss concerns of the disabled person.

## Outline

Activity is a basic human need. Research indicates that beginning at birth, activity is essential for optimum development. Without physical activity, a child's muscles, joints, and bones will not develop to maximum size and strength; the circulatory system will fail to develop the extensive network of small vessels that provides for additional circulation to meet stressful situations; and the respiratory system will not develop additional lung capacity. Insufficient physical activity causes muscles to atrophy, joints to become stiff, and internal organs to function less effectively. And the diminished strength of atrophied muscles undermines the systems they support. For example, weakened back muscles make the spine more liable to injury; weak abdominal muscles cause the bowel to function less effectively.

Rest can be thought of as the opposite of activity. It is not the same thing as sleep (see Chapter 20). All body parts need regular rest, just as they need activity. Overused muscles are unable to rid themselves of all waste products and thus become painful and nonfunctioning. For example, using one's eyes to do detail work for long hours may make them ache and temporarily impair one's vision. Thus a balance between activity and rest is necessary for optimum health.

Muscle tone, posture, and body mechanics are the fundamentals of physical activity. Exercise may be either active or passive. We will discuss the various types of exercise and explore the role of activity in physical and mental well-being.

## Muscle Tone

Muscles are composed of bundles of cells able to contract and expand. In their most expanded state, muscles are relaxed. However, well-conditioned muscles maintain a state of minimal contraction, or *tonus*, even when relaxed. This minimal contraction renders the muscle strong and prepared to act when called upon. It also enhances circulation in the muscle. The healthy muscle maintains enough tonus to be firm to the touch. *Atony* is complete lack of muscle tone, which sometimes accompanies paralysis of central nerv-

ous system origin. The atonic muscle is very flaccid. A muscle with some tonus that is not fully firm is termed *hypotonic*; hypotonic muscles result from inactivity and insufficient exercise or from illness and fatigue. A hypotonic muscle is weak and easily injured. *Hypertonic* muscles are very firmly contracted even when they are ostensibly at rest. They promote fatigue and muscular aches and pains and contribute to joint deformities. Hypertonic muscles may result from tension, disease, or injury.

## Posture

*Posture* is the position of the body parts relative to one another. In order to maintain posture, muscles must be constantly at work, balancing and adjusting. Ideal posture is that which puts the least strain on body parts and is most functional. It is usually described with reference to the standing position.

The feet (in low-heeled or flat shoes) are placed

slightly apart to provide a wide *base of support* for the body's weight. The abdominal muscles are contracted, supporting the abdominal organs. The buttocks are tucked in and down, somewhat flattening the curve of the lower back. Since the muscles support the abdomen and buttocks as a girdle does, this state is sometimes compared to "wearing an internal girdle."

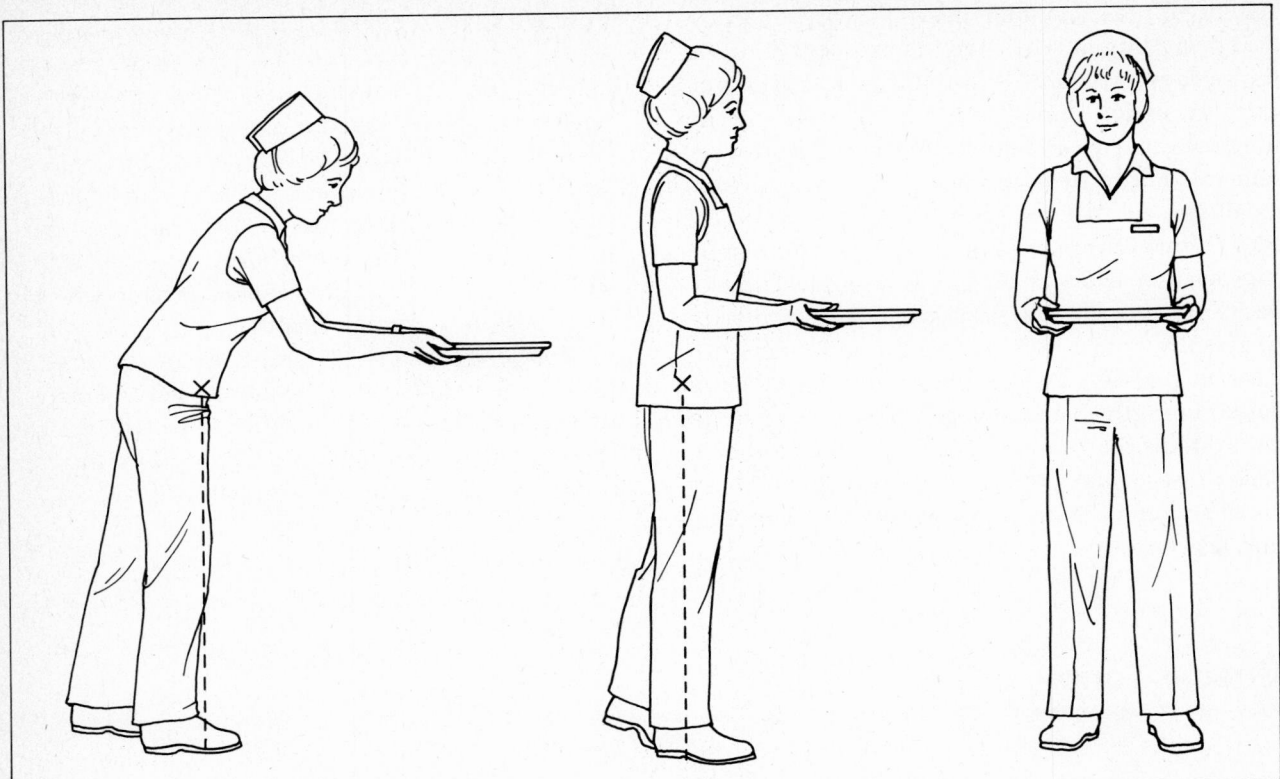

**Figure 19.1   Using the base of support**
*Left:* Center of gravity (X) not over base of support (incorrect). *Center:* Center of gravity (X) over base of support (correct). *Right:* Good posture.

The alignment of body parts in relation to the spine is a critical aspect of good posture. Twisting the pelvis, shoulders, or head to the side would also twist the spine. Instead, the head is held erect over the shoulders and faces straight ahead. The shoulders are held straight (often best achieved by pulling them back and then dropping them). In this position, the body's *center of gravity*—the point at which gravitational pull functions as if the body's entire weight were concentrated at that single point—is directly above the base support (see Figure 19.1). The center of gravity in the human body is approximately at the level of the pelvis.

Maintaining appropriate posture while sitting and lying down—usually spoken of as proper *alignment*—is particularly important for the hospitalized patient. Proper alignment is essential to rest.

An understanding of appropriate posture will prove important to you in your own work and in assisting and teaching patients. Good posture helps prevent muscle strain and back injury and minimizes the fatigue associated with infrequent changes of position.

It is the nurse's responsibility to maintain correct body alignment in the patient confined to bed. In order to approximate optimal erect body posture when lying, it is necessary to use pillows, sandbags, and other supportive devices. The spine is thus positioned in its optimal S-curve without twisting or torsion. The shoulders and hips must be squarely aligned, and the arms and legs should be supported parallel to the spine. This may be accomplished in a variety of positions: back-lying, side-lying (Figure 19.2), or on the abdomen.

Sitting posture is also important for the ill person. The back muscles need to be well supported and the body should be flexed at the hips, not slumped along the spine. The patient's feet should have a firm support, either the floor or a footstool, to prevent excess pressure behind the knees and to allow them to remain in a functional position.

Arms need support so that their weight does not pull on the shoulders. The head must be either positioned vertically over the neck or supported, since the neck muscles are not strong enough to support the head adequately against the pull of gravity. Module 12, "Moving the Patient in Bed and Positioning," demonstrates how to help a patient achieve good alignment.

## Body Mechanics

*Body mechanics* is the application of mechanical principles and knowledge of human anatomy to the action of body parts during activity. It usually involves learning appropriate ways to move the body in order to accomplish tasks without stress or injury. Correct body mechanics helps protect joints and muscles from being pushed beyond their capacities while allowing them to be used for maximum effectiveness. Body mechanics is particularly important to those who perform physical work and those who already have musculoskeletal injuries. Exhibit 19.1 outlines basic principles of body mechanics, which are discussed more thoroughly in Module 4, "Basic Body Mechanics." Let us review the major principles of body mechanics.

### Maintaining Center of Gravity Over Base of Support

The spine is a shallow S-curve that balances the body's weight evenly over its base of support. When the spine is not balanced vertically, the muscles are unduly strained by the task of supporting the body's weight. As we have seen, weight is balanced best when the center of gravity is directly above the base provided by the feet. This relationship may be preserved when moving by bending from the knees, rather than the waist, or by placing one foot in the direction of the bending to enlarge the base of support and provide stability.

### Avoiding Twisting

Twisting, or *torsion,* of the spine lessens its ability to function effectively and makes it more susceptible to injury. Rather than maintaining a twisted position, the entire body should be turned in one plane as shown in Figure 19.3.

### Using Leg Muscles

The broad, flat muscles of the back are weakest when stretched and flattened, and are susceptible

---

Exhibit 19.1
**Basic Principles of Body Mechanics**

1. Weight is balanced best when the center of gravity is directly above the base of support.
2. Enlarging the base of support increases the body's stability.
3. A body or object is more stable if its center of gravity is close to its base of support.
4. Enlarging the base of support in the direction of the force to be applied increases the amount of force that can be applied.
5. Tightening the abdominal muscles upward and the gluteal muscles downward before undertaking any activity decreases the likelihood of strain or injury.
6. Facing toward the task to be performed and turning the entire body in one plane, rather than twisting, lessens the back's susceptibility to injury.
7. Lifting is better undertaken by bending the legs and using the larger leg muscles rather than by using the back muscles.
8. Moving an object on a level surface requires less effort than moving it against the force of gravity.
9. Less energy is required to move an object when friction between the object and the surface on which it rests is minimized.
10. It takes less energy to hold an object close to the body than at a distance from the body.
11. The weight of the body can be used to facilitate lifting and moving.
12. Smooth, rhythmic movements at a moderate speed require the least energy.
13. When a soft object is pushed, it absorbs part of the force being exerted; pulling a soft object subtracts less of the force from the movement.

---

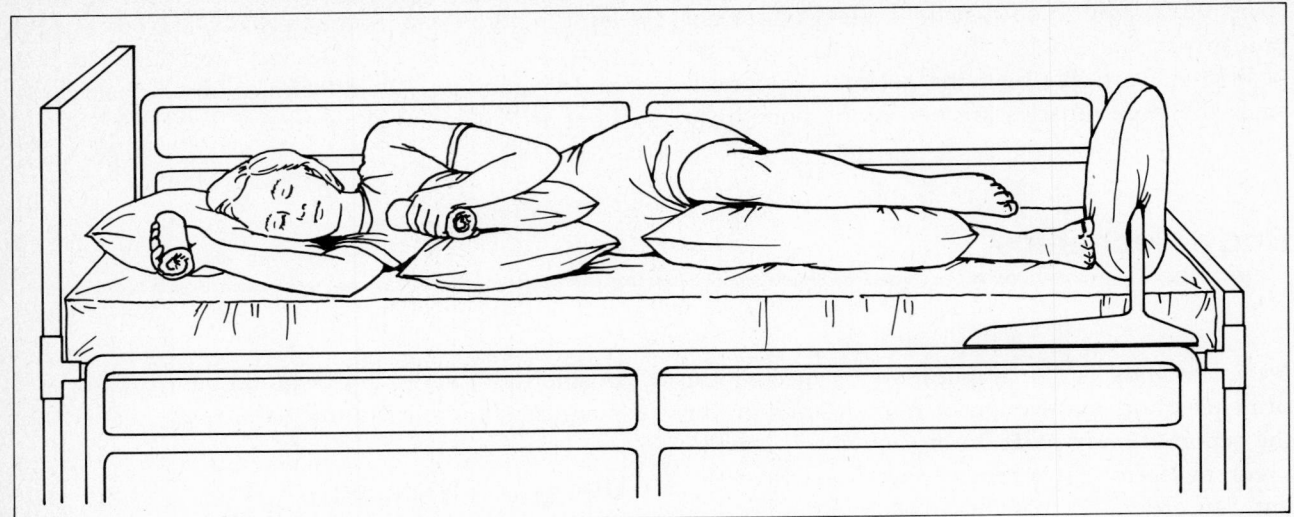

**Figure 19.2**
Pillows and other supportive devices are used to maintain correct alignment in the side-lying position.

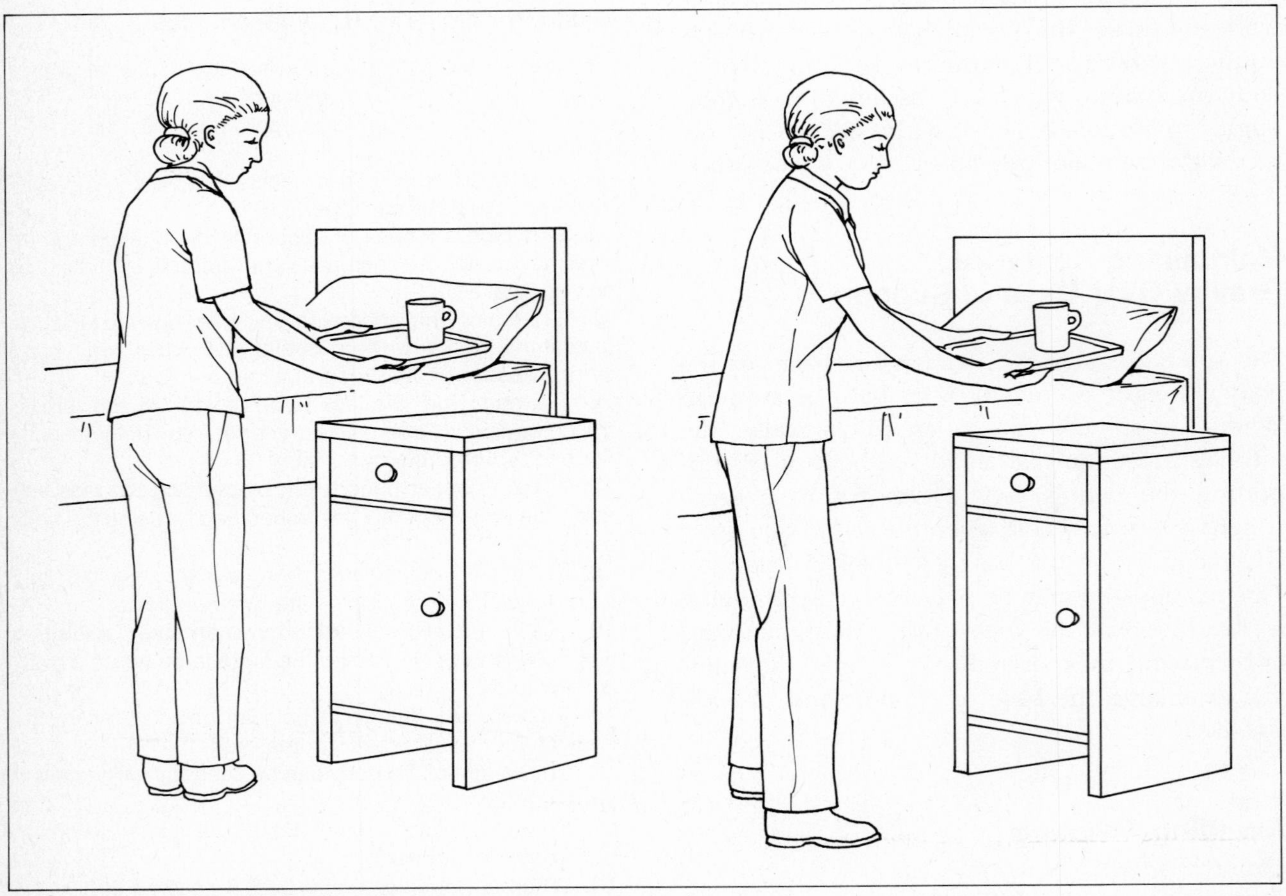

**Figure 19.3   Avoid torsion of the spine**
*Left:* Nurse twisting to lift tray from bed to table (incorrect). *Right:* Nurse turning whole body to lift tray from bed to table (correct).

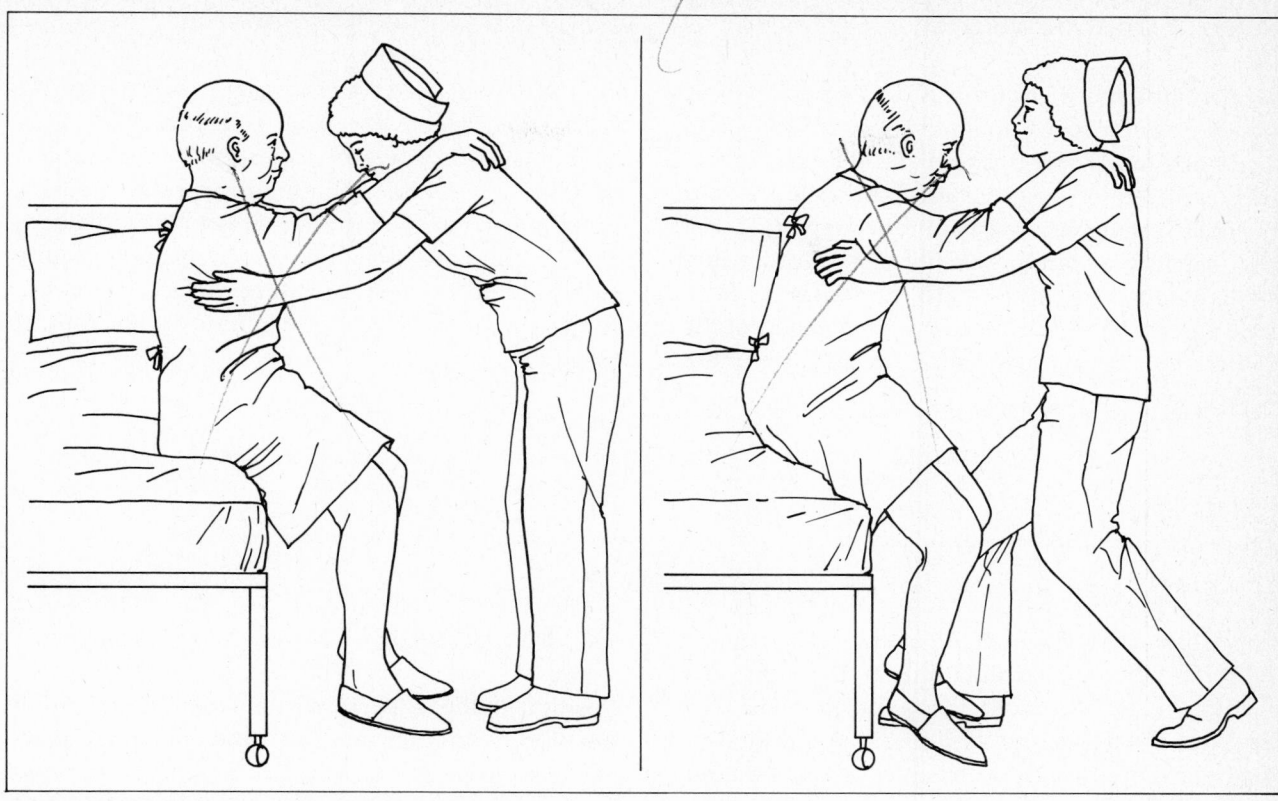

**Figure 19.4   Lifting with the leg muscles**
*Left:* Nurse assisting patient to stand, hands under patient's arms, body bent over from waist (incorrect). *Right:* Nurse assisting patient to stand, hands under patient's arms, back straight, knees flexed (correct).

to injury when lifting heavy objects. The large, thick muscles of the legs are better able than the back muscles to tolerate heavy loads. Therefore, lifting is best undertaken by bending the legs and using the leg muscles (see Figure 19.4). By lifting excess weight or bending from the waist, it is possible to injure not only the back muscles but also the spine itself, which can cause lifelong disability.

## Pulling or Sliding Instead of Lifting

Before moving an object or a patient, consider whether the weight might be pulled or slid, rather than lifted, to the new position. Both alternatives require less strength. Friction of the surface under the object or person can be minimized by providing a smooth surface (such as tight bedsheets) and/

or a lubricating substance (such as talcum powder). A turning sheet placed under a patient is an effective aid, since there is less friction between two dry sheets than between the bottom sheet and the patient's skin, which is moist. Because movement against the force of gravity requires more strength than horizontal movement, it will be less difficult to reposition a patient if the bed is first returned to a flat position (see Figure 19.5).

## Contracting Abdominal Muscles

Undue strain on the abdominal muscles when lifting can tear the muscle along a weakened point, causing a *hernia*. This outcome can be avoided by contracting the abdominal muscles—referred to earlier as "wearing an internal girdle"—before undertaking any effort.

## Using a Counterweight

Your weight and that of the object or person to be moved may be used to assist movement. Hold your body in a stable position and then rock back, using your entire weight, rather than simply your muscular strength, as a counterbalance to assist the patient to a standing position. This procedure is illustrated in Figure 19.4. To turn a patient from back to side, bend the knees up. The weight of the legs turning to the side will help pull the entire body over.

## Body Mechanics for Patients

Patients often need to be taught how to move safely and effectively. This is especially true of those with disorders of the musculoskeletal system. The nurse can promote proper body mechanics by means of such measures as placing the bedside stand in a position that does not require twisting and by demonstrating correct techniques for moving in bed and for getting in and out of bed.

# Exercise

Exercise is active movement of the body beyond the requirements of maintaining muscle tone and posture. Exercise maintains joint mobility and function, as well as muscle strength and flexibility. Furthermore, physical exercise enhances the functioning of the gastrointestinal system by increasing appetite and promoting elimination. The metabolic rate increases during activity, exercising the temperature-regulating mechanisms and a wide variety of other physiological processes.

Exercise seems to enhance the ability to think clearly by stimulating circulation and promoting optimum ventilation. Activity also serves as an outlet for tension and anxiety. A game of tennis or a long walk may reduce tension and anxiety to manageable levels and permit one's energy to be focused on problem-solving. Even asleep we are physically active, moving our extremities, turning from side to side, and changing position repeatedly.

The following types of exercise are normal components of daily living and may be adapted to the special needs of those with decreased energy and ability.

## Active Exercise

Active exercise involves voluntary movement of a body part by means of muscular contraction and relaxation.

## Position Changes

Position changes, such as from one sitting or lying position to another, are fundamental components of our exercise baseline. When we are well, we do not even think about our constant shifts and changes of position. Position changes serve to alleviate pressure on supporting body parts, such as the buttocks, feet, and sacrum, and enhance circulation. Position changes also facilitate drainage from the kidneys, deep respirations, drainage of lung secretions, and gastrointestinal functioning.

## Activities of Daily Living (A.D.L.s)

A.D.L.s include feeding oneself, caring for one's own hygiene and elimination needs, dressing oneself, and performing other tasks necessary to meet one's basic needs. Performing A.D.L.s will usually provide a minimum baseline of activity for avoiding illness. It also supports self-esteem and a self-image as a competent individual. For these reasons, activities of daily living tend to be the first active exercises a recuperating patient is encouraged to perform, the most likely to be allowed during the course of illness, and the first taught in the course of rehabilitation.

## Ambulation

Ambulation is walking. Though a simple exercise, walking very effectively accomplishes all the pur-

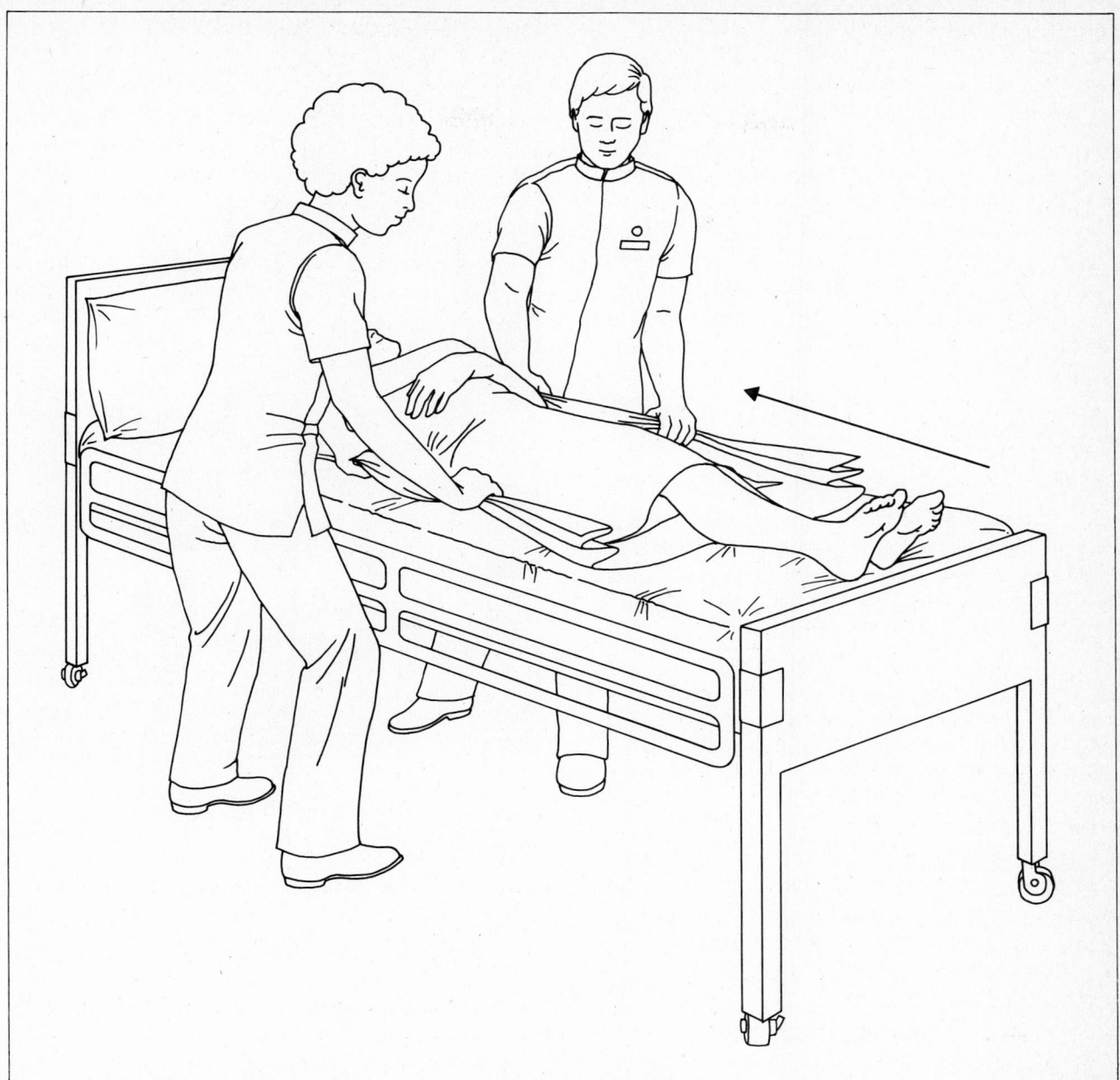

**Figure 19.5  Moving a patient up in bed using a turn sheet**
Both nurses face the foot of the bed. Knees and hips are slightly bent and backs are straight. Feet are spread to form a wide base of support.

*Sci Rat for Amb.*

poses of exercise. It not only keeps joints flexible and strengthens muscles but also stimulates the entire circulatory, respiratory, and gastrointestinal systems. Walking uses almost all the body's muscles. As an exercise, it can be varied in speed and distance to accommodate the abilities of a wide variety of people, even those with severe disabil-

ity. Hospitalized patients often require support or the use of such devices as walkers and crutches in order to ambulate. Considerable care must be taken to prevent an ill person from falling while ambulating. Module 16, "Ambulation," describes how to help a patient ambulate and use assistive devices.

## Isometric Exercise

*Isometric exercises*—also called static exercises—involve contracting a muscle, holding it tightly, and then relaxing it without moving the joint. Isometric exercises strengthen muscles and effectively stimulate circulation, especially venous return. They are particularly useful when joint mobility is not possible or desired, such as in the case of a person with a joint disability. Isometric exercises may also be used to strengthen muscles in preparation for more active exercise.

## Isotonic Exercise

*Isotonic exercise* is any exercise involving movement. However, the term is most often used to refer to planned active movement. The ordinary daily activities of people with sedentary occupations may not be adequate to meet all the body's needs for exercise. Maximum health of the cardiovascular and respiratory systems requires exercise that causes the pulse to rise and respirations to increase, at least three times a week on a regular basis. Calisthenics, jogging, and tennis are examples of isotonic exercise.

## Resistive Exercise

*Resistive exercise* is a special type of isotonic exercise performed against resistance, such as a weight. Weightlifting is resistive exercise. Resistive exercise builds muscle volume and strength faster than more active isotonic exercise. In women, resistive exercise produces strong muscles but, because of differing hormonal responses, of a different shape and contour than in men. Resistive exercise is a preferred mode of treatment in physical therapy when muscle strength is poor.

## Range-of-Motion (R.O.M.) Exercise

Each joint in the body is capable of certain types of movement, and some joints can perform more than one type of movement. The full extent to which a joint can move in any direction is called its *range of motion*. Types of joint movement are illustrated in Figure 19.7 and defined in Exhibit

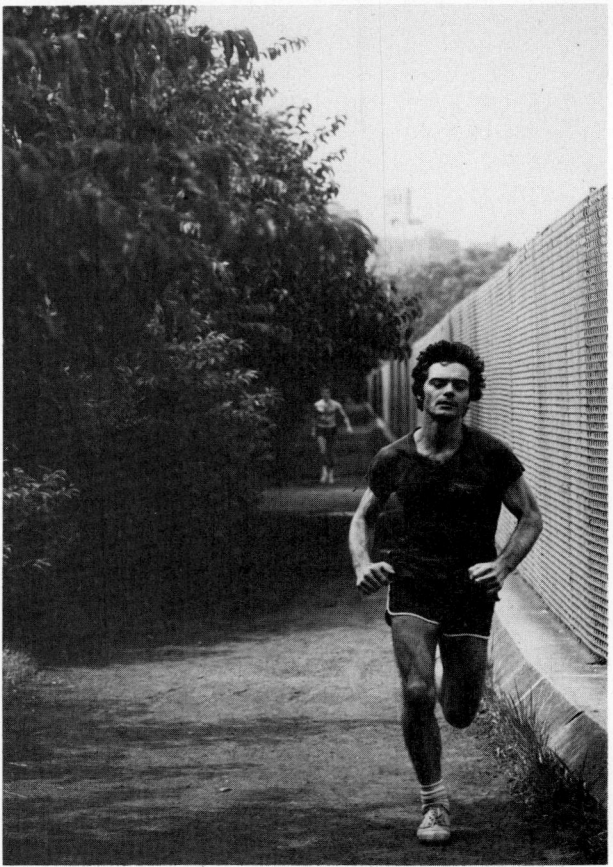

**Figure 19.6**
Jogging is a popular isotonic exercise. (R. D. Ullmann/Taurus Photos)

19.2. Range-of-motion exercises are typically recommended when a person is in danger of losing the full extent of joint motion due to disease process or weakness.

The range of a joint may be determined by measuring the degree of the angle formed by the joint at each end of its movement. A joint in which structural changes (shortened muscles and tendons and inflexible skin) have occurred, preventing full range of motion, is termed a *contracture*. If bone deformity has also occurred, and the two bones are fused together, the joint is termed *ankylosed*.

Range-of-motion exercises are designed to maintain maximum joint mobility. The joints are moved to their full range or as far as possible without causing pain. A severely disabled person might need to do so several times a day in order to maintain functional ability.

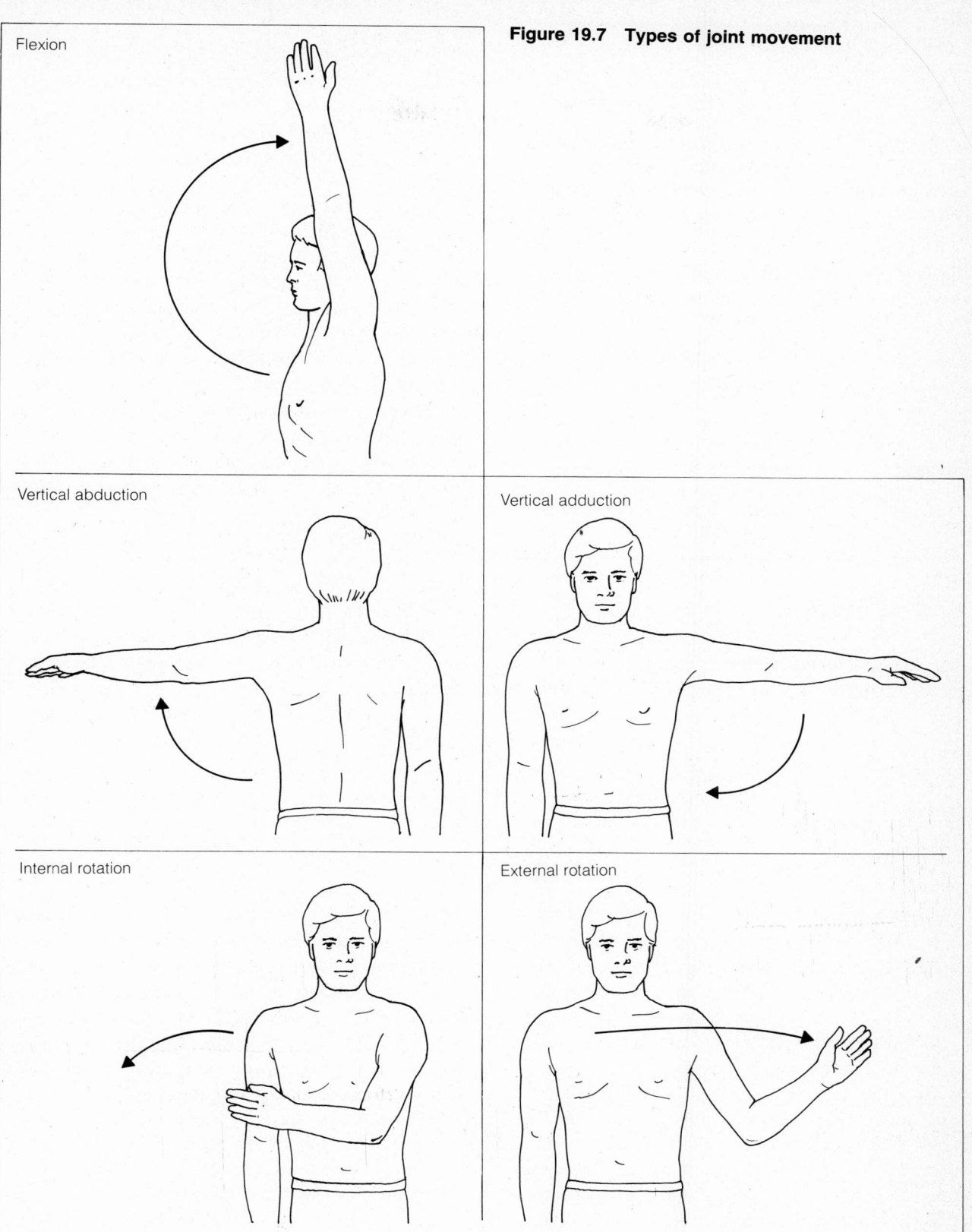

Flexion

Vertical abduction

Vertical adduction

Internal rotation

External rotation

**Figure 19.7 Types of joint movement**

## Exhibit 19.2
## Types of Movement

| | |
|---|---|
| Abduction | Drawing away from the median line or center of the body. |
| Adduction | Drawing toward the median line or center of the body. |
| Circumduction | Circular movement of a body part. |
| Extension | Straightening or extending a limb. |
| External rotation | Moving a body part outward on an axis. |
| Eversion | Turning the feet so that the toes point away from the median line of the body. |
| Flexion | Bending a joint. |
| Inversion | Turning the feet so that the toes point toward the median line of the body. |
| Inward rotation | Moving a body part inward on an axis. |
| Pronation | Turning the palm of the hand or forearm downward. |
| Supination | Turning the palm of the hand or forearm upward. |

## Passive Exercise

Any exercise in which the energy and movement are provided by a person other than the person exercising is called *passive exercise* (see Figure 19.8). Passive exercise is usually performed to increase range of motion and joint flexibility. Needless to say, passive exercise serves fewer of the purposes of exercise than does active exercise, but it is a valuable alternative.

When an individual can perform some joint motion independently but needs help completing the motion, such help is termed *active assistive range-of-motion exercise*. Active and active assistive R.O.M. provides for more complete exercise than does passive R.O.M., which provides only for joint mobility. Module 14, "Range-of-Motion Exercises," provides complete directions for performing passive R.O.M.

By changing a person's *position*, it is possible to alter circulatory patterns. Raising a person to a sitting position, for example, will tend to increase the heart rate and facilitate general circulation. Respiration is also enhanced. Sometimes a person can be helped to perform activities of daily living in a passive manner. To help a patient wash his or her chest, for example, place the washcloth in the patient's hand and help move the hand in washing strokes. This exercise is used in an effort to rehabilitate a patient to greater independence in A.D.L.s.

# Rest

Rest is a period of inactivity. Either the entire body or a single body part may be rested. A sprained ankle, for example, is supported by elastic bandages and walking is curtailed to allow the ankle to rest.

Rest affords the body the opportunity to use all its resources to repair damaged cells, remove waste products, and restore tissue to maximum functional ability. Ideally, rest should be alternated with activity to allow the various body parts to recover completely from one activity before another is begun. This is preferable to planning a lengthy, strenuous period of activity followed by a long rest.

If a physician prescribes rest as part of the plan of care, it is very important to distinguish between rest of a specific body part and rest of the entire body. The patient on bedrest for a broken leg is still able to move the arms and the other leg; indeed, he or she should be encouraged to do so. However, the patient on bedrest after a heart attack is discouraged from moving since all body activity requires increased heart activity. Clarifying the exact meaning of a prescription for rest is the responsibility of the nurse. The meaning of any prescription for activity or rest must also be carefully explained to the patient, and arrangements should be made for the assistance necessary to adhere to the prescription.

# The Effects of Immobility on the Body

Mobility may be restricted by the illness itself or by the physician's prescription for rest. Since both activity and rest are basic needs, restricting mobility has profound and far-reaching effects. Immobilization causes changes and deterioration in even a healthy person; the axiom "that which is not used is lost" is apt. However, nursing measures can help prevent such deterioration. Common problems resulting from immobility will be discussed in terms of the affected body systems. It is important to remember that no system is affected independently and that preventive measures addressed to one body system may also help prevent problems in others. You may wish to refer to the chapters focusing on particular physiologic needs to review normal functioning.

## The Musculoskeletal System

Muscle *atrophy* due to lack of exercise causes the muscles to become weaker, smaller, and even shorter. If this situation persists for a long enough period (variable from person to person), it can limit the joint's range of motion and eventually cause a contracture of the joint. Because flexor muscles are stronger than extensors, the atrophied joint has a tendency to remain flexed. The flexor muscles then become shortened and the extensors lengthened.

When the stresses and strains imposed on the bones by normal movement and weight-bearing are suspended, the body begins to reabsorb calcium and *osteoporosis*—weak and porous bone—occurs. This condition may cause pain on stress and can result in easily fractured bones.

## The Integumentary System

The skin and subcutaneous tissue are not equipped to tolerate continued pressure in one area. Small blood vessels become occluded (blocked off) by such pressure, and cells begin to suffer from *ischemia* (lack of blood supply to a tissue). When pressure is alleviated, blood supply is restored and the cells recover; however, if the blood supply is interrupted too long, cells are unable to recover and *necrosis* (cell death) sets in. This situation is the origin of most *pressure ulcers*, commonly called bedsores. Sometimes the term *decubitus ulcer* is used to refer to any pressure ulcer; correctly speaking, however, a decubitus ulcer is one that results from the decubitus, or lying-down, position. Pressure ulcers may occur on any body surface as a result of any position maintained for too long.

A pressure ulcer usually begins as an area of reddened skin. If it disappears when massaged, permanent tissue damage has not yet occurred. If

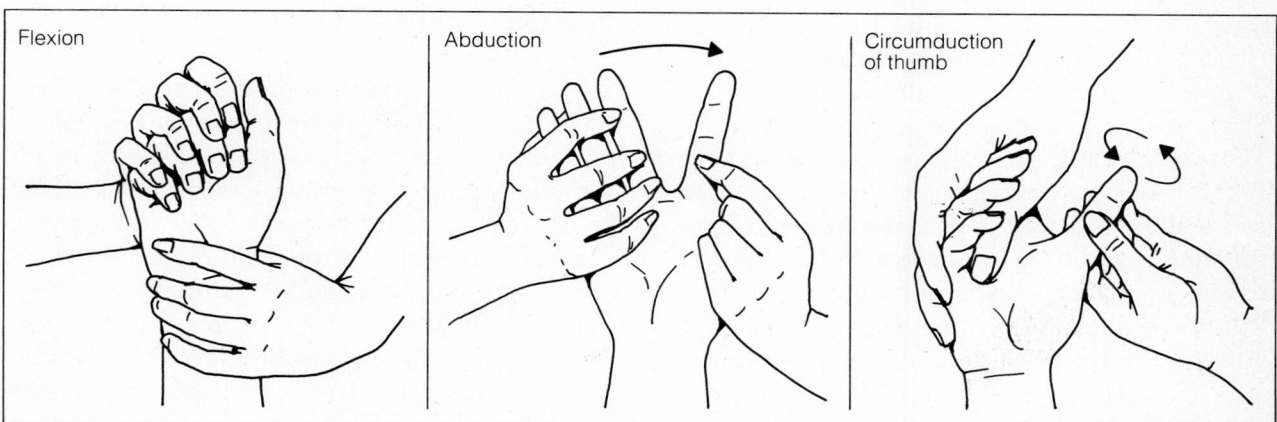

**Figure 19.8   Performing passive range-of-motion exercises on the hand**

the redness does not disappear, some tissue damage has occurred, and an *incipient pressure ulcer* is present. Further breakdown may be prevented by aggressive nursing care, but damage to deeper tissues may have already taken place. If so, surface tissue may continue to break down in spite of intensive nursing action.

Other factors that contribute to the formation of pressure ulcers are the presence of moisture, which tends to *macerate* (soften) the skin, decreasing its resistance; shearing forces, which catch the soft tissue between bone and another surface (such as a sheet) and tear or bruise the underlying tissue; and chemical irritation from stool and urine, which tends to break down the skin. Friction may cause abrasion of the skin and begin the breakdown process.

People with decreased awareness of peripheral sensation, such as diabetics and those who have suffered strokes, have a high risk of pressure ulcers. Unable to perceive discomfort in the affected tissue, such individuals do not respond to it by correcting its cause. Those with impaired circulation also develop pressure ulcers rapidly because the cells cannot recover from minor damage.

Pressure ulcers are most common over bony prominences, such as the coccyx, trochanters, scapulae, ankles, and elbows. An ulcer may occur over ischial spines due to prolonged sitting or on the ankle bone due to a prolonged side-lying position. Ulcers are less likely to occur when there is adequate soft subcutaneous tissue to pad the bone, and correspondingly more likely when the person is thin. Adequate nutrition, especially enough protein and fluids, promotes prevention by providing the means for cells to repair themselves.

Treatment of a decubitus ulcer is a serious medical problem. A culture is usually taken if infection is suspected; preventing and treating infection is a primary concern. A variety of agents have been used in treatment. Enzymatic ointments are often used to remove dead tissue, and heat lamps have been employed to dry the surface of the ulcer and increase circulation. Adsorbent granules, such as Debrisan, may be placed in the open wound to adsorb moisture and bacteria. Vegetable-gum wafers, such as Stomadhesive and karaya, are sometimes used over the ulcer to prevent further irritation from urine and stool. Healing can occur underneath these substances. In addition to these treatment methods, which have been verified by research, you may hear of other treatment methods that nurses have found successful. The reported success of some of these alternative methods may be due more to the accompanying attention given the problem than to the specific agent used. In other instances, the agent used may be effective, though formal research has not been conducted to verify its effectiveness. In extreme cases, surgical debridement and skin grafting may be needed. All the preventive measures discussed on pages 319–321 are also used in treatment.

## The Urinary System

Some people's ability to void is impaired by lying down. This is especially true of men, who are accustomed to urinating in a standing position. If a person cannot maintain a normal position to urinate, the bladder may not empty completely and urinary retention may occur. The overdistended bladder may also overflow, causing incontinence. Both of these situations may predispose to infection (see Chapter 22).

Normal kidney drainage is maintained by gravitational flow. If a person must remain prone, urine may pool in the kidney pelvis, creating a climate for infection. Furthermore, the stagnant urine may be a source of kidney stones, which are minerals precipitated out of the urine. This problem is aggravated by the excess calcium excreted when the body is reabsorbing it from inactive bone.

## The Gastrointestinal System

The progress of food through the digestive system is also facilitated by gravity and the normal movement of abdominal muscles. When these forces are not functioning, the entire digestive process may be slowed. This situation can result in increased gas formation and the retention of stool for such a long time that excess fluid is reabsorbed, making the stool dry and hard. If a patient is required to use a bedpan, the normal position for defecation cannot be achieved. Lack of privacy also inhibits bowel function. Together, these factors may lead to constipation and even *impaction* of hardened feces in the rectum (see Chapter 22).

## The Respiratory System

Secretions in the lungs are usually moved from the alveoli by changes in gravity due to position change and the pressure of moving air. Once the secretions are in the bronchioles, cilia move them upward and out of the respiratory passages. When movement and position changes are minimal, secretions tend to pool in the dependent sections of the lungs, where they consolidate and can cause *hypostatic pneumonia.* This condition decreases the surface available for oxygen exchange and can be life-threatening.

## The Circulatory System

Although the heart pumps blood through the arterial system to the tissue, there is no pump to return blood to the heart. This return blood flow depends greatly on movement and pressure from muscles surrounding the veins, aided by a system of valves that maintains one-way flow. When muscle movement is decreased, blood moves sluggishly in the large veins, predisposing to *thrombus* (clot) formation and *phlebitis* (inflammation of the vein). Clots dislodged by rubbing the muscles become *emboli* (moving particles in the bloodstream), which can move through the circulatory system to the heart and out into pulmonary arteries, where they lodge in the small vessels and block circulation. Called *pulmonary embolism,* this situation is a serious threat to lung function and possibly to life. In order to prevent embolism, the leg muscles of immobilized patients are not massaged.

Ordinarily, the body compensates for changes in position, and the resulting changes in the effect of gravity on circulation, by constricting and dilating vessels as necessary to maintain constant blood flow. After a period of bedrest, during which these mechanisms are not used, they do not function as effectively. Thus, if the circulation is unable to make the rapid adjustment to first arising, blood pools in the lower extremities, causing *hypotension* (low blood pressure), diminished blood flow to the brain, dizziness, or fainting. Low blood pressure caused by position change is called *postural* or *orthostatic hypotension.*

## Psychological Effects

A person who is immobilized may suffer emotionally in a variety of ways. First, the need for belongingness is interfered with. When an individual is not able to join in the mainstream of life, he or she may feel that life is passing by. Loneliness or a sense of isolation from others is not uncommon.

Self-esteem may suffer, possibly severely. In our society people are usually valued for their accomplishments, and an immobilized person is unable to *do* anything. He or she cannot work, take care of family responsibilities, or socialize with friends. Suspension of these activities may diminish self-esteem and contribute to depression.

Perception may also be affected. Decreased sensory input may make it difficult to remain oriented in terms of time: a few minutes may seem like half an hour to an immobilized person. If stimuli are greatly reduced, sensory deprivation can occur (see Chapter 28).

Dependence on others can create a host of additional problems. Resultant anger may be directed at care givers, who serve as constant reminders of dependence. Some people, on the other hand, submit to dependence so completely that they do not undertake independent activities of which they are capable. Such patients may exhibit an apparent lack of motivation either to work toward improvement or to learn (see Chapter 15).

When care givers recognize these responses and continue to be accepting and supportive, a climate of trust is established in which constructive communication can help alleviate the immobilized patient's distress.

## Assessing the Patient's Activity and Rest

In assessing a patient's status with regard to activity and rest, the following aspects of the musculoskeletal system and its condition should be considered: posture, muscle tone, joint mobility, body mechanics, and ability to perform such activities as turning, sitting, standing, and walking. Attention should be paid to the relation between activity and need for rest, and to the patient's capacity to recognize the need for rest.

Assessment involves thinking in terms of past, present, and future. Previous level of activity will affect the patient's physical condition, as well as feelings and attitudes about activity. Consider both what the patient was able to do and what he or she actually did. Knowledge of the patient's prognosis will help you plan for the future with the patient and take into account any adaptations that must be made. Current activity level will govern your current nursing actions.

The physician's current prescription for activity and rest is a major determinant of what the patient should be encouraged to do. Sometimes this prescription is very specific, such as "Up in chair twice a day." In other cases, a prescription is very general: "Activity as tolerated."

## Planning to Meet Activity and Rest Needs

When planning a patient's activity and rest, you will need to plan (1) the type of activity to be undertaken, (2) its frequency, and (3) a method of evaluation. Your efforts will ordinarily be aimed at attaining and/or maintaining an activity level as near to normal as possible.

### Type of Activity

The various kinds of activity—range-of-motion exercise, ambulation, activities of daily living, and the like—have already been described. In some instances a physician will write orders specifying a particular activity in accord with the prescription for care. More frequently, the physician's orders indicate the maximum activity that can be undertaken but do not specify each activity. For example, a person unable to move his or her joints will require range-of-motion exercises to maintain joint mobility unless there is a specific medical contraindication. However, the physician will not usually order range-of-motion exercises. As a nurse, it will be up to you to determine that range-of-motion exercises are needed and not contraindicated by the patient's condition. As a beginning student, you will not know enough about specific diseases and pathological problems to make this decision, so you will need to consult with your instructor or another registered nurse.

Activities of daily living should be encouraged whenever possible. The goal here is not to save the nurse time; in fact, it may be far more time-consuming to help patients feed themselves or perform some aspect of personal hygiene than to do it oneself. The point is that self-care promotes self-esteem.

Sitting in a chair is valuable even if the patient must be lifted into the chair. Sitting in a chair for meals often enhances appetite as well as providing for activity. At times you will need to choose from among several activities the one or two most valuable for the patient, since performing all of them would be too fatiguing. For example, you might choose to bathe a patient so as to conserve his or her energy for sitting in a chair if you consider the change in posture and position more important for the patient than self-care. The skills needed to transfer a patient from a bed into a chair are outlined in Module 15, "Transfer."

When the goal is to increase activity progressively, a gradual approach is used. The first step may be *dangling*—that is, sitting with the legs over the edge of the bed. Simply standing at the bedside, which requires balance and strength, may be the next step. Then ambulation can begin, increasing only a few steps each time until the patient has achieved an optimal level of activity. Sometimes patients need to remain at a given level of activity for an extended time before proceeding further, or they may have to regress temporarily due to other problems associated with their illnesses. Helping such a patient remain motivated to increase activity and not become discouraged by the slow pace of progress is a very challenging task. A patient who is responding well to treatment, such as a person recovering from a common intestinal upset, may be able to make advances in activity at four-hour intervals during the day.

In helping a patient ambulate, you may need to use such assistive devices as a walker, a cane, or crutches. Usually the physical therapist initiates instruction of the patient at the time the device is issued. The nurse is then responsible for continuing assistance to the patient and monitoring progress. Module 16, "Ambulation," explains the use of walkers, canes, and crutches.

Observation is essential at each step so that the effectiveness of the plan for the patient's activity can be evaluated and revised as needed.

## Frequency of Activity

Activity is most effective when it is attempted with adequate rest periods. If a patient is to sit in a chair three times a day, a sound distribution of the activity might be once each morning, afternoon, and evening.

Ideally, passive range-of-motion exercises would be performed four times a day or more. Realistically, it may be possible to schedule full R.O.M. only twice a day.

Position changes are traditionally scheduled every two hours. The adequacy of this interval should be verified by carefully checking the appearance of the patient's skin. If the reddened pressure areas blanch when rubbed, and there is no residual reddening at the next position change, the tissue is recovering from the pressure. If, when it is time to return the patient to a position

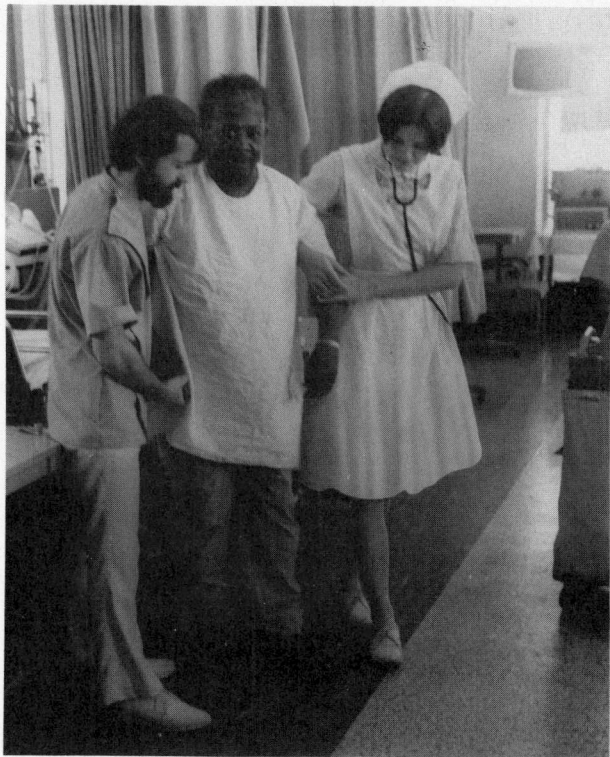

**Figure 19.9**
Ambulation effectively combats the effects of immobility.
(Elizabeth Wilcox)

that pressures those areas, the tissue is still red or fails to blanch at all with rubbing, the length of time between positions needs to be reduced. It may be that two hours can be tolerated on the sides but not on the coccyx. It is important to individualize planned position changes, which are as critical for the person immobilized in a wheelchair as for the person in bed. Even very slight movement can change the focus of pressure. Whenever position is changed, massage of the pressured area will help restore the tissue more rapidly.

## Planning Additional Intervention for Immobility

The best means of combating the effects of immobility is activity—whatever activity the patient can pursue. When activity is not possible, alternative measures can be taken to combat the effects of immobility.

There are many devices that help prevent pres-

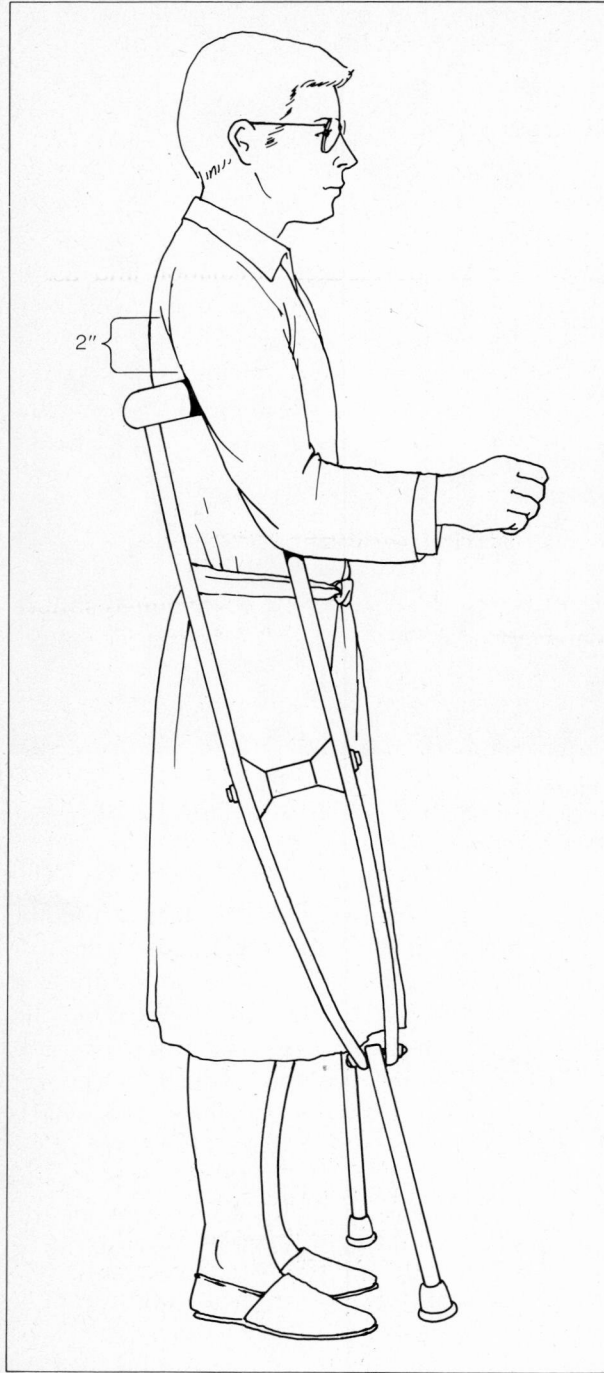

**Figure 19.10  Measuring crutches**
The top of the crutch should fall 2 inches below the axilla.

sure sores. Though all of them have demonstrated value, they must be used in conjunction with appropriate position changes and exercise. Such devices in no way replace basic activity.

## Hygiene

The importance of hygiene for an immobilized patient cannot be overemphasized (see Chapter 18). Perspiration and incontinence are much more complex problems when a patient is immobilized since they increase the likelihood of skin breakdown. Careful bathing after each episode of incontinence is crucial to prevent skin breakdown. Use of an absorbent powder after a bath may help alleviate maceration in a person who perspires heavily.

## Massage

Each time a patient is turned, all bony prominences should be massaged until the redness begins to fade. If the patient was lying on his or her side, the shoulder, hip, and ankle should be rubbed. The shoulders, coccyx, and heels may need particular attention when the patient has been supine.

## Bridging

*Bridging* is the use of pillows and cushions to support the body in such a way as to distribute weight and pressure over areas not normally exposed to pressure and reduce pressure on areas usually subject to maximal pressure. The customary pressure points literally form a bridge between two pillows. For example, when the person is in the back-lying position, pillows and cushions are placed underneath the legs, back, and head, but a space is left under the sacrum. The weight is thus distributed on the pillows and the sacrum is entirely free of pressure. When a person is in the side-lying position, pillows may be placed under the leg, side, head, and arm; the hip and shoulder are bridged to remove pressure. The criteria for correct position are the same as usual; the only difference is the support points.

## Coughing and Deep Breathing

Frequent deep breaths and coughing at intervals can be effective in preventing *atelectasis* (collapse of lung segments) and hypostatic pneumonia.

These measures help move secretions in the lungs and fully expand all alveoli.

## Increased Fluid Intake

A high fluid intake—3000 ml or more—if feasible in light of the patient's condition, will help keep minerals in suspension and guard against stones in the urinary tract. A dilute urine also helps protect against infection, and ample fluid intake keeps the skin and mucous membranes moist and lessens the risk of their breaking down. High fluid intake also combats the tendency toward constipation and enhances bowel function.

## Nutritional Support

A well-balanced diet provides the nutrients necessary for the body to repair and maintain tissue, especially the integument (skin). Particular care should be taken to provide adequate fruits and fiber, which tend to combat constipation. If the patient is troubled by digestive upset and gas, foods that cause gas or increase digestive problems should be eliminated.

## Special Devices

### Alternating-Pressure Mattress

An alternating-pressure mattress is a plastic mattress whose air-filled tubes are attached to a motor that automatically inflates and deflates them. Alternating tubes are connected to different outlets, with the result that one set of tubes is inflated while the other set is deflated. The pressured areas thus constantly change, helping to prevent pressure ulcers. The effectiveness of such a mattress is diminished if there is more than one layer of bedding between it and the patient because fabric packs into the spaces left by the deflated tubes and equalizes pressure. Sheets pulled tightly across the surface of the mattress have the same effect, so sheets should not be taut. To protect a patient who perspires freely from a damp sheet on top of the plastic mattress, a cotton blanket may be used in place of the sheet.

### Silicone-Gel Pads

Silicone-gel pads are used most frequently under the buttocks. These devices, very similar in density to body fat, provide padding and distribute pressure across the entire body surface, preventing its concentration on any one point. Lessened pressure prevents blocked circulation and tissue damage. The pad must usually be rotated regularly to prevent permanent ridges from occurring on the surface. Such pads are encased in easily cleaned plastic and may be covered with protective padding.

### Foam-Rubber Mattress Pads

A soft foam-rubber pad with a convoluted surface characterized by many small (about 1-inch-high) fingerlike projections (often called an egg-crate mattress) may be placed over the regular mattress. The pad's irregular surface allows air to circulate near the skin, helping alleviate skin maceration due to perspiration. Its softness allows pressure to be distributed over a wider area, thus relieving some of the pressure on bony prominences. Such pads are produced in small sizes to fit under the buttocks or in wheelchairs and in large sizes to cover the entire bed.

### Sheepskin Pads

Sheepskins, both natural and synthetic, have been used under bony prominences to provide a soft surface that does not abrade (rub open) the skin. The furry surface also allows for air circulation and distribution of weight. Natural sheepskins have the added advantage of surface lanolin, which softens and protects the skin; however, they are difficult to clean and quite expensive. Artificial sheepskins are completely washable. Both kinds are effective only in direct contact with the patient's skin.

### Water Beds

Water beds have proven successful for patients who need to be immobilized for prolonged periods. Because the patient literally floats on the surface of the bed, pressure is distributed evenly over the entire body.

## Turning Frames

Special beds (Stryker, Foster, or Bradford frames and CircOlectric beds) are sometimes used to facilitate position changes for immobilized patients.

The bottom mattress or support is suspended in a frame. When it is time to turn the patient, an alternate mattress or support is fastened in place above the patient. With both the top and bottom supports in place, the entire frame is rotated, repositioning the patient from the abdomen to the back or vice-versa. The top mattress is then removed until the patient is to be turned again.

# Implementing Activity Plans

In order to implement activity plans effectively, you will need to develop many direct-care skills. You will need to be able to move a patient in the bed using good body mechanics. You will need to be able to help transfer a patient from bed to a chair, wheelchair, or stretcher. Assisting with ambulation and using assistive devices are also essential skills. You must be familiar with range-of-motion exercises so you can perform them or teach the patient to do them independently.

# Evaluating Activity

Whatever the prescription, the nurse is responsible for thorough observation of the patient's response to any activity undertaken. Measuring vital signs before and after activity may yield important information on the patient's response or tolerance. If pulse, respiration, and/or blood pressure rise considerably and do not return to the preactivity level within a few minutes, the activity may have been too strenuous. Excessive dizziness may indicate that the activity was performed too rapidly. If severe fatigue occurs, you may be increasing the amount of activity too rapidly. Evaluation of the patient's response will enable you to replan your nursing actions.

# Rehabilitation

*Rehabilitation* is the process by which an individual affected by a disabling condition returns to as nearly normal functioning as possible. In its most comprehensive sense, rehabilitation begins the moment the disabling illness begins. Care that is planned from the outset with the person's eventual return to autonomy in mind is rehabilitation. When you preserve joint function through range-of-motion exercises, encourage each small increment in self-feeding, or help a person keep track of his or her own intake and output, you are participating in rehabilitation.

Comprehensive rehabilitation may require extensive team efort. In cases of major disabling illness, rehabilitation may be planned by a team composed of physicians, nurses, social workers, occupational therapists, physical therapists, and dieticians. The patients may be transferred to a special unit or even a special hospital whose staff has particular expertise in rehabilitation and whose facilities are especially designed for this purpose. In such a setting, the disabled person is helped to pursue independence and autonomy in all aspects of life. For example, the paraplegic, paralyzed from the waist down, may learn new ways of managing elimination and skin care as well as moving about. Vocational counseling and job placement may be an important part of the rehabilitation process as the patient progresses. Education for an occupation that can be pursued from a wheelchair may be undertaken. Personal counseling to help the patient resolve feelings about the tremendous changes in his or her body and life is an essential part of a major rehabilitation program.

## The Disabled Person

Many people have disabling conditions, including congenital disabilities related to neuromuscular functioning, such as cerebral palsy; paraplegia or quadriplegia due to spinal-cord injury; hearing and vision impairment; and a host of other conditions.

People with such problems do not usually consider themselves ill; they see themselves as having special conditions that necessitate special adaptations in daily life. Until very recently society was unsupportive of the efforts of many disabled people to function independently. However, recent federal legislation (and state legislation in some jurisdictions) has opened doors to fuller participation on the part of the disabled person. Public buildings are being designed (or remodeled, when possible) with disabled people in mind. Schools now allow disabled children to attend regular classes whenever possible (called "mainstreaming"). Some employers are adapting the work environment by means of devices that print messages for the deaf and telephones with desk speakers for the quadriplegic, enabling the disabled to become economically independent.

When a person with a disability is admitted to a hospital for an illness or surgery, it is common for the staff to impose more dependence than necessary. In fact, the disabled person may have a greater need than any other patient to maintain autonomy since that autonomy is often the result of arduous work. Assessment of the disabled person should involve determining what he or she

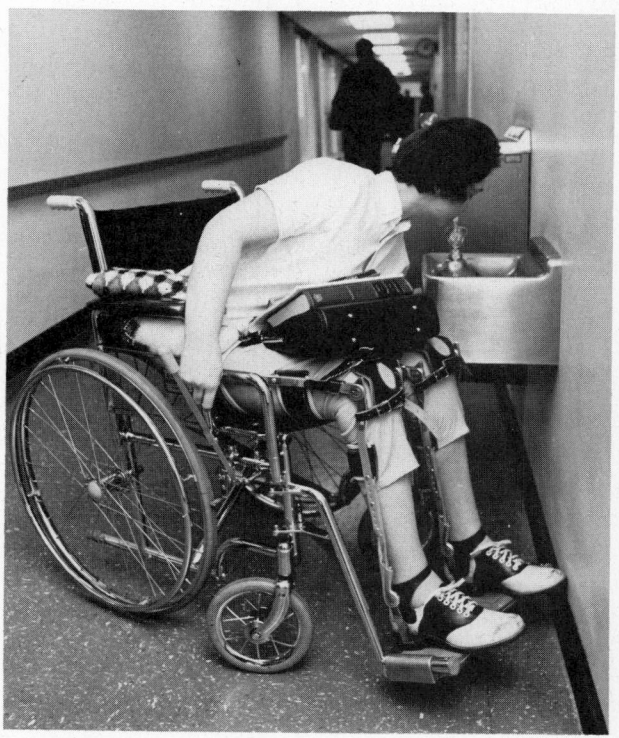

**Figure 19.11**
The disabled person can function independently. (Southern Illinois University, Carbondale; staff photo)

can do independently and what adaptations can be made in the environment to facilitate independence. For example, crutches should not be stored in a closet but placed where they can be reached when needed. The quadriplegic who manages personal skin and bowel care at home should be allowed to continue to do so. If the person reports that bowels are kept functional by means of stool softeners daily and the use of a glycerin suppository every other day, your plan of care should provide for continuation of that routine. With regard to each activity of daily living, you should consult with the individual and plan together for the adaptations that will be necessary in the hospital.

## Conclusion

Activity and rest may be profoundly affected by any illness. Often the patient experiences some degree of immobility, and the nurse must assume a major role in maintaining the patient's ability and functioning. As you assess the patient's activity and rest status, identify particular problems and needs, and undertake those nursing actions that will be most supportive, keep in mind that your goal is the optimal activity level for the patient.

## Care Study   An immobilized patient

John Taylor, a student nurse, was assigned to care for Sarah Mitchell, a ninety-two-year-old woman completely immobilized due to a cerebral vascular accident (stroke).

In the course of his assessment, John noted that, though one leg and arm did flex slightly, Mrs. Mitchell did not change her position in bed at all. Her joints were somewhat stiff although there did not appear to be any deficit in range of motion. The physician's order for Mrs. Mitchell was "activity as tolerated."

After consulting with his instructor, John decided to do complete passive range-of-motion exercises during bathing. Doing so would also present an opportunity to assess joint range accurately. After a rest period, he would obtain assistance and move Mrs. Mitchell into a chair. He arranged for adequate pillows to support her position and decided that a two-person lift would be needed for the transfer.

John carried out his plan for Mrs. Mitchell. As he observed her in the chair, he noted that her respirations were deeper than they had been in bed and that for the first time all morning she opened her eyes and was looking around as if interested in her surroundings. He concluded that this level of activity was beneficial to her and decided to consult with the team leader about entering it on the nursing care plan.

## Study Terms

| | |
|---|---|
| active exercise | immobility |
| active assistive exercise | impaction |
| activities of daily living (A.D.L.s) | incipient pressure ulcer |
| alignment | internal girdle |
| ambulation | ischemia |
| ankylosed | isometric exercise |
| atelectasis | isotonic exercise |
| atony | masceration |
| atrophy | necrosis |
| base of support | osteoporosis |
| body mechanics | passive exercise |
| bridging | phlebitis |
| center of gravity | position changes |
| contracture | postural hypotension |
| dangling | posture |
| decubitus ulcer | pressure ulcer |
| disabled | pulmonary embolism |
| emboli | range-of-motion (R.O.M.) exercise |
| hernia | rehabilitation |
| hypertonic | resistive exercise |
| hypostatic pneumonia | thrombus |
| hypotension | tonus |
| hypotonic | torsion |

## Learning Activities

**1.** For an entire day concentrate on bending from the knees, not the waist.

**2.** Stand in front of a mirror (full-length, if possible) and analyze your posture from the front and from the side. Which features of your posture are correct? incorrect? Try to correct your posture.

**3.** In the clinical area, help to position a patient in bed, both lying and sitting.

**4.** Try using crutches and a walker as if you did not have the full use of one leg.

**5.** In the clinical area, visit the physical therapy department and observe the exercises and activities.

## Relevant Sections in
## Modules for Basic Nursing Skills

| Volume 1 | Module |
|---|---|
| Basic Body Mechanics | 4 |
| Moving the Patient in Bed and Positioning | 12 |
| Range-of-Motion Exercises | 14 |
| Transfer | 15 |
| Ambulation | 16 |

## References

Brower, P., and Hicks, D. "Maintaining Muscle Function in Patients on Bed Rest." *American Journal of Nursing* 72 (July 1972): 1250–1253.

Browse, N. L. *The Physiology and Pathology of Bed Rest.* Springfield, Ill.: Charles C. Thomas, 1965.

Carnevali, D., and Brueckner, S. "Immobilization: Reassessment of a Concept." *American Journal of Nursing* 70 (August 1970): 1502–1507.

Ciuca, R., *et al.* "Active Range of Motion Exercises: A Handbook." *Nursing '78* 8 (August 1978): 45.

Drapeau, J. "Getting Back Into Good Posture: How to Erase Your Lumbar Aches." *Nursing '75* 5 (May 1975): 63–65.

Ford, J. R., and Duckworth, B. "Moving a Dependent Patient Safely, Comfortably: Part 1: Positioning." *Nursing '76* 1 (January 1976): 27–36.

Foss, G. "Body Mechanics: Use Your Head and Save Your Back." *Nursing '73* 3 (March 1973): 25–32.

———. "Breaking Architectural Barriers with Crutches, Wheelchairs, Walkers." *Nursing '73* 3 (March 1973): 16–31.

Gordon, M. "Assessing Activity Tolerance." *American Journal of Nursing* 76 (January 1976): 72–75.

Hoover, S. A. "Job-Related Back Injuries in a Hospital." *American Journal of Nursing* 71 (November 1971): 2078–2079.

Hrobsky, A. "The Patient on a CircOlectric Bed." *American Journal of Nursing* 71 (December 1971): 2353.

Jordan, H. S., and Kauchak, M. A. "Transfer Techniques." *Nursing '73* 3 (March 1973): 19–22.

Kamentetz, H. L. "Exercise for the Elderly." *American Journal of Nursing* 72 (August 1972): 1401.

Olson, E. V., ed. "The Hazards of Immobility." *American Journal of Nursing* 67 (April 1967): 779–797. Supplement.

Works, R. F. "Hints on Lifting and Pulling." *American Journal of Nursing* 72 (February 1972): 260–261.

Young, C., Sr. "Exercise: How to Use It to Decrease Complications in Immobilized Patients." *Nursing '75* 5 (March 1975): 81.

tions decrease; digestive juices subside to some degree; and the kidneys become less productive. The basal metabolism rate (BMR) decreases as muscle relaxation increases. Most of the reflexes weaken or disappear entirely, with the important exception of the cough reflex. The cough reflex protects the sleeping person from foreign bodies lodging in the respiratory tract. During sleep, the mind focuses on its internal environment. The activities of the mind during sleep will be considered in detail shortly.

## The Causes of Sleep

Just what causes sleep is unknown. Though not crucial to the provision of care, theories of sleep hold considerable interest. Theorists have differed in characterizing the origins of sleep as primarily chemical, vascular, pituitary, neurohormonal, feedback-related, or instinctual.

The *chemical* theory holds that sleep is brought on by an increase of carbon dioxide in the blood, which affects brain functioning. However, decreased physical activity could in turn account for the increase in carbon dioxide. Although it is commonplace for drowsiness to develop in inadequately oxygenated surroundings, the chemical theory has proved inadequate in explaining the more complex findings about sleep.

The *vascular* theory rests on the assumption that the fall in blood pressure that occurs during sleep decreases the flow of blood within the brain, sustaining the state of unconsciousness. Current studies clearly show, however, that the opposite is the case: cerebrovascular blood flow increases during sleep.

It has long been thought that the *pituitary*, a small gland at the base of the brain, is a regulator of sleep, if not its primary activator. Nevertheless, people whose pituitary glands are removed surgically do not experience great changes in their sleep habits.

Neurophysiologists, working on the *neurohormonal* theory, have singled out the neurohormone serotonin as a possible causative agent of sleep. When this substance is injected directly into the cerebral vascular system of an animal, sleep immediately ensues.

One of the most promising theories to date— and a very complicated one—is the *feedback* theory, which proposes that, after a period of neuronal activity during which electrical impulses are relayed throughout the system, fatigue occurs at the synapses, or connections between nerve cells, bringing on sleep.

Finally, some dismiss the entire controversy by stating plainly that sleep is *instinctual*.

## The Stages of Sleep

To the person who awakens in the morning feeling fairly well rested, sleep may seem no more or less than a period of unawareness and quiescence, highlighted by an occasional dream and the sensation of turning. However, sleep researchers have demonstrated that the nature of sleep is far more active and complicated than had been supposed.

Dement, Kleitman, and Oswald, three prominent researchers working separately, have found that the character of sleep changes during a given sleeping episode, progressing through sequential stages. Their findings are based on the use of the *electroencephalograph* (EEG), a machine that measures and records the electrical energy produced by the *cortex*, or thin outer layer of the brain (see Fig-

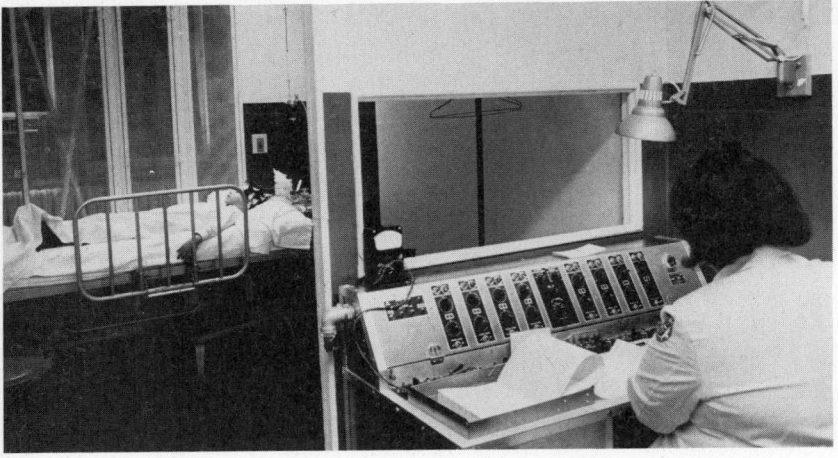

**Figure 20.2**
The electroencephalograph measures
sleep patterns. (Elizabeth Wilcox)

ure 20.2). The recording is called an *electroencephalogram,* or tracing.

According to Dement, Kleitman, and Oswald,
a typical episode of sleep consists of from four to
six complete cycles, each of which is composed of
five stages. Each of the five stages has its own
special characteristics. The sleep cycle is illustrated
in Figure 20.3.

## Stage I

Stage I most closely resembles wakefulness and
produces a recording of brain activity similar to
that of a person who is awake, except for a few
slow waves on the tracing. Muscles retain their
tone, though a slow rolling of the eyes takes place.
If aroused during this stage, a person will often
deny having slept, saying that he or she was "just
drifting off"—though sleep had actually begun.

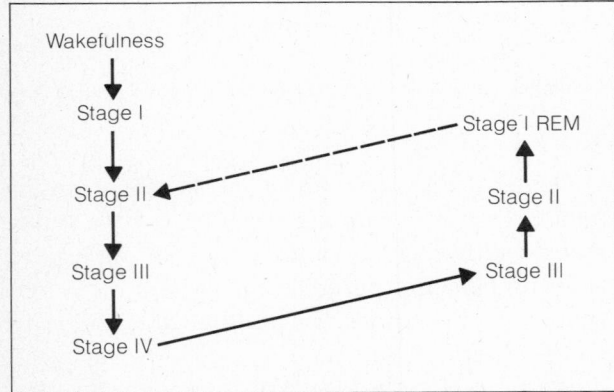

**Figure 20.3   The sleep cycle**

## Stage II

Stage II marks the beginning of muscle relaxation.
The EEG waves become more regular and rounded.
The person appears asleep but can still be aroused
by calling his or her name. Considerable turning
and shifting in bed accompanies progression toward the next stage.

## Stage III

Stage III consists of deeper sleep, manifested in
further slowing and rounding of the EEG tracing
and loss of muscle tone. Some reflexes diminish
at this point, and snoring may occur. The person
no longer responds to name call and can be
aroused only by touch.

## Stage IV

Stage IV, the period of deepest sleep, is characterized by total relaxation and the onset of dreaming. The EEG tracing appears as very large, slow
waves. The muscles are in their most relaxed state
since the onset of sleep. The dreams that occur
during this stage have a conventional, everyday
quality and are typically extensions or revisions of
the preceding day's events or familiar experiences.
This is in distinct contrast to the dreams that occur
in REM sleep.

Twenty to thirty minutes elapse between initially falling asleep and Stage IV. At this point the
process is reversed: the sleeper begins an ascent

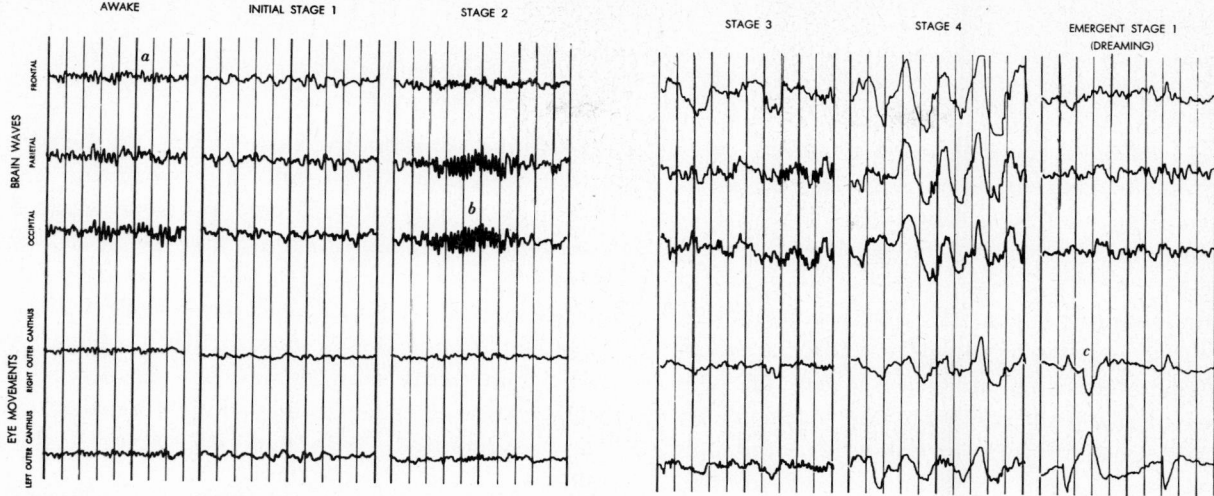

**Figure 20.4  Electroencephalographic tracings of sleep stages**
From Nathaniel Kleitman, "Patterns of Dreaming," Scientific American, November 1960, pp. 46–47. Courtesy of William Dement, Stanford University School of Medicine.

from Stage IV through Stage III to Stage II and then enters the most profound stage of sleep, REM sleep.

## REM Sleep

Although sometimes referred to as Stage I REM (rapid eye movement), REM sleep is a distinct phenomenon and quite different from Stage I. The characteristics of REM sleep are dramatic. Both eyes move rapidly back and forth horizontally. One observer has reported occasional twitching of the ears, and body twitching is not uncommon. With the exception of the eyes, the muscles are almost totally relaxed. Reflexes are even more diminished than in Stage IV. However, both blood pressure and respirations increase. Although the muscles are completely relaxed, cortical activity (activity in the outer, or thinking, portion of the brain) is high. The tracing is varied and quite active, not unlike that of waking. The dreams that take place frequently during REM sleep are much more vividly detailed than those of Stage IV and may be colorful, violent, or erotic. The contradiction between the relaxation of the muscles and the extreme activity of the brain leads some to refer to REM sleep as *paradoxic sleep*. This term is used interchangeably with REM and Stage I REM.

With the end of REM sleep, one sleep cycle has been completed. The entire cycle usually takes about ninety minutes. The next cycle begins with entry into Stage II sleep. As the night progresses, Stages III and IV decrease in length and REM increases. Though scientists dispute the precise purpose of REM sleep, they seem to agree that it is essential.

Some of the findings of sleep research may well have significance for nurses. First, people suffering from schizophrenia experience much less REM sleep than do nonschizophrenics. Second, a recent investigation of the causes of SIDS (sudden infant death syndrome) has led to the theory that respiratory failure in infants is caused by neurological dysfunction during Stage IV or REM sleep.

Sleep-deprivation studies appear to demonstrate that the duration of REM sleep is even more important than the total hours of sleep. Whether REM sleep serves as a psychic outlet for stress and tension accrued during the waking hours or as a data-processing mechanism that establishes new neural pathways is an interesting question. However, these conjectures are less important to you as a nurse than is understanding that both Stage IV and REM sleep are essential to human functioning in a manner that is not fully understood.

New findings suggest that we also have "waking cycles" that correspond to sleep cycles. The human brain appears to become more active for a short period approximately every ninety minutes (Chase, 1979). Minor variations among individuals do occur.

# Insomnia

*Insomnia*—inability to sleep—is a relatively common problem. Patients with insomnia tend to fall into two categories: those who have difficulty falling asleep and those who have trouble staying asleep.

Some insomnia is caused by such contributing factors as pain, emotional upset, and poor sleeping conditions. Eliminating the cause of such sleeplessness usually brings about relief. However, as much as 10 to 15 percent of the population suffers from chronic insomnia, a more troublesome phenomenon whose cause is not so evident.

It is often a longstanding sleep pattern on the part of the individual. The resulting fear of being unable to sleep only intensifies the problem. Medical intervention, including drugs, may be necessary until new patterns are established. If used, sleep-inducing drugs should be carefully selected for suitability to the patient's particular problem. A short-acting drug may be sufficient for a patient who cannot fall asleep, while a longer-acting drug may be required for a patient unable to stay asleep.

# Age and Sleep

Almost as if resting in preparation for life's journey, the infant spends many more hours of the day sleeping than does the adult. Of this time, approximately 50 percent is spent in REM sleep. During the REM stages, grimacing, twitching, and sucking movements are frequent.

The adult, on the other hand, experiences four to six sleep cycles per night, averaging a total of 7.9 hours of sleep. Of this time, 23 percent is REM sleep. There are no appreciable differences between males and females with regard to sleep.

Elderly people experience less Stage III, Stage IV, and REM sleep than do infants and adults. As little as 15 to 18 percent of total sleep may be REM. Nurses should keep in mind that, though the aged may appear to sleep a great deal, they experience less total sleep than younger people because of frequent awakenings. The discomforts associated with many degenerative conditions are not conducive to sleep. Arthritic pain can cause frequent interruptions in the sleep pattern. The patient with respiratory problems is often forced to sleep in an almost upright position, which interferes with sleep. And urinary urgency in the elderly also interrupts sleep.

# Sleep Deprivation

*Sleep deprivation* can occur when the duration of sleep is inadequate or when sleep time is repeatedly interrupted, especially during Stage IV or the REM stages. Any individual who must work variable shifts with intervening days off, such as a nurse, may experience sleep deprivation. Patients may be sleep-deprived due to pain, drugs, or the requirements of constant nursing care.

Sleep deprivation studies employ willing subjects to sleep in the laboratory. When the EEG indicates that the person is dreaming, usually during Stage IV or REM, the subject is awakened and then allowed to return to sleep. This arousal at the onset of dreaming is repeated over and over until certain signs and behaviors indicate that the subject is experiencing sleep deprivation. Some studies do not allow the subject to sleep at all for long periods of time.

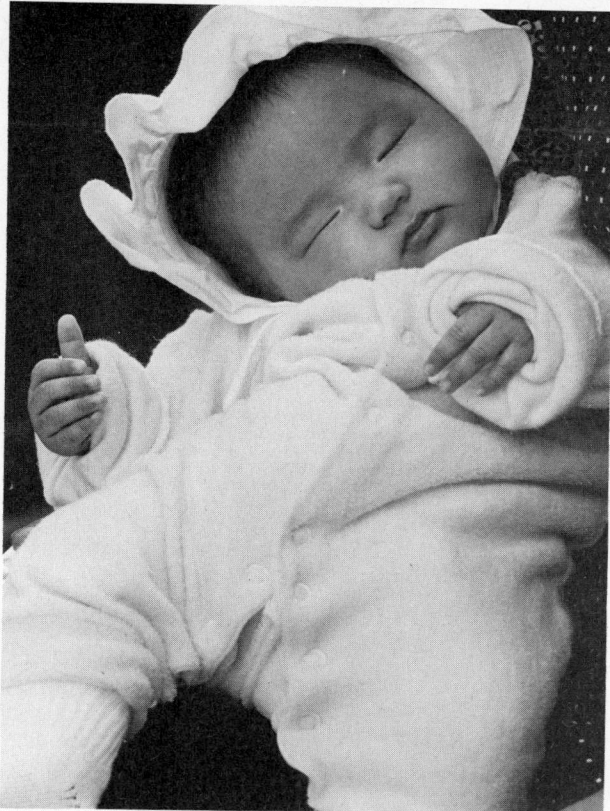

**Figure 20.5**
Infants' sleep patterns differ from those of adults. (David Austen/Stock, Boston)

previous few days. Has the patient been in intensive care for some time, experiencing numerous interruptions of sleep? Has the patient recently been placed on REM-inhibiting drugs? Does the chart indicate several nights of poor sleep due to pain or stress?

Such information enables you to consider signs and symptoms that might indicate the patient is sleep-deprived. Irritability, intermittent dozing, frequent complaints of pain inconsistent in degree with the underlying condition, and complaints of fatigue are all noteworthy.

Hallucinations have been reported in cases of extended periods of sleeplessness. Studies also show that prolonged sleep deprivation lowers the seizure threshold as well as the pain threshold. People with seizure disorders, such as epilepsy, may have convulsions. Thus nurses who do health teaching should caution epileptic patients against undue sleep loss or jobs that require frequent changes in schedule. It is an interesting peripheral fact that for several days after a seizure, epileptics appear to experience much less REM sleep than usual. Perhaps the seizure serves in some fashion as a substitute for the REM sleep the individual usually needs.

## Sleep Deprivation and Nursing Care

Knowledge of the effects of sleep deprivation can guide us in the care of patients. Because of heightened sensitivity to pain, you should closely monitor the discomfort of sleep-deprived patients. Since concentration is impaired to some degree, the sleep-deprived patient may be resistant to health teaching. You may thus wish to delay teaching until the patient is more rested. Moreover, the "irritable" patient may be simply a tired patient who needs understanding and better planning to allow for sufficient sleep.

Studies have repeatedly shown that at least some of the confusion and disorientation displayed by patients in intensive-care units is caused by sleep deprivation resulting from continual interruption of Stages III and IV and REM sleep for vital-sign monitoring, procedures, and treatments. Careful planning so that nursing care can be performed in specified time blocks enables patients to sleep for longer uninterrupted periods.

Initially, sleep deprivation causes a decrease in attention span, irritability, slowed reactions, and heightened sensitivity to pain or a lowered pain threshold. These reactions are significant for nurses responsible for alleviating the pain of their patients. Sleep deprivation also results in an inability to perform repetitive tasks. As deprivation becomes more pronounced, the behavioral and physiological signs intensify. The subject may become confused or even manifest disorientation or psychosis (a state of being out of touch with reality).

Many objective signs also accompany sleep deprivation. Body temperature fluctuates and the body's chemistries are variant. For example, the potassium in the urine is elevated by sleep loss.

## Assessment of Sleep Deprivation

To assess sleep deprivation accurately, one must be familiar with the patient's situation during the

# Drugs and Sleep

The work of Evans (1970) and others reveals that *hypnotics*—drugs used to induce sleep—shorten the REM sleep stage, though the total duration of sleep may be lengthened. Many sleep medications, including the group called barbiturates, decrease REM sleep. None of the hypnotics induces natural sleep.

Amphetamines also inhibit REM sleep. This class of drugs, known colloquially as "speed" or "uppers," figures prominently in drug abuse, and much of the aberrant behavior of "speed freaks" may be attributable to long-term REM sleep deprivation.

To a lesser degree, the use of alcohol also shortens REM sleep. People who consume large quantities of alcohol over an extended time experience some of the same symptoms of REM deprivation as people on other drugs.

Discontinuing any of these drugs causes abnormally extended periods of REM sleep, which is probably a catch-up mechanism. This phenomenon is called *REM rebound*. It is very important for the nurse to know that the patient withdrawing from these drugs also frequently experiences vivid, frightening nightmares. If the person is made so uncomfortable by these episodes as to feel a need to return to the drug, a cycle of drug dependence can begin. Fortunately, the withdrawal period is relatively short. Talking with the patient about the feelings that accompany withdrawal and their cause may be a highly valuable service. Offering emotional support may prevent the patient from using drugs unnecessarily.

# Nursing Intervention

The hospital is not conducive to sleep. It is unfamiliar and full of strange sounds, odors, and people. The bed, furniture, and room itself are far different from what the patient is used to. Accompanying all this is the patient's illness or prospective surgery and the attendant anxiety. Because

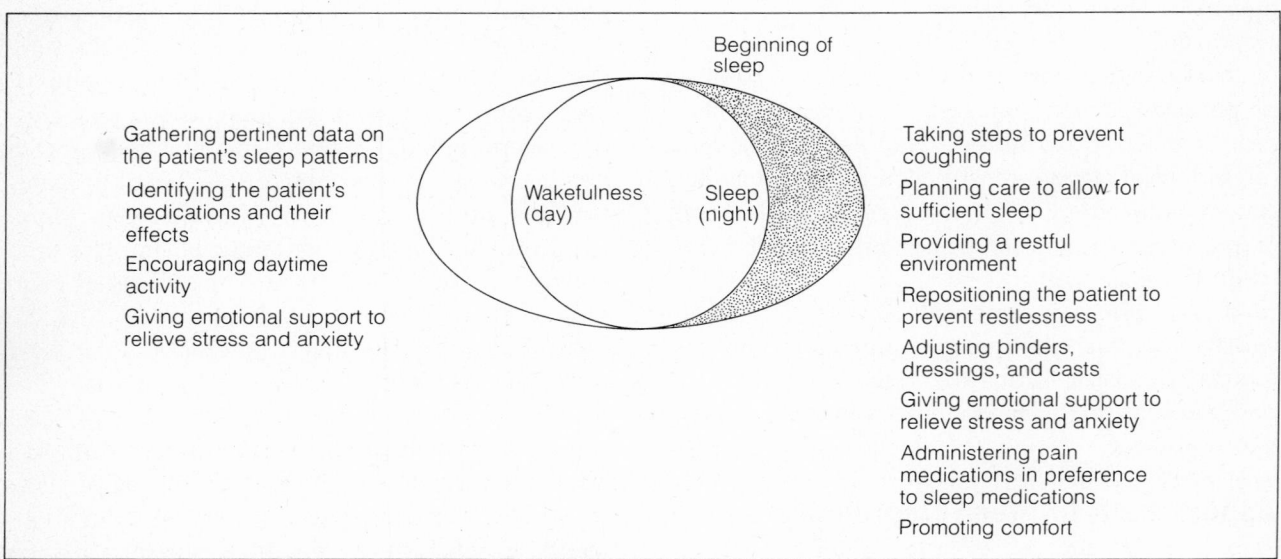

**Figure 20.6  Nursing actions that promote sleep**

adequate sleep is so important for an ill person, nurses should make every effort to assess, identify problems, intervene, and evaluate the patient's basic need for sleep. There are many actions nurses can take to help the patient sleep (see Figure 20.6).

## Gathering Pertinent Data on the Patient's Sleep Patterns

Few nursing history forms ask about the patient's sleep patterns. One might add such information as the number of hours of sleep the patient normally needs, usual bedtime, and factors conducive or disturbing to the patient's sleep. For example, a ticking clock soothes some people and irritates others.

## Identifying the Patient's Medications and Their Effects

Awareness of medications being given or withdrawn enables the nurse to observe for signs of sleep problems and to offer reassurance if unpleasant dreams or other side effects occur. Although nurses do not order medications for patients, our assessments of possible drug effects, particularly with relationship to sleep, can be very helpful to the physician when the patient's drugs are reviewed for renewal.

## Taking Steps to Prevent Coughing

If the patient has been troubled by a cough, it is sometimes helpful to instruct him or her to deep-breathe and cough in the high Fowler's or sitting position (see Module 12, "Moving the Patient in Bed and Positioning"), just before sleep. It is desirable to cough up and expectorate any secretions.

The recumbent position can increase bronchial and nasal secretions, aggravating a cough. Anticipating this outcome in the case of the respiratory patient, and securing an order for an appropriate cough medication before the patient's bedtime, may prevent hours of sleeplessness.

## Planning Care to Allow for Sufficient Sleep

Whether to facilitate an uninterrupted night's sleep or a daytime nap, care can be carefully planned in blocks to allow for complete sleep cycles. For critically ill patients, of course, this may prove less feasible.

## Encouraging Daytime Activity

Boredom often causes bedridden patients to sleep intermittently throughout the day, becoming wakeful and demanding at night. You might contact the family or occupational therapy department or, on your own initiative, plan interesting activities and/or exercises for such a patient during the day. A patient who is alert and active in the daytime tends to sleep more soundly at night.

## Providing a Restful Environment

Eliminating or minimizing disturbing factors in the hospital environment is also helpful. Unpleasant odors, excessively warm or cool temperatures, and unnecessary lights and noises—including conversation in proximity of the patient—may all prove distracting and interfere with sleep.

## Repositioning the Patient to Prevent Restlessness

The non-ill person is very active throughout the sleeping period and has frequent turnings. Thus some patients may sleep restlessly or sporadically simply because of their inability to turn. Repositioning the restless patient can often help promote sound sleep by lessening muscle fatigue.

## Adjusting Binders, Dressings, and Casts

Binders, dressings, and casts also cause discomfort and restlessness. Rewrapping a binder, reinforcing or replacing dressings, and padding or repositioning casts can easily alleviate or prevent such a problem.

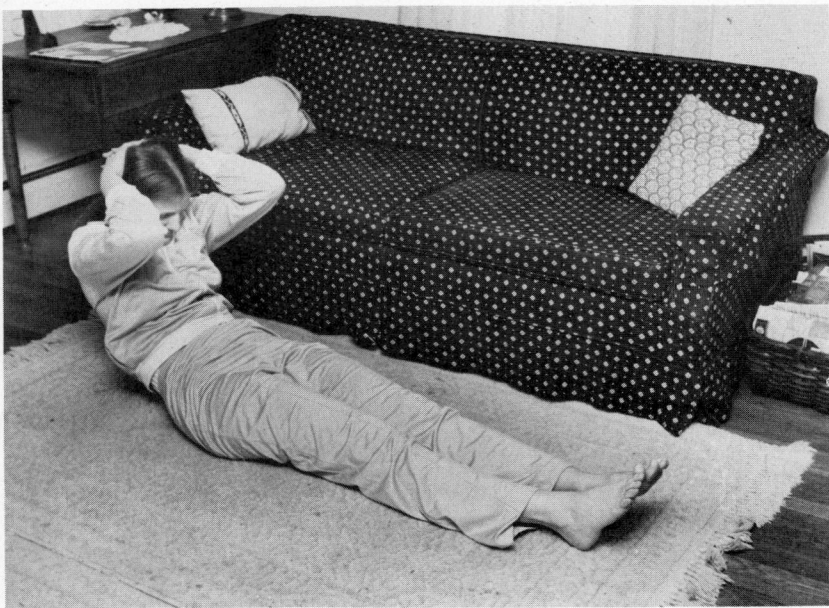

**Figure 20.7**
A nurse working on the night shift may need to exercise to relax prior to sleep. (Russ Kinne/Photo Researchers, Inc.)

## Giving Emotional Support to Relieve Stress and Anxiety

As well as providing physical comfort, the nurse strives to provide for maximum peace of mind, remembering that stress and anxiety frequently cause restlessness and/or insomnia. Such anxiety could be related to tests just performed or about to be performed, apprehension over the condition, or the strangeness of the hospital environment. The nurse who listens and discusses such concerns with the patient is promoting sleep by providing maximum peace of mind.

## Administering Pain Medications in Preference to Sleep Medications

If sleep is disturbed due to pain, it is much more sensible and helpful to administer the prescribed pain medication than a sleeping medication. It is undesirable to give medication known to interfere with REM sleep since relief of pain often allows sleep to ensue naturally.

## Promoting Comfort

The value of comfort-promoting measures cannot be underestimated. The nurse who spends time providing care before the patient's bedtime may considerably minimize the need for sleep medications. An unhurried backrub, the straightening or replacement of wrinkled or soiled linens, and perhaps a warm, noncaffeinated beverage all enhance the ability to sleep. Offering the bedpan or urinal at bedtime prevents sleep from being interrupted.

## Nurses and Sleep

Nurses are themselves susceptible to sleep disturbances and sleep deprivation due to irregular hours and shift changes. Some nurses adjust more easily than others. A nurse who has worked the night shift for a number of years may slip more easily into a pattern of night work punctuated by a two-days-off rotation than a nurse who works four nights consecutively and then shifts back to the day shift after two days off. Studies show that it takes as long as ten days for some individuals who have worked night shifts to revert to normal daytime body temperatures and urine potassium levels (Felton, 1976). It is also known that nurses who transfer from the night shift to day work experience less REM sleep for a while (Lanuza, 1976). We must be cognizant of our usual sleep patterns and how we react to sleep disturbances. Mild depression is quite common. Irritability may strain interpersonal relations. Medication errors and deviations from aseptic technique, which can endanger the patients, can occur if the nurse is overly tired.

There are some measures that can be taken to lessen the effects of sleep deprivation on shift nurses. If possible, begin gradually adjusting your sleeping hours several days in advance of a shift change. Go to sleep an hour or two earlier or later, depending on what your new shift will be. Be sure to keep up your nutritional level and exercise.

As a nurse you should be particularly vigilant about any effects of fluctuating working hours that may jeopardize you or the patient. Avoiding sleep loss as much as possible promotes safe practice.

## Conclusion

Illness causes stress and places undue demands on both the physiological and psychological response systems of the individual. Thus sleep is even more important than usual to people who are ill. To provide for adequate sleep when planning nursing care and to intervene appropriately when sleep problems arise are essential elements of good nursing practice.

## Care Study   A patient with sleep deprivation

Mrs. Julie Stafford is a fifty-seven-year-old patient with bronchitis and emphysema. A long-term heavy smoker, Mrs. Stafford has experienced increasing respiratory difficulty over the past few years. In recent weeks the infection has made breathing so difficult that Mrs. Stafford has become dependent on frequent use of an IPPB (Intermittent Positive Pressure Breathing) apparatus.

On admission Mrs. Stafford reported feeling anxious as well as "generally tired" and appeared pale. Her respirations were shallow and rapid. Mr. Stafford said his wife had been sleeping poorly for two to three weeks.

The physician's orders include bedrest, an antibiotic, a mild tranquilizer, pain medication, and IPPB treatments every two hours.

The staff nurse assigned to Mrs. Stafford begins her assessment by reading the data in the record, which notes the history of sleeping poorly, tiredness and anxiety, and the physician's orders. A visit to Mrs. Stafford confirms the persistence of the same concerns. The nurse notes the patient's exhausted appearance. A menu order lies on the bedside table unmarked. When asked if she would like to complete the form or needs help to do so, Mrs. Stafford replies, in a mildly irritated manner, "I really don't care what I eat. I just want to be left alone." When asked if her husband has left the hospital, she replies, "I really can't remember." She requests pain medication every three hours. Her medical and nursing management is such that Mrs. Stafford's sleep is interrupted about once an hour. Mrs. Stafford appears to be experiencing sleep deprivation.

The staff nurse determines that nursing intervention is needed. Knowing that the normal sleep cycle lasts about ninety minutes, she thinks the patient needs an extended period of uninterrupted sleep. The nurse arranges to talk with the physician, to whom she describes the patient's sleep history and behavior. The physician and nurse examine the current blood gas reports and, noting improvement, decide that the 2:00 p.m. IPPB treatment might be omitted. The physician writes the order to omit the treatment, and the plan is explained to the patient. Mrs. Stafford seems to welcome the intervention. At 12:00 she receives her noon meal, medications, IPPB treatment, and a relaxing backrub. The hospital telephone operator is instructed not to put through calls to the patient for four hours. The room is darkened. A sign noting the period during which the patient is not to be disturbed is attached to the closed door of the room. At 3:00, the plan is explained to the p.m. staff nurse.

Evaluation by the staff nurse at the 4:00 p.m. report is positive. Mrs. Stafford awakens from four hours of deep sleep stating that she feels "so much better." She appears to breathe more easily and requests a colorful gown in preparation for evening visiting hours.

## Study Terms

chemical theory of sleep
circadian rhythm
cortex
cough reflex
electroencephalogram
electroencephalograph (EEG)
feedback theory of sleep
hypnotics
insomnia
instinctual theory of sleep
neurohormonal theory of sleep
paradoxic sleep
pituitary theory of sleep
REM (rapid eye movement) sleep
REM rebound
sleep cycle
sleep deprivation
sleep stage
vascular theory of sleep

## Learning Activities

1. Keep a record of your hours of sleep per night for one week. What is your nightly average? Is this pattern representative of your sleep habits? If not, why?

2. Read at least one current article on drugs and sleep.

3. Write out questions that might be used in taking a patient's sleep history.

4. Record a seriously ill patient's sleep time, using your own observation and the record, over a forty-eight-hour period.

5. How do you assess the sleep status of the patient in Activity 4? What intervention would you recommend, if any?

## References

Chase, Michael H. "Every Ninety Minutes, a Brainstorm." *Psychology Today* 13 (November 1979): 172.

Evans, J. I., and Ogunremi, O. "Sleep and Hypnotics: Further Experiments." *British Medical Journal* (August 1970): 310–312.

Felton, Geraldine. "Body Rhythm Effects on Rotating Work Shifts." *Nursing Digest* 4 (April 1976): 29–32.

Garner, Howard G. "You May Have to Leave the Hospital to Get Well." *Supervisor Nurse* 9 (September 1978): 76–79.

Grant, Donna Allen, and Klell, Cynthia. "For Goodness Sake—Let Your Patients Sleep." *Nursing '74* 4 (November 1974): 54–57.

Kales, A., *et al.* "Hypnotics and Altered Sleep–Dream Patterns." *Archives of General Psychiatry* 73 (September 1970): 211–218.

Klein, K. E., *et al.* "Circadian Rhythm of Pilot's Efficiency and Effects of Multiple Time Zone Travel." *Aerospace Medicine* 41 (1970): 125–132.

Kleitman, N. *Sleep and Wakefulness*, rev. ed. Chicago: University of Chicago Press, 1963.

Lanuza, Dorothy M. "Circadian Rhythms of Mental Efficiency and Performance." *Nursing Clinics of North America* 11 (December 1976): 583–593.

Lavie, P., *et al.* "Ultradian Rhythms: The 90-Minute Clock Inside Us, Part 2." *Psychology Today* 8 (May 1975): 54–56.

Long, B. "Sleep." *American Journal of Nursing* 69 (September 1969): 1896–1899.

Luce, G. G. "Internal Tempos: To Live in Harmony With the Earth, Trust Your Body Rhythms, Part 1." *Psychology Today* 8 (May 1975): 52–53.

O'Dell, M. L. "Human Biorhythmology: Implications for Nursing Practice." *Nursing Forum* 14 (January 1975): 43–47.

Oswald, I. "Human Brain Protein, Drugs and Dreams." *Nature* 233 (1969): 893–897.

———. "The Biological Clock and Shift-Work." *Nursing Times* 67 (September 1971): 1207–1208.

Owen, M., and Bliss, E. "Sleep Loss and Cerebral Excitability." *American Journal of Physiology* 18 (January 1970): 171–179.

Wyeth, R. J. *Treatment of Insomnia.* National Institute of Mental Health. Washington, D.C.: U.S. Government Printing Office, 1973.

Zelechowski, Gina Pugliese. "Helping Your Patient Sleep: Planning Instead of Pills." *Nursing '77* 7 (March 1977): 81–84.

# Chapter 21
# Nutrition

## Objectives

After completing this chapter, you should be able to:
1. Define good nutrition, describing in detail how to evaluate a diet.
2. Discuss the role of sociocultural factors in dietary intake.
3. List information necessary for nutritional assessment.
4. Outline a variety of ways the nurse can help the patient meet nutritional needs.
5. Outline ways the nurse can help the patient with fluid intake.
6. Describe nursing approaches to malnutrition, obesity, nausea, and vomiting.

## Outline

Food and water are among human beings' most basic needs. A person cannot go without water for more than a few days; the body soon becomes unable to function. One can survive somewhat longer without food, because the body can consume its own stores of fat and protein to provide for its most essential functions. But this supply is limited, and very soon the body cannot function.

Even those who nursed in antiquity, without education or an understanding of disease processes, were aware of the value of nourishing food. Through trial and error, they had found some foods more helpful than others in restoring health. They also recognized that, in certain illnesses, some foods are better tolerated than others. Many nineteenth-century home nursing manuals focused mainly on the preparation of special broths and other foods for the sick person. Awareness of invalids' need for fluids is long-standing, and most such foods were in liquid or semiliquid form.

## Basic Nutrients

In the broadest sense, good nutrition consists of eating foods that provide all the nutrients needed by the body in amounts adequate for *energy, maintenance, repair, replacement* of tissue, and—in the young—*growth*. It also involves avoiding an excessive amount of any nutrient that can damage the body.

As our knowledge of body physiology and our understanding of foods have grown, the definition of good nutrition has expanded. We now recognize as essential a wide variety of nutrients and are beginning to ascertain the optimum amount of each that is needed for good health.

### Carbohydrates

*Carbohydrates* are the starches and sugars in the diet. All fruits and vegetables have some carbohydrate content, but cereal grain products are the major source. Carbohydrates have roughly the same caloric value as proteins (four calories per gram), but because they require less extensive metabolism, they are available more quickly for energy. A majority of the calories in most diets are consumed in the form of carbohydrates, because they are low-cost, readily available foods. This is appropriate, because most primarily carbohydrate foods also contain needed vitamins, minerals, and even some plant proteins. The only exceptions are refined simple sugars, which do not have other food value. Providing additional carbohydrate is a way of increasing calorie level to meet the special requirements of growth or unusual activity. Carbohydrate intake exceeding current need is converted in limited amounts to glycogen (an animal starch) for storage in the liver. Carbohydrate in excess of that level is converted to fat for long-term storage.

### Proteins

*Proteins* are the basic material for building and repairing body tissue. Amounts in excess of these needs are broken down into carbohydrates and nitrogen; the nitrogen is excreted and the carbohydrate is used just as is dietary carbohydrate. It is important to understand this process when advising people on their diets. Protein foods are usually the most expensive items in the diet, but large amounts are not necessary. Although protein needs may rise due to illness or injury, you will find that some people have exaggerated views of how much protein is required. When money is limited, it is quite satisfactory to consume only the necessary amount of protein, deriving additional calories from carbohydrate. Proteins do have an additional value when calorie control is necessary, in that their slow digestion and metabolism makes for long-sustained calorie availability. Proteins are found in large quantities in meat, eggs, fish, and milk products. Some vegetables—especially legumes such as dry beans and peas—and nuts and whole grains also contain proteins.

## Fats

*Fats* are the most concentrated form of food energy. Though necessary to the diet because they serve as building blocks for essential body components and as vehicles for the transport of certain fat-soluble vitamins, large amounts of fats can quickly raise the calorie value of the diet to an undesirable level. Excessive fats, especially saturated fats, are also receiving attention as contributory factors in coronary artery disease. Therefore, it is currently recommended that no more than 25 percent of dietary calories be derived from fats. Butter, margarine, and cooking oils are a major source of fat. There is also significant fat content in such protein foods as meat, cheese, and whole milk.

## Minerals

*Minerals* are present in a number of foods. Some, such as calcium and iron, are needed in fairly large amounts; others, such as copper and zinc are needed in only minute traces. Excesses and deficiencies of these trace minerals are receiving increasing attention for their possible role in the origin of illness. Probably the most common mineral deficiency is iron deficiency in women who are in the reproductive years, since the loss of menstrual blood increases the body's need for iron. The most effective means of supplying it is to consume adequate dietary iron. Iron appears in large quantities in red meats and liver, and it is also found in dark green leafy vegetables, whole-grain cereals, and some dried fruits such as raisins.

## Vitamins

*Vitamins* are minute organic substances essential to body processes. The list of vitamins is still growing, as more are discovered. Vitamins are found in a variety of foods. Fat-soluble vitamins are stored by the body, allowing for intake to fluctuate. The majority of vitamins, however, are water-soluble, and must be ingested daily because amounts not currently needed are rapidly excreted. A well-balanced diet is the best source of vitamins. The routine use of vitamin supplements is not necessary for individuals in good health.

## Fiber

The need for nondigestible *fiber* in the diet has recently begun receiving increased attention. Fiber, or roughage, is composed mainly of cellulose and is found in fresh fruits and vegetables and in whole-grain cereal products, both raw and cooked. These fibers increase the bulk of the stool, making it pass along the bowel more easily, which helps to prevent constipation. Recent research has also demonstrated a higher incidence of certain diseases of the bowel in those who eat highly refined diets lacking fiber or roughage. Though the exact relationship has not been determined, this finding underlines the need for a highly varied diet, restricted only when absolutely necessary. A wide range of foods makes probable an adequate intake of needed nutrients of which science is still ignorant.

# Recommended Diet

The Food and Nutrition Board of the National Research Council has established a standard called the *Recommended Dietary Allowance* (RDA) for most nutrients. Differing recommendations are made for different age levels and, after age nine, for males and females. There are also special recommendations for pregnant women and nursing mothers. The exact recommendations may be found in a nutrition textbook. They are very generous, providing for considerable variance among individuals and for changes in needs due to minor illness. They do not, however, allow for needs caused by major illness or trauma. Recommendations are given for all nutrients on which there

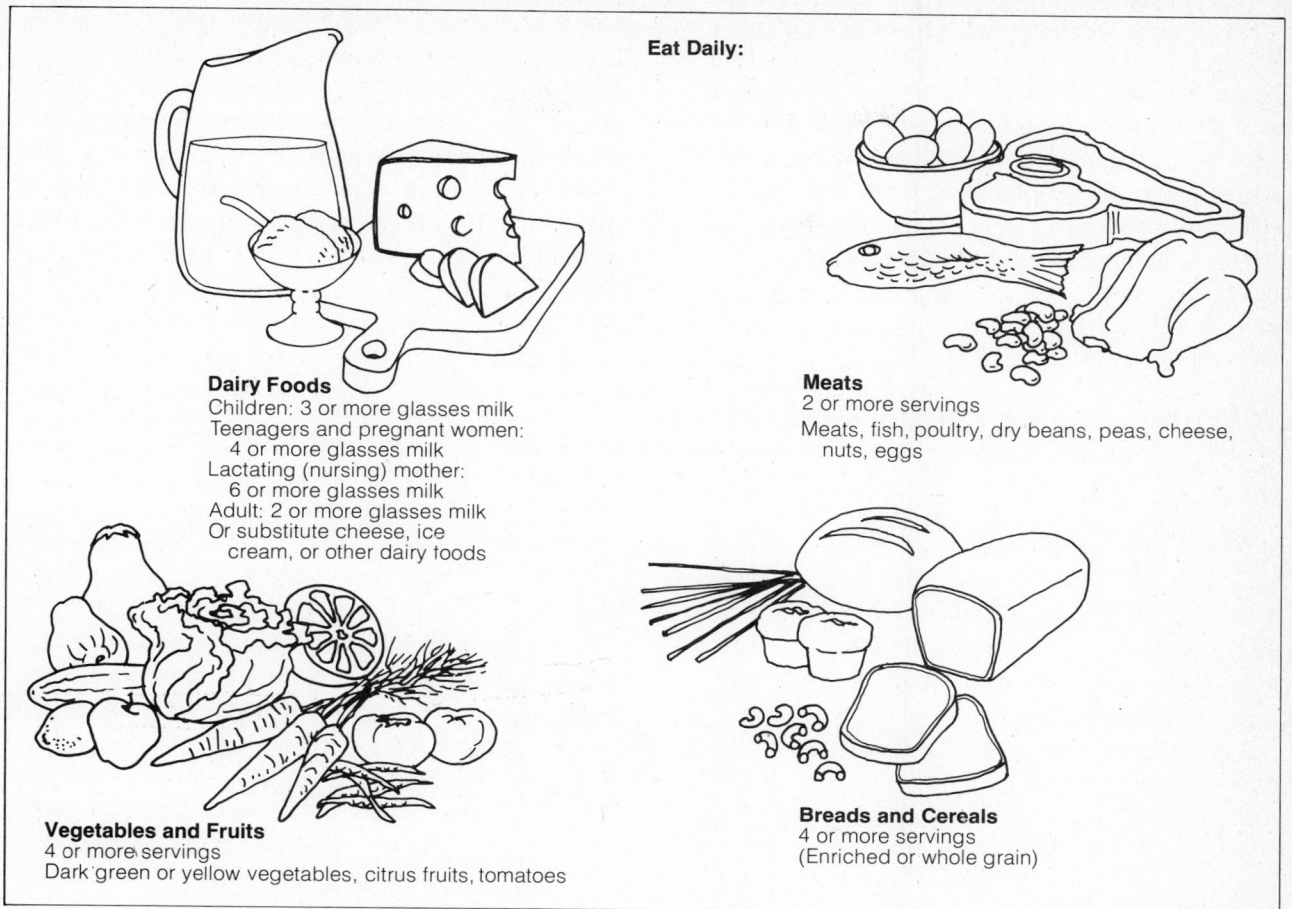

**Eat Daily:**

**Dairy Foods**
Children: 3 or more glasses milk
Teenagers and pregnant women:
    4 or more glasses milk
Lactating (nursing) mother:
    6 or more glasses milk
Adult: 2 or more glasses milk
Or substitute cheese, ice
    cream, or other dairy foods

**Meats**
2 or more servings
Meats, fish, poultry, dry beans, peas, cheese,
    nuts, eggs

**Vegetables and Fruits**
4 or more servings
Dark green or yellow vegetables, citrus fruits, tomatoes

**Breads and Cereals**
4 or more servings
(Enriched or whole grain)

**Figure 21.1   The four basic food groups**

exist sufficient research data to establish need. Thus there are no recommendations for nutrients necessary in very small amounts or those for which the exact need has not yet been established.

The RDA standard may not be attainable by low-income persons or those who live in parts of the world where food supplies are limited. Minimum daily requirements have been established by some official groups, including the Canadian government. Because these standards do not take individual variations into consideration, they are of limited value. However, they may be useful in evaluating diets to establish gross deficiency or malnutrition.

Nutritionists at the U.S. Department of Agriculture have devised a simple way to plan meals that supply the RDA, called the *Basic Four* (see Figure 21.1). This approach is based on the prevailing American dietary pattern, and meal patterns that do not conform to the standards of the Basic Four may be very nutritious and supply all the RDA. Thus it is much more accurate (though far more complex) to evaluate a diet in terms of the RDA than of the Basic Four.

Recent research reveals that individual variations in need may be much greater than was previously thought. The predominantly European background of most Americans has meant that the universal value of milk has gone undisputed. Now we have evidence that some people, primarily of Asian and African origin, do not have the digestive enzymes necessary to utilize milk properly after the age of three or four years. For these people, milk is not merely of little value but actually harmful, causing gas, diarrhea, and digestive upsets. Thus the concept of good nutrition must be constantly modified in light of the latest knowledge.

Interest in vegetarian diets is widespread, for a combination of religious, economic, and philosophic reasons. A vegetarian diet can be well balanced and supply the basic nutrients if it is very carefully planned and if it incorporates a wide range of plants and plant products. It is easier to supply all nutrients if milk is included; such a diet is known as a *lacto-vegetarian* diet. If eggs are also eaten—the *ovo-lacto-vegetarian* diet—it is still easier. The key is careful planning. Lifelong vegetarians have been found to have excellent health and longevity records. Certainly, the typical American diet contains more meat than is needed, and health is in no way jeopardized by decreasing meat intake if other protein sources are included in the diet.

## Determinants of Food Intake

*Hunger* is the physical sensation of discomfort caused by an empty stomach. Hunger also seems to be affected by some poorly understood central nervous system mechanisms, and such factors as blood sugar level may play a part in the sensation of hunger.

*Appetite*—the desire to eat—is affected by both physical and emotional factors. Growth, physical activity, and large body size tend to increase appetite in order to meet body needs. Appetite can be limited in focus to a specific food or group of foods and may cause a person to eat far more than the body needs. This kind of appetite usually arises from psychological feelings, not body needs.

Likewise *anorexia*—the loss of appetite—can prevent a person from eating even though the body requires more food.

*Satiety* is the feeling of having eaten a sufficient amount. Some foods, such as fats, promote satiety because they are digested slowly and thus remain in the digestive tract a relatively long time. Satiety may also be affected by central nervous system controls, blood sugar levels, and perhaps other unknown factors, as is hunger. Some people seem not to experience satiety even when the stomach is full and thus consistently overeat.

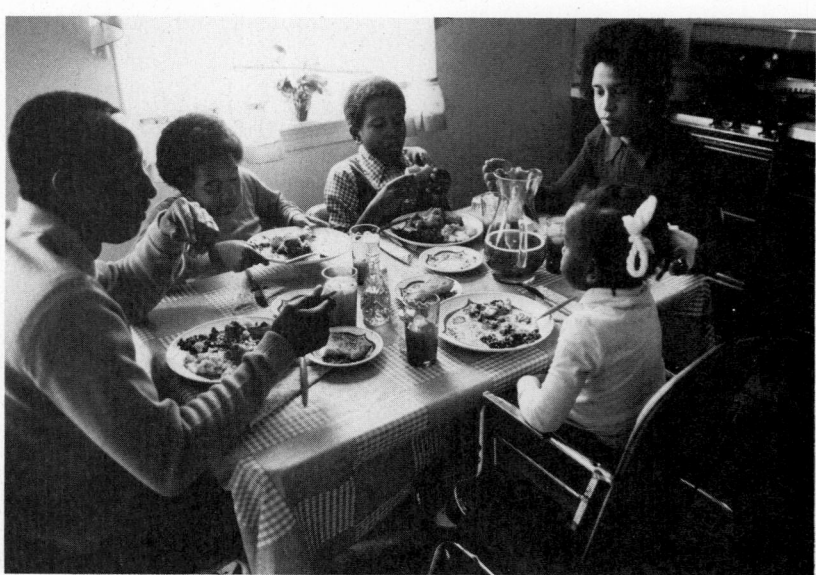

**Figure 21.2**
Culture affects people's eating habits.
(Owen Franken/Stock, Boston)

# Sociocultural Influences on Diet

## Culture

All societies impose values on food, making some foods more acceptable or desirable than others. Puréed foods are regarded as infant foods in the United States, as is milk in some African nations. Other foods, such as lobster and caviar, are accorded prestige or status. Food that is familiar and typical of one's family or social group may arouse feelings of warmth and belonging. For example, a person from a traditional German background may derive feelings of security and comfort from dishes like sauerbraten and veal stew with dumplings because they are reminiscent of the comfort and security of the home. During illness, what is familiar may be a remedy in itself. For this reason, one person will prefer chicken soup when ill while another considers tea the perfect remedy. The feelings associated with a given food may render it tolerable to the digestive system when nothing else is acceptable.

Some foods, though very nutritious, are simply not acceptable in certain cultures. In fact, cultural aversion to a food can be so great as to cause nausea and vomiting. Fish eyes elicit this response from many people brought up in Western cul-

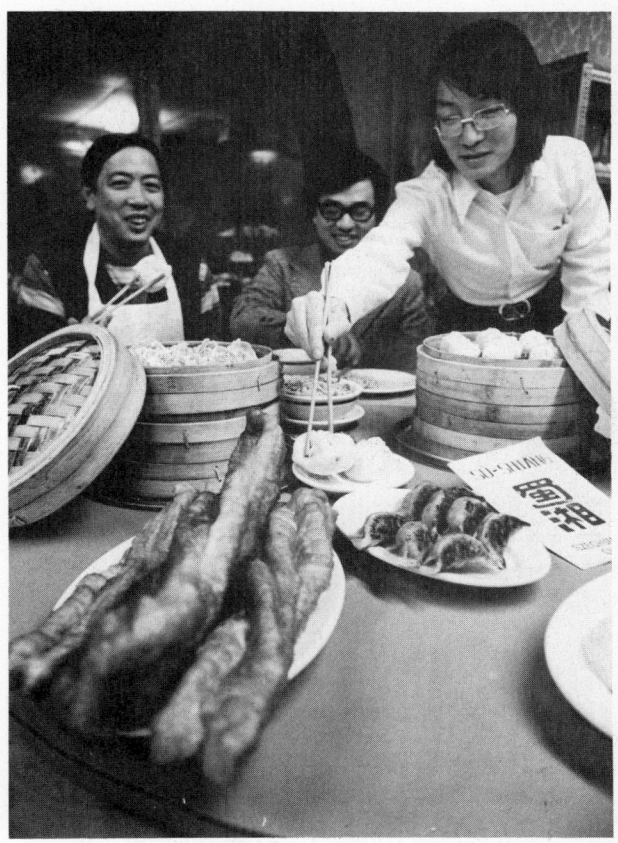

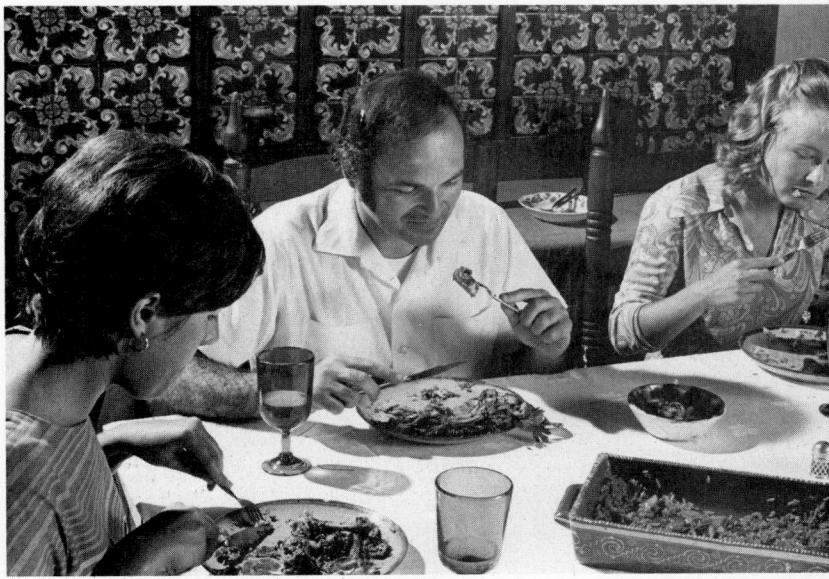

**Figure 21.2  (continued)**
(*Top:* Peter Southwick/Stock, Boston; *bottom:* John Urban)

tures, although they are nutritious and considered a delicacy in Asia. The most extreme manifestation of cultural aversion is a taboo or forbidden food, such as pork for Orthodox Jews and devout Muslims.

The patterns of meals are also cultural in origin. American travelers to Europe find that breakfast is coffee and a bread-type roll in one country, a large and hearty meal in another. The main meal may be eaten at noon, at 6:00 p.m., or at 10:00 p.m. In the United States we are accustomed to three meals a day, while in England a fourth small meal called "tea" is served in the late afternoon. People become used to a given meal pattern and tend to become hungry at the usual time.

## Religion

Some religions have dietary rules that are an aspect of religious observance. Orthodox Jewish law, for example, requires that all foods be obtained, prepared, and served according to specific rules. For example, meat and milk products are kept completely separate, and pork, scaleless fish (like eels), shellfish, and other foods are not eaten. Food that conforms to Jewish dietary rules is called *kosher*. Hospitals in areas where there are many Orthodox Jews may be equipped to provide kosher food. If you work in such a setting, you will need to be familiar with the rules for serving kosher food. If such food is not available, the Orthodox Jew will usually eat nonkosher food as long as foods specifically prohibited by Jewish law are omitted. Such a person might be expected to eat poorly while hospitalized because of emotional aversion to nonkosher food.

Some Christians omit certain foods from their diets during the Lenten (pre-Easter) season. Many Roman Catholics still omit meat on Friday, though it is no longer required by the Church. Such customs may usually be set aside during periods of illness, but some people prefer to maintain them regardless of circumstances. The individual's wishes are of primary significance, regardless of policy.

Adherents of many Eastern religions, such as Hinduism, are vegetarian. Eating flesh is so repugnant to such people that even suggesting they do so may cause them to be ill.

## Income

A family's income largely determines its diet. Because meat and fresh fruits and vegetables tend to be expensive, people with limited finances eat more of such less expensive foods as bread, potatoes, and other starches. Such a diet might cause one to be overweight and undernourished. Severe economic deprivation usually restricts the quantity of food available, which can result in severe underweight and inadequate growth and development in children.

## Personal Preference

Everyone has likes and dislikes with regard to food. Given the variety of foods available in the United States, it should be possible to plan nutritionally adequate diets composed only of foods a person likes. When a person's likes and dislikes are taken into account in planning meals, he or she is more likely to eat well. However, extreme and numerous dislikes may interfere with good nutrition, especially when a special diet is needed.

## Emotional Attitudes

In addition to culturally induced attitudes toward certain foods, food in general may evoke strong feelings. Food is often used to reward children, and the resulting attitudes persist into adulthood. When food is withheld, for example, one may feel punished. Or one may want to reward oneself for enduring illness by eating favorite foods, even when they are contraindicated. The person responsible for withholding desired foods may be seen as antagonistic and punishing.

Being fed, or having to eat what is typically considered baby food, may make a person feel dependent and inadequate and may result in anger toward the person who provides such food. Recognizing the emotional importance of food will enable you to recognize these problems when they occur and to plan effective action. Intervention is based on skills of therapeutic interaction (see Chapter 12).

# Nutrition and Illness

Illness generally increases nutritional needs. Healing requires greater numbers of calories, more protein, and more vitamins and minerals than does maintenance of health. A fever raises the metabolic rate and increases the body's caloric requirements. And certain illnesses, such as hyperthyroidism, also increase metabolism, which in turn increases the calories needed by the body.

When a person is ill, appetite is often adversely affected. Food in general is less appealing, and fatigue may make eating an effort. Many illnesses cause unpleasant odors or tastes in the mouth, decreasing the desire for food. Furthermore, in some illnesses specific nutrients are not digested or metabolized in the normal way, necessitating special modifications of the diet.

The simplest such modification involves the *form* or *texture* of the food served. A general diet in which all foods are chopped is of special value to those without teeth, those whose dentures fit poorly and make chewing difficult, and those with very carious teeth. It is usually also possible to order all foods puréed for the person who cannot manage solid foods at all. The nurse often recognizes a need for dietary modification and is generally free to order it. The physician may also order such dietary changes. In facilities where only the physician may order dietary modifications, the nurse provides the relevant information to the physician and requests that an order for a change in form be written.

Other dietary modifications involve the overall *content* of the diet. Certain nutrients may be omitted or decreased, as in a low-sodium diet; nutrients may be carefully controlled as to type and timing, as in a diabetic diet; or nutrients may be added, as in a high-protein diet. Many other diets also restrict or increase nutrients in light of needs created by a specific illness or disease process. A nutrition text or diet manual should be consulted for detailed information on the many special diets that may be ordered by the physician as part of the medical treatment plan. The nurse should not revise them at will.

Patients' diets may also be modified in response to personal likes and dislikes. The nurse may communicate the patient's preferences to the dietitian so they can be considered in planning menus. The dietitian may make a personal visit to the patient in order to plan an appealing diet. This often proves especially helpful when the patient has not been eating well.

# Assessing the Patient's Nutritional Status

## Appearance

The first step in assessing an individual's nutritional status is to observe his or her general appearance closely. Is the weight/height ratio appropriate, indicating neither too few nor too many calories for the person's needs? Is the skin color clear and the skin texture smooth? Many nutritional deficiencies are first evident in changes in the skin and mucous membranes. Is the hair thick and glossy? Are the lips and gums intact, or are they reddened, pale, or swollen? Many factors other than nutrition can affect a person's general appearance, but such observations may indicate a need for more complete investigation.

## Dietary History

The patient's *dietary history*—information on the usual meal pattern, types of foods usually eaten, likes and dislikes, and allergies—is then gathered.

This information will enable you to ascertain whether or not the patient maintains a sound diet at home. It will also help you plan a present and future diet that will be most acceptable and involve the least disruption in the patient's pattern of living. Information on the patient's sociocultural group and its attitudes and preferences with regard to food can also be helpful in diet planning.

## Current Needs

Assessment of nutrition also involves consideration of current needs. Is the person growing? Are special needs created by tissue repair and healing? Is the person underweight and in need of weight gain, or overweight and in need of weight reduction?

## Ability to Eat

The patient's physical ability to eat is especially important in nutritional assessment. A wide variety of factors, ranging from muscle strength and hand coordination to discomfort in the mouth, may affect ability to eat. Some common problems faced by hospitalized people are immobilization in a position that does not allow easy eating or swallowing, restraint or immobilization of the dominant hand with an IV, and extreme physical fatigue and weakness. Paralysis of one hand and arm sometimes occurs in elderly patients who have suffered cerebrovascular accidents (strokes). After the basic aspects of nutritional status have been examined, special needs related to specific diseases—including information on the diet ordered by the physician—are considered.

## Level of Knowledge

Another important aspect of nutritional assessment is the extent of the patient's knowledge about nutrition. Does the patient know what constitutes a good diet? Does he or she know where to seek information about nutrition? If a special diet is indicated, does the patient understand the diet and its purpose? Does he or she have enough depth of understanding to make appropriate modifications for such circumstances as eating out or attending a party? This information is needed to adequately plan for intervention.

## Current Intake

It may be necessary for you to gather information about what a patient is currently eating and drinking. Almost all charts have a place to record each meal and the approximate amount eaten (¼, ½, or all). If more detailed knowledge is needed, it might be appropriate to design a special chart to record everything the patient eats. This chart might later be analyzed by the dietitian to determine caloric intake, patterns of eating, and what foods the patient likes and dislikes.

Measuring all fluids ingested may be important to assessment. In such cases, output must also be measured so the two can be compared. Measured intake will include all oral fluids, foods that would be liquid at body temperature (such as gelatin desserts and ice cream), intravenous fluids, and irrigating fluids that are not returned. Output measurement includes urine, liquid stool, and all drainage. Profuse perspiration is also noted. See Module 11, "Intake and Output," for directions on measuring "I & O" (intake and output).

# Meeting the Patient's Nutritional Needs

## Positioning the Patient

People who are ill often have special needs with regard to the eating process itself. Positioning is one factor that may make eating a problem. It is easiest to eat in a sitting position, with the food placed directly in front in one's line of vision. If this position can be maintained, it is important to position the patient before the meal. If this position is impossible, the nearest approximation of it is most desirable. The very weak or disabled person may need pillows or other supports on each side and under the arms to maintain correct posture for eating. If the patient is not permitted to sit up, a side-lying position may be used for meals.

People usually use both hands to feed themselves, the dominant hand performing the most skilled tasks. If only one hand is available, the patient will have great difficulty with such tasks as opening a milk carton. If only the nondominant hand is available, even one-handed tasks may require more dexterity than that hand possesses. Planning placement of IVs and turning the patient so that the dominant hand is free for eating can avoid this problem. You may have to offer to perform some tasks, such as opening a milk carton or cutting meat. However, patients should always be asked whether they want help, the kind of help they want, and how such help is to be given. Independence in eating fosters self-esteem and should be encouraged. Module 5, "Feeding Adult Patients," provides more information on this topic.

## Stimulating the Patient's Appetite

Environmental factors are important in promoting appetite. Control of odors and unpleasant sights is often difficult in the hospital, but any such steps that can be taken may help the patient retain a minimal appetite or regain a lost appetite. Removing soiled linen, opening a window, or using air freshener may be appropriate nursing actions in such a situation.

Personal comfort can promote appetite and may be enhanced by bathing, washing the hands and face, straightening the bed, giving pain medications, or in myriad other ways.

Stressful events tend to decrease appetite and should be avoided immediately before meals are served. Many pieces of equipment found in a hospital (such as those used for a venipuncture) are stress-producing to observe, and removing them from the patient's presence during meals will decrease anxiety.

Interaction with family and friends is typical of mealtimes for most people. If visitors can stay during the meal, or even order a tray and eat with the patient, a more congenial mealtime atmosphere is created. Sometimes several patients can sit together to visit during a meal, or a staff member might sit with a patient for a few minutes to make the meal a special event. Company is especially helpful when the meal itself is less than tasty due to the omission of seasonings or salt: the interaction replaces the bland food as the focus of attention.

## Helping the Patient Eat

Special feeding devices and methods are often used to help patients maintain independence in eating. The use of such equipment—which includes utensils with shaped handles, devices to keep a plate or dish in place, and special straws— needs to be carefully evaluated for each individual. One person may appreciate such an aid, while another prefers to eat more slowly and with greater difficulty using conventional utensils.

Feeding a patient is sometimes necessitated by muscle and joint disability that prevents movement, neurological involvement that prevents muscle function, or extreme weakness. Many patients are able to feed themselves partially if the nurse helps with difficult tasks. Sometimes a patient can manage finger foods, such as bread and butter, but must be fed foods requiring more dexterity, such as soup. If weak vision is the problem, a description of the items on the tray, and their location, may enable the patient to eat without help. Because maximum independence increases the patient's self-esteem, time and effort expended toward this end are well spent.

## Alternative Feeding Methods

A nasogastric tube is a long flexible tube with a diameter narrow enough to pass through the nose to the nasopharynx and then through the esophagus to the stomach. The nurse inserts such a tube only on the order of a physician. A nasogastric tube is frequently used to aspirate stomach contents, and may in some circumstances be attached to a low suction to remove gas and gastric contents. Here, however, we are concerned with its use to deposit food in a liquid form directly into the stomach. Some tubes with small diameters are weighted so they will move into the duodenum; this allows feeding directly into the small intestine, which may benefit the patient with nausea. Special pumps often have to be connected to these small tubes to aid in the flow of formulas through them.

*Nasogastric tube feedings* are performed for a variety of reasons, most frequently because the person is unable to swallow or lacks a gag reflex to prevent aspiration of food or fluids. A commercially prepared liquid formula may be used for the feeding. Such formulas vary in nutrient content and are ordered by the physician. Alternatively, a carefully planned combination of regular foods is liquified in a blender, and liquid is added to achieve the appropriate consistency. The commercial preparations are easily controlled and convenient, but many patients suffer fewer digestive disturbances, such as diarrhea, when a blenderized formula is used. Additional water must always be given with tube feedings to meet the body's needs, and the exact amount may be ordered by the physician. Because tube feedings are meals, they should be served as such. If the patient is aware of the surroundings, a pleasant atmosphere will increase the flow of digestive juices and thus enhance digestion.

There are dangers in nasogastric tube feedings. If the tube is malpositioned, fluid could be deposited in the lungs or nasopharynx, allowing aspiration to occur. Excessive pressure may cause gastric irritation, gas, and reflex vomiting, and excessive rapidity may also precipitate vomiting. Allowing air into the tube will cause distention and discomfort and possibly vomiting. Food is ordinarily moderated in temperature in the mouth and esophagus before it reaches the stomach. Temperature extremes can irritate the gastric mucosa, making it essential that the formula is of moderate temperature before instillation. Thus any procedure for nasogastric tube feeding should take into consideration tube placement, prevention of air ingestion, the temperature of the fluid, and the force and speed of the fluid as it enters the stomach.

Patients receiving tube feedings frequently experience diarrhea. This phenomenon has been attributed to a variety of factors, including too concentrated a solution, inappropriate temperature, bacterial contamination of the feeding, and the unfamiliar consistency. Such diarrhea may decrease over time. If care is taken with regard to the other possible causes of diarrhea, the patient usually adjusts to the consistency of the formula. (Some new commercial formulas are especially devised to minimize diarrhea.)

A surgically produced opening from the abdomen directly into the stomach is called a *gastrostomy.* A tube is inserted into the opening and a liquid feeding instilled, just as is done through a nasogastric tube.

*Elemental feedings* consist of basic nutrients that need not be digested but can be directly absorbed. One such commercial product is called Vivonex. A very narrow-diameter feeding tube may be inserted into the small intestine through the nose. Because the diameter of the tube is so small, a pump is often used to facilitate movement of the solution through the tube. This process is sometimes termed *enteral feeding.* Elemental feedings leave no residue to be eliminated by the large intestine, which allows that organ to rest. Since digestion is not required, the energy that would ordinarily be expended on that process is saved.

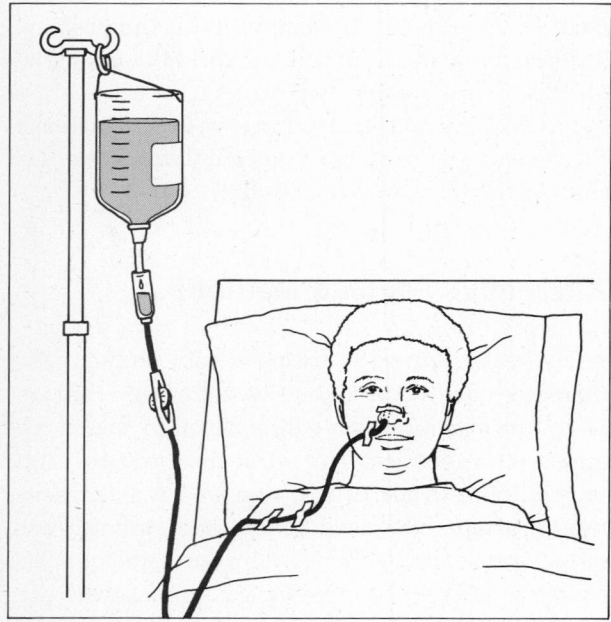

**Figure 21.3  Burette method of tube feeding**

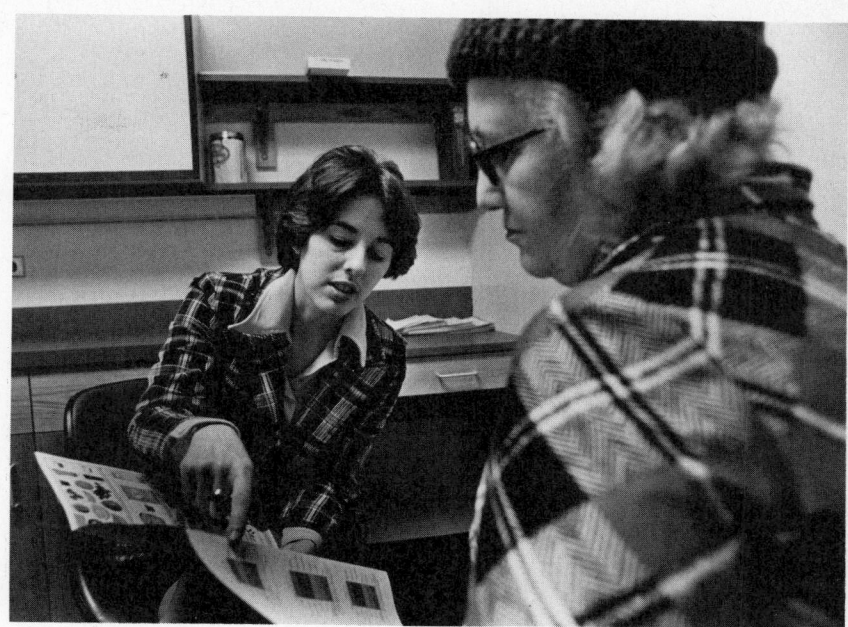

**Figure 21.4**
Health teaching is an important part of nutritional intervention. (Chris Maynard)

In cases of extreme need, elemental feedings may be given throughout a twenty-four-hour period to maximize caloric intake.

## Hyperalimentation

*Hyperalimentation*, or *total parenteral nutrition* (TPN) is a method of providing nutrients intravenously. In conventional intravenous fluids, which will be discussed in Chapter 24, 5 percent dextrose is the source of calories. This solution provides approximately 170 calories in 1000 ml, which is not adequate for nutritional needs. When a patient cannot take oral food and fluids for a prolonged period, healing may be severely compromised due to a lack of nutrients. In total parenteral nutrition, all types of nutrients are given intravenously.

Dextrose may be given in concentrations of 10–20 percent. In these concentrations, dextrose is very irritating to veins and causes them to sclerose (become inflamed and close due to scarring). Therefore, a large central vein with a high blood flow, in which the solution can disperse rapidly— most commonly the subclavian vein—is used to administer high concentrations of dextrose.

Protein may be given in the form of simple amino acids or simple proteins. If very dilute, the amino acids may sometimes be given in peripheral veins. Proteins and the amino acids in higher concentrations must be given in a large vein with a high blood flow.

Lipids in a special emulsified form may also be given intravenously. The lipids are not irritating and are often given in a peripheral vein.

Vitamins, minerals, and trace elements are added to the feedings in amounts determined by the physician. These may be given either peripherally or in central veins.

*Complications* of hyperalimentation are many and potentially serious. *Infection*, either at the site of administration or systemic (affecting the whole body), is the most common complication. To prevent infection, most facilities have established a strict routine for care of the hyperalimentation site. This regimen usually includes a cleaning procedure and special care in dressing changes. In addition, no medications are added to the hyperalimentation line. Each needle puncture of the line increases the potential for contamination. Tubings and solutions are changed on a rigid schedule so that organisms will not have time to reproduce if contamination occurs.

*Fluid overload*, which strains the heart and may cause respiratory distress, can occur if the fluid is given at too rapid a rate. For this reason, a special intravenous pump that measures the flow rate and monitors the line is usually used.

*Hyperglycemia* (high blood sugar) may occur if dextrose is given more rapidly than the body can utilize it. Urine may be checked for the presence of glucose to determine whether blood glucose is so elevated that the kidneys are excreting the sugar. It is sometimes necessary for the physician to order the hormone insulin to be given to facilitate use of the glucose.

If *allergic reactions* to the protein occur, the fluid must be discontinued. Another brand or type of nutritional solution may be substituted.

In spite of the potential complications, some patients who cannot take oral foods are now being discharged to receive total parenteral nutrition at home. With careful teaching, patients and their families can become very skillful at this type of care.

## Health Teaching

Health teaching about nutrition-related problems is a very common need. When you have determined through assessment that dietary teaching is needed, your task will be to combine your knowledge of nutrition with your knowledge of health teaching (Chapter 13) in planning your instruction approach. You may find it necessary to teach the patient about normal nutrition before you can teach about special diets.

# Assisting the Patient with Fluid Intake

## Increasing Oral Intake

Many ill people need to consume large quantities of fluid to allow for excretion of excess waste products or to combat fever. The physician may thus order *force fluids*. This order means not that you literally force the patient to drink but that you exert maximum effort to encourage the patient to consume fluids. Simply reminding the patient to drink frequently may be all that is needed.

Because patients are likely to consume more of fluids they enjoy, it is fruitful to take time to learn likes and dislikes and to order what the patient prefers. And because people are more likely to reach desired goals if they receive feedback on their progress, you might design a method of recording intake or graphing it on a wall chart. Furthermore, behaviors that are reinforced (rewarded) tend to be repeated. Thus praise or even marks on a chart for ingesting certain amounts of fluid may have the effect of increasing intake. Setting a specific goal for the twenty-four-hour period and ascertaining when fluid should be taken help the nursing staff to organize its efforts. If the goal is 3000 ml per twenty-four-hour period, a realistic plan acknowledges that the patient sleeps during the 11 p.m. to 7 a.m. shift and therefore will usu-ally take less than 200 ml if offered fluids only when awakened in the morning. If medications are given during the night, fluid intake at these times may be encouraged. The plan might provide for 2000 ml to be taken from 7:00 a.m. to 3:00 p.m. That period of time includes two meals and two snacks, and if the patient also drinks fluids between meals, the goal can be reached. If the mechanics of drinking are a problem, special straws and cups are available to assist the patient.

## Limiting Fluids

A physician may occasionally order that fluids be limited. Fluids are often withheld for short periods before procedures that require general anesthesia or slight dehydration as well as when disease necessitates it. This is very trying for the patient, and careful planning with the patient is needed to space the allowable intake throughout the day and to provide for fluid to accompany oral medications. The patient will also need support from others to tolerate fluid deprivation. When the limitation is very severe, close supervision may be necessary: it is difficult to maintain self-control when one's thirst is extreme. Ice chips often serve to minimize the desire for fluid and provide greater relief than the same amount of water; remember that they too must be counted as intake. Allowing responsible patients to perform mouth care and to rinse the mouth may promote a feeling of well-being during this time. If a patient cannot be expected to refrain from drinking fluid while performing mouth care, you may moisten the lips and provide mouth care for the patient.

## Special Problems Related to Nutrition

### Malnutrition

*Malnutrition* is literally ''bad'' nutrition, the opposite of good nutrition. Malnutrition has two components: the first is lack of adequate calories to meet the body's needs, which results in weight loss, decreased resistance to infection, inhibited healing, and general malaise (lack of energy). Second, malnutrition is characterized by insufficient quantities of some essential nutrients, which can occur even when calories are adequate and the person is of normal weight or even obese. Lack of nutrients may produce deficiency diseases such as scurvy, which arises from a lack of vitamin C.

The most common cause of malnutrition is poverty—insufficient money to buy appropriate foods. Some parts of the world also suffer severe shortages of food. In the United States, many cases of malnutrition are due to lack of knowledge about nutrition and poor budgeting. For example, many people believe that meat is needed and purchase it in large quantities, forgoing other more nutritious foods. In fact, the RDA for protein can be met with very modest amounts of meat or with inexpensive foods such as grains and legumes. Low-income people may not be aware of programs that can help maintain nutritional levels, such as food stamps and inexpensive meals at community centers for the aged.

Health teaching in response to poor nutrition must be done with sensitivity and care. It is important not to undermine the self-esteem of a family that is already struggling with other difficulties. In planning with them to achieve a better diet, take into account their cultural and ethnic food preferences, access to grocery stores and transportation, and individual likes and dislikes. Sometimes you may need to refer to a social worker or some other person who can help the family with its income problems. If help with budgeting is needed, consumer credit counseling services provide this service without charge. (These organizations should be differentiated from commercial credit counseling agencies.) You can find ways to teach about appropriate nutrition that will help enhance people's self-esteem and pride in their ability to care for themselves and their families.

### Obesity

*Obesity* is usually defined as body weight of 15 percent or more above the ideal weight for height, frame, and age. (Occasionally 20 percent is considered the baseline for obesity.) Obesity poses health hazards. For example, an obese person is at increased risk during surgery because greater technical skill is required to cope with the fatty tissue, the anesthetization is prolonged by the need to dissect and repair the fatty tissue, healing is slowed because fatty tissue has poor circulation, the risk of infection is greater for the same reason, and the obese person is less likely to be active during the postoperative period. Obesity has also been linked with a variety of illnesses, such as heart disease and diabetes mellitus.

Another way of defining obesity is to calculate the percentage of body weight accounted for by fat. This may be done with precision by the complex process of weighing in water, or it may be estimated by using calipers to pinch and measure subcutaneous fat. In women, 25–30 percent of body weight is typically fat; men have more muscle and bone mass and thus usually only 14 percent fat. Higher percentages indicate excess fat.

Obesity is not necessarily synonymous with ov-

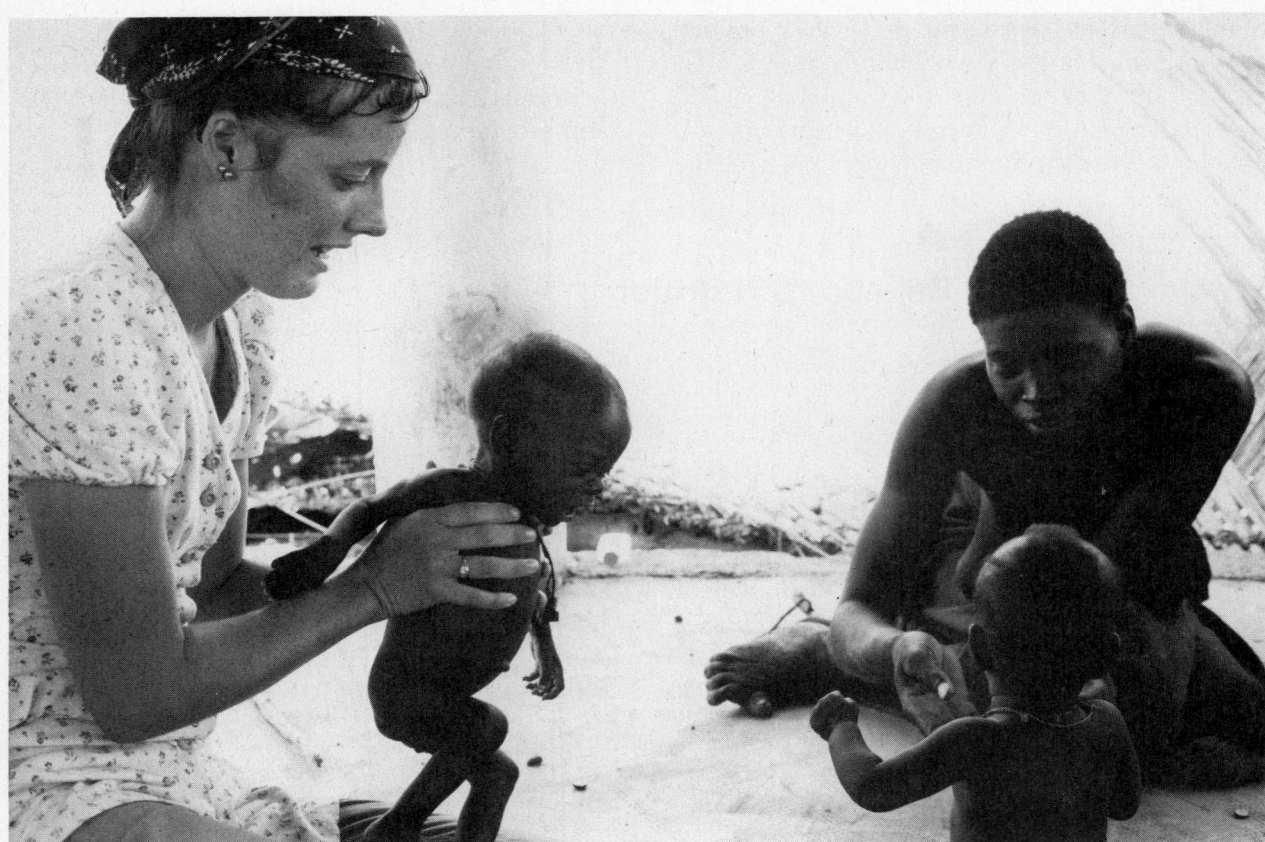

**Figure 21.5**
Malnutrition is common throughout the world. (Photograph by Kay Chernush, courtesy of Action)

erweight, which is a matter of individual perception. In modern industrial societies, the fashion ideal for women tends to be a very slim figure. Thus a woman might perceive herself as overweight in light of fashion without being obese or at risk of health problems associated with obesity.

## Causes

The immediate cause of all obesity is intake of more calories than the body can use, and these excess calories are then stored as fat. The underlying causes may be more diverse. Some people need fewer calories than the norm and thus gain weight on an ordinary dietary intake. This group includes people with hormonal deficiencies that reduce metabolic rate as well as others whose normal metabolism appears to be very efficient. Another reason for needing fewer calories is a lower-than-usual activity level. People with sedentary jobs, those who dislike sports, and those whose

lives do not include any regular physical exertion may become obese for this reason.

In the United States, excessive intake of calories is most often the reason for obesity. The pattern of excessive dietary intake is reinforced socially: most social occasions include food and caloric beverages, and as a nation we consume large per capita quantities of simple sugar in desserts, snacks, and beverages. Advertising promotes keen interest in and desire for food unrelated to actual needs. Some people habitually overeat for psychological reasons: food may represent security and love or serve as a defense against the need to relate to others.

## Related Factors

The development of fat cells in infancy and early childhood is being studied in relationship to obesity. It is known that individuals who are obese as infants are more likely to be obese as adults and that those who were obese as infants have a greater number of fat cells as adults.

Obesity does seem to characterize some families more than others. This pattern may be influenced by heredity, acquired eating habits, and/or the psychological meanings attached to food in a particular family—factors that cannot be effectively separated.

Obesity increases in frequency with age, usually due to decreased activity levels. Changes in metabolic patterns associated with aging may also have a contributory effect.

## Assessment

To assess an individual's weight status, you must know both height and weight and carefully observe bone structure. Wrists and ankles are often the best indication of whether a person's frame is large or small. When you have gathered all three pieces of information, consult a height-weight table to determine whether the person is obese.

Physical assessment should be accompanied by assessment of the person's mental health. A person's attitude or state of mind will greatly influence his or her interest in and willingness to participate in a weight-control plan. A person with serious mental health problems may not be able to tolerate the added stress of strenuous weight control until adequate psychological support is available.

## Planning

A goal for weight loss should be realistic, and it should be set jointly with the patient. It is often helpful to set short-term goals as well as an overall long-term goal; a single ultimate goal can be discouraging.

An effective weight-control program has two major components: planning actual food intake and helping the person stay on the prescribed diet. Let us first examine the wide variety of ways to plan intake, all of which have had some success.

*Calorie counting* relies on looking up the caloric value of foods and choosing a diet whose total calories are within the guidelines. Stress is put on maintaining a nutritious and well-balanced diet. Although this method works well, it is time-con-

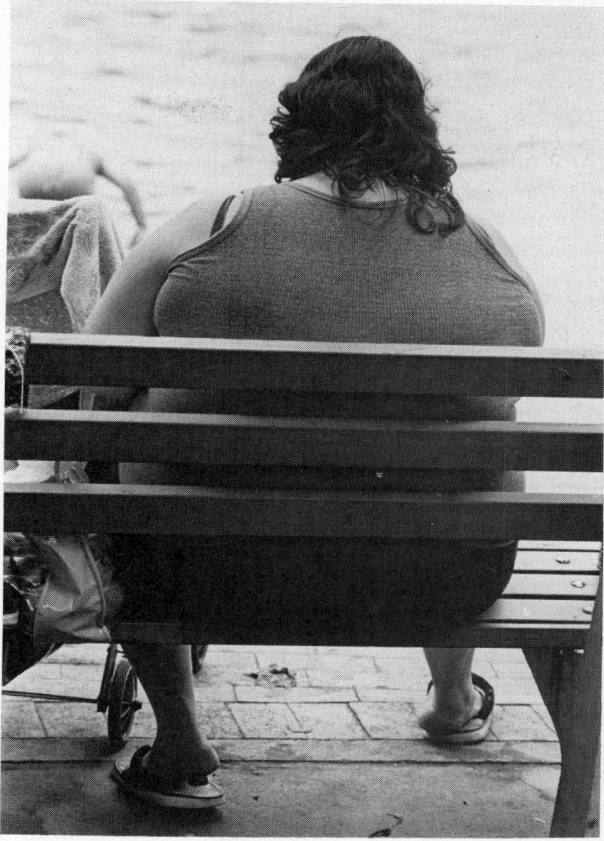

**Figure 21.6**
Obesity exists among children as well as adults. (Ira Kirschenbaum/Stock, Boston)

suming and involves careful planning and figuring, and some people find it tedious.

*Exchange menus* consist of a basic diet plan that specifies a given number of servings of several types of food—meat, bread or bread substitutes, low-calorie vegetables, high-calorie vegetables, fruits, and milk products—and provides lists of foods that are calorically interchangeable and can be used to fulfill the diet's specifications. This approach has the advantage of greater simplicity than direct calorie counting. Though less exact, it is sufficiently so.

*Carbohydrate counting* is performed in an effort to limit calories from carbohydrates, on the assumption that the high satiety value of the fat and protein eaten in place of carbohydrates will naturally limit their intake. This approach can be effective, but some people gain the mistaken impression that protein foods cannot contribute to obesity.

*Ketogenic diets* are those that limit carbohydrates so severely that the body becomes glucose-depleted. In order for the body to get the energy it needs for basic functioning, fat is burned in large quantities. Since the body is not equipped to burn fat rapidly, the metabolism is incomplete, resulting in ketone bodies as waste products. These ketone bodies are acidic in nature and therefore cause a mild metabolic acidosis (see Chapter 24). Though such diets are effective in quick weight loss, even their proponents recommend limiting them to one or two weeks. There is controversy over whether mild metabolic acidosis is of danger to the well person. It is essential to be under medical care when undertaking this type of diet.

*Starvation* has been used to enforce weight loss in some severely obese people. No food at all is allowed (though the person may have water). However, starvation causes the body to break down muscle stores as well as fat and is therefore not recommended.

*Liquid protein diets,* which are commercially prepared, were until recently being aggressively promoted as the solution to weight-control problems. Then, after major weight losses, some people who used these products suddenly died. The exact cause of death has not been determined, but as a result, liquid protein diets are allowed to be recommended only as supplements to food, not as total replacements.

*Liquid diets* containing a variety of nutrients owe their popularity to the assumption that an all-liquid diet must have fewer calories than a diet containing solids. Needless to say, a liquid diet's caloric value depends on the types of liquids allowed. When the liquids allowed consist primarily of vegetable juices, with some fruit juices and broths, such a diet may indeed be low-calorie, but liquid diets are rarely well balanced and should be used with caution.

The second major aspect of weight control is promoting adherence to the prescribed diet. Many different approaches have been employed.

*Group support* has proven quite successful. A group of people, all of whom have or have had weight problems, meet regularly to discuss common concerns and ways of coping and to encourage one another to stay on the diet.

*Behavior modification* is often used to help obese people establish new eating habits. The hypothesis underlying this approach is that overeating is learned behavior and that one can thus learn not to overeat. A system of rewards for appropriate food intake may be used to reinforce desired behavior.

*Free foods*—that is, foods that have very few or no calories and may be eaten in unlimited quantities—are often used to help people stay on a diet. Artificially sweetened beverages are popular free foods, but recent reports about the health hazards of artificial sweeteners have led some people to give them up. Others believe the risk is small compared with the risk of obesity.

*Medications*—primarily the amphetamines—have the effect of decreasing appetite. However, amphetamines have such side effects as insomnia, irritability, nervousness, and drug dependence and thus are recommended only in rare cases. There have been instances of hormones, such as thyroid hormone, being given for weight loss, but by upsetting the body's own hormonal balance, this regimen may create long-term problems. In general, medications are not recommended for weight loss.

Another aspect of weight control is *activity level.* If a person's activity level is low, an increase in exercise may help weight loss occur more rapidly. Paradoxically, increased activity may also help decrease appetite in the person who has been overeating.

Whatever plan is pursued, it must be one the obese person feels comfortable with and is determined to follow through on. An encouraging and supportive approach is usually more helpful than a critical attitude. When lapses from the diet occur (and they usually do), the person needs reassurance that one slip does not mean failure. Each pound lost should be treated as a significant accomplishment.

## Nausea and Vomiting

*Nausea* is the subjective feeling that one might vomit. Discomfort is often localized in the stomach and back of the throat. Increased salivation, headache, and general malaise may accompany the nausea. Vomiting usually but not always follows nausea.

*Vomiting* is the forceful ejection of the contents

of the stomach. Severe vomiting may be accompanied by reverse peristalsis, which brings material from far down in the intestine up to the stomach for expulsion. The force expelling the vomitus may be great enough to eject it several feet from the mouth; this phenomenon is called *projectile vomiting*.

## Causes

Vomiting is initiated by a center in the medulla of the brain, in response to a wide variety of stimuli: irritation in the stomach, stimulation of the gag reflex in the back of the throat, emotional stress, and chemicals in the blood, such as certain drugs, toxins released by bacteria, and body waste products that are not eliminated. Other organs that can stimulate the vomiting center include the kidneys, the duodenum, the uterus, and the heart. Motion sickness causes nausea and vomiting by disturbing the semicircular canals in the ears, which in turn sets up a chain of nerve impulses that stimulate the vomiting center.

## Assessment

Initial assessment usually involves gathering *subjective information* from the patient: how he or she feels, for how long that feeling has persisted, any causative factors the patient perceives, what the patient has done to try to relieve the nausea and/ or vomiting, and the effectiveness of that action. Data about the person's overall level of stress are also highly desirable.

*Objective information* includes the state of the mouth and teeth, ability to swallow, the person's behavior when food is presented, and actual amounts eaten at any time. Look for pallor, perspiration, increased salivation, and changes in the vital signs (increases in pulse and respiration and elevated temperature are common).

Encourage the patient to use a basin when vomiting, not to go to the bathroom. If the person actually vomits, observe the amount, color, consistency, and contents of the vomitus. For example, blood in the vomitus may be bright, indicating that it is fresh, or it may be reddish-brown and of the consistency of coffee grounds, indicating di-

gested blood. If you or someone else observed the vomiting, note whether or not it was projectile. Ask the patient whether nausea preceded the vomiting.

The person's *general condition* is also important: note weight loss, constipation, dehydration, and electrolyte imbalance (see Chapter 24).

## Planning

A variety of possible goals might be appropriate for the person with nausea and vomiting. In some cases the goal might be limited to maintenance of personal hygiene and comfort. In other instances your goals might be that serious sequelae such as dehydration and electrolyte imbalance not occur. Or, finally, your goals might be that the nausea and vomiting cease and that the person eat an adequate diet.

## Implementing Nursing Actions

First, try to identify the *cause* of nausea and vomiting and seek to eliminate it. In order to do so, you should investigate the medications the patient is receiving, consider his or her stress level, and investigate the disease process. If, for example, you believe a drug to be causing the problem, it is appropriate to withhold the drug and consult with the physician before giving another dose.

*Environmental control* may be very beneficial to the person who is nauseated: make the room neat and clean, eliminate odors and unpleasant sights, adequately ventilate the room, and in general make the setting as pleasant as possible.

*Personal hygiene* helps prevent vomiting as well as promote comfort after vomiting has occurred. Oral hygiene is especially important.

*Emotional stress* should be lessened whenever possible. It is especially important that mealtimes not be associated with stress. In order to accomplish a lowered stress level, you may need to schedule tests and procedures away from the mealtime, and family members and staff should be asked to assist in keeping conversation away from stressful topics during the mealtime.

*Meal management* includes discussing with the patient what foods might be acceptable. The cen-

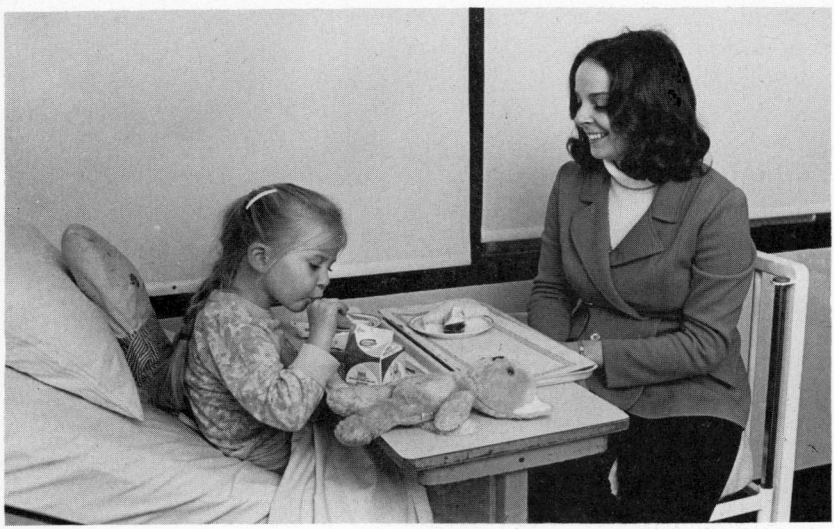

**Figure 21.7**
Meal management may help combat nausea and vomiting. (Dan Bernstein)

tral role of emotions in nausea makes this process potentially very effective. Some people may tolerate dry toast even when very ill; others find tea or broth acceptable. When regular meals are served, small portions make the meal seem less forbidding and often serve to increase intake; large portions may simply be rejected out of hand.

*Antiemetic drugs* may be ordered by the physician. If so, you will need to exercise careful judgment about when to give them. Administering the medication approximately half an hour before the patient's mealtime allows adequate time for it to take effect before the food is served. If the medication is effective, it will render the sight of food less distasteful and enable the person to eat. The duration of action of the antiemetic drugs is such that the effect will persist long enough for the food to be digested. Medication may also be administered when nausea is first felt and after the patient vomits. Giving the medication only after the patient actually vomits causes fatigue and increases the chance of complications, such as dehydration.

*Support while vomiting* is also important. If the person is very young, weak, or debilitated in any way, he or she should be positioned on the side to allow the vomitus to drain from the mouth, preventing aspiration. Suction is sometimes needed to remove vomitus from the mouth of the unconscious person. Whenever possible, screen a vomiting person to provide for privacy and to protect other patients from the unpleasant sight. Usually a person who is vomiting will wish to be positioned on the side or abdomen to facilitate expulsion of vomitus from the mouth. An emesis basin is ordinarily used for vomitus, but it is sometimes not large enough and in cases of projectile vomiting may not contain everything. In such an instance, you might want to obtain an extra washbasin to use. After the episode of vomiting is over, the person will need to rinse his or her mouth, have soiled linen changed, and be allowed to rest.

## Conclusion

Providing food and fluids for patients is an emotional experience as well as a nursing task. Your role may seem pleasant when you are a provider, but it is difficult when you must withhold or limit these essentials of life. Helping the patient understand and participate actively in this essential aspect of care and treatment requires skillful nursing.

## Care Study  An obese child

Martha Brown, R.N., was working in a well-child clinic, where she assisted with the screening of children and counseling for health maintenance. Observing the first child for the morning, six-year-old Billy, she noted that he appeared plump and had trouble bending over to pick up a toy he had dropped on the floor. She greeted the mother and introduced herself to Billy.

As part of the standard well-child examination, Ms. Brown weighed and measured Billy. His weight was far above the norms for his height on the growth chart. Interviewing the mother, she asked carefully about Billy's eating habits and was told that Billy was always a good eater and liked to snack a lot too. Questioned further, the mother reported that Billy liked potato chips and pop for snacks and also ate lots of her homemade cookies.

Ms. Brown asked the mother if she had noticed that Billy was quite heavy for his height. In doing so, Ms. Brown pointed out his place on the growth chart and explained what the graph meant. The mother answered that she had thought about it but figured that Billy "would outgrow being fat." Ms. Brown explained that this was a common assumption but that in fact children who were overweight were quite likely to be overweight as adults. She also pointed out that being overweight compromised Billy's ability to participate in games and sports as well as his acceptance by other children.

"I suppose I should see if he could lose some weight, shouldn't I?" said Billy's mother. "It would be good for Billy's health," Ms. Brown replied. Mother: "Would I have to put him on a diet? He wouldn't like not being able to eat. I'd have a cranky kid on my hands." Ms. Brown: "The clinic has a special diet you could use. But it's planned so that there are things available for snacks and so the children on it don't have to be hungry. Would you like to look it over?" Mother: "Sure."

Ms. Brown got out the printed explanation of the diet and sat down to talk with the mother about it. As they discussed the diet, Billy's mother became more positive about her ability to use it for Billy. The diet took into account carrying school lunches and substituted fruits and vegetables for high-calorie snacks. Ms. Brown encouraged the mother to try the diet and to call if she encountered problems. She set up an appointment for Billy to be checked again the following month. Ms. Brown encouraged the mother to try to involve Billy in the plan and perhaps to offer Billy some nonfood rewards for staying on the diet.

After Billy and his mother had left, Ms. Brown reviewed what she had done. She had obtained information about Billy's eating habits as well as his current height and weight. She had provided information to the mother, who had in turn acknowledged that a problem existed. The mother had been encouraged to make a personal decision to put Billy on a diet. Ms. Brown had performed health teaching about the diet itself and methods of helping Billy stick to the diet. An appointment had been made for follow-up and evaluation. Ms. Brown felt pleased with her efforts.

## Study Terms

anorexia
antiemetic
appetite
Basic Four
calorie counting
carbohydrate counting
carbohydrates
deficiency
dehydration
diet
  content
  form
  texture
dietary history
elemental feeding

enteral feeding
exchange menus
fats
fiber
fluid overload
force fluids
free foods
gastric
gastrostomy
hunger
hyperalimentation
hyperglycemia
ketogenic diet
kosher
malnutrition

mineral
minimum daily
  requirement
nasogastric tube
  feeding
nausea
normal saline
nutrition
obesity
projectile vomiting
proteins

Recommended Dietary
  Allowances (RDA)
satiety
starvation
total parenteral
  nutrition (TPN)
vegetarian
  lacto-vegetarian
  ovo-lacto-vegetarian
vitamins
vomiting

## Learning Activities

1. Record your own diet for twenty-four hours. Compare it to your RDA and to the Basic Four. Evaluate your diet.

**2.** Plan and conduct a dietary history for a patient in the clinical area.

**3.** Assess a patient to determine his or her level of knowledge about "normal nutrition." If any learning needs are apparent, plan health teaching to meet those needs. After consulting with a clinical instructor, carry out your health teaching plan.

**4.** Keep track of your own intake for twenty-four hours. Devise a plan to increase your intake to 3000 ml per day. Be very specific.

## Relevant Sections in
## Modules for Nursing Skills

| Volume 1 | Module |
|---|---|
| Feeding Adult Patients | 5 |
| Intake and Output | 11 |

## References

Caly, J. C. "Helping People Eat for Health: Assessing Adults' Nutrition." *American Journal of Nursing* 77 (October 1977): 1605.

Colley, R., *et al.* "Helping With Hyperalimentation." *Nursing '73* 3 (March 1973): 6–17.

Dudrick, S. J., and Rhoads, J. E. "Total Intravenous Feeding." *Scientific American* 226 (1972): 73.

Dwyer, L. S., *et al.* "Simplified Meal-Planning for Hard-to-Teach Patients." *American Journal of Nursing* 74 (April 1974): 664–665.

Fenton, M. "What to Do About Thirst." *American Journal of Nursing* 69 (May 1969): 1014–1017.

Fleshman, R. P. "Eating Rituals and Realities." *Nursing Clinics of North America* 8 (March 1973): 91–104.

Gormican, A., *et al.* "Nasogastric Tube Feedings: Practical Considerations in Prescription and Evaluation." *Nursing Digest* 2 (January 1974): 59–63.

Grant, J. A. "Patient Care in Hyperalimentation." *Nursing Clinics of North America* 8 (March 1973): 165–181.

Howard, L. "Obesity: A Feasible Approach to a Formidable Problem." *Nursing Digest* 4 (November-December 1976):86–90.

McCarter, D. "Nourishing the Solute-Sensitive Patient." *American Journal of Nursing* 73 (November 1973): 1935–1936.

Nelson, A. H. "Self-Recorded Diet Histories." *American Journal of Nursing* 72 (September 1972): 1601.

Newton, M., and Falta, J. "Hospital Food Can Help or Hinder Care." *American Journal of Nursing* 67 (January 1967): 112–113.

# Chapter 22
# Elimination

## Objectives

After completing this chapter, you should be able to:

1. Describe the urinary system and define the eleven terms used in assessment.
2. List normal and abnormal characteristics of urine.
3. Discuss objective data, intake and output, and collection of urine specimens in relation to assessment of urinary problems.
4. Discuss treatments appropriate for the patient with urinary problems, such as catheterization, health teaching, and replacement procedures.

5. Describe general nursing care for patients with urinary problems.
6. Describe the intestinal system and define the six terms used in assessment.
7. List normal and abnormal characteristics of feces.
8. Discuss objective data and collection of stool specimens in relation to assessment of intestinal problems.
9. Discuss general nursing care, including enemas, appropriate for the patient with intestinal problems.

## Outline

Fluids are eliminated from the body through the urinary system, the lungs, and the skin. Solid wastes are excreted exclusively through the intestines. In this chapter, we will consider the elimination processes of the urinary and intestinal tracts.

Elimination is a taboo topic in our society. So-called bathroom jokes are more prevalent in American culture than in many others, and public rest rooms in the United States provide much more privacy than is characteristic in most countries.

Although people treat the subject of elimination with some embarrassment, it engenders much interest. One need only listen to the radio or watch television to be reminded that "regularity" is considered highly desirable and "irregularity" is regarded as cause for concern.

Urinary or intestinal problems tend to be very upsetting to people because they not only interfere with daily living but also arouse a sense of being unwell or suffering from a disturbance of the body's vital systems.

## Excretory Organs

Most of the body's elimination of liquids and waste products involves the urinary and intestinal systems. A brief survey of all the body's organs of excretion will shed light on the interrelationship of the several systems involved. The *kidneys* excrete most of the fluids being eliminated in the form of water containing nitrogenous wastes from protein metabolism, toxins from bacteria, and mineral salts. Through perspiration, the skin also excretes water containing nitrogenous wastes and mineral salts, though in lesser quantities. The lungs take oxygen into the body and excrete carbon dioxide and water. Carbon dioxide is produced by the process of catabolism. The gas is dissolved in the plasma and excreted by the lungs.

Solid wastes from the processes of digestion are excreted by the *intestines*. Fecal material contains small amounts of water.

It is important to note that water is used by all these systems as a medium to facilitate elimination of other waste products. Water is also a medium for ingestion; the moisture components of most foods make them receptive to digestion, and the saliva and gastric juices contain large amounts of water and enzymes. These facts will become very important when we consider the water balance of patients with elimination disturbances. See Chapters 21 and 24 for discussions of body water balance as it relates to homeostasis.

## The Urinary System

Basically, the urinary system consists of the kidneys, ureters, bladder, and urethra. This system promotes homeostasis by means of its delicate filtration process: substances needed by the body are retained by the kidneys and filtered back into the circulation, while those that are not needed are excreted in the urine (see Figure 22.1).

### Kidneys

The two *kidneys* are located posteriorly outside the peritoneum (the membrane lining the abdominal cavity), just above the waistline, and are suspended by connective tissue. Each kidney is approximately 3 inches by 4 inches and bean-shaped. Kidney tissue is composed of tiny units called *nephrons*, intricate structures of convoluted blood vessels that have the ability to filter the blood and excrete urine. An almost unbelievable amount of blood is estimated to pass through the kidneys every minute—over 125 ml. Each day 190 liters are filtered, and 189 liters are reabsorbed. Each nephron has its own collecting tubule, which carries minute droplets of urine into the pelvis of the kidney. Urine drains from the kidney pelvis in response to certain pressures and, through gravity, passes into the ureter.

## Ureters

Leading downward from each kidney is a *ureter*, a tube some 10–12 inches in length. The ureters are quite slender, ranging from 1/16 inch to 1/2 inch at the point of attachment to the kidney. A peristaltic or wavelike action causes urine to pass downward into the urinary bladder, and a mucous-membrane valve prevents backward flow of urine into the ureter.

## Bladder

The urinary *bladder* is a storage organ for urine. It normally holds about 500 ml before emptying but has been known to hold upwards of 2000 ml. The bladder provides a sterile environment for the urine. There are three openings on the posterior floor of the bladder: two from the ascending ureters and a descending one for the urethra.

## Urethra

The length of the *urethra* depends on the person's sex. In the female it is a slender tube, 1½ inches in length, which passes behind the pubic bone anterior to the vagina. In the male the urethra is approximately 8 inches long and is threaded through the prostate gland before entering and passing through the penis. Urine is finally excreted through an opening called the *urethral meatus*.

# Assessing Urination

*Urination*, also called *voiding* or *micturition*, is both voluntary and involuntary. A sufficient amount of urine in the bladder—approximately 100 to 500 ml—activates the stretch receptors in the bladder wall; this is called the *stretch reflex*. In response to this reflex, parasympathetic (involuntary) nerve impulses cause the bladder to contract and the internal sphincter of the bladder to relax. The external sphincter, or urethral meatus, is controlled by the cortex or higher centers of the brain, allowing for voluntary control. Thus a person can postpone voiding for some time after the internal sphincter relaxes, although there may be some discomfort. A child learns to control urination by about age three.

## Oliguria

*Oliguria* is scanty formation of urine by the kidneys, which may occur in patients suffering from dehydration or blood loss. The healthy adult kidney secretes approximately 50 ml per hour. As a general guideline for assessment, any amount less than 30 ml per hour is considered insufficient to eliminate body waste and can result in damage to the kidney itself. When a seriously ill patient has a catheter, you may use a special device called a *urimeter*, which measures urine in a small calibrated cylinder as it flows through the tubing before entering the collection bag. For accurate assessment, you may be required to measure the urine every hour.

## Anuria or Suppression

The terms *anuria* and *suppression* both refer to the same condition, total absence of formation of urine by the kidneys. No output will be observed and the patient will not feel distended since there is no urine in the bladder. "Complete kidney shutdown" (a commonly used phrase) is sometimes referred to as *renal failure*.

## Polyuria

*Polyuria* is an excessive amount of urine. A patient who excretes more than 1500 to 1800 ml of urine in twenty-four hours might be said to have polyuria. Though often simply a result of high fluid

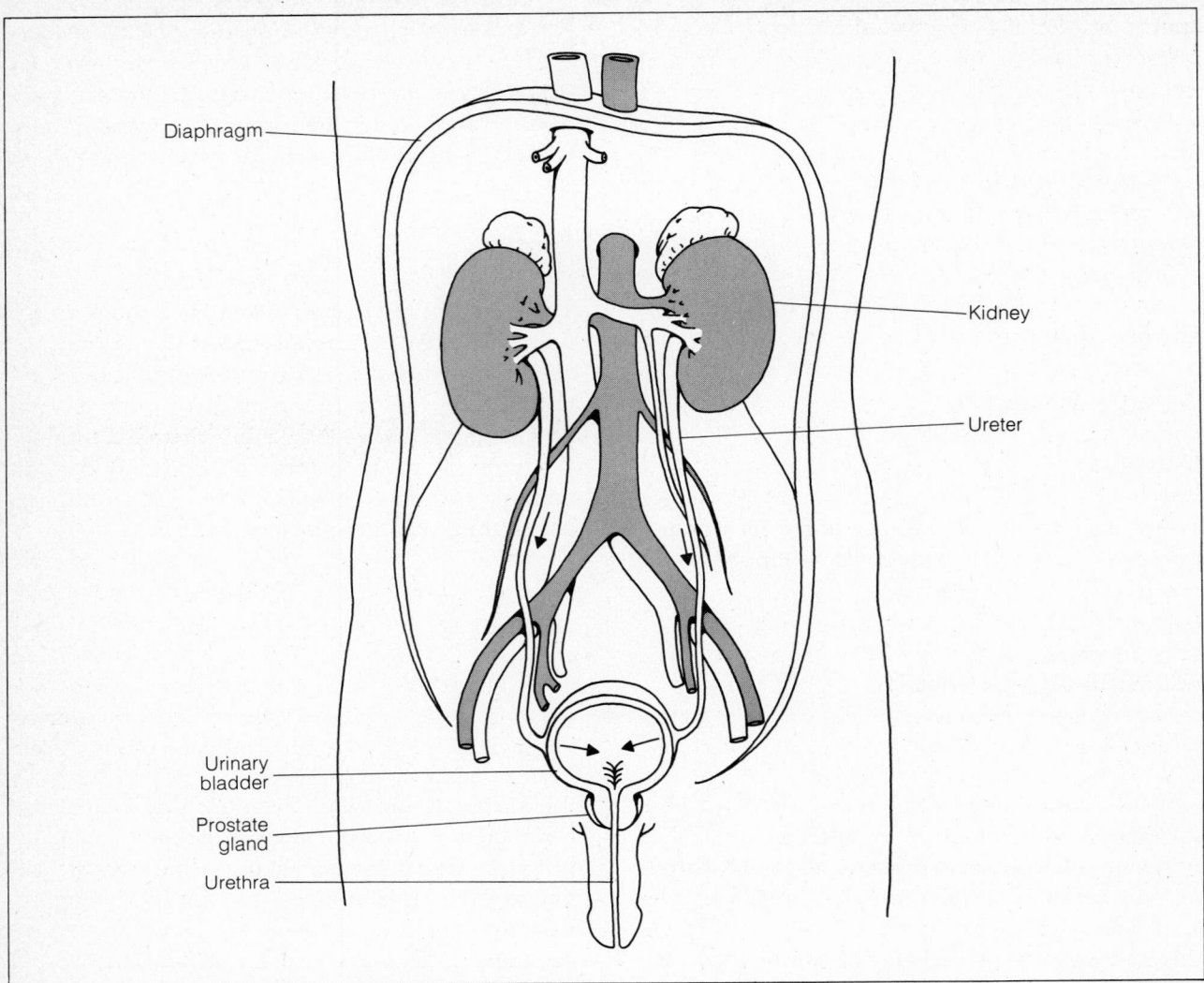

**Figure 22.1   The urinary system (male)**

intake, this condition also characterizes hormonal disturbances. Both diabetes mellitus (a disease of carbohydrate metabolism) and diabetes insipidus (a pituitary disorder) cause polyuria.

## Frequency

*Frequency* is the need or desire to void at more frequent intervals than usual. Each voiding may produce as little as 50 ml. Pressure on the bladder, stress, or infection of the urinary tract can cause frequency.

## Urgency

*Urgency*, which often accompanies frequency, is the inability to postpone urination. The diminished sphincter control of some elderly people and some women who have borne a number of children leads to urgency, as do stress and infection.

## Retention

Urinary *retention* is the holding of urine within the bladder due to inability to void. This condition often occurs in the patient whose urinary system is obstructed, as well as in the postoperative patient as an effect of anesthesia or local trauma. If a patient who has received adequate fluid fails to void within eight hours of surgery, you should consult the physician, who may decide that catheterization is needed. Palpating with care over the bladder area will indicate the extent of retention.

## Urinary Incontinence

Urinary *incontinence,* or involuntary micturition, is not a simple problem. It has variants: inability to hold urine in the bladder at all is called *complete incontinence; partial incontinence* is occasional or infrequent inability to retain urine in the bladder. Complete urinary incontinence causes "dribbling," which is particularly stressful. Incontinence calls for special nursing actions since it is not only distressing to the patient but also a hazard to skin integrity. Many incontinent patients could be continent if appropriate toileting devices or facilities were always near at hand.

# Urine

Urine is normally sterile and consists of approximately 95 percent water. The remaining 5 percent is made up of nitrogenous wastes, diluted toxins, and mineral salts. The characteristics of urine can indicate homeostatic balance or imbalance (see Figure 22.2).

## Normal Characteristics of Urine

In order to identify abnormal characteristics of urine, you should be familiar with what is considered normal. Module 27, "Common Laboratory Tests," will familiarize you with testing methods used to determine the characteristics of urine.

### Amount

The amount of urine excreted varies, depending on many factors, but normally approximates 1500

## Dysuria

*Dysuria* can mean either difficulty urinating or pain on urination. Strictures (narrowing) of the urethra and infection of the urinary tract are causative factors.

## Burning

A burning sensation accompanying urination is one type of dysuria. Because it is a common occurrence, the more specific term *burning* is typically used. Infection is the most frequent cause.

## Nocturia

*Nocturia* is urination during the night, either voluntary or involuntary. Involuntary urination during sleep is called *enuresis*. Common causes are infection and high fluid intake during the evening. In the elderly, nocturia is often caused by diminished bladder tone and/or control of the sphincter.

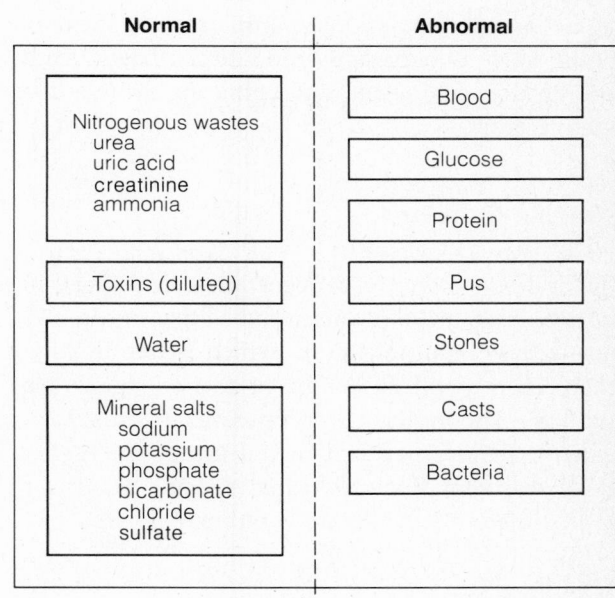

**Figure 22.2 Normal and abnormal characteristics of urine**

ml in twenty-four hours. Fluid intake, environmental temperatures, and perspiration have an influence on the volume of urine.

## Color

The varying shades of normal urine can be described as "pale yellow" (dilute), "straw" (less dilute), and "amber" (concentrated). These differences in coloration are normal. Not only concentration but also certain foods (beets give a reddish tinge) and drugs affect color. Some drugs turn the urine blue, some brown, and others orange.

## Clearness

Urine should be clear or transparent. Allowed to stand, however, cloudiness may occur because of precipitation of phosphates and urates (salts) and bacterial growth. Some drugs, such as the sulfonamides, may give a hazy appearance to the urine.

## Odor

A faint aromatic odor is normally present. If allowed to stand, urine will give off the odor of ammonia due to formation of ammonia salts. Some foods, such as asparagus, and some drugs, such as high dosages of thiamine, give the urine a distinctive odor.

## Specific Gravity

The *specific gravity*, or concentration of wastes, in the water of urine is measured with a hydrometer—a glass bulb on a stem, which, when floating freely in a small container of urine, registers a number. The hydrometer operates by displacement: the more particles in the urine, the higher the instrument floats. Normal specific gravity is approximately 1.010 to 1.025 (French, 1980).

## pH

*pH* is a measure of the acidity or alkalinity of a solution. Neutral pH is 7; usually the urine is slightly acid (about 6), though it may vary from 4.8 to 7.5. The intake of certain foods, primarily vegetables, may render the urine temporarily alkaline. The pH of urine is usually measured with a dipstick, a litmus-impregnated plastic strip. Again, see Module 27, "Common Laboratory Tests."

## Abnormal Characteristics of Urine

The following are abnormal characteristics of urine.

## Blood

Bleeding may occur anywhere in the urinary tract and be detected in the urine. Blood in the urine is called *hematuria*. Blood in the urine that is not observable is called *occult*, or hidden. You should always consider menstrual flow as a possible source of hematuria in female patients of childbearing age.

## Glycosuria or Glucosuria

Sugar is an abnormal finding in urine. It can be attributable to an abnormally high intake of sugar or to infectious, metabolic, or inflammatory diseases.

## Protein

Although small amounts of protein are sometimes present in otherwise normal urine, amounts large enough to measure are considered abnormal. Protein in the urine can be indicative of bleeding, infection, or inflammation. This condition is called *proteinuria* or *albuminuria*.

## Pus

The presence of pus in the urine, called *pyuria*, indicates the presence of a highly infectious process. The person will probably have other signs and symptoms, such as fever, flank or back pain, and difficulty or pain when voiding.

## Stones

Stones that originate in the kidney, called *renal calculi,* are formed from various kinds of salts that precipitate. Smaller stones, often resembling sand, may pass out of the body in the urine. It is not uncommon for larger calculi to lodge in the pelvis of the kidney or in the urethra, causing inflammation; these stones sometimes have to be surgically removed.

## Casts

*Casts* are small hardened dish-shaped mucus particles that are "casted" in the tubules and discarded in the urine. It is not unusual to find a limited number of casts in urine that is otherwise normal in character. Such a condition is not considered harmful.

## Bacteria

In cases of infection, bacteria can be found in the urine. The term for this condition is *bacteriuria.* A specimen of urine can be sent to the laboratory, where the organisms are grown in a culture for purposes of identification.

# Urinary Problems

Because all the systems of the body are interrelated, disturbances of other systems can cause urinary problems. Localized problems can also occur in specific parts of the urinary tract, such as the kidneys, ureters, bladder, or urethra.

As for localized factors, *obstruction* may occur anyplace within the urinary system. Abnormal cell growth, benign or malignant, may occur in the kidney, ureters, bladder, or urethra. Stones can also form, causing obstruction. Localized trauma may be evident in the form of bruising, hemorrhaging, or swelling of localized parts of the system. Because the urinary tract is lined with mucous membrane, the urinary system is particularly prone to infection; such infection travels readily throughout the system.

A number of systemic factors can cause urinary problems. Heart disease and complications of the circulation cause urinary disturbances due to the decreased flow of blood to the kidneys. Without sufficient blood to process, the body retains fluid and substances, and the kidney tissue may be damaged. The patient may show signs of electrolyte imbalance, such as muscle weakness, lassitude, and even confusion. Fluid is also retained in the tissue, resulting in edema, most commonly in the lower part of the sacrum and the ankles. Hormonal factors can also cause problems. Because certain hormones, such as aldosterone, have a regulatory effect on the kidneys, a disturbance of the pituitary or adrenal glands that produce these hormones can cause urinary disturbance.

Severe dehydration, regardless of cause, may bring about serious kidney problems due to the decreased blood flow to the organs. Any overwhelming generalized trauma to the body has a systemic effect, causing kidney dysfunction. Generalized infection depletes body fluid due to elevated temperatures, affecting kidney function. Loss of muscle tone, often seen in the elderly and in patients suffering disease of the muscular system, may bring about an inability to exercise muscular control over urination. Conditions of the central nervous system and spinal cord may also directly influence urinary efficiency through interruption of innervation. The interplay between urinary function and other systems can greatly complicate assessment.

The anatomical differences between males and females make for some differences in the prevalence of specific problems. The female is more prone to infection because of the shortness of the urethra relative to that of the male. The male may, however, be more susceptible to obstruction: because the *prostate* gland surrounds the male urethra, any hypertrophy, or swelling, of this gland will cause some degree of obstruction. And, of course, the male is more vulnerable to trauma of the urethra due to its external position.

# Assessing Urinary Function

Three general considerations are central to the assessment process. First, it is important to know something about the patient's *condition* and *diagnosis*. The female patient with an infection of the vagina can readily develop an infection of the bladder as well because of the close proximity of the organs. The male patient with an enlarged prostate may have difficulty voiding. Any surgical patient who is to spend a relatively long period under anesthesia should be assessed for urinary retention.

Second, the patient's *subjective symptoms* are instructive to the nurse. A patient who trusts the nurse is more likely to discuss his or her urinary problems. If the patient does not volunteer such information, the nurse might without embarrassment ask one or two direct questions. Patients often spontaneously report changes in the color or odor of urine. A change in amount is sometimes mentioned, if the patient becomes concerned. And the patient who experiences pain or burning on micturition will usually report it, since this symptom is very disturbing.

Third, the nurse relies heavily on *objective observations*. Nursing data adds important information in assessing urinary function. Does the patient have any of the conditions described on pages 366–367? The patient should excrete approximately 1000–1800 ml of urine in twenty-four hours (though many factors influence output, such as the amount of fluid consumed). Some fluids, such as coffee, beer, and wine, are *diuretic*—that is, they stimulate the production of urine. Medications may either decrease or increase the production of urine. A large, general classification for drugs whose purpose is to increase the amount of urine is *diuretic*. Some pain medications decrease urine production. Testing the urine for the presence of abnormal substances is also an aspect of assessment. Some such tests can be performed on the nursing unit; others require laboratory processing.

# Intervention for Urinary Problems

The three most common procedures in intervention for urinary problems are intake and output, collection of urine specimens, and catheterization.

## Intake and Output

In assessing urinary function, the physician may order the patient to be placed on *intake and output*. If nursing assessment so indicates, you may also initiate this procedure on your own, noting it in the record. Output—the fluid excreted from the body—is measured in conjunction with intake. *Intake* involves measuring and recording all fluids ingested orally or intravenously, including water and solidified fluids, such as gelatin dessert and ice cream. Data are usually recorded on an appropriate form and totaled every eight or twenty-four hours, depending on the policy of the facility.

Most of the water excreted from the body is in the form of urine. Thus, to assess the functioning of the urinary system, urinary *output* must be accurately measured. This measurement can prove meaningless without careful recording of input to determine water balance of the patient (see the section on water balance in Chapter 24, "Circulation").

If the patient is able, it is essential to include him or her in the plan. First, explain why the procedure is important and how it is performed. A measuring container can be kept in the bathroom or, if the patient uses a bedpan or urinal, you may do the measuring. Writing down the finding immediately on the appropriate form at the bedside prevents the loss of valuable information. Module 11, "Intake and Output," outlines how to compute these measurements.

## Collecting Urine Specimens

Urine may be collected for any of several reasons. It is routine to collect a voided specimen upon a patient's admission to the hospital, regardless of the diagnosis; this procedure is often referred to as a *UA* or *routine urinalysis*. If the physician wants a "clean-catch" or "clean-voided" specimen, the patient's external urethral meatus is cleansed and he or she is instructed to begin urinating, "catch" a portion of the flow in a sterile container, and finish voiding.

A "twenty-four-hour urine" specimen is one that contains all urine voided for a twenty-four-hour period. At the specified starting hour, the patient voids and discards the specimen. All subsequent urine is saved in a large container. At the end of twenty-four hours, the patient voids a last time, adding this urine to the container. In order to prevent chemical deterioration of the urine over the twenty-four-hour period, a preservative substance may be added to the container, or the container may be refrigerated or kept in a pan of ice.

## Catheterization

If a sterile specimen of urine is ordered by the physician, a *catheterization* is performed: a small tube or catheter is inserted through the male or female urethra and into the bladder, and urine is withdrawn for the specimen. When a catheter is already in place, it should not be disconnected to secure a urine specimen, since each time the system is interrupted there is a chance of introducing pathogens that may cause a urinary-tract infection. Instead, the nurse should clamp the distal (farthest from the body) portion of the catheter for twenty minutes to allow a small amount of urine to collect in the catheter. Then, after the surface of the catheter is cleansed with an alcohol sponge, the needle is inserted through the catheter wall and urine is withdrawn into the syringe. If the insertion is performed carefully and at an angle,

the catheter will reseal. The insertion should be made between the end of the catheter and the tubing that connects to the catheter balloon so as not to aspirate the sterile water in the balloon and cause the catheter to come out.

Whatever method is used to obtain a urine sample, it is the nurse's responsibility to see that the specimen is labeled properly, usually by attaching the appropriate laboratory slip. The urine should either be sent to the laboratory reasonably promptly or refrigerated to prevent the character of the urine from changing as it stands. For the specific techniques of collecting urine specimens, consult Module 18, "Collecting Specimens."

Very large amounts of urine should not be drained from the bladder all at once, since doing so can cause local trauma to the bladder or a mild-to-severe systemic reaction characterized by symptoms of shock. This outcome is due to autonomic nervous system reactions as a result of pressure changes in the abdomen. The patient may be catheterized with a "straight" catheter, which is removed from the bladder at the end of the procedure, or, in cases of incontinence, a catheter that remains in the bladder due to the inflation of a 5–30 ml balloon filled with sterile water. Such a catheter is called an *indwelling, Foley,* or *continuous-drainage catheter,* depending on the facility (Figure 22.3 shows a Foley catheter in place in a male pa-

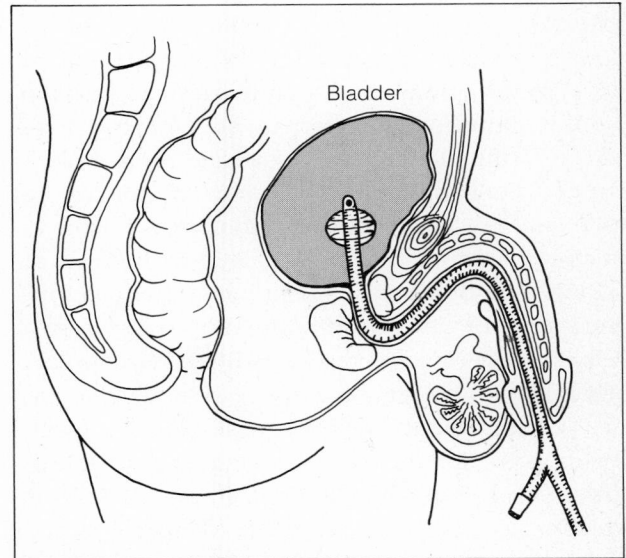

**Figure 22.3  Foley catheter in place**

tient). For specific aspects of the skill of catheterization, Module 39, "Catheterization," should be consulted.

Because of the danger of infection, catheterization is usually performed only when essential for diagnosis or treatment. A physician may order a catheterization either to secure a sterile specimen of urine, relieve a distended bladder, or instill a bladder medication. A person who, because of spinal-cord injury, has a *neurogenic bladder* (partial paralysis of the bladder musculature that prevents sufficient emptying) can be taught self-catheterization. Catheterization is also performed in order to instill a dye that can be visualized by x ray in order to detect structural problems of the urinary tract, but this procedure is done in the x-ray department rather than the nursing unit. Strict sterility must be maintained when catheterization is performed, since the urine and urinary tract are normally sterile and all efforts must be taken to avoid infection.

## Initiating Bladder Rehabilitation for the Patient With a Catheter

When a patient has an indwelling catheter, a bladder rehabilitation program can be initiated to help the bladder return to normal functioning after the catheter has been discontinued. The goal is to restore the normal elasticity of the bladder for proper emptying. A physician may order a "clamp and release" routine before the catheter is removed, which means that the catheter is clamped for a period of time and then released so that the bladder empties. The alternate stretching and relaxing of the bladder walls simulate normal bladder-wall functioning and help maintain or restore tone. At first, the conscious patient may be able to tolerate clamping only as long as thirty minutes at a time. The duration of clamping is gradually increased until the patient can tolerate it for two hours. After removal of the catheter, the bladder rehabilitation program continues in the same manner. The unconscious patient who has an indwelling catheter should also be placed on such a program. One word of caution: if the patient is unconscious and cannot voice discomfort, the nurse must be scrupulously conscientious about releasing the catheter clamp at the designated

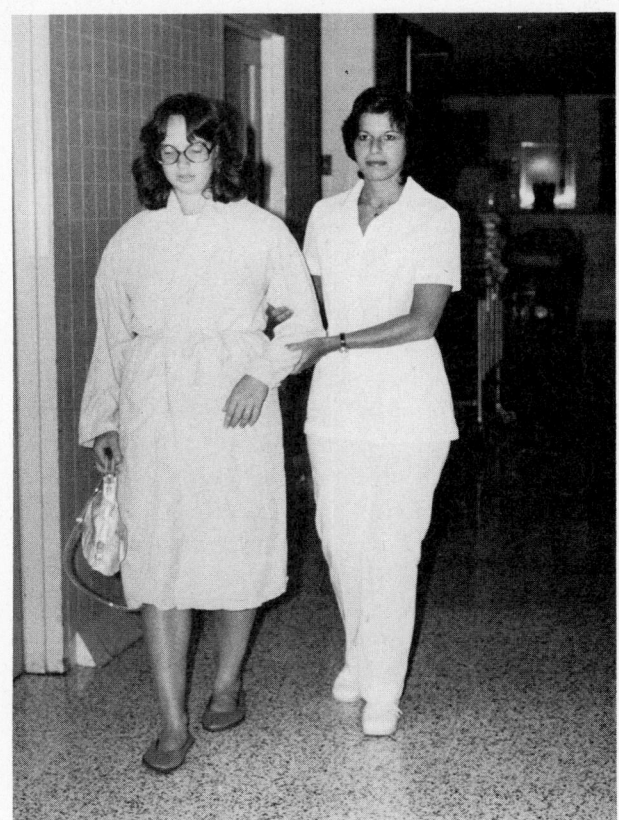

**Figure 22.4   A patient ambulating with a catheter in place**
Lawrence Cherkas

time. Serious injury can occur to the bladder if proper drainage does not take place.

## Catheter Removal and Health Teaching

The patient who has had an indwelling catheter is in need of health teaching when it is removed. It is unusual for a patient who has an indwelling catheter for a long time to be completely free of urinary-tract infection. For this reason, the importance of consuming large amounts of fluid is stressed before, during, and after the insertion of an indwelling catheter. A high fluid intake "flushes" the system and prevents the pooling of urine in the bladder. It is sometimes recommended that the patient drink cranberry juice, which tends to render the urine more acid, discouraging the growth of pathogens. The patient may be warned that a mild burning sensation might occur initially upon urination. Very frequent urination may also be necessary at first. To help the nurse observe, assess, and plan care of urinary problems, the patient should be asked to tell the nurse when voiding occurs, the amount voided, and whether discomfort occurs.

## Replacements for Kidney Function

When complete renal (kidney) failure occurs, there are a number of procedures for replicating kidney function; these are called *dialysis* procedures. Two such methods are currently in use, and research is continuing to refine them. One is *hemodialysis*, which is circulation of the patient's blood through a filtering or "kidney" machine. The blood is drawn and returned through a venous-arterial shunt, usually just above the inner wrist. The semipermeable membranes of the machine remove waste products. Because hemodialysis is increasingly being performed on nursing units, you should be aware that the shunt arm must never be used to draw blood, start an intravenous infusion, or take blood pressure measurements. The veins must be protected from any compromise or injury.

The second dialysis method is *peritoneal dialysis*, whereby carefully measured amounts of a special dialyzing solution are introduced into and withdrawn intermittently from the peritoneal cavity through a small incision and cannula. The patient's blood pressure must be constantly monitored during the procedure.

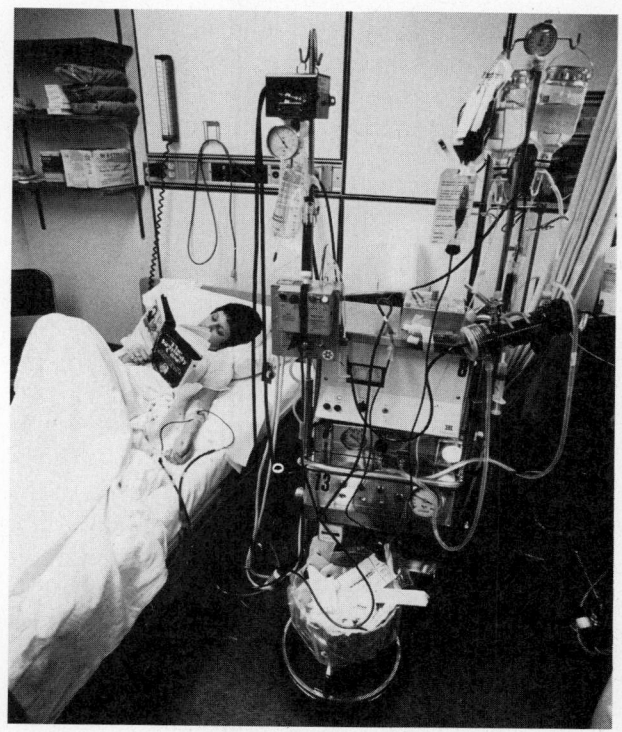

**Figure 22.5  A patient on a hemodialysis "run"**
Dan Bernstein

## Nursing Care for Urinary Problems

Whatever the patient's particular urinary problem, good general nursing care is imperative. Encouraging fluids provides the water needed for more efficient filtration. Adequate nutrition is essential to overcome infection and build tissue. Exercise stimulates output, and rest provides for needed relaxation of the organs of urination.

If the patient has an infection or needs increased output, you may be required to administer special medications. Knowledge of these specific drugs will allow you to inform the patient about their actions and uses. Patients with urinary infections also need health teaching about special measures for personal hygiene.

Because urinary problems cause the patient not only physical pain but also embarrassment and anxiety, a confident and accepting attitude on your part can be of the utmost value in comforting the patient.

Two of the most common and difficult problems, for both the nurse and the patient, are inability to urinate and urinary incontinence.

## Encouragement of Voluntary Urination

It is distressing to the patient to feel the need to void but be unable to do so. There are several ways the nurse can promote adequate emptying of the bladder. First, the patient needs privacy and benefits from an unhurried attitude on the part of the nurse. Adequate fluid intake is essential, since sufficient urine must be present before the bladder reflex is activated: only when the bladder contains at least 300 ml is the desire to eliminate usually activated. Placing the patient's hands in a pan of warm water, pouring warm or very cold water over the perineum, running tap water within the patient's hearing, or putting pressure on one side of the urinary meatus may facilitate voiding. Manually exerting pressure on the bladder to force urine out, known as *credé,* should be avoided; this procedure does not allow the elasticity of the bladder wall to function and may cause damage to the sphincter. However, credé may be used appropriately in some rehabilitation settings, on the order of a physician, with a patient who has lost and is not expected to regain voluntary bladder control. If all methods to encourage and help the patient to void voluntarily within eight hours of the last voiding fail, the physician may have to be contacted to order a catheterization.

## Bladder Rehabilitation

General bladder rehabilitation, frequently called bladder training, is different from the bladder re-habilitation of the patient with a catheter. It is an important undertaking planned and carried out by the nurse for the patient suffering from urinary incontinence. Like any health teaching, it must be a cooperative effort on the part of both patient and nurse. The nurse should explain the program and its goals to the patient. Patients who fully understand that the goal is more normal functioning of the bladder usually become highly motivated. Sufficient fluid intake, usually from 2000 to 4000 ml daily, is essential. The patient is encouraged to retain the urine as long as possible, not exceeding two hours. Use of the bathroom toilet to void is preferred; however, a commode or, if neither of the two is feasible, a bedpan (the patient in the upright position) may be used. Any of these approaches, along with a provision for the male patient to stand, approximates normal voiding conditions. Positioning, of course, is contingent on the patient's physical condition. Voidings are spaced increasingly far apart, from the duration that can initially be tolerated up to two hours. The stretching-relaxing sequence of this process reinstates bladder muscle tone, eventually affording the patient more voluntary control.

Although incontinence usually has a physiological basis, it also has overtones of dependency. With older patients, it has been demonstrated that getting up out of bed, dressing in their own clothing, and being offered bathroom accommodations on a regular schedule can often reverse a trend toward incontinence.

Whether the patient has difficulty voiding or controlling voiding, the nurse's attitude is crucial. It is understandable for the patient to be noticeably embarrassed and upset over such a situation, and the nurse should exhibit an understanding attitude.

# The Intestinal System

The function of the intestinal system is to eliminate solid wastes from the body. Although the intestinal system has many parts, it is sufficient for our purposes to consider the small intestine, the large intestine, and the rectum.

## Small Intestine

Partially digested food passes from the stomach into the first part of the small intestine, the *duodenum,* and then along 20 or more feet of small intestine, whose diameter is about 1 inch. The duodenum (10 inches long) is followed by the *jejunum* (about 8 feet in length) and, finally, the ileum (12 feet) (Anthony and Kolthoff, 1978).

Digestion is completed when the small intestine absorbs any nutrients needed. It also secretes hormones, which in turn stimulate other digestive juices.

## Large Intestine

The large intestine, or *colon*, stores and transports waste products. It has a larger diameter than the small intestine, a little over 2 inches, and is only 5 to 6 feet in length. The first portion of the large intestine is the *cecum*, a short pouchlike structure that attaches to the second part, or colon (the same term is applied to this segment alone and to the entire large intestine). The colon ascends, transverses, and then descends, and the corresponding parts are known, respectively, as the *ascending colon, transverse colon,* and *descending colon* (see Figure 22.6). The fourth portion of the large intestine, the *sigmoid,* is somewhat flexed and attaches to the rectum.

## Rectum

The *rectum,* a vascular, muscular structure, expels feces out of the body through an opening called the *anus.*

# The Process of Defecation

*Defecation* is the expulsion of solid wastes in the form of *feces,* also called *stool.* After the essential nutritional components have been extracted from the ingested food, the solid wastes are propelled through the large intestine by peristalsis.

The massive movement of feces into the rectum from the colon by means of peristalsis stimulates the receptors in the walls of the rectum. Reflex (involuntary) relaxation of the internal sphincter of the anus expels the feces. Because the external sphincter is voluntarily controlled, the person may strain and relax to expel feces or inhibit the sphincter to withhold defecation.

Thus defecation, like urination, is both voluntary and involuntary. The parasympathetic nervous system carries the rectal sensation of fullness to the sacral area of the spinal cord and stimulates peristalsis and muscle tone. The sympathetic nervous system has the opposing effect. The alternating effects of these two systems allow the rectal sphincter to relax and the fecal contents of the rectum and large bowel to pass. Voluntary control can also be exerted to delay defecation. Most children have control of bowel function by age three.

The frequency of stools varies a great deal from individual to individual. Some people defecate on a regular daily basis, while others have bowel movements as infrequently as every three to four days. Each pattern is normal for a given individual. Thus it is prudent to talk about frequency in terms not of what is "normal" but of what is usual for the person in question.

## Assessing Defecation

### Constipation

*Constipation* is the retention of fecal material within the rectum. This condition may be characterized merely by a hardening of the fecal material, which interferes with easy passage, or by the lack of stool for a prolonged period due to the buildup of feces in the rectum. It is important to keep in mind the person's usual pattern of defecation: if the patient usually defecates daily, an absence of stool for several days constitutes constipation; if the person

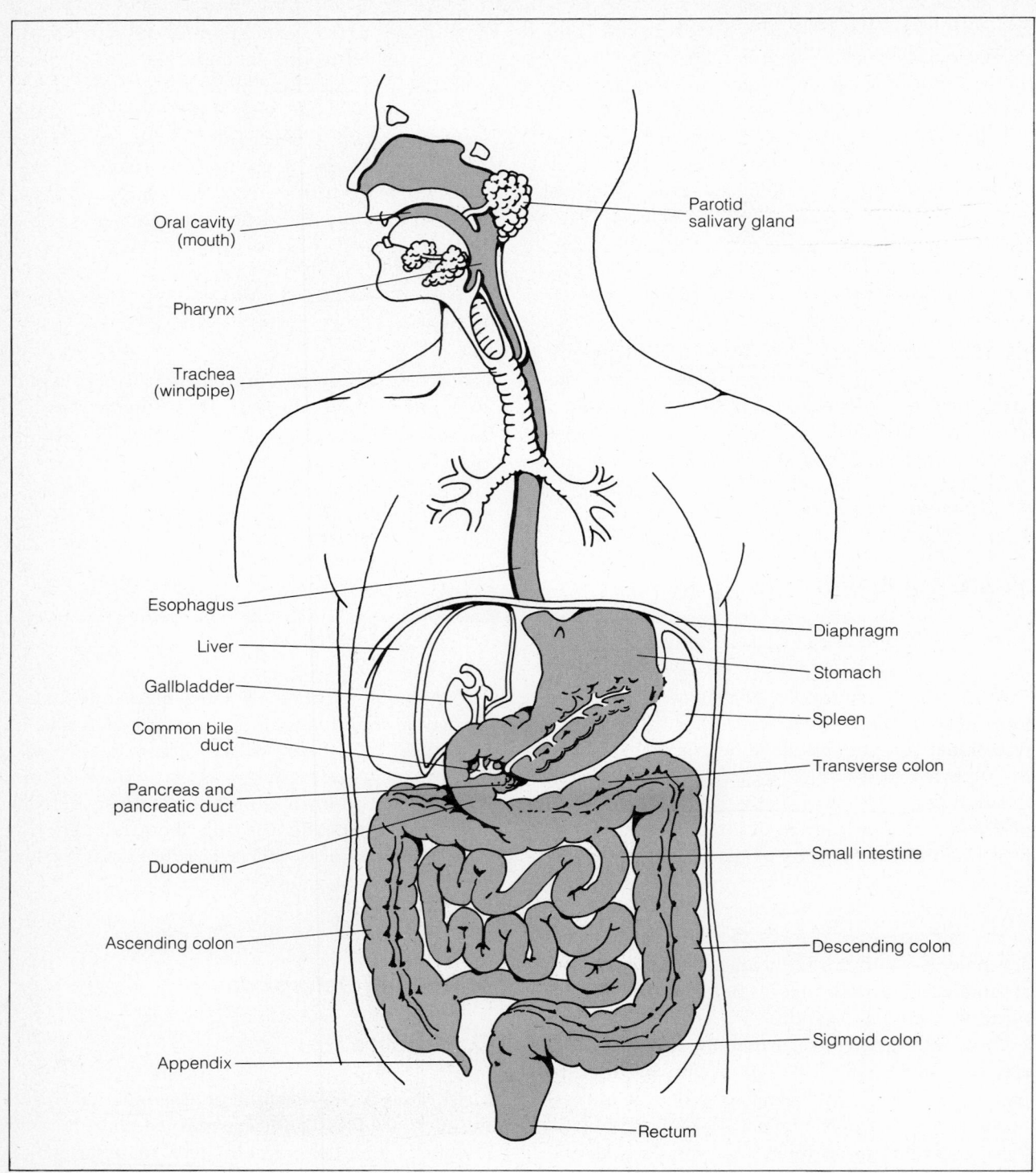

**Figure 22.6 The intestinal system**

Labels on the figure:

Oral cavity (mouth)

Pharynx

Trachea (windpipe)

Parotid salivary gland

Esophagus

Liver

Gallbladder

Common bile duct

Pancreas and pancreatic duct

Duodenum

Ascending colon

Appendix

Diaphragm

Stomach

Spleen

Transverse colon

Small intestine

Descending colon

Sigmoid colon

Rectum

defecates less frequently, more days must elapse before assessing the person as constipated.

## Impaction

*Impaction* is a different and more severe condition than constipation: a *bolus,* or rounded stone-hard stool, becomes lodged in the lower bowel and cannot be passed. The patient may have frequent small amounts of liquid stool due to seepage around the irritation of the very hard stool mass. To assess for an impaction in the lower bowel, you can put on a clean glove and insert a lubricated finger into the rectum, feeling for and possibly removing an impaction. When the impaction is high in the bowel, this is not possible. A high impaction will usually eventually move downward, where it can be felt and removed.

## Diarrhea

*Diarrhea* is the frequent passage of unformed or liquid stool, which can become so profuse that defecation becomes involuntary.

## Flatulence

*Flatus* is gas in the intestinal tract, usually expelled through the anus. Gas can be caused by many factors, including diet, emotions, and the swallowing of air.

## Steatorrhea

*Steatorrhea* is a condition caused by malabsorption and characterized by stool containing large amounts of fat. Such stools have a foul odor and an oily, fatty appearance. The malabsorption that gives rise to steatorrhea can result from such diseases as sprue, a tropical disease, and enzyme deficiencies of the pancreas.

## Fecal Incontinence

*Fecal incontinence* is inability to control defecation. Though the term does not describe the characteristics of the stool, it is usually more liquid than solid in consistency.

# Feces

Unlike urine, fecal material is not sterile; it contains certain bacteria that make up the normal flora of the intestinal tract. The characteristics of the feces, too, can help us assess the patient's state of homeostasis.

## Normal Characteristics of Fecal Material

Fecal material is normally soft but formed and contains a variety of organisms as well as other substances. It is important to know the characteristics of normal fecal material in order to make accurate assessments.

## Water

Some percentage of fecal matter is water. The proportion of water varies, depending on the firmness of the stool. Patients who have fever or are dehydrated may have less water in the stool, causing constipation.

## Color

Normal stool is a medium-brown color, though it may vary somewhat in tone. Foods can influence color: green vegetables may lend a green tint, and beets a reddish color. The unabsorbed portion of oral iron medications makes the stool black.

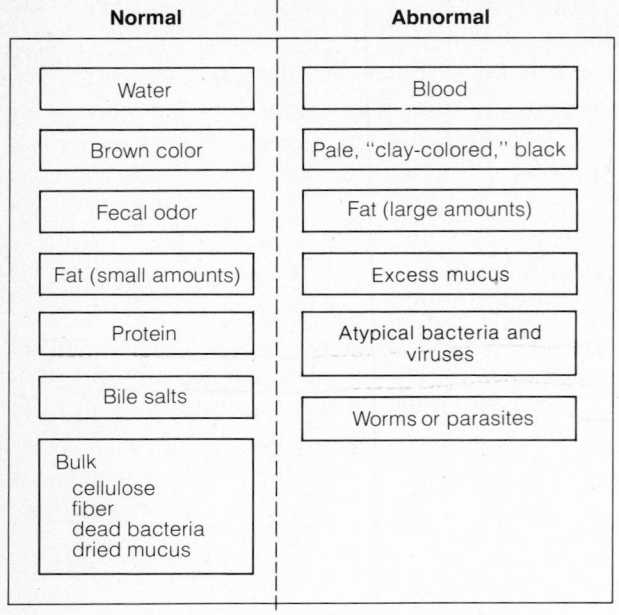

| Normal | Abnormal |
|---|---|
| Water | Blood |
| Brown color | Pale, "clay-colored," black |
| Fecal odor | Fat (large amounts) |
| Fat (small amounts) | Excess mucus |
| Protein | Atypical bacteria and viruses |
| Bile salts | Worms or parasites |
| Bulk<br>  cellulose<br>  fiber<br>  dead bacteria<br>  dried mucus | |

**Figure 22.7  Normal and abnormal characteristics of feces**

## Odor

Feces have a distinctive odor, which varies depending on the kinds of foods ingested.

## Fat

A small amount of undigested fat is a normal constituent of the feces.

## Protein

A small percentage of fecal matter is protein.

## Bile Salts

The bile salts in the feces give it its normal brown color.

## Bulk

Bulk—the waste products of digestion—is composed primarily of cellulose and fiber. Dead bacteria and dried mucus particles are also present.

## Abnormal Characteristics of Fecal Material

### Blood

Blood in feces is abnormal. Fresh blood, which is bright red, indicates bleeding low in the intestinal tract. Old (coagulated) blood, which has gone through the process of digestion and appears black, may have come from a source high in the intestinal tract.

### Fat

Certain diseases make for large amounts of excreted fat, giving the stool a frothy appearance. The term for this is steatorrhea.

### Mucus

Several types of a condition called colitis, or inflammation of the colon, are characterized by large amounts of mucus in the feces.

### Color

Feces of an abnormal color may indicate disease. Very pale "clay-colored" stools may accompany disease of the biliary system; very dark stools may contain increased bilirubin due to liver impairment.

### Atypical Bacteria and Viruses

In cases of intestinal infection, atypical bacteria or viruses can be found in the fecal matter.

### Parasites and Worms

The warmth and nourishment provided by the intestinal environment invite infestation if a person is exposed to parasites or worms. Many of these organisms can be seen without the aid of a microscope.

## Defecation Problems

As is true of urination, there are numerous factors that can cause bowel problems. Because of the innervation of the tract by both sympathetic and parasympathetic nerve pathways, emotions can play a direct part in bowel disturbance. Though the effect of emotions on intestinal function is not simple, it has been suggested that overstimulation of the parasympathetic nervous system due to emotional stress results in diarrhea and that excessive stimulation of the sympathetic nervous system results in constipation. Studies show that both chronic and acute diarrhea and constipation can be caused by emotional factors. Anxiety and stress can alter patterns of defecation (Farrar, 1973; Connell, 1973).

Fecal elimination is directly related to diet. Lack of roughage, which characterizes bland or liquid diets, usually causes diarrhea because such substances pass through the intestinal tract very rapidly. Other patients develop constipation due to stagnation of the waste material in the tract. A certain amount of roughage seems essential to maintain regularity.

Because increasing the water in the intestine causes the stool to soften, drinking sufficient fluid is an important aspect of avoiding constipation. Many physicians recommend at least 2800–3000 ml of fluid per day. Conversely, dehydration causes constipation; in an effort to provide itself with water, the body reabsorbs fluid from the bowel, leaving hard, dry feces that are difficult to expel.

The effects of drugs on ability to defecate and on stool consistency have long been known. The psychotropic drugs, iron preparations, and some medications for pain, such as morphine, cause constipation.

Structural conditions such as loss of tone in the intestinal wall and partial or complete obstruction interfere with the passage of solid waste products. Inflammatory or infectious conditions, various types of colitis, and the presence of parasites can alter intestinal function. Damage to the brain or spinal cord can interrupt nerve impulses, causing either fecal retention or fecal incontinence.

Exercise is very important to bowel function. Lack of exercise decreases abdominal muscle tone and slows peristalsis, resulting in constipation. Regular exercise promotes regular bowel elimination.

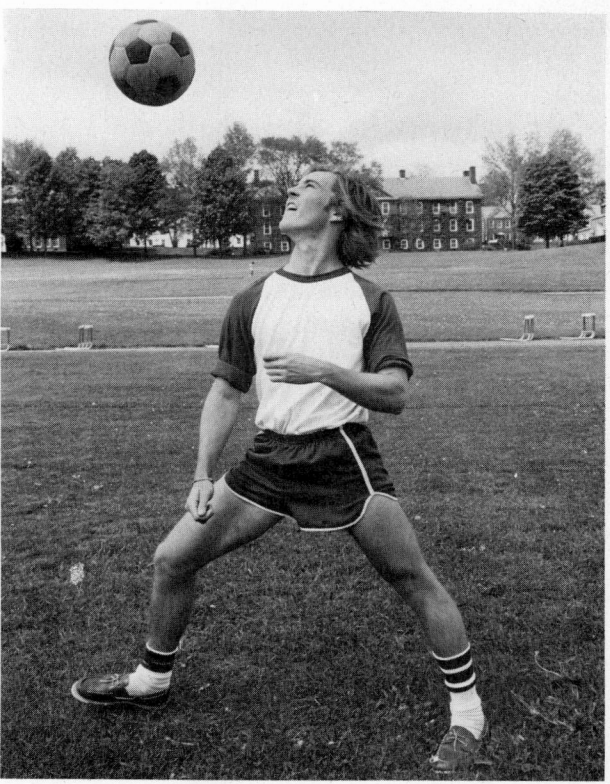

**Figure 22.8  Exercise promotes elimination**
J. D. Sloan/Global Focus

## Assessing Intestinal Function

Several factors should be considered in an assessment. The patient's *condition* is important in that a patient who is immobilized or on bedrest is prone to constipation. Lack of exercise diminishes the tone of the intestinal wall. Abdominal or pelvic surgery has a direct effect on defecation because of the mechanical manipulation of the intestinal structures. The patient's *diagnosis* is also crucial to assessment. For example, a patient with ulcerative colitis is observed and assessed for the frequency and character of stools and for intestinal bleeding. *Subjective data*—what the patient tells the nurse about bowel problems or habits—enhance assessment. Such information is usually requested when a nursing history is taken on admission to the hospital.

Again, objective data are very important. An accurate record of the frequency and character of the patient's stools is necessary to plan care. Very often patients in hospitals have standing orders for a laxative or antidiarrheal drug to be provided at the discretion of the nurse, and such a record helps the nurse to gauge the administration of such drugs and to promote a regular pattern of defecation. Stools are usually described as small, moderate or medium, or large, though you may wish to be more explicit in unusual cases. To describe consistency, terms such as "formed," "semi-formed," and "liquid" are employed. Unusual color or odor, such as "green," "yellow," or "clay-colored," should also be noted. Occasionally, a stool requires such special terms as "frothy" or "mucoid" (containing mucus).

It is also important to look for unusual or foreign substances in the stool. If frank, bright red blood is present, it should be so described. Some foods and drugs may turn the stools reddish, but this phenomenon does not resemble fresh blood. Tests must be performed to identify the substance. Black tarry stools are caused by blood that has been passed through the stomach and small intestine and been digested.

## Intervention for Defecation Problems

Two procedures widely used for purposes of assessment and/or treatment are collection of stool specimens and enema administration.

### Collecting Stool Specimens

Examination of stool specimens in the laboratory is an adjunct to diagnosis and measurement of a patient's progress. Some tests for the presence of *occult* (hidden or invisible) blood in the stool, such as the *guaiac* test, are usually performed in the laboratory. Another test for blood in the stool is the "Hematest," for which the directions on the package should be consulted. Tests for parasites require that the stool specimens be sent to the laboratory promptly or kept warm so that any parasites present will be viable and observable. Stool cultures reveal the presence or absence of bacteria. It is the nurse's responsibility to see that specimens are collected and cared for properly. Consult Module 18, "Collecting Specimens," for specific directions on collecting stool specimens.

### Enema

An *enema* is a procedure whereby a fluid is injected or instilled into the colon through the rectum. It is usually done for cleansing purposes, either to allow for the passage of hard stool or in preparation for tests. Large-volume enemas typically use tap water or mild soap suds (though soap-suds enemas are infrequently performed because of their irritating quality). Smaller-volume oil-retention enemas are used to soften hardened feces and to help the patient pass the stool. Most commonly used are commercial premeasured hypertonic disposable enemas. After a small amount of fluid has been instilled into the colon by squeezing the container, a chemical reaction occurs that stimulates peristalsis and defecation. The procedure is explained in Module 19, "Administering Enemas."

Medications are occasionally delivered by means of an enema, using a small amount of fluid. An enema is a clean but not sterile procedure, relatively free of discomfort if good technique is observed. A physician's order is needed. Many physicians leave standing orders for bowel care, allowing the nurse to exercise independent judgment as to a particular patient's needs.

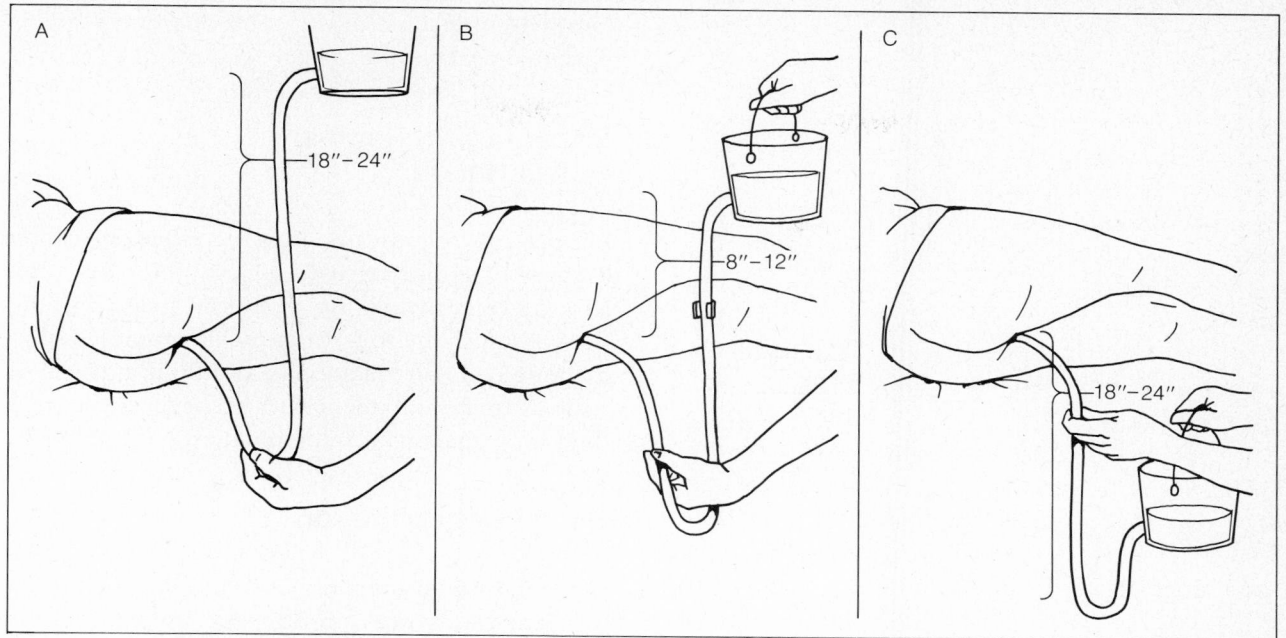

**Figure 22.9 Regulating fluid pressure by height of container**
A: Moderate pressure; B: low pressure; C: negative pressure, for siphoning.

## Nursing Care for Intestinal Problems

As a nurse you will encounter a variety of types of intestinal dysfunction. By far the most common are constipation and diarrhea. It is not unusual for a patient to experience alternating episodes of constipation and diarrhea during an illness. The nurse must thus vary nursing actions in response to the immediate situation.

Unless specially prescribed by the physician, laxatives should be avoided as the principal treatment for constipation because of their habit-forming and irritating characteristics. Often physicians leave standing orders for laxatives to be used at the request of the patient or at the discretion of the nurse. It is better to increase fluid intake, supply adequate roughage in the diet, and provide sufficient exercise if the patient's condition warrants. Private toilet facilities and sufficient time to relax are a great help to the patient; patients are too often hurried because of the demands of care

or procedures to be performed. If the patient is made anxious by the busy hospital environment, defecation becomes difficult.

The patient with diarrhea has multiple problems. Within a very short time, profuse diarrhea can cause dehydration. The patient soon becomes debilitated and exhausted, and adequate rest must be allowed for. Losing liquid stool can cause disturbances in the electrolyte and acid-base balance, with dire consequences for the very young and very old. Skin care becomes a major concern, due to excoriation or redness and irritation of the skin in the rectal area. Encouraging fluids prevents the effects of dehydration, and good skin care and the application of protective emollients restore the skin. The nurse may also administer drugs ordered by the physician.

Abdominal pain and cramping can occur in conjunction with both constipation and diarrhea. The

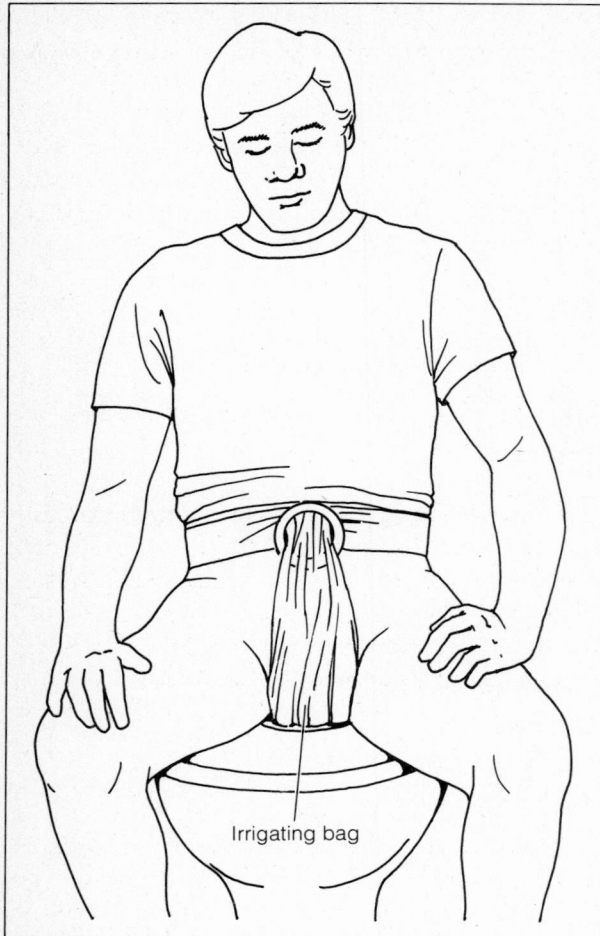

**Figure 22.10 Patient sitting on a commode for irrigation of a colostomy**
A lap drape has been omitted to make the position of the drainage bag clear.

Irrigating bag

application of heat and medications ordered by the physician are often used to relieve such symptoms.

Although impaction most frequently afflicts the elderly patient, it can occur at any age, particularly in cases of immobilization. An oil-retention enema is frequently administered to soften the impaction and lubricate the intestinal wall, facilitating passage of the impaction. After the oil-retention enema, a cleansing enema may be ordered. If this procedure is not successful, the impaction may need to be broken up and removed with a gloved, lubricated finger. Good general nursing care supportive of all body systems is essential to the pa-

tient with intestinal dysfunction of any type, as is psychological support.

## Encouraging Regular Bowel Habits

For patients who can no longer control defecation because of age or disease (such as neurologic deficit), there are ways the nurse can help. Helping the patient to the toilet after meals promotes elimination, as do adequate bulk and fluid in the diet. Always treat the patient with respect, never belittling incompetencies in elimination.

## Bowel Rehabilitation

Although urinary incontinence is a more common problem than bowel incontinence, involuntary defecation may characterize patients suffering from chronic illness, particularly of a neurologic nature. The paraplegic patient—who is capable of little or no sensation and/or movement in the lower portion of the body—can often neither feel nor control bowel movements. However, bowel rehabilitation, sometimes called bowel training, is usually successful. As is true of bladder rehabilitation, the patient's understanding and cooperation are essential even though the program is initiated by the nurse, usually on the order of the physician. The patient is given extra fluids, often prune juice, with the morning meal. Approximately thirty minutes after breakfast, a glycerine *suppository* is inserted into the rectum. The action of the medication causes peristalsis to begin shortly thereafter, and the patient is placed on the commode or bedpan to defecate. Bowel rehabilitation sometimes also employs the technique of digital stimulation: shortly after the suppository is inserted and before defecation takes place, the nurse, wearing a clean glove, inserts the middle finger into the rectum to stimulate peristalsis. Another method is to give a small cleansing enema after the morning meal. The amount of solution used is gradually decreased each morning until the enema is no longer needed. Regardless of the method used, the goal of causing the bowel to empty of its own volition at approximately the same time each day is usually attained.

## Colostomy Care

A colostomy is an opening of the bowel onto the abdominal wall. Since there is no sphincter and therefore no control over defecation, special care is needed. Dressings and bags may be placed over the opening. Irrigation, which is similar to an enema, may be needed. Module 30, "Ostomy Care," gives complete directions on caring for a colostomy.

## Conclusion

The processes of elimination are important, both physically and psychologically, throughout our lives. Development of the ability to control elimination provides infants and young children a feeling of independence and a degree of power. The adult in full control of such mechanisms recognizes the relationship of healthy functioning to the sense of well-being. In later life, some compromise may become necessary, and older people may feel they are once again becoming dependent. Knowledge and understanding of the impact and connotations of elimination on individuals of various ages helps us to afford maximum comfort to patients.

## Care Study  A patient with constipation

Mr. Jensen is an eighty-eight-year-old recently admitted to the chronic-care facility where Judy Gomez is a student nurse. Ms. Gomez's assignment is to develop a nursing care plan on a patient's primary need. She notices, while caring for Mr. Jensen, that he is very preoccupied with bowel function and asks several times to be assisted to the bathroom. Each time he is unable to defecate. He refuses to go to morning activities because he might want to go back to the bathroom. She decides to collect data and carry out a plan on constipation.

The nursing history reports that Mr. Jensen has been living alone and eating prepared meals only sporadically, resulting in an insufficient diet. He states that he has had hard, difficult-to-pass bowel movements every three to four days and has frequent abdominal distention with pain. She also notices that the physician has written an order for glycerine suppositories q.o.d., p.r.n.

Ms. Gomez consults her resources and learns that increased bulk in the diet, extra fluids, and exercise are the best measures to combat constipation. With the dietitian, the head nurse, and the patient, she completes her plan:

1. One tablespoon bran over warm cereal each morning.
2. Prune juice with breakfast.
3. Use of the bathroom one-half hour after breakfast.
4. Extra juices and fluids at midmorning and midafternoon.
5. Attendance at the morning exercise program and ambulation with assistance each afternoon and evening.
6. A glycerine suppository if defecation does not take place in two days.

When Ms. Gomez assures Mr. Jensen that this plan represents a positive step toward solving his problem, and that he can play an active role in it, he eagerly accepts.

At the end of the fourth day, Ms. Gomez writes that her plan is partially successful, since only one suppository has had to be given. By day eight, Mr. Jensen is having bowel movements regularly after breakfast. The distention and pain have disappeared. The plan is added to the patient's card index (Kardex) and progress is recorded daily in the record.

## Study Terms

URINARY SYSTEM

albuminuria
anuria
bacteriuria
calculi
casts
catheterization
colostomy
credé
dialysis
diuretic
dysuria
emesis
enuresis
frequency
glycosuria
hematuria
hemodialysis
incontinence
lassitude
meatus
micturition
neurogenic bladder
nocturia
oliguria
peritoneal dialysis
pH
polyuria
prostate
proteinuria
pyuria
renal failure
retention
specific gravity
sphincter
stretch reflex
suppression
UA
ureter
urethra
urgency
urimeter
urinalysis
urination
voiding

INTESTINAL SYSTEM

colostomy
diarrhea
duodenum
enema
fecal incontinence
feces
flatus
guaiac
impaction
occult blood
peristalsis
steatorrhea
stool
suppository

## Learning Activities

1. Visit a drugstore and note the many preparations on display for regulation of the urinary and intestinal tracts.
2. Familiarize yourself with the intake-output recording procedures in the facility with which you are affiliated.
3. With a particular patient in mind, write a nurs-

ing plan for bladder training, including health teaching.

4. With a particular patient in mind, write a similar nursing plan for bowel training.

## Relevant Sections in
## Modules for Basic Nursing Skills

## References

Anderson, E. "Women and Cystitis." *Nursing '77* 7 (April 1977): 50–53.

Anthony, Catherine P., and Kolthoff, Norma J. *Textbook of Anatomy and Physiology.* St. Louis: C. V. Mosby, 1978.

Bass, L. "More Fiber—Less Constipation." *American Journal of Nursing* 77 (February 1977): 254–255.

Beaumont, E. "Urinary Drainage Systems." *Nursing '74* 4 (April 1974): 52–60.

Butler, P. A. "Assessing Urinary Incontinence in Women." *Nursing '79* 9 (March 1979): 72–74.

Connell, Alastair M. "Functional Aspects of Colonic Motility: Constipation." *Emotional Factors in Gastrointestinal Illness,* A. E. Linder, ed. Excerpta Medica International Congress series no. 304. Amsterdam: Excerpta Medica Foundation, 1973.

Corman, Marvin L., et al. "Cathartics." *American Journal of Nursing* 75 (February 1975): 273–279.

DeGroot, Jane, and Kunin, C. M. "Indwelling Catheters." *American Journal of Nursing* 75 (March 1975): 448–449.

DeGroot, Jane. "Catheter-Induced Urinary Tract Infections: How Can We Prevent Them?" *Nursing '76* 6 (August 1976): 34–37.

DiPalmo, J. "Drugs That Induce Changes in Urine Color." *RN* 40 (January 1977): 34–35.

Farrar, John T. "Functional Aspects of Small Bowel and Colon Motility: Diarrhea." *Emotional Factors in Gastrointestinal Illness.* A. E. Linder, ed. Excerpta Medica International Congress series no. 304. Amsterdam: Excerpta Medica Foundation, 1973.

French, R. M. *Guide to Diagnostic Procedures,* 5th ed. New York: McGraw-Hill, 1980.

Garner, J. S. "Urinary Catheter Care: Doing It Better." *Nursing '74* 4 (February 1974): 54–56.

Habeeb, M., and Kallstrom, M. "Bowel Program for Institutionalized Adults." *American Journal of Nursing* 76 (April 1976): 606–608.

Hogstel, M. "How to Give a Safe and Successful Cleansing Enema." *American Journal of Nursing* 77 (May 1977): 816–817.

Khan, A. J., et al. "Urinary Tract Infection in Children." *American Journal of Nursing* 73 (August 1973): 134–136.

Lewis, D. "Care of the Constipated Patient." *Nursing Times* 72 (25 March 1976): 444–446.

Maney, J. "A Behavioral Therapy Approach to Bladder Retraining." *Nursing Clinics of North America* 11 (March 1976): 179–188.

McGuckin, M. "What You Should Know About Collecting Stool Culture Specimens." *Nursing '76* 76 (March 1976): 22–23.

Nickerson, D., et al. "Two-drop and One-drop Test for Glycosuria." *American Journal of Nursing* 72 (May 1972): 939.

Whyte, J., and Thistle, N. "Male Incontinence: The Inside Story of External Collection." *Nursing '76* 76 (September 1976): 66–67.

Willington, F. "Incontinence: Psychological and Psychogenic Aspects." *Nursing Times* 71 (13 March 1975): 422–423.

———. "Incontinence: The Nursing Component of Diagnosis and Treatment." *Nursing Times* 71 (29 March 1975): 464–467.

———. "Incontinence: The Prevention of Soiling." *Nursing Times* 71 (3 April 1975): 545–548.

———. "Incontinence: Training and Retraining for Continence." *Nursing Times* 71 (27 March 1975): 500–503.

Wilson, M. F. "Bladder Training for the Chronically Ill." *RN* 38 (June 1975): 36–37.

# Chapter 23

# Oxygenation

## Objectives

After completing this chapter, you should be able to:

1. Briefly describe the respiratory system and the process of oxygenation.
2. Explain in simple terms the relationship of respiration to acid-base balance.
3. Describe normal respiration with regard to rate, depth, rhythm, breath and chest sounds, and comfort.
4. State normal arterial blood gas values.
5. Discuss assessment of cough and methods of intervention.
6. Name the common acute and chronic respiratory problems discussed in the chapter.
7. Discuss nursing intervention in respiratory problems, including psychological comfort.
8. Briefly describe ways that health teaching and participation in community programs can help prevent respiratory disease.

## Outline

All body cells need oxygen for survival. Oxygen depletion can cause death of organs and body parts or the death of the patient. For this reason, the respiratory system may be the most important system of the body. Its function is oxygenation through ventilation, which occurs through an intricate exchange of two gases, oxygen and carbon dioxide. The acid-base balance of the body is maintained by the properly balanced exchange of oxygen and carbon dioxide brought about by respiration.

## The Respiratory System

The respiratory system is composed of several structures whose purpose is the exchange at several levels of the nutrient gas oxygen, which nourishes body cells, and the waste gas carbon dioxide, given off by the cells (see Figure 23.1).

### Nose, Pharynx, and Larynx

Air enters the body through the nose, where it is warmed and particles are filtered out. It then flows through the pharynx into the larynx, or voice-box. From there, the air moves downward to the trachea.

### Trachea

The *trachea* is a tube, composed of a number of horseshoe-shaped cartilaginous rings, leading from the larynx to the bronchi.

### Lungs

The *lungs* are two cone-shaped structures, one on the left and one on the right side of the chest. They differ slightly in shape: the left is more concave to allow room for the heart. The lungs have lobes to allow for greater surface exposure to the inspired air. The left lung has two, the upper and the lower. The right lung has three lobes: superior, middle, and inferior. The round-pointed top of each lung is called the *apex*; the lower flattened portion is called the *base*.

### Bronchi

Uniting the lungs in the middle are the *bronchi*, often referred to as "the bronchial tree" because their structure resembles an inverted tree. The trunk or main bronchi, right and left, composed of cartilaginous rings, are the "pipes" through which air enters the lungs. The right is larger and straighter than the left. Branching off the bronchi are the smaller bronchioles, which form a network of passages through which the air reaches large portions of lung tissue. The muscular walls of the bronchioles can constrict to decrease the air flow or relax to increase it.

### Alveoli

After many subdivisions, the bronchioles are connected to millions of *alveoli* by the alveolar ducts. The alveoli are highly vascular air sacs surrounded by a thin single-layer membrane through which gases can flow. It is here that the exchange of gases takes place.

### Diaphragm

The *diaphragm* is a broad, flat, elastic muscle that stretches across and seals off the lower thoracic cavity, enclosing the lungs. It maintains pressure, facilitating the movement of gases, and is innervated by the phrenic nerve.

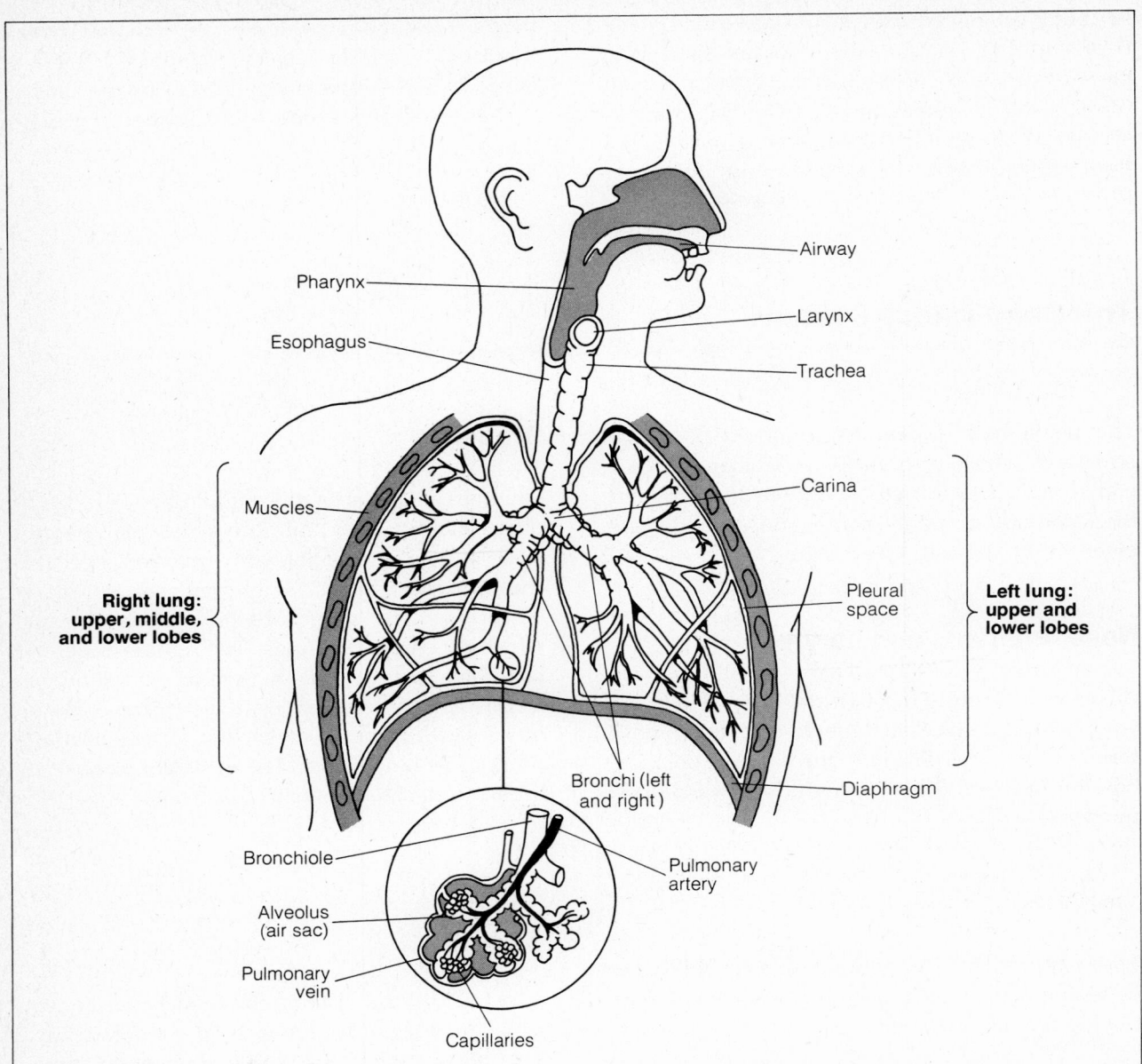

Figure 23.1   The respiratory system

## The Process of Oxygenation

Ventilation takes place because of pressure changes in the chest. When the diaphragm drops and the thorax expands, the pressure of the air in the alveoli falls below atmospheric pressure. As a result, air rushes down the bronchi; this process is called *inspiration*, or the breathing-in of air. *Expiration* is the exhaling or breathing-out of air, which normally occurs due to the elastic recoil of the lungs and chest.

Room air, which is approximately 20 percent

oxygen, continues down the bronchial tree until it reaches the millions of alveoli, where the first exchange of gases takes place. This exchange is called *external respiration.* Oxygen is transported into the blood by means of *diffusion,* or movement from an area of greater pressure to an area of lesser pressure. At the same time, carbon dioxide is released or given off.

The circulation of blood throughout the body carries the oxygen to individual cells in the tissue. At the cellular level there occurs another exchange, called *internal respiration,* whereby the cells take up oxygen and give off carbon dioxide. Traveling by way of the circulatory system, the carbon dioxide finds its way back to the lungs for expiration. Again, this expiration takes place when the pressure in the alveoli is greater than atmospheric pressure (see Chapter 24 and Figure 23.1).

With every inspiration, some air remains in the nose and passageways, including the bronchi. Because the oxygen in this air does not reach the alveoli and is not exchanged, it is called "dead air."

## Effects of Respiration on Acid-Base Balance

The pH, or acidity-alkalinity balance, of the arterial blood must remain within a very narrow range—7.4 or a few hundredths below or above—for the body to function optimally. Thus the arterial blood is slightly alkaline. Any factor that alters this level produces a state of either acidosis or alkalosis in the body. One such factor is respiration. Acid-base balance is discussed more fully in Chapter 24. You will also study it in more detail in your medical-surgical nursing course. We will confine ourselves here to a general overview of acid-base balance as it relates to respiration (see Figure 23.2).

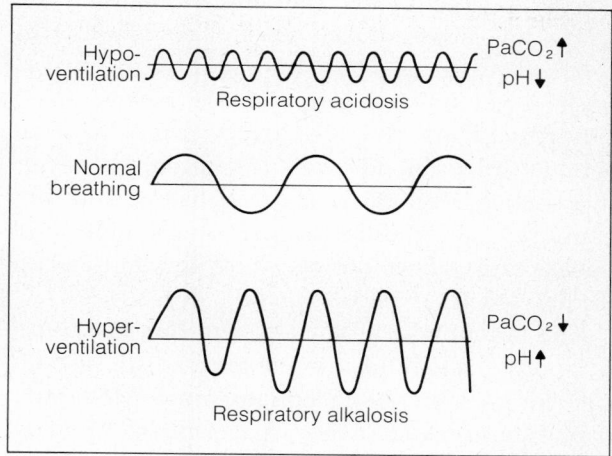

**Figure 23.2    Effects of respiration on acid–base balance**

### Respiratory Acidosis

When a patient is *hypoventilating* (breathing shallowly) for any reason, excess carbon dioxide is retained. This carbon dioxide is converted to carbonic acid, and the pH falls as the partial pressure of carbon dioxide in the arterial blood ($PaCO_2$) rises. Respiratory acidosis can occur in patients with central nervous system depression, perhaps due to drug use, and in patients with pulmonary disease that prevents full ventilation. (See Chapter 24, "Circulation," for a more complete discussion of respiratory acidosis.)

### Respiratory Alkalosis

Conversely, when a patient is *hyperventilating* (breathing abnormally deeply) for any reason, excessive amounts of carbon dioxide are exhaled. The lowered level of carbonic acid in the blood causes the pH to rise. Hyperventilation, which may accompany fever or anxiety, can lead to respiratory alkalosis. (See Chapter 24, "Circulation," for a more complete discussion.)

## Measuring Air Volume

The volume of air that moves in and out of the lungs must be sufficient to maintain all the tissues of the body. There are two ways of measuring volume.

*Tidal volume*—the amount of air exchanged with a single ordinary breath—is measured with an instrument called a spirometer. In adults, the expired air measures approximately 500 ml.

*Vital capacity*—the largest possible amount of air that can be exchanged with a single breath—is also measured with the spirometer. This time the patient inspires as deeply as possible and then expires as much as possible. The expired air may reach, in the adult, 3000 ml.

## Factors Influencing Oxygenation

Many factors influence oxygenation. The neurologic system is involved since respiration is controlled by the respiratory center in the medulla of the brain. The primary stimulus to breathing is a rise in the carbon dioxide level of the blood. This mechanism is sensitive to minor changes and keeps the blood level fairly stable by means of regular respiration. The respiratory center also responds to low blood levels of oxygen. However, this backup mechanism is less sensitive and, operating alone, produces irregular respirations and "peaks and valleys" of blood oxygen and carbon dioxide levels.

The autonomic nervous system can also affect respiratory rate, and it is the mechanism responsible for the increasing respiratory rate that accompanies tension and anxiety. It also causes the body to change breathing patterns with changes in air temperature.

Respiration can also be voluntarily controlled. With conscious attention, a person can temporarily stop breathing or change the pattern of breathing. This control is secondary to the involuntary controls and can be maintained only while the body is receiving adequate oxygen supplies. Thus

an angry child may hold his breath until he loses consciousness, but involuntary control then causes him to resume breathing.

*Age* also influences oxygenation. A newborn may breathe as many as 30–50 times per minute, while a normal adult breathes 16–20 times per minute. The depth of respirations may also vary with age: the diminished resilience of older people's rib cages can cause shallow breathing, as can anything that constricts the free movement of the chest, including clothing, poor posture, and position. Because of their larger stature, males tend to have greater vital capacity than females.

*Respiratory disease* affects oxygenation. Upper-respiratory-tract infections (URI), pneumonia, and influenza decrease volume. *Chronic obstructive pulmonary disease* (COPD) and other conditions are obstructive; *emphysema*, another chronic lung disease, diminishes the elasticity of the alveoli and interferes with exchange. The presence of secretions anywhere in the respiratory tract is a hazard to good ventilation and a matter of concern for the nurse. Lung tumors can have a profound effect in all the above ways.

## Nursing Assessment of Respiration

Rate of breathing is a vital sign. You should also become familiar with the many parameters of respiratory assessment and the terms assigned to them. The procedure for measurement of respirations is described in Module 20, "Temperature, Pulse, and Respiration."

## Rate

The first task in respiratory assessment is to measure the rate of respiration. A single cycle of inspiration and expiration is counted as one respiration. It is usually easiest to count inspirations. Because it is difficult for a patient to maintain a normal breathing pattern knowing he or she is being watched, the nurse often counts by resting the patient's arm across the chest with the nurse's hand in place as if feeling for the pulse. The risings of the chest can thus be felt and counted. Beginning at zero will make for a more accurate count. Count for a full thirty seconds. If the respirations are irregular, however, it may be desirable to count for a full minute. The respiratory rate is highest in the newborn—35–40 respirations per minute—and gradually decreases, reaching the adult level of 14–20 respirations in adolescence. Respiratory rate is increased by activity, fever, anxiety, and all the factors that affect the pulse rate. Many health problems create rises in respiratory rate; others cause the rate to decrease. Very rapid respiration is called *tachypnea*. Unusually slow respiration is called *bradypnea*. Absence of respiration is called *apnea*.

## Depth

The extent to which the whole lung is involved in respiration is called the depth of respiration. A shallow respiration is one characterized by minimal chest movement and thus minimal air exchange. A deep respiration is one in which the rib cage is fully expanded and the diaphragm descends to create maximum lung capacity. Shallow respirations are not effective, even at a rapid rate, because they produce air movement in the physiologic dead space where no gas exchange with the blood can take place and inadequate air movement in the alveoli where gas exchange does take place. Sighing and yawning are automatic mechanisms to increase ventilation by forcing deep breaths. In addition to the lack of oxygen exchange, hypoventilation—shallow respiration—causes secretions to accumulate and alveoli to collapse. This problem, common to immobilized patients, can be combated by encouraging movement, deep breathing, and coughing. Chronic anxiety may be accompanied by hyperventila-

tion—breathing with rapid, deep inspiration. Excessive carbon dioxide loss causes respiratory alkalosis, an acid-base disturbance, discussed more fully in Chapter 24, "Circulation."

## Rhythm

Healthy respirations are characterized by a regular rhythm of expirations twice as long as inspirations (a 1:2 inspiration-expiration ratio). Irregularities in rhythm may indicate the presence of illness. A cycle of respirations that are very deep (hyperpnea) and rapid (tachypnea), gradually tapering off to the point of cessation (apnea) and then gradually becoming deep and rapid again are called *Cheyne-Stokes respirations*; they usually indicate that the patient is in very critical condition.

*Kussmaul's respirations* are deep and rapid. Their extreme depth resembles blowing and gasping.

*Biot's respirations* resemble Cheyne-Stokes except that the respirations between the episodes of apnea appear normal. Certain references may describe this term in slightly different ways. In assessing rhythm, always check for yourself; never rely entirely on someone else to monitor for potentially serious signs.

## Breath Sounds

Breath sounds are very helpful in assessing pulmonary status but require a trained ear. You will become more proficient as you listen to a number of patients. Breath sounds are usually easily discerned without a stethoscope merely by standing near the patient in a quiet room.

*Wheezing* is a clearly audible whistling sound particularly characteristic of the patient suffering from asthma. It can also be present in other respiratory conditions. *Snoring* is a breath sound normal in deep sleep but possibly indicative of coma in the neurological patient. The child with croup may have a crowing sound called *stridor*; this sound can also occur with laryngospasm, a serious complication of second-stage anesthesia. *Sighing*, *hiccoughs* (singultus), and *yawning* are all familiar breath sounds: sighing can be a sign of anxiety, hiccoughs frequently occur after anesthesia, and yawning can indicate narcolepsy (a sleep disorder).

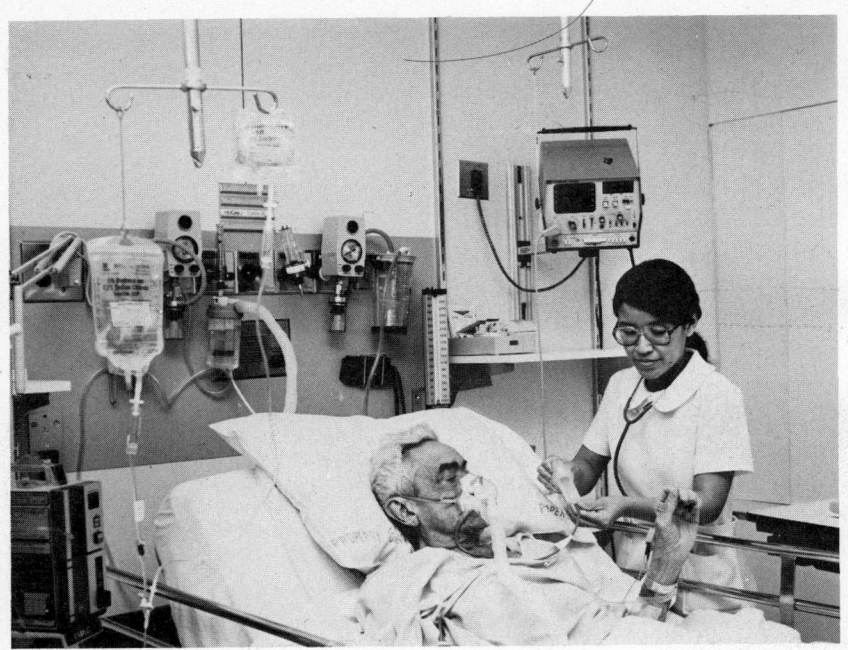

**Figure 23.3 Respiratory assessment and treatment of the critically ill patient.**
Russ Kinne/Danbury Hospital/Photo Researchers, Inc.

## Chest Sounds

There are several standard terms used to describe chest sounds. In preference to these terms, however, it has recently been suggested that the use of ordinary descriptive words promotes accuracy and minimizes the subjectivity of listening. Try to characterize the sound you hear as descriptively as possible. You might say, for example, "a soft rustling" or "a loud crackling." A stethoscope is used to listen to chest sounds.

*Râles* are crackling or bubbling sounds made by air moving through moisture or secretions in the bronchioles or lungs. *Rhonchi* are lower pitched and drier sounding than râles. *Wheezes* sound very much like the sound made by a toy whistle. Some whistling sounds are interrupted and some continuous. *Pleural rub* is a distinct grating or rubbing sound as the pleurae rub together; "friction rub" is another term used for this sound.

*Adventitious* is a general term for *any* abnormality, commonly used in the negative; that is, the nurse might record, "no adventitious sounds heard." The skills needed for listening to breath and chest sounds are described in Module 32, "Inspection, Palpation, Auscultation, and Percussion."

## Comfort

If the patient reports subjective discomfort—difficult or painful breathing—the term used is *dyspnea*. Normal painless breathing is *eupnea*.

# Blood Gases

In conjunction with objective nursing observation, you should also be able to distinguish normal from abnormal *blood gas* values, which signify the partial pressure of gases in arterial blood. Arterial $O_2$ is written $PaO_2$. The symbol for partial pressure of carbon dioxide in arterial blood is $PaCO_2$. Though you may see these symbols written as $PO_2$ and $PCO_2$, it is preferable to add the a, which indicates arterial blood, since the figures are different for venous blood. Normal values for arterial blood gases are: $PaO_2$, 95–100 mmHg; $PaCO_2$, 35–45 mmHg. For venous blood, the values are $PO_2$, 35–40 mmHg; $PCO_2$, 45 mmHg.

In many facilities, the respiratory therapy department is responsible for drawing blood gases. In others, the laboratory is responsible. Only rarely is it a nursing procedure. The radial artery is located by palpation (feeling). After cleansing, a long, thin-gauged needle is inserted straight downward until bright red blood appears in the barrel. After a sufficient amount has been collected, the needle is withdrawn and firm pressure applied for five minutes to prevent bleeding from the artery. Some degree of pain accompanies insertion of the needle, and ice applied a few minutes before the procedure can be helpful. A heel stick is usually done in newborns and small infants since the radial artery is too small to enter. Because this method produces capillary blood, however, the values will be lower than arterial blood and higher than venous blood; they are usually evaluated in light of the individual infant's circulatory status. The pH of the blood is always reported with blood gases.

## Cough

The cough center, located in the medulla, is activated by any threat of obstruction of the respiratory tract. A foreign body, such as dust, will activate the cough reflex. Cough is an important protective mechanism and remains active even during sleep.

In the patient with respiratory problems, such as an infection with irritation or the buildup of secretions not normally present, coughing is persistent.

### Assessment of Cough

Simply to say that the patient is coughing is inadequate assessment. Consider the persistence of the cough and when it occurs. It is common for children and some adults to cough upon arising, when secretions have accumulated during the night, and/or at night when in the horizontal position. How does the cough sound? Is it a moist or dry cough?

Cough is described as *productive* or *nonproductive*, depending on whether or not the patient is coughing up and expectorating (spitting) sputum or phlegm. *Sputum* is predominantly composed of mucus, epithelial cells, and microorganisms. It is usually tenacious in consistency. When you state that a patient has a productive cough, you should assess the character of the sputum being expectorated. *Quantity* may be described as small, moderate, or large. *Color* may vary: some sputum may be red-tinged, indicating that it contains blood, or green, indicative of a bacterial infection. Other words that may be appropriate are "thick," "clear," "frothy," and "stringy."

### Intervention for Cough

The nursing measures for cough include control of the environmental temperature, since coughing increases if the patient is too warm. The room should be comfortably cool and excess blankets should be removed from the patient's bed. Helping the patient cough and deep-breathe to bring up secretions may decrease the patient's need to cough. Other nursing actions include avoiding unnecessary exertion, which stimulates coughing, and, if appropriate, administering medications to control the cough.

## Respiratory Problems

Respiratory problems may be either acute or chronic. Acute respiratory problems require immediate assessment and intervention in order to sustain life. Chronic respiratory problems are often irreversible and necessitate changes in life style.

## Acute Respiratory Problems

Acute respiratory distress is a medical emergency. Certain body tissues, especially brain cells, die within minutes with no oxygen. In an emergency involving both acute respiratory distress and hemorrhage, therefore, respiratory distress must receive attention first. Cardiopulmonary resuscitation (CPR), the procedure for maintaining vital respiratory and circulatory vital function, is discussed in Chapter 24, "Circulation," and described in Module 26, "Cardiopulmonary Resuscitation."

The patient in acute distress may be gasping for air; the nostrils flare and the mouth is open. Because of the gasping respirations, the area of the chest just below the sternum may sink deeply on inspiration; this phenomenon, called *retraction*, is particularly noticeable in oxygen-deprived newborns due to the softness of the rib cage (see Figure 23.4). The patient is in a state of *hypoxia* (low body oxygen), detectable in the skin color: the extremities may be bluish or the entire body and face a dusky or blue color; this condition is called *cyanotic*. If the patient is conscious, he or she may be extremely apprehensive and anxious. As consciousness lowers, thrashing and irrationality set in due to oxygen hunger. If intervention does not take place, death will ensue.

Common causes of acute respiratory failure are heart attack, drug overdose, trauma (injury), diabetic acidosis, other serious medical diseases, and obstruction by large foreign bodies. Inhaled food, particularly large pieces of meat, can suddenly halt breathing. In the case of children, toys, marbles, and peanuts can also obstruct. A quick method of assessment is to ask the person to speak. If he or she cannot, the airway is obstructed.

The *Heimlich maneuver*, developed by a University of Cincinnati physician to expel foreign bodies from the larynx and posterior pharynx, has saved countless lives. This procedure is accomplished by standing behind the victim, placing one's arms about the victim's body with the hands clasped just above the epigastrum and delivering a quick thrust. The object is expelled by the force of expelled air.

Because the Heimlich maneuver has caused damage to internal organs (particularly liver lacerations), a *modified Heimlich maneuver* is now recommended. After identifying that the victim has a blocked airway, you first deliver *four back blows* in succession. These blows may be enough to dislodge the object. If the airway is still obstructed, you then administer a *chest thrust* by standing behind the victim, placing your arms around the victim's body with the hands clasped over the chest and giving a quick, hard thrust. A chest thrust may also be performed by delivering the thrust from above with the victim lying down with the head turned to the side. The chest thrust may be repeated four times if the object is not expelled. Further repetitions are not recommended since they would increase the likelihood of rib damage without increasing the potential for successful removal of the obstruction. Along with external cardiac massage and rescue breathing (CPR), everyone should know how to perform this emergency procedure.

## Chronic Respiratory Problems

As a student nurse, you are more likely to care for a patient with chronic than acute respiratory problems. There are many categories of patients with chronic respiratory problems. Some are postsurgical, having had a lobectomy or pneumonectomy (removal of a lobe or an entire lung). Patients with pulmonary infections, such as pneumonia, may have respiratory problems over an extended period of time, which are considered more chronic than acute. Cardiac disease, liver impairment, and cancer in the terminal stages bring about long-

**Figure 23.4  Chest retraction with oxygen depletion**

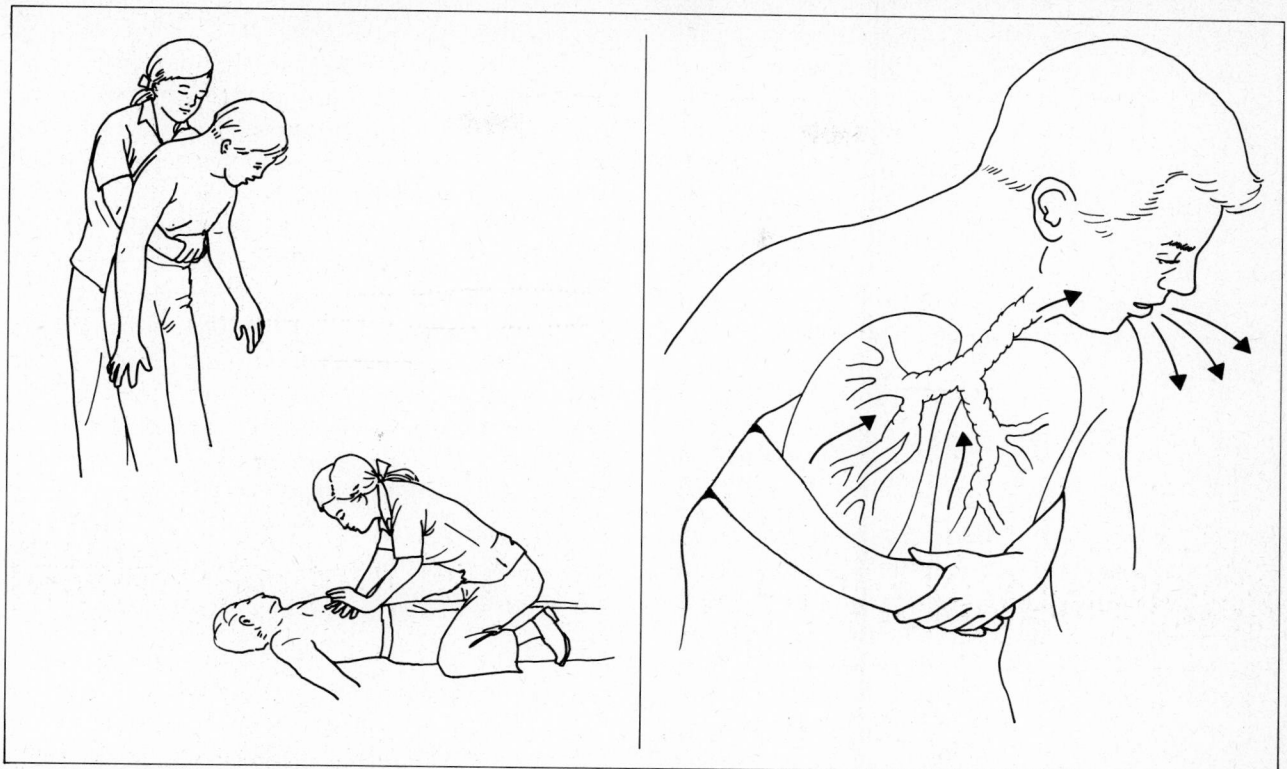

**Figure 23.5  The modified Heimlich maneuver**

term pulmonary compromise. Early respiratory failure has chronic symptoms.

Patients with chronic respiratory illness may yawn or sigh frequently in an attempt to take in more oxygen. The underlying pathology can cause hypoventilation such that the patient breathes rapidly and shallowly. The skin is often pale (*pallor*) and the extremities, particularly the nail beds, are blue in color. The patient may exhibit signs of irritability or restlessness. Low body oxygen causes fatigue.

In patients who have had increasing respiratory problems over many years, clubbing of the fingers can occur. The fingernails become thicker and much broader. If the respiratory condition persists, the tips of the fingers themselves flatten and broaden. In patients of long chronicity, the chest becomes barrel-shaped because of the loss of elasticity of the thorax and the fixed expansion of the chest.

## Nursing Intervention for Respiratory Problems

In many respiratory conditions, the underlying causes may be irreversible. However, this should never keep us from inventive, knowledgeable nursing care. There are many actions we can take to improve pulmonary function and make our patients more productive and comfortable.

### Position

The upright position appears to aid breathing in patients with respiratory problems; this is called the *orthopneic position,* and the patient who is comfortable only in this position is said to have *orthopnea.* The patient may tell you which position is optimal. It is important, however, to stress change of position. It is never wise to sacrifice healthy skin because the patient insists on assuming a single position that puts pressure on bony prominences. Health teaching should emphasize the importance of ambulating and changing position in bed, both of which stimulate circulation to lung tissue and move accumulated secretions into areas where they can be coughed up and expectorated.

## Oxygen

The physician usually orders the amount of oxygen and the route of administration. The amount of oxygen is measured in either liters per minute (l/min) or percentages. The newer ventilating equipment tends to use percentages.

We now know that too much oxygen can be not only harmful to some patients but also potentially fatal. The patient who has had long-term pulmonary compromise with serious breathing problems has adjusted to an abnormally high $PaCO_2$ in the blood (see Figure 23.2) due to habitual hypoventilation. In such a patient, lack of oxygen is actually the stimulus for breathing; it is the trigger mechanism to the medulla for respiration. Giving this particular patient high concentrations of oxygen thus eliminates the trigger for respiration, and acute respiratory failure may result. Though this is fortunately an uncommon occurrence, it should alert us to be cautious in delivering oxygen to patients in this category.

There are other dangers in oxygen administration. Oxygen is not in itself combustible or explosive, but it greatly accelerates burning. Signs should be posted prohibiting smoking near oxygen, and any equipment or objects that could produce sparks should be removed.

Oxygen may come from a central reservoir or tank or may be piped in to individual patient units. Whatever its source, the techniques of administration are the same. Oxygen may be delivered by mask, catheter, cannula, or tent. The mask is used primarily for short-term or emergency consumption. Catheters are irritating to the nose and uncomfortable for the patient and thus used infrequently. The nasal cannula is used most commonly because it has prongs that fit the nostrils and is much more comfortable than other devices. Even if the patient mouth-breathes with the cannula in place, the oxygen is taken up by the mouth since it is heavier than air. Tents are expensive, difficult to clean, and need high concentrations of oxygen to maintain ordered levels. Except for pediatric use, they too are rare.

Although usually a physician orders the amount of oxygen and method of administration, it may become necessary for you to initiate the administration of oxygen to a patient if you assess a threat to patient safety or extreme discomfort. After starting the oxygen, immediately consult with the physician for further instructions. For the specifics of oxygen administration, see Module 31, "Administering Oxygen."

## Postural Drainage

*Postural drainage* is a nursing procedure to bring about drainage of secretions from various lung segments by placing the patient in different positions. Gravity will drain secretions from a segment if it is positioned higher than the rest of the chest (see Figure 23.7). Before the treatment, bronchodilating drugs are sometimes given by inhalation to further promote drainage. While the patient is in the prescribed position, the nurse may perform percussion (tapping) over the chest area to loosen secretions. Vibration has the same effect (see Module 33, "Respiratory Care Procedures").

## Oral Care

Oral care is very important for the patient with respiratory problems. Mouth-breathing causes crusts to build up, accompanied by *halitosis* (unpleasant mouth odor).

## Fluids

Encourage the patient to drink more fluids than usual. Fluids help liquefy secretions, making them easier to move upward and out of the congested

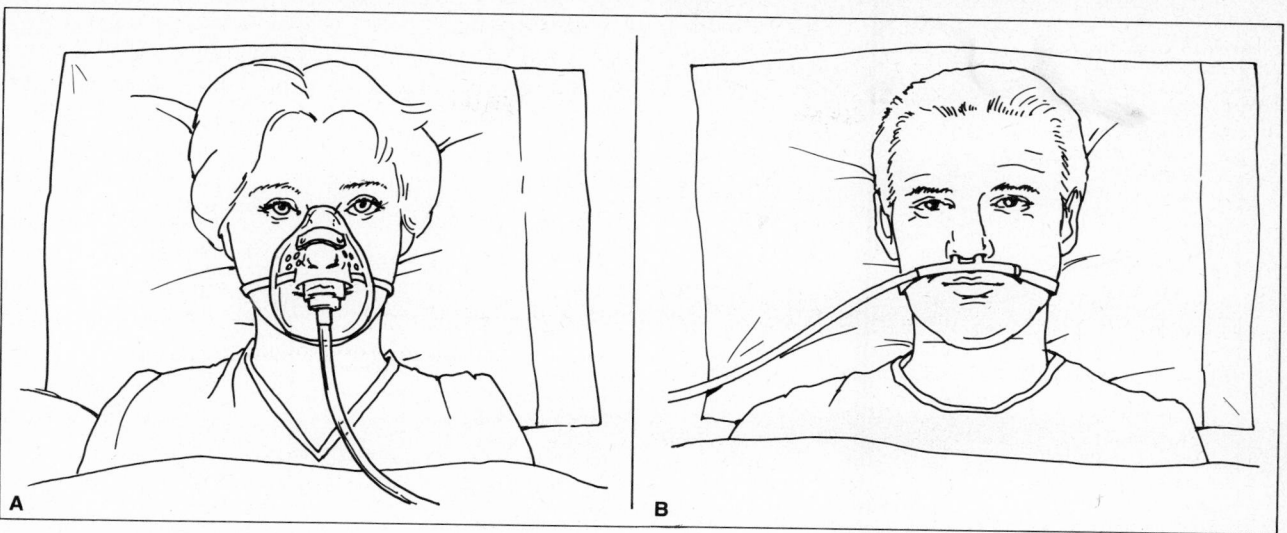

**Figure 23.6   Oxygen mask (A) and nasal cannula (B)**

lungs. Though it has been said that the patient should desist from milk products because they tend to increase the production of secretions, there is no scientific evidence to support this contention.

## Humidification and Nebulization

*Humidification*—increasing the amount of water vapor in the air—helps tissue stay moist and lessens irritation. It is for this reason that adding moisture to the room air has long been a treatment for respiratory difficulty. A humidity tent is commonly used with children who have croup. A portable misting device is used with adults. These machines can deliver either warm or cool mist depending on the physician's order; some combine the mist with oxygen. Hot steam devices require particular attention to safety, especially if the patient is a child.

*Nebulization* is a type of humidification in which small particles of moisture are dispersed into the air with a hand-held device containing water or medication. It is either manually operated or attached to a ventilating machine of some type. Unless the patient can breathe voluntarily only through the nebulizer, a plastic nose clamp is usually applied so all the mist or medication is received as forcefully as possible into the respiratory tract.

## Deep Breathing and Coughing

All respiratory patients benefit from learning the technique of combined deep breathing and coughing: after three very deep breaths, the patient coughs forcefully. This combination, which should be performed three to five times and repeated after a short rest, serves two purposes. It encourages fuller inflation of the lungs and raises secretions. The patient should be in the sitting position with hands on thighs. The nurse should demonstrate first and then ask the patient to do the same. Postoperative patients routinely perform this exercise, and the technique is typically discussed in the section of medical-surgical texts devoted to the postoperative patient. It is also described in detail in Module 33, "Respiratory Care Procedures."

## Cough Medications

Cough medications are typically administered by the nurse in accordance with the physician's prescription. These medications, often given p.r.n. (when necessary), should be used with discretion. There are several categories of such drugs.

*Suppressants* suppress cough by depressing the cough center in the medulla. If you wanted your patient to rid the lungs of excessive secretions by

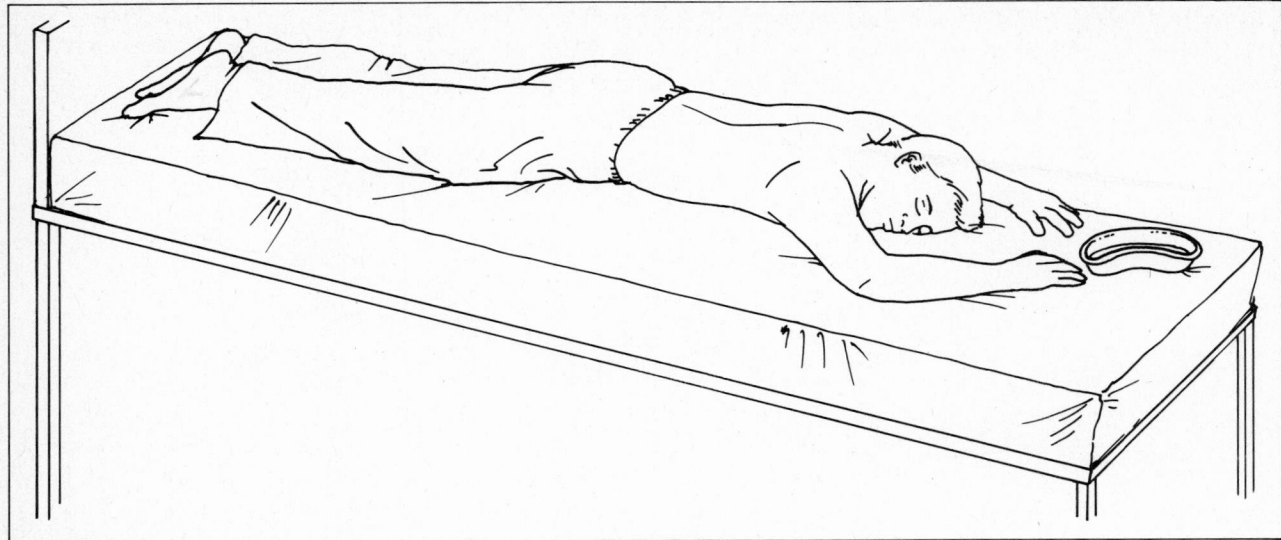

**Figure 23.7  A common position for postural drainage**

coughing, the use of these drugs would be inappropriate and, indeed, harmful to the patient.

*Expectorants* are drugs that promote cough and expectoration. They are used for patients who have audible secretions but little cough activity.

There are a number of nonprescription cough preparations whose action is basically to soothe the pharynx, or upper respiratory tract. These preparations may be adequate for the patient who describes the cause of his or her cough as "a tickle in my throat," if the patient does not need to raise secretions and a dry cough is interfering with sleep or activity.

Many cough medications, particularly those used to soothe the throat, are elixirs containing sugar. Keep their sugar content in mind if the patient is a diabetic on sugar restriction.

*Antihistamines*, though not cough medications, depress the production of secretions and may thus lessen the patient's need to cough in order to expel sputum.

## Nasal and Oropharyngeal Suctioning

If the patient cannot raise and expectorate secretions efficiently and breathing is hampered, the patient may have to be suctioned. This is done using either a portable suction machine or a wall suction. A catheter is connected to the suction source and, using sterile technique, inserted through the nose or mouth (nasally or oropharyngeally) downward into the pharynx to remove secretions emerging from the bronchi. Because the respiratory tract is very susceptible to infection, sterility should always be maintained. For the patient in acute distress, a *tracheostomy*—a surgical opening into the trachea that bypasses upper airway obstruction—may have to be performed to allow for direct removal of secretions by suction (see Figure 23.8). These techniques are described in Module 41, "Oral and Nasopharyngeal Suctioning," and Module 42, "Tracheostomy Care and Suctioning."

## Intermittent Positive Pressure Breathing (IPPB)

In some facilities, *intermittent positive pressure breathing* (IPPB) is performed by the respiratory or inhalation therapist; in others, it is a nursing function. The procedure is ordered by the physician, usually to be administered for about fifteen minutes several times a day. Its purpose is to help

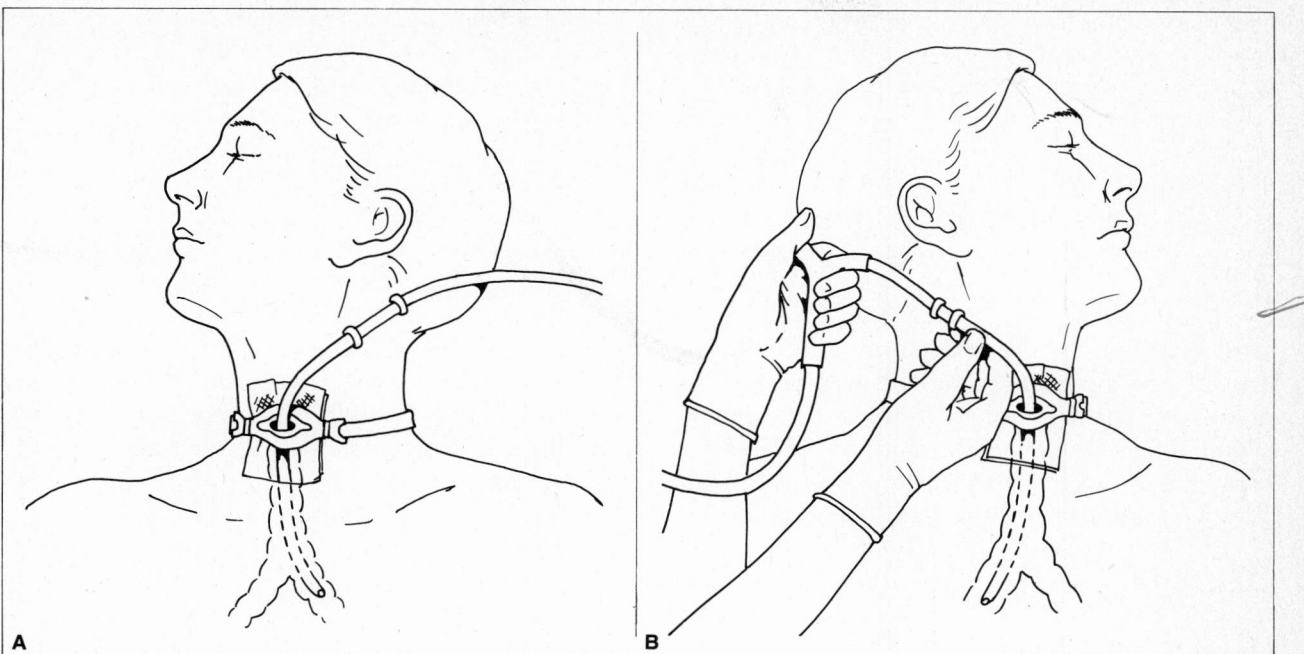

**Figure 23.8   Alternate positions for bronchial suctioning**
*A*: Suctioning left bronchus; *B*: suctioning right bronchus.

inflate the lungs more fully. IPPB can be used postoperatively to prevent respiratory problems or as a treatment for any patient who cannot fully expand the lungs and who has or may develop *atelectasis*, a condition in which a number of alveolar sacs have collapsed, thus preventing adequate oxygenation.

The principle underlying IPPB is positive pressure. Because the air is delivered to the lungs under positive pressure, all the alveoli are more fully inflated. The machine can be set to deliver a preset *volume* of air, to deliver air until a preset *pressure* is reached in the lungs, or to deliver air for a preset *time.* IPPB machines are quite versatile and can greatly help the patient with a breathing problem. There are several commercial IPPB machines. The Bird and Bennett brands are widely used and similar in performance.

## Rest

Because pulmonary problems limit the oxygen available for use by vital tissues, rest is extremely important. The nurse must plan care with this in mind. Interspersing activity with rest periods helps the patient conserve needed energy. A rest period accompanied by a brief period of oxygen (if ordered) may enable the patient to participate in a planned activity or a special visit without respiratory distress.

## Psychological Comfort

Oxygen is a basic, primary need of all humans. To be deprived of oxygen, even briefly, is a profound threat to survival. Try holding your breath for just a few moments; you will probably begin to experience the fear that would accompany a delay in resumption of breathing. The patient who has difficulty breathing or getting enough air for comfort can experience anxiety to the point of panic if the situation is not relieved.

When you are with a patient experiencing respiratory distress, any appropriate actions you take to help the patient will also assure him or her that help is possible. Touching or holding the patient's hand indicates that you are near, aware of what he or she is experiencing, and can help. Asking the patient to try to relax and conserve energy is helpful. Coaching the patient in deep breathing enhances relaxation and may calm the patient.

## Respiratory Therapy Departments

Most large hospitals have departments devoted to the care and treatment of patients with respiratory problems. The personnel of these departments may hold associate or baccalaureate degrees or may have received on-the-job training. Some are called respiratory therapists and some inhalation therapists; the title does not reflect the level of education. Depending on the facility, these care givers may perform all respiratory care, including health teaching, or may share such responsibility with nurses.

## Health Teaching

As health-care providers, nurses are in a position to teach by example and by sharing knowledge. Health maintenance and prevention of illness are two of the most important components of health teaching.

Because poor posture and obesity can both cause difficulty in breathing, nurses should encourage correct posture and weight control. The federal government has amassed clear evidence that cigarette smoking and air pollution are among the causative agents of lung cancer and serious pulmonary disease. Clearly, nurses should not smoke and should encourage others not to do so. National and regional programs to minimize air pollution merit the support of health-care personnel. The American Lung Association offers respiratory patients and their families a wide variety of services.

People afflicted with respiratory problems may have to revise their patterns of daily living. Avoidance of pollutants in the air, such as smoke, is essential, and conserving energy for important tasks may prove necessary. Some patients who live at home keep portable liquid oxygen on hand in a canister; by breathing it as it converts back to a gas, they are able to extend their activities of daily living.

## Ventilators

A number of complicated ventilators are used in intensive-care units to aid or sustain respiration for the critically ill patient. These ventilators work on the same principle as the IPPB—positive pressure to inflate the lungs—but can be set to meet the individual needs of a particular patient with regard to rate and depth of respirations, as well as the concentration of oxygen needed at a given time. Close monitoring of the blood gases allows constant assessment and readjustment of the ventilator. Operating ventilators requires a high level of critical-care nursing expertise.

# Conclusion

The universal human need to maintain respiration—and life—requires special skills on the part of the nurse. Accurate assessment is essential since emergency situations can arise quickly. Nursing actions must be carefully planned to maximize the patient's respiratory capacity. Allaying psychological discomfort is a challenging part of care planning and intervention. Recognition that any patient can develop respiratory problems and that the number of persons suffering from chronic lung disease is steadily increasing places great responsibility on the nurse to gain knowledge and skill in this area.

## Care Study    A patient with emphysema

Edna Donner, R.N., got up from the nursing station to help transfer the new admission from the stretcher to her bed. She knew that Mrs. Alder, a fifty-one-year-old woman, had emphysema, a condition characterized by loss of elasticity of the alveoli leading to inefficient oxygenation. An oxygen mask was in place, with 3 liters of oxygen per minute running. Mrs. Alder was attempting to pull off the mask and moving her head from side to side as she cried out, "Oh, please, please, somebody help me!"

Mrs. Donner made a quick assessment. The mask seemed to be complicating matters, giving Mrs. Alder the sense of being suffocated. The transfer to the bed appeared to have taxed Mrs. Alder's energy reserves and she lay back, restless but exhausted. Her color was slightly dusky.

A plan formed in Mrs. Donner's head. With words of assurance and explanation as to what she was doing and why, she held Mrs. Alder's hand as she raised the bed with the electric control. She then placed a pillow under Mrs. Alder's shoulders and head so as to elevate the thorax. A nursing assistant who entered the room to take Mrs. Alder's vital signs was sent to obtain a nasal cannula with prongs. As soon as it arrived, Mrs. Donner, continuing to reassure the patient, changed the oxygen from the mask to the prongs. Mrs. Alder's head-twisting movements stopped. Mrs. Donner quietly spoke to Mrs. Alder: "Try to breathe more deeply and evenly now. Concentrate on your muscles, and feel them begin to relax. Notice how much easier you are able to breathe now." Mrs Donner repeated this message over and over, until Mrs. Alder became calm and relaxed and her duskiness disappeared. An hour later, as Mrs. Donner again sat with Mrs. Alder, Mrs. Alder said, "Thank you, I really thought I was going to die until you helped me breathe."

Back at the nursing station, Mrs. Donner noticed the blank nursing history form. She had forgotten all about it during Mrs. Alder's crisis. "Well," she thought, "that will just have to wait."

## Study Terms

acid-base balance
adventitious sounds
alveoli
antihistamine
apnea
atelectasis
Biot's respirations
blood gases
bradypnea
Cheyne-Stokes
    respirations
COPD (chronic
    obstructive
    pulmonary disease)
cyanotic
diaphragm
diffusion
dyspnea
emphysema
eupnea
expectorant

expiration
external respiration
halitosis
Heimlich maneuver
    (modified Heimlich)
humidification
hyperventilation
hypoventilation
hypoxia
inspiration
internal respiration
intermittent positive
    pressure breathing
    (IPPB)
Kussmaul's
    respirations
nebulization
nonproductive cough
orthopnea
orthopneic position
pallor

pleural rub
postural drainage
productive cough
râles
respiratory acidosis
respiratory alkalosis
retraction
rhonchi

singultus
sputum
stridor
suppressant
tachypnea
tidal volume
tracheostomy
vital capacity

## Learning Activities

1. In the clinical facility, visit the respiratory therapy department. If possible, have a respiratory therapist demonstrate the types of care provided.
2. Identify a patient in the clinical area who has a respiratory problem. Write out your complete assessment and plan for supporting respiratory function.
3. Check your facility's policy regarding the level of autonomy nurses have in initiating oxygen therapy.

## Relevant Sections in
## Modules for Basic Nursing Skills

## References

Chrisman, Marilyn. "Dyspnea." *American Journal of Nursing* 74 (April 1974): 643–646.

Chusid, E. L., *et al.* "When Your Patient Is on Respiratory Therapy." *Nursing Digest* 4 (Summer 1976): 43–46.

Felton, Cynthia L. "Hypoxemia and Oral Temperatures." *American Journal of Nursing* 78 (January 1978): 56–57.

Fuchs, Patricia L. "Understanding Continuous Mechanical Ventilation." *Nursing '79* 9 (December 1979): 26–33.

Graas, Suzanne. "Thermometer Sites and Oxygen." *American Journal of Nursing* 74 (October 1974): 1862–1863.

Herron, C. "Home Care for the Patient With C.O.P.D." *Nursing '76* 6 (April 1976): 81–86.

Mechner, F. "Patient Assessment: Examination of the Chest and Lungs." *American Journal of Nursing* 76 (September 1976): 1–23.

Moody, L. E. "Primer for Pulmonary Hygiene." *American Journal of Nursing* 77 (January 1977): 104–106.

"Programmed Instruction: Blood-Gas and Acid-Base Concepts in Respiratory Care." *American Journal of Nursing* 76 (June 1976): 1–30.

"Programmed Instruction: Patient Assessment: Examination of Chest and Lungs." *American Journal of Nursing* 76 (September 1976): 1–23.

Rau, Joseph, and Rau, Mary. "To Breathe or Be Breathed: Understanding IPPB." *American Journal of Nursing* 77 (April 1977): 613–617.

Sandham, G., and Reid, B. "Some Q's and A's About Suctioning." *Nursing '77* 7 (October 1977): 60–65.

*Smoking and Its Effects on Health.* World Health Organization Technical Report 568. Geneva: WHO, 1976.

Stanley, L. "You Really Can Teach COPD Patients to Breathe Better." *RN* 41 (April 1978): 43–49.

Sweetwood, H. "Acute Respiratory Insufficiency: How to Recognize This Emergency . . . How to Treat It." *Nursing '77* (December 1977): 24–31.

Traver, G., ed. "Symposium on Care in Respiratory Disease." *Nursing Clinics of North America* 9 (March 1974): 97–207.

Waterson, Marian. "Teaching Your Patients Postural Drainage." *Nursing '78* 8 (March 1978): 613–617.

Worthington, Laura. "What Those Blood Gases Can Tell You." *RN* 42 (October 1979): 23–27.

Zavala, I. "The Threat of Aspiration Pneumonia in the Aged." *Geriatrics* 32 (March 1977): 46–51.

# Chapter 24
# Circulation

## Objectives

After completing this chapter, you should be able to:

1. Briefly discuss the function of the heart, blood vessels, and blood.
2. Outline information necessary for basic circulation assessment.
3. Define the terms used to report on pulse and blood pressure.
4. Explain the processes involved in basic life support (CPR).
5. List data necessary for basic assessment of fluid and electrolyte balance.
6. Define and describe the major types of fluid and electrolyte imbalance.
7. Explain acid-base balance and the principal factors responsible for its control.
8. Define and describe the four major acid-base imbalances discussed in the chapter.
9. Outline the nurse's role in fluid therapy.
10. List and describe adverse reactions to blood administration.
11. Outline the nurse's responsibility in the administration of blood.

## Outline

The Circulatory System
  Heart
  Vessels
  Blood
Basic Assessment
  Pulse
  Blood Pressure
  Skin Color and Temperature
  Fatigue Level
  Fluid Retention
  Complete Blood Count
Basic Life Support
  Recognizing the Need for Life Support
  Administering Emergency Life Support
Fluid and Electrolyte Balance
  Body Fluid Compartments
  Movement of Electrolytes
  Movement of Water
  Control Mechanisms for Fluid and Electrolyte Balance
  Measuring Electrolytes

Assessment of Fluid and Electrolyte Balance
Common Fluid and Electrolyte Problems
  Potassium Imbalances
  Calcium Imbalances
  Sodium Imbalances
  Fluid Imbalances
Acid-Base Balance
  Body Mechanisms for Maintaining pH
  Common Acid-Base Imbalances
  Using Laboratory Records
Fluid Therapy
  Types of Solutions
  Assessment in Fluid Therapy
  Caring for the Intravenous Line
Blood Transfusions
Types of Blood Products Used
Adverse Reactions to the Administration of Blood or Blood Products
Nursing Responsibilities
Care Study: A Patient With Electrolyte Imbalance

# The Circulatory System

The circulatory system is composed of the heart, which pumps blood throughout the system; the vessels, which carry the blood; and the body fluid, composed of blood and other body liquids, which carries oxygen, nutrients, and wastes to appropriate parts of the body.

## Heart

The heart is a muscular organ located in the middle of the chest. The wide upper end is called the *base*. The more pointed lower end, called the *apex*, extends to the left in the chest. The heart is contained in a membranous sac called the *pericardium*. The central space in the center of the chest occupied by the heart, great vessels, and trachea is called the *mediastinum*.

The heart has four chambers. The left and right *atria* both receive blood into the heart: the left from the pulmonary vein, which comes directly from the lungs; and the right from the great vessels, which come from the rest of the body. The right and left ventricles are strong pumps, which propel the blood forward in the system. The right ventricle pumps blood to the lungs and the left pumps blood to the rest of the body.

There are valves between the atria and corresponding ventricles and at the entrance to the great arteries from each ventricle. The purpose of the valves is to prevent blood from flowing backward when the ventricles contract.

Cardiac rate and rhythm are controlled by autonomic nerves and also by a conduction system intrinsic to the heart muscle itself. For further explanation of the functioning of the heart, consult your physiology text.

## Vessels

There are three distinct types of blood vessels. The *arteries* carry blood away from the heart. They decrease in size from the large aorta and pulmonary artery to ever smaller arteries. All arteries have muscular walls and are able to constrict.

*Capillaries* are located at the end of the arteries and join them with the veins. Capillaries extend to each body cell and have thin permeable walls. It is through the capillaries that all exchange of oxygen, nutrients, and wastes takes place. The permeability of the capillary walls varies with the stimulation of various body chemicals and in response to toxins.

*Veins* return blood to the heart. Tiny in the periphery of the body, the veins gradually become larger and larger as they near the heart. There is,

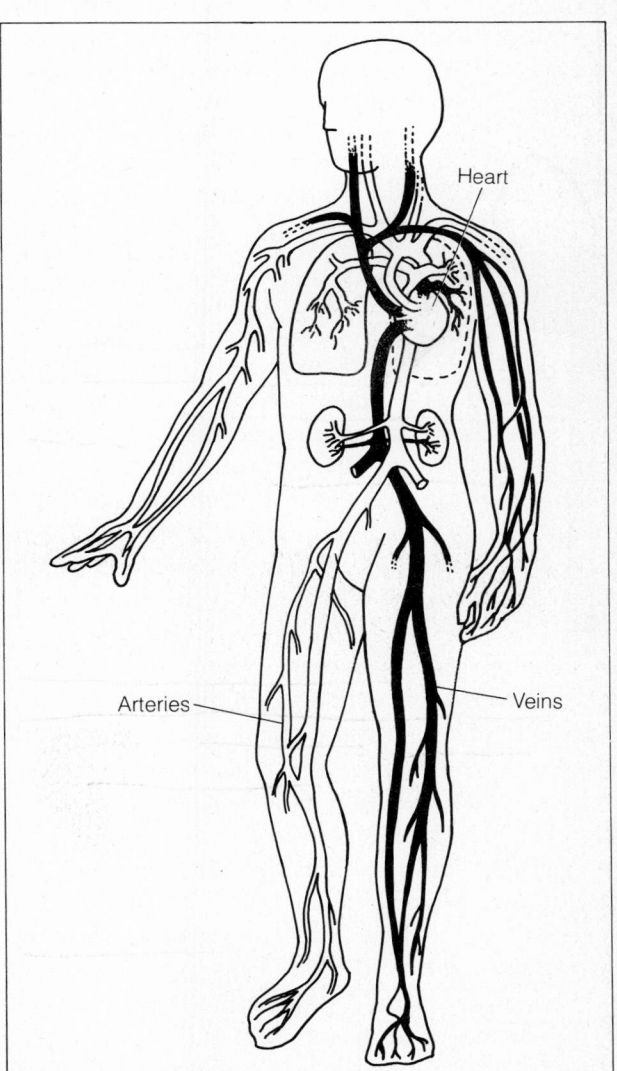

**Figure 24.1   The circulatory system**

of course, no pump propelling blood through the veins, as there is at the starting point of the arteries. Blood flows through them in response to several forces: the pressure of more blood entering from the arterial end, the pumping action of skeletal muscles around the veins, and changes exerted by gravity when the position of the body is changed. Valves in the veins prevent blood from flowing backward and maintain flow toward the heart.

## Blood

Blood is a complex body fluid. Its basis is *plasma*, which is composed of water, chemicals, and circulating proteins. In addition to the plasma itself, a variety of specific blood cells are suspended in the plasma. Let us look at some of the important components of blood. The normative amounts of each component are listed in Table 24.1 on page 411.

## Red Blood Cells

*Red blood cells (RBCs)*, also called *erythrocytes*, contain *hemoglobin*, an iron-based compound that gives blood its oxygen-carrying capacity. A person's red blood cell count specifies the number of red blood cells per 100 ml (a decaliter) of blood. The norms for women are lower than those for men due to blood loss through menstruation. Scarcity of red blood cells may indicate bleeding or a deficit in the body's ability to produce red blood cells.

Hemoglobin is measured in terms of the weight of the hemoglobin contained in the red blood cells in 100 ml of blood. Hemoglobin will, of course, be reduced if the number of red blood cells is low. It is also reduced if there is a deficiency of iron in the diet, which results in inadequate hemoglobin production, and if various disease processes such as anemia are present.

*Hematocrit*, the percentage of the whole blood accounted for by red blood cells, is expressed as a volume per 100 ml. Hematocrit is lowered by the same factors that lower hemoglobin and RBC count and by the presence of excessive fluid in the body. Dehydration increases hematocrit.

## White Blood Cells

*White blood cells (WBCs)*, or *leukocytes*, contain and destroy anything that is a threat to the body. There are several types of white blood cells, each with a specific function. White blood cells are able to move under their own power.

The white blood cell count is measured in terms of the number of cells per 100 ml of blood. A *differential* (often called a "diff") is a further analysis of the leukocytes that differentiates the percentage of cells of each type.

## Platelets

The third major type of blood cell is the *platelet*, which initiates the formation of blood clots. Whenever an injury or irregularity occurs in the lining of a blood vessel, the platelets adhere to the edges of the injury and begin the clotting process. The normal platelet count is approximately 150,000 to 300,000 per cubic millimeter.

## Blood Typing

Protein substances called *antigens* may be attached to the red blood cells. Though there are several groups of these antigens, the two of common clinical significance are the ABO group and the Rh group.

The ABO group includes two different antigens, called A and B. A person whose red blood cells contain only the A antigen has Type A blood. If the red blood cells contain only the B antigen, the blood is Type B. If the red blood cells contain both A and B antigens, the blood is Type AB. If the blood cells contain neither antigen, the blood is termed Type O.

The Rh group consists of only one antigen, the Rh factor. If the red blood cells contain this factor, the blood is termed Rh positive; if not, it is Rh negative.

A person is capable of producing antibodies against any antigen his or her own blood does not contain. Thus a person with Type-A Rh-negative blood would be capable of producing antibodies against Type-B blood and against any Rh-positive blood. In the event of a blood transfusion, exactly matching the recipient's blood type prevents the production of antibodies against unfamiliar antigens. However, there are several instances in which blood that does not exactly match can be safely transfused. This is the case, for example, if the blood given simply does not contain any antigens capable of causing a reaction. Since Type O does not contain any antigen in the ABO group, it can be given to people with any ABO blood type. In the same way, Rh-negative blood can be given to people who are Rh negative or Rh positive because it contains no antigen in the Rh group. Thus a person with Type-O Rh-negative blood is called a universal donor.

## Basic Assessment

Assessment of circulatory status is an essential aspect of basic assessment. To do so correctly, you must master a considerable body of knowledge as well as skills. Specific directions for performing these skills are found in Module 20, "Temperature, Pulse, and Respiration," and Module 21, "Blood Pressure."

### Pulse

The *pulse* is a shock wave produced within the artery as the heart beats. It can be felt as an increase in the size of the artery each time the heart contracts. Thus counting the pulse rate (beats per minute) is an indirect means of counting the heart rate. Though present in every artery, the pulse is counted at those points where a large artery passes close to the surface near a bone and can be easily palpated.

### Counting the Pulse

For reasons of convenience and accessibility, the pulse is most commonly counted at the radial artery in the wrist. It may be counted at other points if the wrist is inaccessible because of a cast or intravenous line; if the radial pulse is weak and hard to find, such as in an infant or critically ill person; or to assess circulation to a particular body part, such as using the femoral pulse to check circulation to a leg (see Figure 24.3).

It has been variously recommended that pulses be counted at fifteen, thirty, and sixty seconds. At least one study (Jones, 1967) found that the short-

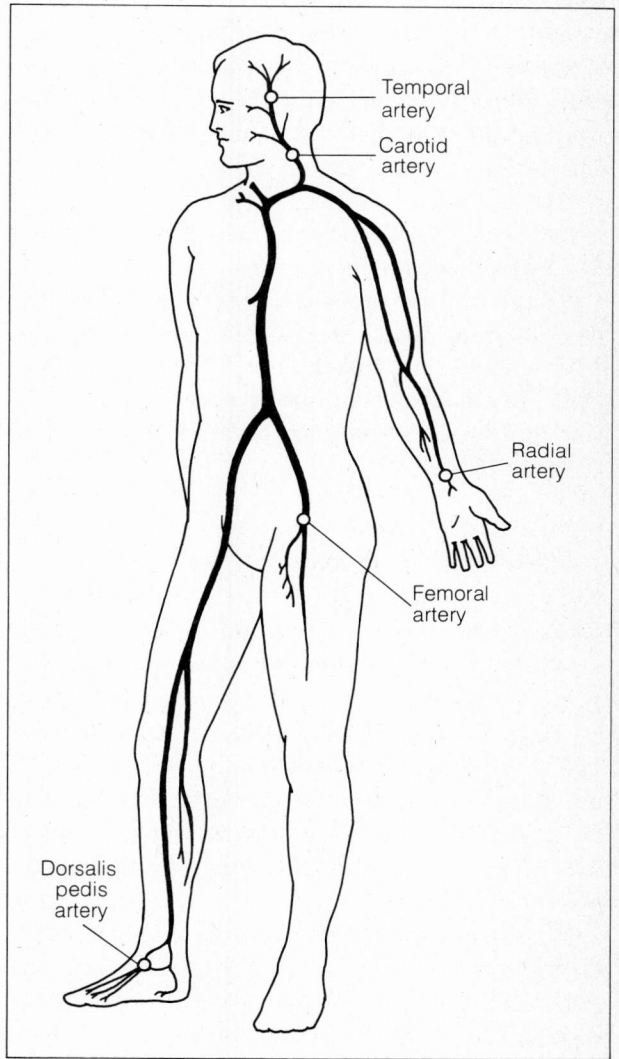

**Figure 24.2  Common locations for taking the pulse**

est duration is the most accurate for regular pulses, probably because it allows for fewer counting errors. Irregular pulses may need to be counted for sixty seconds in order to compensate for irregularities over time. Apical pulses (direct heart rate) are also usually counted for a full minute. Because all manually counted pulses deviate somewhat from direct readings taken by an ECG (electrocardiogram), the pulse rate should be considered approximate. If gross abnormalities are found, the pulse should be rechecked. An effort should be made to use a consistent technique so that trends and changes may be noted. It is advisable to check the policy of a facility when you begin working there so that your technique will be consistent with that of others who are checking a patient's pulse rate. One source of counting error can be avoided by beginning the count at 0 instead of 1 so that you are counting the beats that actually occur within a given period. For a patient whose condition is such that even small changes in rate and rhythm are serious, an electronic monitoring system is used.

Electronic pulse counters are now in limited use. Some function by sensing pulse in the earlobe, some in the tip of a finger. The accuracy of these devices makes it possible to identify even slight changes in pulse rate. Cardiac monitors, which maintain a continuous surveillance of the heart's action, also monitor heart rate.

## Apical Pulse ~ heart

Heart rate may also be counted directly over the apex of the heart by using a stethoscope. The apex of the heart is usually located on the left side of the chest at the fifth interspace between the ribs, directly below the arch of the clavicle. In the elderly person with an enlarged heart, the apex may be further to the left and lower. In the infant or young child, it is usually located closer to the midline and higher. You may need to listen at a number of spots throughout the general area to identify the site where the beat is heard most clearly. The heart rate counted in this way is called the *apical pulse*. Often the apical pulse must be counted for a full minute before the administration of drugs that affect cardiac rate (such as digitalis products);

such a drug may be withheld if the rate is too slow or too fast.

## Pulse Deficit

On occasion, some heartbeats are so weak that the waves they produce in the artery cannot be felt in the periphery. In such a case, the heart rate will be greater than the peripheral pulse. The difference between the apical and radial pulse rates, measured simultaneously, is called the *pulse deficit*. The pulse deficit represents the number of weak, ineffective beats per minute.

## Pulse Rates

Pulse rates vary greatly and are affected by such factors as activity, eating, emotional tension, drugs, and illness. Mild to moderate activity usually raises the rate 20 to 30 beats per minute. In the healthy individual, the rate will return to normal within two minutes after discontinuing such activity. Age is also an important determinant of pulse rate: pulse rate is very rapid in the infant—120 to 140 per minute—and decreases throughout life to approximately 80 per minute in the adult.

Consistent strenuous exercise will cause the heart to enlarge and to beat more slowly and forcefully. Thus a normal resting pulse rate for an athlete may be 50 to 60 per minute.

An adult pulse rate below 60 per minute is referred to as *bradycardia*, while a pulse rate that is above 100 is called *tachycardia*. Because these are relative terms, the heart rate itself is a more accurate way of characterizing heart function.

## Rhythm

It is also important to observe the *rhythm* of the pulse. A normal pulse has a regular beat. When the beat is irregular, the specific type of irregularity should be noted, since it may be of diagnostic significance. For example, double beats (bigeminy) may occur, either occasionally or at frequent regular intervals. The rate may vary from rapid to slow and back, or beats may be "skipped." Any such pattern needs to be recorded.

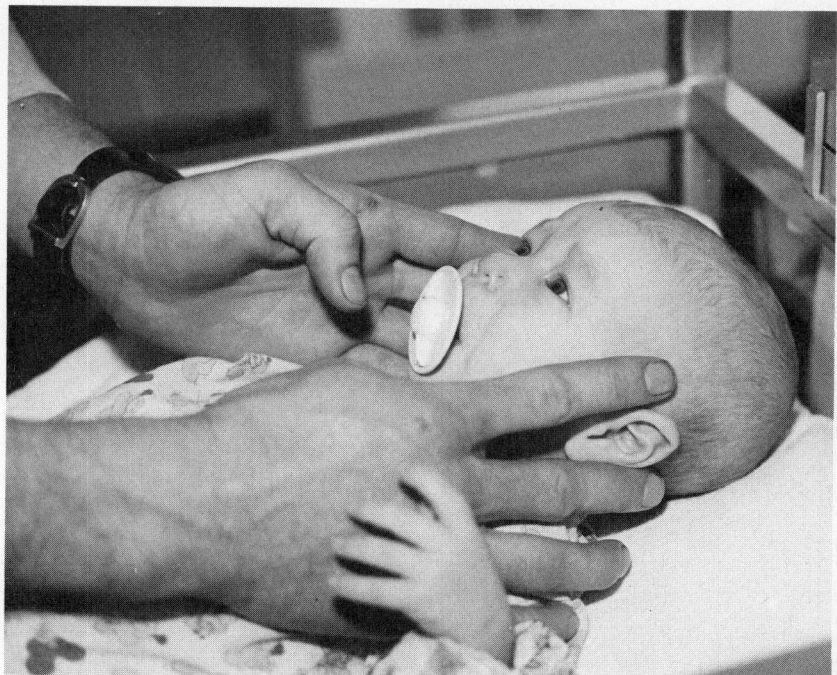

**Figure 24.3**
The temporal pulse is convenient for a small infant. (Russ Kinne/Danbury Hospital/Photo Researchers, Inc.)

## Strength

*Pulse strength* may be weak, thready, or strong; a pulse may also be said to be bounding. The strength of the pulse reflects the strength of the heart contraction. When no cardiac pathology exists, strength may not be recorded on the patient record; when there is cardiac pathology or an abnormality, pulse strength should be included in the chart.

## Blood Pressure

The pressure of the circulating blood is a significant indication of the effectiveness of heart action and of the adequacy of the blood supply to the tissue. The term *blood pressure* usually refers to arterial pressure measured in millimeters of mercury. However, the pressure in the largest veins—central venous pressure (CVP)—is also an important indicator of circulatory efficiency.

## Measuring Blood Pressure

An indirect measure of blood pressure using a sphygmomanometer (blood pressure cuff) and a stethoscope is commonly performed over the brachial artery at the elbow. It is also possible to measure blood pressure over the popliteal artery behind the knee, using a large cuff on the thigh. The principle underlying indirect measurement is that blood flowing through healthy arteries does not make sounds audible through a stethoscope. When the flow of blood in the artery is occluded by external pressure, and the pressure is then reduced until the heart is again able to pump blood through the artery past the point of occlusion, a sharp sound called a *Korotkoff sound* is produced with each contraction. The pressure at which the blood is first able to push past the point of occlusion and make a sound is equal to the *systolic* pressure, or the maximum pressure extended by the heart during a contraction.

True *diastolic* pressure is the lowest pressure maintained in the artery between heart contractions. Indirect measurement of this pressure has been the subject of some difference of opinion. As the pressure applied by the blood pressure cuff continues to decrease after the first sounds are heard, a change or "muffling" of the sounds occurs. Then, as the pressure decreases more, the sound disappears entirely. Direct measures of blood pressure reveal that neither of these points, the muffling or the cessation of sound, is consis-

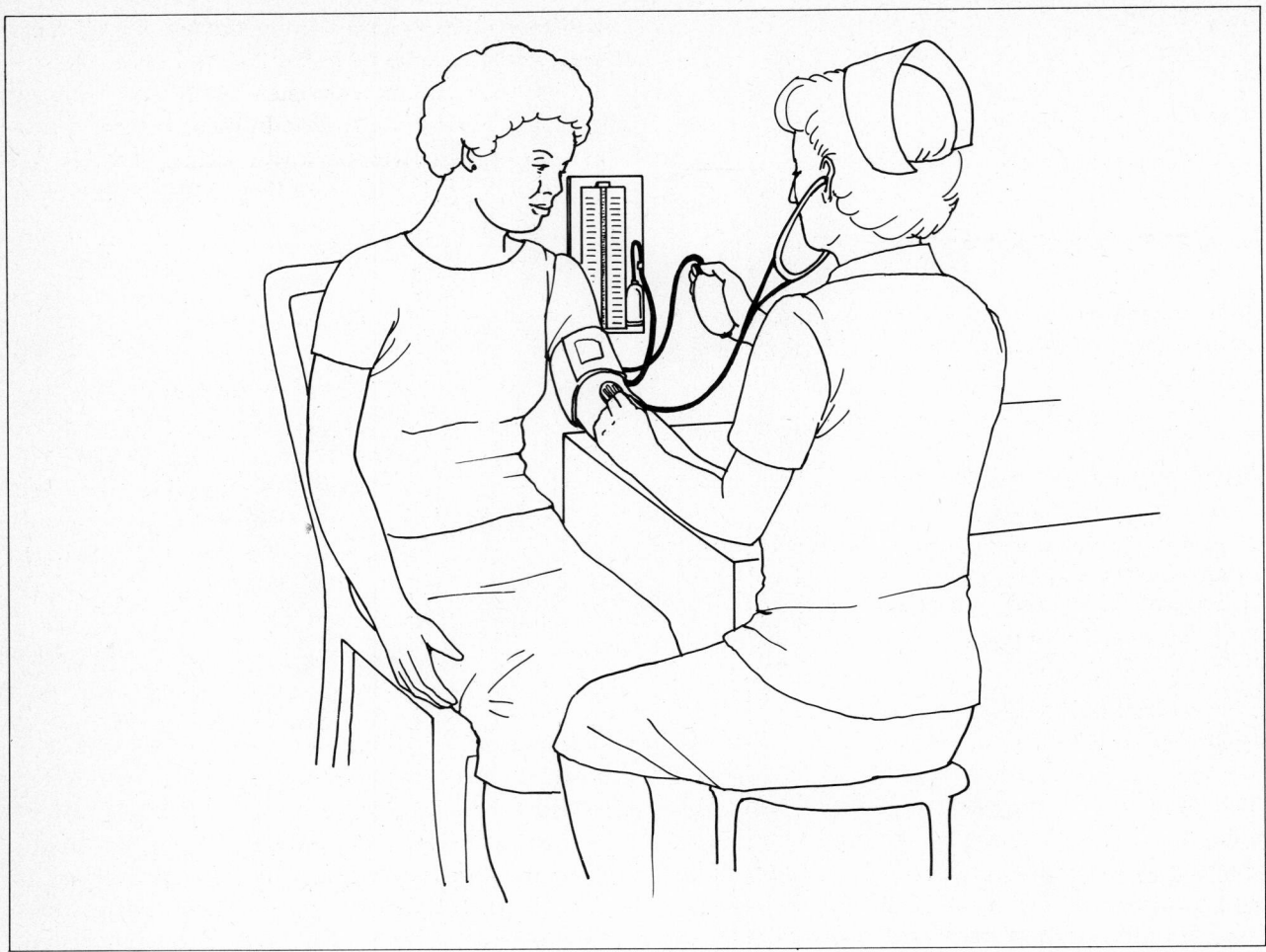

**Figure 24.4**
Taking the blood pressure is an important component of circulatory assessment.

tent with true diastolic pressure. In healthy arteries, the true diastolic pressure is usually 10 mm below the muffling and may coincide with the cessation of sound. However, in arteries diseased due to atherosclerosis, the sound may continue to be heard far below the true diastolic due to turbulence in the vessel. At present, the American Heart Association recommends that a blood pressure reading consist of three figures: (1) the first sounds heard, (2) the muffling of sound, and (3) the cessation of sound (even if this figure is zero). The AHA labels these figures the systolic, the first diastolic, and the second diastolic. When a muffling is not detected, a dash may be drawn to indicate the lack of a figure. (See Figure 24.5.) If the facility where you are working records only two figures, be sure to check the policy to determine whether to measure the first or second diastolic. If only one is to be recorded, it is usually the second. (See Module 21, "Blood Pressure," for specific directions for measuring blood pressure.)

Blood pressure measurements are sometimes made by people with minimal training, and there are many possibilities of error in selection of cuff size, acuity of hearing, and reading of the instrument. When a gross abnormality is reported, it is wise for the nurse to recheck the measurement.

Direct measurement of arterial blood pressure is ordinarily performed in special care units. A special catheter must be inserted into an artery, and equipment that permits direct readings of blood pressure is then attached. Various new elec-

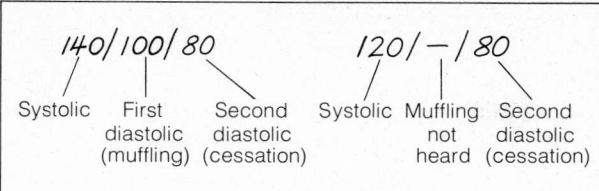

**Figure 24.5 Recording blood pressure readings**

tronic machines for the indirect measurement of blood pressure have been invented but are not yet in general use.

## Blood Pressure Levels

Blood pressure is lowest in the newborn—approximately 40/20—and gradually increases to the adult level—approximately 120/80—during adolescence. Statistically, blood pressure rises as the individual grows older. However, recent evidence suggests that this phenomenon may be due not to aging but to decreasing physical activity. Those who maintain regular physical activity and do not gain excessive weight are less apt to experience increases in blood pressure with aging. As is true of all other body measures, there are wide individual variations in blood pressure. The usual range for adults is 110–140/60–90. Pressures above 160 systolic and/or 100 diastolic are labeled *hypertensive*. A systolic pressure below 100 is labeled *hypotensive*. Such judgments must not be made, however, without gathering baseline data on the individual to determine whether the blood pressure reading represents the person's usual blood pressure or is an isolated instance.

## Factors Affecting Blood Pressure

Many factors affect blood pressure. Activity, drugs, anxiety, anger, joy, or any strong emotion can cause a sharp rise in blood pressure. Anything that dilates blood vessels or causes blood loss will result in a fall in blood pressure. The pattern of rising or falling blood pressure is important to the diagnosis of many pathological conditions.

If the circulatory system is functioning correctly, there will be relatively little difference in blood pressure when body position changes.

However, illness and certain medications render the system unable to make the rapid changes required to maintain consistent blood pressure in the face of position change. In these instances, the blood pressure will be lower sitting than lying, and still lower upon standing. This condition is called *postural hypotension.*

## Frequency of Measurement

When changes are noted in blood pressure and when medications are given to alter blood pressure, measurements may be taken at frequent intervals, in some cases as often as every five minutes. For other patients, such as those in rehabilitation, blood pressure may not be measured after an admission screening. The physician may make a decision on the frequency of blood pressure checks, but it is the nurse's responsibility to recognize any situation that demands closer monitoring and to act independently as necessary.

## Pulse Pressure

Another important indicator is the difference between the systolic and the diastolic readings, which is called the *pulse pressure.* An increasing pulse pressure may indicate a serious problem, such as an increase in intracranial pressure (pressure on the brain). Average pulse pressure is 40 mm of mercury. A pulse pressure of greater than 60 mm of mercury is considered elevated.

## Central Venous Pressure

*Central venous pressure (CVP)* is measured by a catheter inserted into a large peripheral vein and threaded into a large central vein. This catheter is kept open by an intravenous drip, and direct measurement of the pressure may be taken with a special manometer. Normal CVP is 5 to 10 cm of water. Low values indicate a low blood volume; a high value indicates that the circulating volume is increased and the heart is overloaded with fluid to pump. Measuring central venous pressure is an advanced technique, usually performed in special care units by nurses with additional training. More detailed information on the procedure is available in several of the references listed at the end of this chapter.

## Skin Color and Temperature

The color and temperature of the skin reflect the circulation to those areas. It is possible to identify both lack of circulation and lack of oxygenation in the circulating blood by observing skin color.

With good circulation, the extremities are warm and the skin is lent color by the presence of oxygenated blood. White skin has a pink tone, and darker skin has a reddish or warm overtone.

### Cyanosis

Cyanosis is a blue-gray skin color caused by the presence of inadequately oxygenated blood. Easily identified in a person with white skin, it appears as a blue or gray overtone to darker skin. If cyanosis is suspected, examination of the conjunctiva of the eyes, mucous membranes, and nailbeds will indicate the amount of cyanosis present; since these body parts have relatively little pigment, their color derives from the blood itself.

### Pallor

Pallor is paleness of the skin caused by a lack of blood supply to a given area. Pallor signifies that the area is receiving neither oxygenated nor unoxygenated blood. Pallor makes the skin of a white person look white. The skin of a black- or brown-skinned person will lack healthy reddish overtones but will not have the blue-gray overtones characteristic of cyanosis. Again, the areas without pigment most clearly manifest a lack of circulation: the conjunctiva, mucous membranes, and nailbeds will lack their normal healthy pink color.

## Fatigue Level

Cardiac difficulties are a major cause of excessive fatigue in the ill person because the heart is unable to circulate blood adequately to meet cell needs. Fatigue level is assessed by comparing the degree of fatigue experienced with that expected in response to a given activity. In other words, fatigue after strenuous activity is expected; fatigue induced by ordinary activities of daily living may indicate cardiac problems. Since fatigue may also result from respiratory difficulties, it is only a general indicator of potential problems.

## Fluid Retention

Inadequate cardiac function is a major cause of fluid retention, which most commonly takes the form of *edema,* fluid retained in the interstitial spaces between cells. Edema may be identified by the puffiness and swelling of tissues, most commonly in the dependent areas of the body, that is, the legs and sacrum. Edema so severe that the pressure of a finger leaves an indentation is called *pitting edema.* Degrees of edema may be further characterized as 1+ (moderate), 2+ (large amount), 3+ (very large amount), and 4+ (an exceptionally large amount). Needless to say, this is not a precise scale.

Fluid retention may also be identified by an increase in the size of the abdomen due to fluid retained in the peritoneal cavity, a condition called *ascites.* Ascites may be accurately identified by measuring abdominal girth daily. So as to be sure of measuring at the same site, a mark is usually made on the abdomen.

Sometimes fluid is retained in the lungs. This condition, called *pulmonary edema,* is characterized by difficulty in breathing, *orthopnea* (the need to sit up to breathe), and frothy white sputum. Pulmonary edema may be a serious threat to life and is treated by the physician.

Total fluid retention may be measured by weighing the person daily. Weighing for this purpose must be done in a very consistent manner. Usually the person is weighed before breakfast and after emptying the bladder. If possible, the same type of garment should be worn and the same scale used consistently. Each kilogram of body weight added or lost due to fluid equals one liter of fluid (one kilogram is approximately 2.2 pounds).

**Table 24.1**
**Complete Blood Count (CBC) Norms for Adult Men and Women**

| Test | Men | Women |
|---|---|---|
| Hemoglobin* | 14.5–16.5 grams/100 ml | 13–15.5 grams/100 ml |
| Hematocrit* | 45 percent (43–50 percent) | 40 percent (40–45 percent) |
| Erythrocytes (RBC)† | $4.3–5.5 \times 10^6$/cu mm | $4.5–6 \times 10^6$/cu mm |
| Leukocytes (WBC)† | 5,000–10,000 cu mm | 5,000–10,000/cu mm |

*R. M. French, *The Nurse's Guide to Diagnostic Procedures*, 4th ed. (New York: McGraw-Hill, 1978), p. 68.
†*Medifacts* (Indianapolis: Eli Lilly, 1975), p. 4.

## Complete Blood Count

A *complete blood count* (CBC) is usually done for each person admitted to a hospital. It is also a component of many physical examinations. The CBC consists of a red blood cell count, white blood cell count, and a measurement of hemoglobin and hematocrit. Table 24.1 lists norms for each.

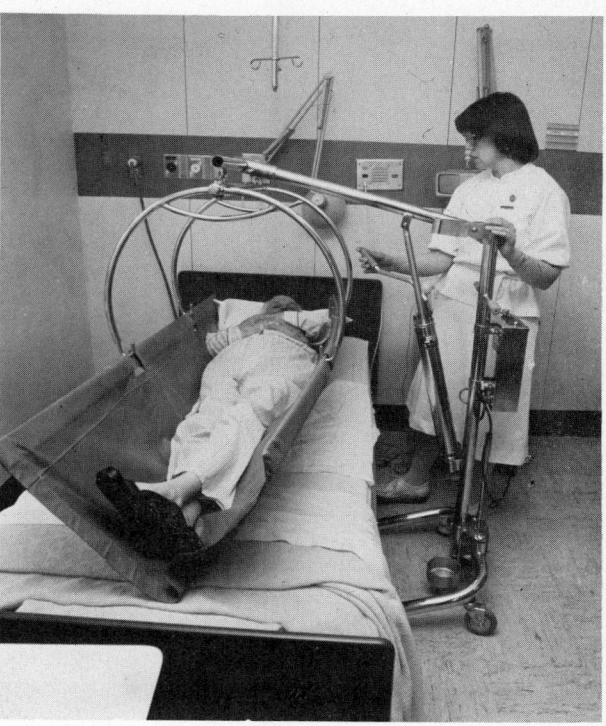

**Figure 24.6**
Fluid retention may be assessed by weighing the patient daily. A bed scale may be used to weigh a patient who cannot stand. (Russ Kinne/Danbury Hospital/Photo Researchers, Inc.)

## Basic Life Support

The National Conference on Standards for Cardiopulmonary Resuscitation (CPR) and Emergency Cardiac Care has recommended that all medical and allied health personnel be trained in techniques of basic life support. These techniques include: (1) recognition of airway obstruction, (2) recognition of respiratory arrest and cardiac arrest, and (3) ability to perform cardiopulmonary resuscitation, which includes rescue breathing and external cardiac massage.

It is necessary for *all* health-care personnel to be so prepared because resuscitation cannot wait for the arrival of special personnel; resuscitation must begin as soon as the need is discovered. Special personnel or teams trained to perform more advanced life-support measures can then be summoned to continue care. Some communities are even establishing extensive programs to teach basic life-support skills to as many citizens as possible. These are not exclusively medical skills.

In an effort to standardize techniques of CPR, "Standards for Cardiopulmonary Resuscitation (CPR) and Emergency Cardiac Care" have been formulated and published in a supplement to the *Journal of the American Medical Association* (see end-of-chapter references). These standards were revised in 1980. Though no training in CPR is adequate unless it provides both a theoretical understanding of the process and mannikins on which to practice one's skills, we shall review some basic concepts here.

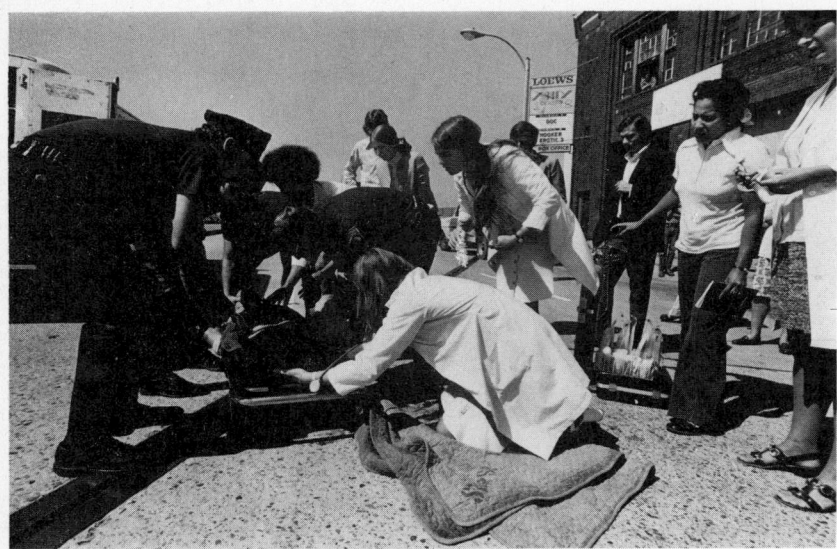

**Figure 24.7**
Emergency life support may be performed in many different settings. (Dan Bernstein)

## Recognizing the Need for Life Support

Because all basic life-support measures have the potential to injure the victim, it is essential that a clear determination of need be made before undertaking them.

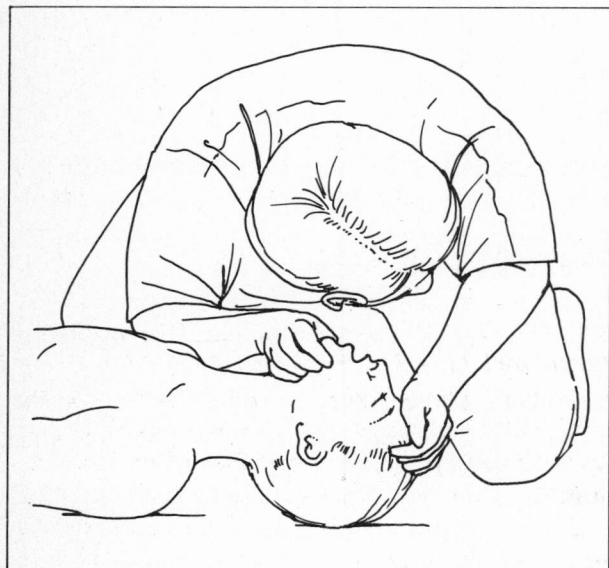

**Figure 24.8  The ABCs of CPR**
Emergency life support can be administered by one or two rescuers. (1) Check, clear, and position the *airway*. (2) Restore *breathing* by mouth-to-mouth resuscitation. (3) Restore *circulation* by chest compression.

The criterion for determining the need for respiratory support is absence of breathing. The absence of breathing is determined by observing for chest movement and feeling for air movement through the mouth and nose. The use of a mirror or glass to check for moisture—and thus breath—has been recommended by some, but taking the time to find such an item could be inadvisable in an emergency. Sometimes chest movement can be felt when it cannot be seen.

The criterion for determining the need for cardiac support is absence of heart action. The absence of heart action is determined by checking for pulse in the carotid arteries. Peripheral pulses are not checked because they may be too weak to be detected, though the heart is still beating. Checking for dilated pupils is sometimes recommended as a means of checking for circulation to the brain. Fixed and dilated pupils may indicate anoxia of the brain but are not used as a criterion for the initiation of action.

## Administering Emergency Life Support

The actions that constitute emergency life support are most easily remembered as "the ABCs," or (1) airway, (2) breathing, and (3) circulation.

The airway is checked and, if necessary, cleared, and positioned to maintain *patency* (open passage).

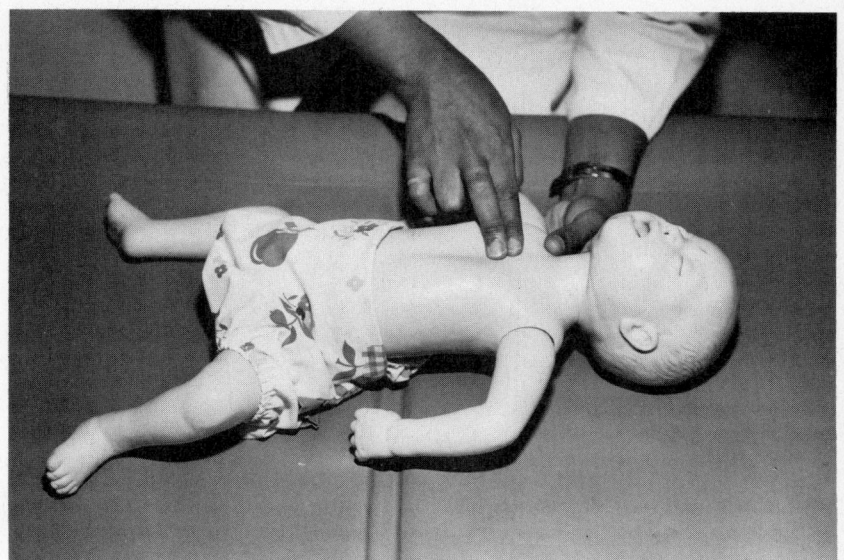

**Figure 24.9  Correct compression for an infant.**
Courtesy Ivan Ellis

Then rescue breathing (mouth-to-mouth resuscitation) is begun. After breathing has been established, circulation is restored by means of external cardiac massage. This process is performed most efficiently by two people but may be accomplished by one.

Your school of nursing or the hospital where you have laboratory practice may train you in emergency life support. Alternatively, such training is available from some fire departments, the Red Cross, and local chapters of the American Heart Association. It is your responsibility to see that you acquire these emergency skills and review them as often as necessary to maintain your proficiency. The directions in Module 26, "Cardiopulmonary Resuscitation," conform to the 1980 recommendations of the American Heart Association.

## Fluid and Electrolyte Balance

*Electrolytes* are chemicals which, when dissolved in water, dissociate (divide) into charged particles called *ions*. The presence of electrolytes enables a solution to conduct electricity. Those ions carrying a positive charge are called *cations* and those carrying a negative charge are called *anions*. The number and types of electrolytes in all the body fluids are critical to the body's biochemical processes.

Water is found in all body tissue. It is the major component of all cells as well as body fluids. As you will note in Figure 24.10, water accounts for an even greater percentage of body weight in infants than in adults. For this reason, infants and children are more susceptible than adults to problems arising from water deficit.

### Body Fluid Compartments

The fluid compartment inside the cell is termed the *intracellular fluid compartment*. Intracellular fluid has a fairly precise composition necessary for the effective functioning of the cells (see Figure 24.11). The major cation of the intracellular fluid is potassium and the major anion is phosphate.

The fluid compartment outside the cell is termed the *extracellular fluid compartment*. Extracellular fluid is further subdivided into the *plasma* (the circulating fluid) and the *interstitial fluid* (that which is between the cells). The composition of the extracellular fluid is not as critical to the body as that of the intracellular fluid. It tends to fluctuate in

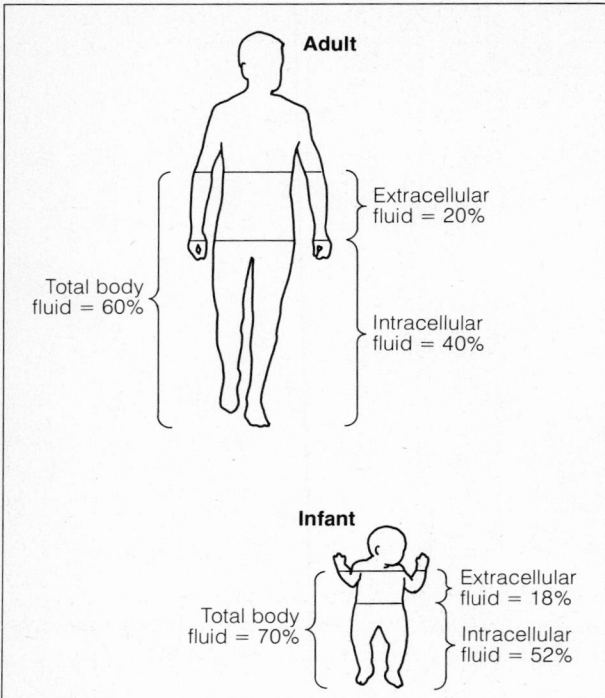

**Figure 24.10   Body water compared to total weight**

## Movement of Water

There are also two processes that move water across membranes. The first is *filtration*: pressure in the arteries creates pressure in the arteriole end of the capillary, which in turn forces fluid through the capillary wall. This pressure is called *filtration pressure*.

The second process responsible for water movement is *osmosis*, a special type of diffusion involving water movement through a membrane rather than the movement of dissolved substances. In osmosis, the fluid on one side of the membrane contains water and particles. Water then moves from an area where the fluid contains relatively more water and fewer particles to the area where the fluid contains less water and more particles

response to food and fluid intake throughout the day. Norms are usually given for fasting levels. The body will also alter the extracellular composition in order to maintain the composition of the intracellular fluid.

## Movement of Electrolytes

Electrolytes move from one fluid compartment to another in two ways. The first process, *diffusion*, is movement of substances from areas of greater concentration to areas of lesser concentration (see Figure 24.12). This process tends to equalize concentration of the electrolytes in all fluid compartments.

Electrolytes are also moved across cell membranes by a process called *active transport*. Active transport is an energy-requiring process of living cell membranes capable of moving electrolytes in the direction needed for optimum cell function, regardless of the concentrations on either side. The active transport system of the cell membrane serves to maintain the difference in composition of the extracellular and intracellular fluids.

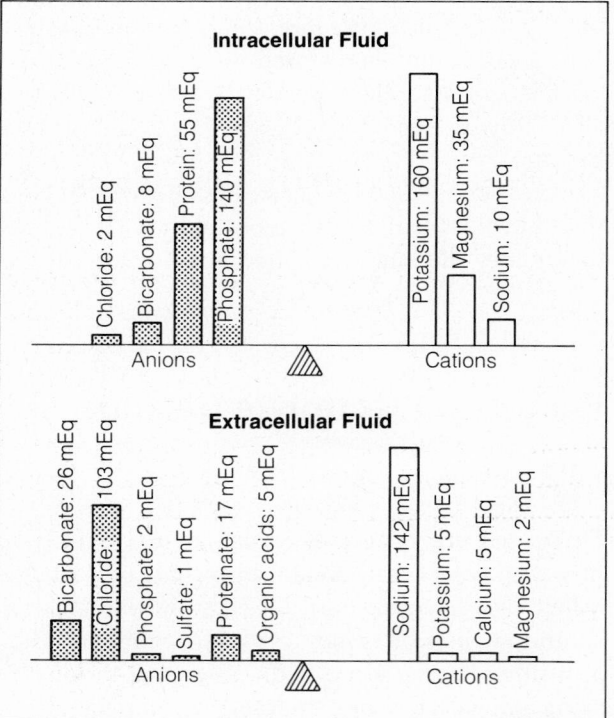

**Figure 24.11   Chemical composition of the body fluids**
Both the intracellular fluid and extracellular fluid of the human body are composed of *anions* (negatively charged electrolytes) and *cations* (positively charged electrolytes). Note that the anions and cations balance each other when expressed in milliequivalents. (Adapted from N. M. Metheny and W. D. Snively, *Nurse's Handbook of Fluid Balance*, 2nd ed. (Philadelphia: J. B. Lippincott, 1974), p. 5. Used with permission.)

(see Figure 24.13). Osmosis tends to move water until the concentration of the fluid is uniform on both sides of the membrane. The osmotic pressure caused by the presence of colloids (large particles that are unable to diffuse through the membrane) is called *colloidal osmotic pressure* (COP) (see Figure 24.14). Electrolytes can also cause osmosis of water to occur.

In summary, water moves in and out of the capillary by means of both filtration and osmosis. Water moves across cell membranes by osmosis. Electrolytes move out of the capillary and across the cell membrane by diffusion. The active transport system of the cell membrane serves to maintain the difference in composition between the extracellular and intracellular fluids.

## Control Mechanisms for Fluid and Electrolyte Balance

The body has a number of different mechanisms that alter fluid and electrolyte balance. *Blood pressure* is critical since all filtration begins with the pressure in the circulating blood. Changes in blood pressure will create changes in fluid and electrolyte balance.

Blood proteins are one of the major dissolved substances in the blood that cause water to move into the capillary from the interstitial space by means of colloidal osmotic pressure. Any disease (such as liver disease) that affects the body's production of proteins and any condition (such as protein starvation) that affects the amount of protein available to the body will affect fluid balance.

The kidneys are able to selectively reabsorb both water and electrolytes according to the body's needs. This process is regulated by a variety of hormonal controls. The *antidiuretic hormone* (ADH) released by the posterior pituitary causes the kidney to reabsorb water. *Aldosterone*, which is secreted by the adrenal cortex, causes sodium and fluid to be retained by the body. These hormonal control mechanisms respond to blood pressure and other changes in fluid and electrolyte balance in the body. Because of their pivotal role, disease of the kidney often creates problems of fluid and electrolyte balance. Other hormones affect specific electrolytes, such as calcium regulation by the parathyroid.

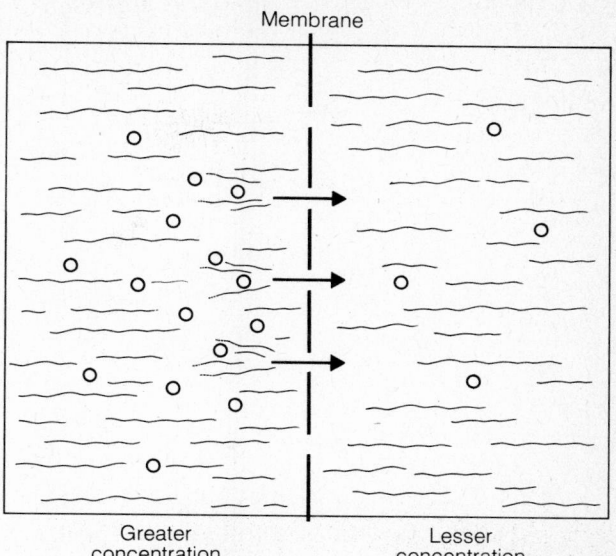

Greater concentration | Lesser concentration

**Figure 24.12  Diffusion of electrolytes**
Dissolved substances move from an area of greater concentration to an area of lesser concentration.

## Measuring Electrolytes

There are three commonly used ways of measuring electrolytes, each of which provides a different type of information.

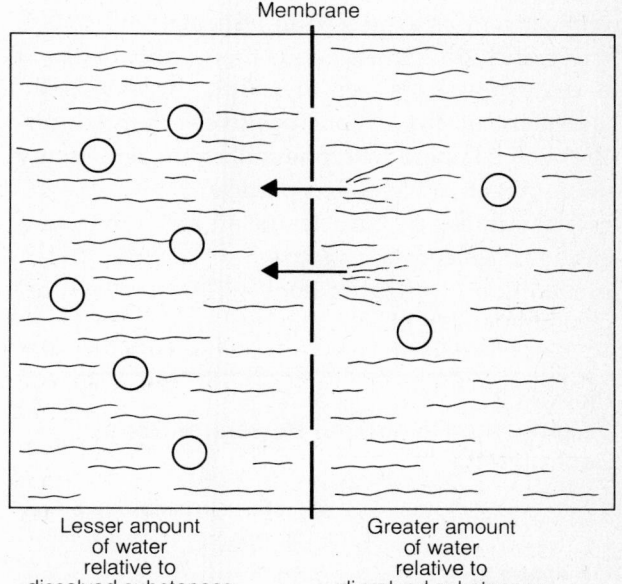

Lesser amount of water relative to dissolved substances | Greater amount of water relative to dissolved substances

**Figure 24.13  Osmosis of water**
Water moves from an area of relatively more water and fewer dissolved substances to an area of less water and more dissolved substances.

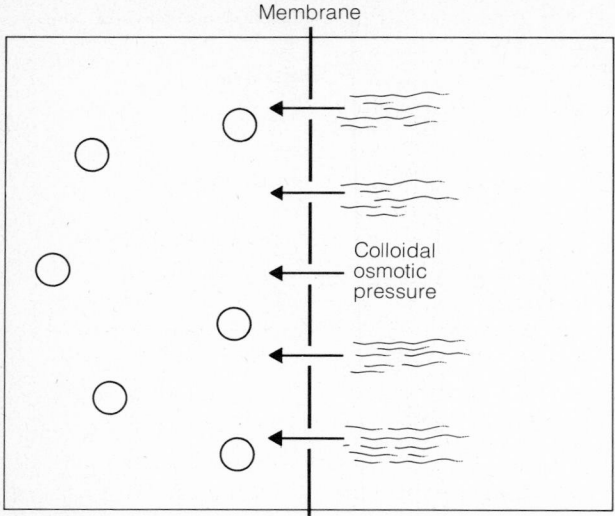

**Figure 24.14**
Large particles that cannot pass through the membrane create colloidal osmotic pressure toward the particles.

The weight of electrolytes is measured metrically, usually in milligrams. When electrolytes are given orally as drugs, they are often measured by weight. In fluids, the number of milligrams per 100 milliliters (mg/100 ml) is most often used as a basis for comparison (see Table 24.2).

The *combining power* of electrolytes is a measure of the number of charges present, either positive or negative; it is expressed in *milliequivalents* (mEq). Fluids, including intravenous fluids, are measured in milliequivalents per liter (mEq/l). One milliequivalent of any cation (positively charged particle) will combine with one milliequivalent of any anion (negatively charged particle).

The number of particles of an electrolyte in a solution, called its *osmolarity* or *tonicity*, determines the movement of body weight through osmosis; osmolarity is usually measured in *milliosmoles* per liter (mOsm/l). Body fluid under normal conditions has an osmolarity of 300 mOsm/l. A fluid with the same osmolarity as body fluid is *isotonic*. One with fewer particles and thus a lower osmolarity is *hypotonic*. One with more particles and thus a higher osmolarity is *hypertonic*. Fluids administered intravenously are usually isotonic in order to avoid potentially dangerous movement of body water across cell membranes.

## Assessment of Fluid and Electrolyte Balance

Though there are many kinds of fluid and electrolyte problems, basic assessment can be approached in a uniform way. You will need to focus on three matters: identification of patients at risk of problems involving fluid and electrolyte balance, observation of key parameters in the patient that are related to cell function, and review of laboratory reports.

### Patients at Risk

There are six categories of patients at particular risk of fluid and electrolyte problems. Any patient who is not receiving any intake is at risk. If fluids and electrolytes are not replaced, the body may quickly become unable to maintain homeostasis.

A patient receiving any type of intravenous fluid is also at risk. Introducing fluids and electrolytes directly into the circulatory system bypasses the gastrointestinal system, which functions to select those items needed by the body. It is possible to provide fluids and electrolytes faster than the body is able to utilize them, which can cause serious and even life-threatening problems.

Any person who experiences excessive loss of body secretions is at risk. Gastrointestinal secretions can be lost through vomiting, suction, or diarrhea. Excessive perspiration due to heat or fever, wound drainage, or moisture lost from the surface of a large burn can also bring about dangerous loss of secretions.

Patients undergoing frequent irrigations of a body cavity are also at risk. The irrigation process can cause electrolytes to move across the walls of

Table 24.2
## Weights and Combining Powers of Some Electrolytes

| | Weight (mg/100 ml) | Combining power (mEq/100 ml) |
|---|---|---|
| Sodium (Na⁺) | 3266 | 142 |
| Potassium (K⁺) | 195 | 5 |
| Calcium (Ca⁺) | 100 | 5 |
| Bicarbonate (HCO₃) | 1546 | 26 |
| Chlorine (Cl⁻) | 3605 | 103 |

the organ being irrigated into the fluid. When the irrigating fluid is removed, electrolytes are removed with it.

People with diseases involving the organs that affect fluid and electrolyte balance are at risk. Diseases of the liver and kidneys are particularly problematic, as are conditions that affect hormonal function.

The last general group of people at risk are those receiving medications that affect fluid and electrolyte balance. Most prominent among these medications are the diuretics, which cause the body to excrete excess fluid and also various electrolytes.

## Observations

There are six general categories of direct observations that will provide evidence of fluid and electrolyte balance. These cues will not reveal the nature of the problem, only that a problem exists.

*Intake and output balance* is indirect evidence of fluid balance. All fluids taken in and output from all sources must be carefully recorded. Intake and output are balanced when the amounts over several days are approximately equal. A short period of time is not adequate to reveal whether intake and output are balanced since the body makes adjustments over time and the bladder is capable of holding up to 500 ml of urine. When intake and output are not balanced, a thorough assessment is necessary to determine the nature of the problem. For example, if the person entered the hospital after several days of vomiting at home, output might be considerably less than intake because

the body is restoring lost fluid. If output is less than intake, the body may be retaining excessive fluid; in such a circumstance, it is appropriate to check for edema. Because intake and output balance are so basic, it is common practice in many hospitals to put all patients identified as being at risk on intake-and-output recording. An alert nurse will independently decide to record fluid intake and output, without waiting for an order from a physician, if the patient is identified as being at high risk.

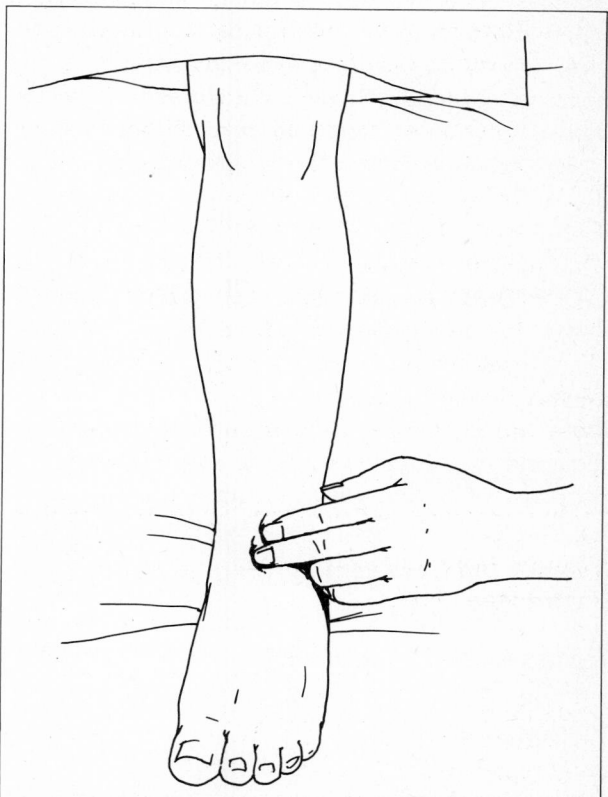

**Figure 24.15 Apply pressure to evaluate pretibial edema**

*Changes in alertness or mental capacity* may be caused by electrolyte imbalance. When such changes as disorientation, depression, and even coma (see Chapter 25) or their opposites—apprehension, hyperexcitability, and delirium—occur rapidly without known neurological disease, you should be alert to the possibility of electrolyte imbalance. Neurological tissue is particularly sensitive to electrolyte concentrations.

*Changes in muscle tone* may also reveal electrolyte abnormalities since electrolyte balance affects the ability of muscle to contract. Muscles may become weak, hypotonic, and even atonic; alternatively, they may become hypertonic, with cramping, tetany, or tremors.

*Changes in respiration* that are unrelated to activity are another cue. When respirations become rapid and deep in the absence of strenuous exercise, or when they become excessively shallow, abnormalities in some key electrolytes may be present or impending.

*Changes in cardiac rate and rhythm* that are not due to heart disease may be caused by electrolyte changes. This reaction is most easily discerned when the person is on a cardiac monitoring device, which allows for precise recordings of the heart's conduction. It can sometimes be detected by auscultation of abnormal heart rhythms.

Finally, *alterations in the fluid present in the tissue* suggest possible fluid imbalance. You will need to check for skin turgor (firmness or fullness). Poor skin turgor, manifested in slow recovery from a pinch, may indicate lack of fluid. The eyes may be dull and lack luster. When fluid deficit is severe, the eyeball itself may lack firmness when palpated. The presence of excessive fluid, in the forms of edema, ascites, or pulmonary edema, has been described on page 410.

## Laboratory Reports

Measurement of serum electrolytes is essential to determining electrolyte and fluid balance. Although laboratory reports specify the serum level, not the intracellular level, of electrolytes, they also may indicate what is occurring in the cell. When fluid and electrolyte imbalances are suspected, the physician will usually order serum electrolytes to be tested. In some facilities, a nurse with appropriate training may also order that a specific electrolyte be checked. Each laboratory publishes a list of the norms for that laboratory based on the specific laboratory methods used. These norms may vary slightly from one facility to another. The norms in Table 24.3 are general and you will need to compare them with those of the facility in which you work.

# Common Fluid and Electrolyte Problems

Fluid and electrolyte problems are often very complex and may involve multiple abnormalities. For purposes of clarity, we will discuss the most common of such problems as they would appear in isolation from other problems.

## Potassium Imbalances

### Hypokalemia

Potassium deficit—serum potassium below 3.5 mEq/l—is known as *hypokalemia*. The most common causes of hypokalemia are the use of diuretic drugs (which cause potassium excretion) and loss of large amounts of gastric secretion. If potassium is not replaced by medication or by foods high in potassium, a deficit may appear.

Because potassium is critical to muscle function, many of the early symptoms of hypokalemia involve lack of muscle function. Fatigue, weakness, and lack of appetite may occur. Due to the importance of potassium in the functioning of the heart muscle, arrhythmias may appear. An electrocardiogram will reveal characteristic signs, which include a flattened T wave and a depressed ST seg-

## Table 24.3
## Serum Electrolyte Norms

| Electrolyte | Normal range |
|---|---|
| Calcium (serum) | 4.5–5.5 mEq/l (9–11 mg/100 ml) |
| Chloride | 100–106 mEq/l (355–376 mg/100 ml as Cl) (585–620 mg/100 ml as NaCl) |
| Magnesium | 1.5–2.5 mEq/l (1.8–3 mg/100 ml) |
| Phosphate (inorganic) | 3–4.5 mg/100ml (in children, 4–7 mg/100 ml) |
| Potassium | 3.5–5.4 mEq/l (14–20 mg/100 ml) |
| Sodium | 136–145 mEq/l (313–334 mg/100 ml) |

ment. (You will learn about electrocardiograph patterns when you study cardiac disease.)

When hypokalemia is identified, the physician will order replacement of potassium by means of intravenous fluids containing potassium or oral potassium supplements.

## Hyperkalemia

Hyperkalemia, or potassium excess, is defined as potassium above 5.6 mEq/l. Potassium excess occurs most commonly in patients being given potassium replacements in larger amounts than necessary, those whose intravenous fluids containing potassium run too rapidly, and those who continue taking a potassium replacement when a diuretic has been discontinued.

The most common symptoms are irritability, nausea, and diarrhea. If hyperkalemia continues, cardiac arrhythmias (peaked T waves on the ECG) may occur. Severe potassium excess can lead to muscle paralysis and cardiac standstill.

Potassium excess is usually treated by restricting potassium intake and allowing the body to restore balance. An oral medication that causes potassium to be excreted into the intestines may be given. In severe instances, kidney dialysis may be used to reduce potassium levels rapidly.

## Calcium Imbalances

### Hypocalcemia

Hypocalcemia, or calcium deficit (serum calcium below 4.5 mEq/l), is most commonly attributable to the body's increased use of calcium due to pregnancy or rapid growth. Less commonly, hypocalcemia can result from disturbance in the parathyroid gland. Tingling of the fingers and extremities is followed by muscle cramping and spasm, and, in extreme cases, grand mal seizures (see Chapter 25).

In cases of mild calcium deficit, the physician may order extra calcium to be taken as tablets. In acute calcium deficit, intravenous calcium in the form of calcium gluconate is usually ordered.

### Hypercalcemia

Hypercalcemia, or calcium excess (serum calcium above 5.8 mEq/l), is uncommon. It occurs when the parathyroid glands are oversecreting or when intravenous calcium is given in excessive quantities. Muscles become hypotonic. Hypotonic muscles of respiration may cause serious oxygenation problems; hypotonic skeletal muscles cause weakness and may contribute to falls. Over a longer term, hypercalcemia can bring about renal stones composed of calcium salts, bone changes and bone pain, and coma. As a palliative measure, dialysis may be undertaken to remove excess serum calcium. Reducing calcium intake may be of value in some instances.

## Sodium Imbalances

Because sodium is the major electrolyte responsible for body-water movement, it is very difficult to distinguish excesses or deficits of sodium from excesses or deficits of water. For example, when serum sodium is low, the true problem may be not a deficit of sodium but an excess of water in the body. Let us look first at genuine disturbances in the sodium level, keeping in mind that they are less common than disturbances in fluid balance, which we shall discuss next.

## Hyponatremia

Hyponatremia, or sodium deficit (serum sodium below 137 mEq/l), occurs when there is a loss of sodium greater than the corresponding loss of water. This may occur when a person perspires excessively, since perspiration has a very high sodium concentration, or when diuretics are used very vigorously and excessive amounts of sodium are excreted. In rare instances, hyponatremia occurs because of excessive water intake, either orally or intravenously.

A person suffering from sodium deficit may have abdominal cramps, diarrhea, and feelings of anxiety. In extreme instances, seizures may occur and death may follow.

People who work in very hot environments and perspire profusely should be encouraged to eat salty foods. In some instances, salt tablets may be taken for replacement. Intravenous solutions containing sodium may be given to people who are acutely ill.

## Hypernatremia

Hypernatremia, or sodium excess, is a serum sodium level above 147 mEq/l. A true excess of sodium that is not a result of changes in body water is rare but may result from excessive ingestion of salt tablets or of sea water in cases of near-drowning. Hypernatremia causes severe nausea and vomiting. Urine output is decreased in an attempt to conserve body water to dilute the sodium. Effects on central nervous system tissue are manifested by agitation, hyperactivity, and sometimes convulsions. Temperature may rise and death can result.

Hypernatremia is treated by providing large amounts of water, orally or intravenously, which the body uses to dilute the sodium and promote its excretion by the kidneys.

## Fluid Imbalances

Fluid imbalances take two general forms. If the total volume of body fluid is abnormal, but its composition is normal, the body functions better than if both volume and composition are abnormal.

Table 24.4
**Laboratory Values for Common Electrolyte Disturbances**

| Electrolyte | Dangerously low | Normal | Dangerously high |
|---|---|---|---|
| **Calcium** | < 6 mg/100 ml | 9–11 mg/100 ml | > 14 mg/100 ml |
| **Potassium** | < 2.5 mEq/l | 3.5–5 mEq/l | > 6.5 mEq/l |
| **Sodium** | < 110 mEq/l | 136–145 mEq/l | >170 mEq/l |

Source: *Medifacts* (Indianapolis: Eli Lilly, 1975), pp. 6–9.

## Fluid Volume Excess

Fluid volume excess can result from excessive amounts of intravenous fluids and from certain disease states. The neck veins will be distended when the head is elevated above 45 degrees because the circulatory system is overloaded. (Module 32, "Inspection, Palpation, Auscultation, and Percussion," demonstrates how to check neck veins for distention.) The body will begin to store the excess fluid in the tissues in order to shift the load away from the circulating plasma so that the heart does not become overloaded. One of the places fluid begins to accumulate first is the base of the lungs because the tissue in that area is characterized by an extensive network of fine capillaries, allowing fluid to move out of the vessels, and the tissue itself is open and does not resist the entry of fluid. This condition is a form of pulmonary edema and can be identified by shortness of breath, orthopnea, and moisture heard on auscultation.

To prevent this condition, intravenous fluids must be monitored with extreme care. Rates of flow should be supervised carefully. If fluid overload occurs, the input must be greatly reduced to give the kidneys an opportunity to excrete the excess fluid. Diuretic drugs may be ordered to increase the rate of excretion.

Slowly occurring fluid volume excess may be caused by a variety of illnesses and situations, including congestive heart failure, excessive administration of adrenal cortical hormones, and renal disease. In such cases the symptoms set in slowly and the circulatory system may not be overloaded.

There may be weight gain, edema of tissues, puffy eyelids, shortness of breath, and a bounding pulse.

When the fluid volume is high, the laboratory report will reveal hematocrit, hemoglobin, and red blood cell count values below normal because of an abnormal amount of fluid relative to the cells. Although electrolytes are being retained, there may initially be a low serum sodium since the body retains water faster than it retains sodium. As the condition progresses, electrolyte concentrations will be normal: the total body content of all electrolytes will be elevated along with the total body water.

Treatment is aimed at correcting the underlying cause of the fluid disturbance. Diuretics may be ordered. If large amounts of fluid have accumulated in the pleural space, restricting breathing, a thoracentesis may be done. If large amounts of fluid have accumulated in the peritoneal cavity, causing severe distress, a paracentesis may be done. In each of these procedures, a large needle is introduced into the cavity to withdraw the fluid. These procedures are avoided if at all possible because they result in the loss of plasma proteins and electrolytes as well as excess fluids. Furthermore, unless the underlying cause has been corrected, fluid will again begin to accumulate.

## Fluid Volume Deficit

Fluid volume deficit is characterized by a deficit of both water and electrolytes. The remaining body fluid is of approximately normal content in terms of electrolytes.

Such a deficit occurs when a person skips drinking fluids or when loss of fluids is greater than intake, as in cases of high fever or diaphoresis (excessive perspiration). At first the extracellular fluid may be hypertonic, but the water is quickly moved out of the cells to establish equilibrium and the body excretes electrolytes to establish the proper level.

The skin and mucous membranes are usually dry, and there may be acute weight loss (a loss of up to 5 percent of body weight in the adult is considered a moderate loss). There may be longitudinal wrinkles in the tongue. Urine output will be decreased or, in severe cases, absent. Laboratory findings will reveal normal electrolyte values. The hematocrit, hemoglobin, and red blood cell count will all be high due to hemoconcentration (concentration of blood cells). Treatment is to provide both fluids and electrolytes so that the body can restore fluid balance. This may be accomplished by oral feeding of water, broth, or soups or by parenteral administration of intravenous fluids.

# Acid-Base Balance

*Acid-base balance*, a specialized kind of electrolyte balance, is the correct balance of hydrogen ions in the body fluids. As the concentration of hydrogen ions in a fluid increases, that fluid becomes more acidic. As the concentration decreases, it becomes more alkaline (basic). Degrees of alkalinity and acidity are measured on a scale from 1 to 14 called a *pH scale*. (For more information on this scale, consult a chemistry text.) On the pH scale, 7.0 is neutral. Numbers above 7.0 indicate a lower concentration of hydrogen ions and thus a more alkaline or basic solution; numbers below 7.0 indicate a greater concentration of hydrogen ions and thus a more acidic solution.

All body fluids are normally basic in pH. The normal pH for arterial blood is 7.45; for venous blood, it is 7.35. The usual norms given for blood pH are 7.35 to 7.45. Any change in body pH below these norms is called *acidosis*. (Strictly speaking, it is only a relative acidosis, since body pH remains above 7.0 and thus remains alkaline.) Any pH above 7.45 is referred to as *alkalosis*, signifying that the body is relatively more alkaline than normal.

## Body Mechanisms for Maintaining pH

The body has many sets of buffers, which serve to maintain acid-base balance. A *buffer* is a chemical

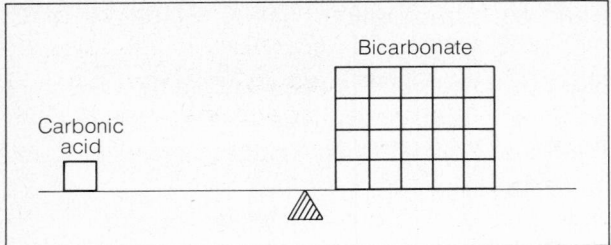

**Figure 24.16**
Appropriate acid–base balance requires a 20:1 ratio of base bicarbonate to carbonic acid.

compound that can combine with a strong acid to make it weaker and with a strong base to make it weaker.

Protein is very important to the body's system of buffers. It is always present, flexible, and capable of handling large quantities of acid or base products. Hemoglobin also serves as a buffer, though not a major one. It too tends to be stable, and problems associated with hemoglobin buffering are rare. The phosphate buffering systems are very active, especially within the cells; these systems can be disturbed by certain poisons but are not of common clinical concern.

The two mechanisms of the greatest clinical concern are the base bicarbonate system (often called the metabolic system) and the carbon dioxide system (often called the respiratory system). These two mechanisms act in relationship to each other.

Essentially, the body is able to maintain acid-base balance when the ratio of bicarbonate and carbon dioxide is 20:1—that is, when there is 20 times as much bicarbonate as carbon dioxide (see Figure 24.16). The bicarbonate ion can be produced by the kidney when it is needed, though this response is not immediate. Carbon dioxide, which dissociates (divides) in solution to form carbonic acid and water, results from cellular oxidation. Constant elimination of carbon dioxide by the lungs maintains the balance.

## Common Acid-Base Imbalances

Acid-base imbalances are analyzed in two different ways: by whether the respiratory mechanism (carbon dioxide level) or the metabolic mechanism (base bicarbonate level) is responsible for the problem; and by whether the change is in the direction of greater acidity or greater alkalinity. Table 24.5 lists laboratory values for common acid-base imbalances.

## Metabolic Acidosis (Base Bicarbonate Deficit)

In metabolic acidosis, the body produces acid end products of metabolism (which must be buffered by base bicarbonate) in quantities so great as to exhaust the body's supply of base bicarbonate. This results in a base bicarbonate deficit.

The first step in assessment is to identify patients at risk of metabolic acidosis. Such people include those in shock (since producing energy without adequate oxygen creates more acid end

Table 24.5
**Laboratory Values in Common Acid-Base Imbalances**

| Imbalance | Plasma pH | Plasma bicarbonate | pCO$_2$ | Urine pH |
|---|---|---|---|---|
| **Metabolic acidosis** (base bicarbonate deficit) | <7.35 (low) | <25 mEq/l (low) | 35–45 mmHg (normal) | <6.0 (low) |
| **Metabolic alkalosis** (base bicarbonate excess) | >7.45 (high) | >29 mEq/l (high) | 35–45 mmHg (normal) | >7.0 (high) |
| **Respiratory acidosis** (carbonic acid excess) | <7.35 (low) | 22–26 mEq/l (norm) or >29 mEq/l (high) | 50 mmHg (high) | <6.0 (low) |
| **Respiratory alkalosis** (carbonic acid deficit) | >7.45 (high) | 22–26 mEq/l (normal) | 30 mmHg (low) | >7.0 (high) |

products) and those who use excessive amounts of fat for energy (people on rigid high-protein diets and diabetics with inadequate insulin to use carbohydrates) since excessive acid end products result from large-scale fat metabolism.

Observation should focus on identifying the effects of low pH: disorientation, drowsiness, stupor, and eventual coma. Respirations may become very deep and rapid as the body tries to compensate for the lack of bicarbonate by eliminating carbon dioxide, which is also an acid.

Laboratory values will show a plasma pH of less than 7.35. The plasma bicarbonate will be less than 25 mEq/l in the adult and less than 20 mEq/l in the child. Urine pH may be less than 6.0. $PCO_2$ is within normal limits.

Intervention by the physician is aimed at correcting the underlying metabolic cause of the problem. Temporary treatment with intravenous bicarbonate is common in cases of severe shock and cardiac arrest.

## Metabolic Alkalosis (Base Bicarbonate Excess)

In this condition, the body has more base bicarbonate than is needed to buffer carbon dioxide and other acid end products.

Particularly at risk are people who are losing large amounts of acid (such as gastric or biliary secretions) from the body, those who take large amounts of bicarbonate of soda for relief of stomach distress, and those with impaired kidney function who drink carbonated beverages in large quantities.

Observation would reveal shallow respirations, as the body seeks to conserve carbon dioxide for its acidifying effect. The muscles would be hypertonic, and tetany and muscle spasms might occur. In severe cases, generalized seizures could occur.

Laboratory findings would reveal a plasma pH of greater than 7.45. The plasma bicarbonate would be greater than 29 mEq/l in the adult and greater than 24 mEq/l in the child. Both the plasma chloride and the plasma potassium would tend to be decreased as the body makes compensatory shifts in electrolytes. Urine pH would be greater than 7.0. $PCO_2$ is within normal limits.

Intervention is directed at correcting the cause of loss of acid, if possible. Vomiting, for example, might be controlled. Fluid and electrolytes would be replaced to offset losses and enable the body to restore homeostasis.

## Respiratory Acidosis (Carbonic Acid Excess)

In respiratory acidosis the level of carbon dioxide rises, most frequently due to a breathing difficulty such as obstructive lung disease. Respiratory acidosis may or may not be associated with hypoxia (lack of oxygen).

Patients at risk are those with ventilation problems, particularly those with respiratory diseases that interfere with exchanges of carbon dioxide and oxygen. Also at risk is the person who has taken or been given excessive narcotics, causing hypoventilation.

Observation may reveal very shallow respirations. Initial disorientation may progress to stupor, coma, and even death, if unchecked. Should hypoxia also be present, its symptoms may intermingle with those of acidosis (see Chapter 23).

Laboratory values reveal a plasma pH below 7.35. The $PCO_2$ will be greater than 50 mm of mercury. Urine pH will be less than 6.0. Bicarbonate may also be elevated, as the body tries unsuccessfully to compensate for the excess acid. The bicarbonate level may be greater than 29 mEq/l in the adult; it may also be within normal limits.

Intervention to remedy the respiratory problem is needed. This might involve breathing exercises to encourage expiration of carbon dioxide or use of mechanical breathing devices, such as intermittent positive-pressure breathing devices, to facilitate air exchange. Medications to help remove secretions blocking the respiratory passages may be needed.

## Respiratory Alkalosis (Carbonic Acid Deficit)

In respiratory alkalosis, the person breathes out excessive amounts of carbon dioxide, leaving the bicarbonate unbalanced. In an effort to adjust, the kidney excretes calcium.

Those at risk include patients on ventilating machines that are set incorrectly and cause excessive expiration. Those who hyperventilate when anxious or hysterical are common victims of respiratory alkalosis.

Such a person might complain of headache, dizziness, faintness, tingling, and abnormal sensations in the lips and the extremities. Tetany (muscle rigidity), muscle spasms, and minor seizures might occur.

Laboratory values include a plasma pH above 7.45 and a urine pH greater than 7.0. Plasma $PCO_2$, though rarely measured, would be low. Plasma bicarbonate would be normal, 22–26 mEq/l.

Treatment, usually quite simple, is aimed at changing the respiratory pattern. If the person is on a breathing device, the settings are corrected. If the person is hyperventilating, efforts are made to slow the respiratory pattern. The person may be encouraged to breathe into a paper bag in order to rebreathe the same air and increase the car-

bon dioxide level. Symptoms usually disappear rapidly.

## Using Laboratory Records

Often the body is able to make adjustments in balance that compensate for a deficit or excess and thereby preserve the body's pH. If so, the condition is known as a *compensated* acid-base balance problem. It is possible, for example, to have a compensated metabolic acidosis or a compensated respiratory acidosis.

The *Davenport Nomogram* is a graph that can be used to plot laboratory values and thus determine the acid-base state (see Figure 24.17). The patient's pH and bicarbonate are the two values plotted. The bicarbonate value is located on the vertical axis and the plasma pH on the horizontal axis. Each of these points is extended into a straight line across the graph, and the point where the two lines intersect represents the person's current status.

## Fluid Therapy

Intravenous fluids are given in many different circumstances. Although ordering the fluid therapy is the physician's responsibility, you need to understand its purposes in order to monitor what is happening to the patient.

## Types of Solutions

### Hydrating Solutions

Hydrating solutions' primary purpose is to provide water. These solutions contain water and either a carbohydrate or sodium chloride; they do not contain any other electrolytes. The most common hydrating solutions are 5 percent dextrose in water and 0.9 percent sodium chloride (normal saline). Hydrating solutions may be used to determine whether kidney function is adequate to allow for rapid replacement of fluids containing

electrolytes. When the adequacy of kidney function is in question, a large volume of fluid is given over a period of forty-five minutes. If kidney function is adequate, the patient will void (or urine will be drained out of the catheter).

Hydrating solutions are also used as diluents for intravenous drugs or to keep an intravenous line open at a slow rate in order to be available for medications or other solutions when ordered.

### Balanced Solutions

Balanced solutions are those containing water, a carbohydrate for basic calorie needs (to prevent muscle tissue wasting), and basic electrolytes. The electrolytes included are sodium, potassium, and magnesium as cations and chloride, lactate, and phosphate as anions. The expectation is that the

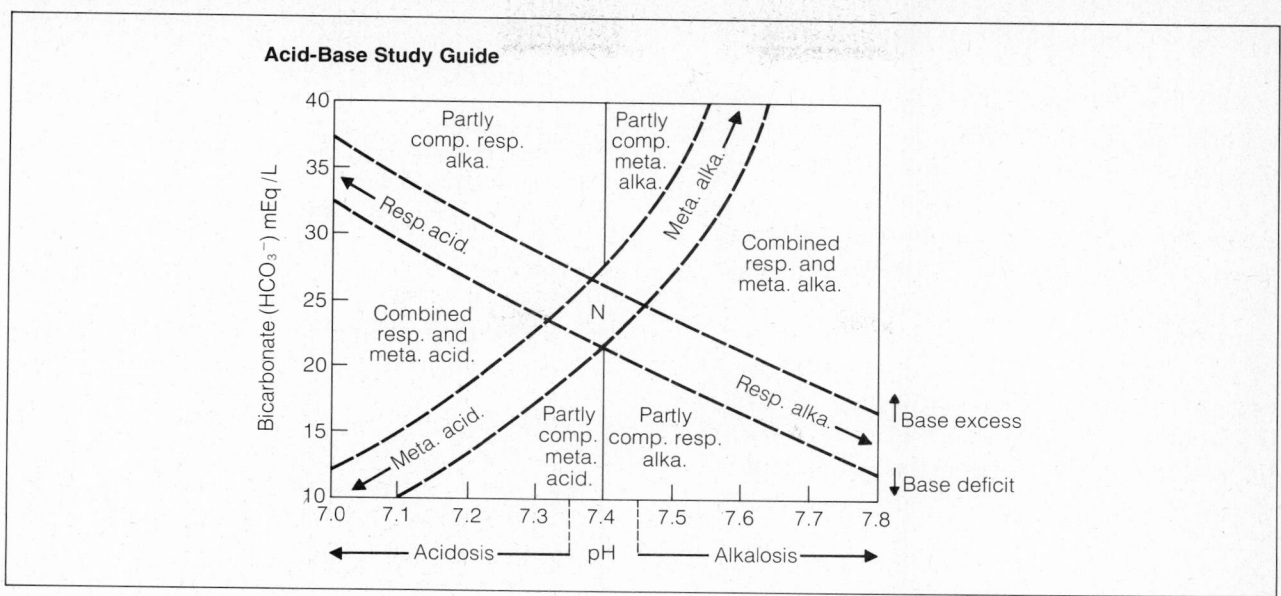

**Figure 24.17 The Davenport Nomogram**
Jones Medical Instrument Co., Oakbrook, Illinois, and Dr. J. D. Hackney.

person's own kidneys will sort, select, and reject electrolytes as needed.

For maintenance when there is no oral intake, a total amount of 1500 ml per square meter of body surface area is given in each twenty-four-hour period.

If a moderate deficit exists, the person will need the maintenance amount plus an additional 2400 ml per twenty-four hours for each square meter of body surface area. A moderate deficit is defined as a weight loss of 5 percent in an adult and up to 10 percent in a child.

If a severe deficit exists, the person will need the maintenance amount plus 3000 ml per twenty-four hours for each square meter of body surface area. A severe deficit is defined as a weight loss of over 5 percent in an adult and over 10 percent in a child.

Balanced solutions are useful for 80–90 percent of patients. They are not used for severely burned persons, those with kidney damage, or those with certain hormonal diseases. Common brand names of balanced solutions are Normosol M and Polyonic M.

## Replacement Solutions

Replacement solutions are used to replace concurrent losses of water and electrolytes in abnormal amounts. The solution used must resemble what is being lost.

Losses due to intestinal suction, vomiting, enterostomy (an intestinal opening) drainage, and diarrhea are replaced with solutions containing additional chloride in the form of ammonium chloride or calcium chloride but no additional sodium. This formula matches the electrolyte concentration of the secretions being lost. Lactated Ringer's solution is often used for this purpose, but because the basic formula for Lactated Ringer's does not contain adequate potassium, extra potassium is often added. Acidifying or alkalinizing solutions may be used to help correct acid-base imbalances.

Replacement solutions are given in addition to needed maintenance solutions in amounts equal to what is being lost. It is common practice to alternate the replacement solution with the maintenance solution.

## Nutritional Solutions

Solutions used to provide for basic nutrition include those with a high percentage of dextrose; protein hydrolysates such as Aminosol, Hyprotigen, and Amigen; amino acids such as Aminosyn, FreAmine, and Travasol; and fat emulsions such as Intralipid. The administration of nutrients by means of hyperalimentation is discussed in Chapter 21.

Ethanol (ethyl alcohol) may also be given intravenously to provide calories. One gram of alcohol yields 6–8 calories and is used first by the body, sparing glucose for use by the brain. If sedation is desired, a 5 percent solution of alcohol may be given at a rate of 200–300 ml per hour for an adult. Be careful to give it slowly enough not to cause inebriation.

Water-soluble vitamins are added to intravenous fluids when the patient will be without oral intake for three or more days. Doing so provides the body with essential compounds necessary for metabolic processes.

## Volume Expanders

Volume expanders are solutions containing large molecules that will tend to increase osmotic pressure and thus maintain the volume of fluid inside the vessels. Volume expanders are used when fluid losses have been massive, such as in severe burns or hemorrhage. Volume expanders may also be used to provide proteins the body is unable to manufacture due to liver disease. The most commonly used volume expanders are plasma, human serum albumin (both prepared from whole blood by the blood bank), and dextran, a product with large carbohydrate molecules. When volume expanders are used, you must be very attentive to the possibility of circulatory overload (fluid volume excess).

## Assessment in Fluid Therapy

A patient receiving fluid therapy requires assessment initially and on an ongoing basis in order to identify problems early and to ensure that the system continues to function correctly.

### Initial Assessment

*Checking the physician's order* for fluid therapy is essential to initial assessment. You will need to know the type of fluid ordered, any additives, and the rate of administration.

Exhibit 24.3
**Basic Assessment in Fluid Therapy**

**Initial assessment**
Check physician's order.
Check nursing record.
Check patient (site, fluid, and rate).

**Routine assessment**
Check patient hourly (site, fluid, and rate).

*Checking the nursing care plan or card index (Kardex)* will reveal whether this is the initial fluid order or one of a series. You will need to find out where the intravenous line is located and any special information about the system being used, such as the presence or absence of a heparin lock. See

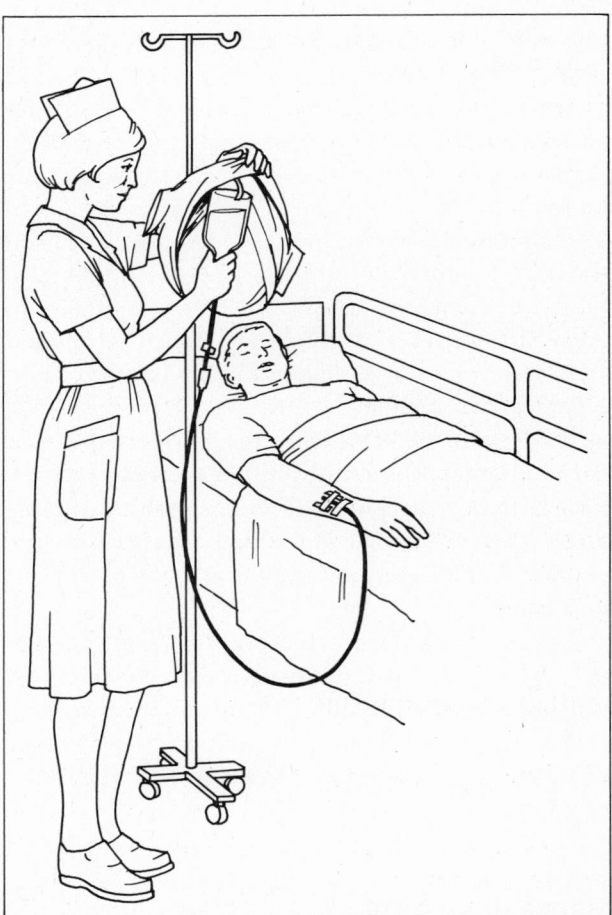

**Figure 24.18 Changing a patient's gown with an IV in place**

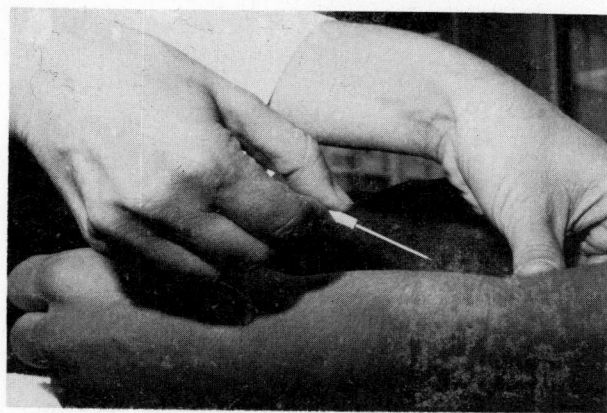

**Figure 24.19    Skin retracted and needle at angle to pierce skin**
Courtesy Ivan Ellis

Modules 46, 47 and 48 for a complete description of intravenous equipment.

*Checking the patient* involves examining the site of the infusion, comparing the rate of administration with the desired rate, and verifying that the correct fluid is being administered. You will want to watch for abnormalities at the site; inflammation, for example, might indicate phlebitis (inflammation of the vein) and cold swelling might indicate infiltration (leakage of the fluid into the tissue around the vein).

## Routine Assessment

After the initial assessment, it is not necessary to recheck the physician's order or the nurse's records each time the intravenous is monitored. The intravenous line itself and the patient should be checked hourly in routine situations and more frequently when the condition of the patient is more serious.

## Caring for the Intravenous Line

### Tubing and Dressing Changes

To lessen the potential for local inflammation of the vein and for infusing contaminated solution, the Center for Disease Control currently recommends that the tubing be changed every forty-eight hours. The dressing over the intravenous

site should also be changed at that time. An iodine-based or antibiotic ointment (depending on the policy of the facility) is applied to the needle entry site, and a new sterile dressing is applied over the site.

## Bottle Changes

In most situations the fluid bottles (or plastic bags) are changed frequently in order to add more fluid. However, when the intravenous is being run very slowly to keep the vein open, a bottle could hang for a long period. The Center for Disease Control recommends that no bottle hang for more than twenty-four hours in order to minimize the potential for infection.

## Changing the Infusion Site

Some publications have suggested that changing the site every forty-eight hours would decrease the potential for phlebitis. Since it is painful to have an intravenous started and many patients have poor veins that offer relatively few sites, some physicians and nurses are unwilling to discontinue a functioning intravenous line in hope of decreasing the incidence of phlebitis. Therefore the line may be left in place until a problem is detected, at which time the site is changed. This approach makes early detection of problems very important.

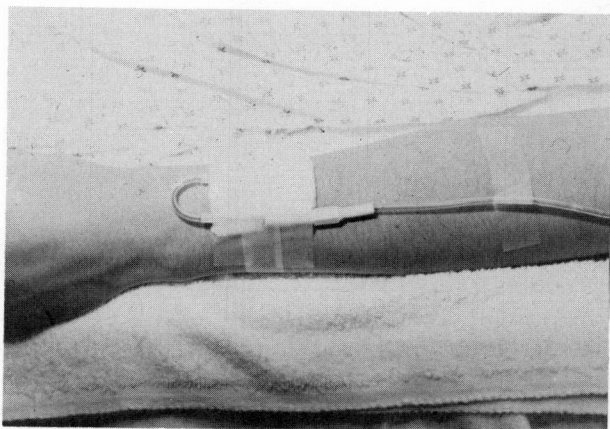

**Figure 24.20    IV dressing and tubing in place**
Courtesy Ivan Ellis

## Regulating the Rate of Flow

The physician may specify the rate of flow in a variety of ways. Often the 1000-ml bottle is used as a standard, and the duration is varied (six hours, eight hours, ten hours, and so on) to provide for the appropriate volume in each twenty-four-hour period. Some physicians order fluids in ml per hour; still others order the total fluid to be run in a twenty-four-hour period.

An intravenous is regulated by adjusting the flow in the tubing in terms of drops per minute. You must therefore be able to translate the physician's order as written into a drops-per-minute figure.

Intravenous tubings are not standardized. Each manufacturer has established its own standard for the number of drops delivered per ml. After checking the package for this information, you may use the following formula to figure drops per minute:

$$\frac{\begin{array}{c}\text{drops per ml}\\\text{of equipment}\end{array} \times \begin{array}{c}\text{number of ml}\\\text{ordered}\end{array}}{\text{number of hours} \times \text{60 minutes}} = \text{drops/minute}$$
$$\text{to run}$$

The rate of flow is important because it is possible to give too little to meet the patient's needs or so much that the circulatory system is overloaded. When electrolytes—especially potassium—have been added, circulatory overload is of particular concern. Sometimes a bottle of intravenous fluid is marked with the approximate level the fluid should reach at specified times to provide the amount ordered. This is a helpful aid in maintaining a general overview of fluid administration but is unsatisfactory as the only method of checking the rate. If the IV is behind schedule, it may be tempting to increase the rate to "catch up," without regard to how fast the fluid is being administered during the catch-up period. As a general guideline, 3 ml per minute is a moderate flow rate for a *healthy adult*, 2 ml per minute is a slow rate, and 4 ml per minute is a rapid rate. If you must readjust an IV, consider the person's age, size, and cardiovascular status to determine a safe speed.

For further information on caring for the patient who needs intravenous fluids and medications, see Module 46, "Preparing and Maintaining Intravenous Infusions"; Module 47, "Administering Intravenous Medications"; and Module 48, "Starting Intravenous Infusions."

# Blood Transfusions

Blood and blood products have many important medical uses and are frequently used in therapy. Though adverse reactions to blood transfusions are not common, they can be very serious.

## Types of Blood Products Used

### Whole Blood

Whole blood is, as its name implies, the entire product obtained from the donor. Blood stored in a blood bank is *citrated*, which involves adding a chemical to prevent clotting on storage. Fresh whole blood may be obtained for use in such special situations as open-heart surgery; this blood has not been treated to prevent clotting. Regular whole blood is most often used to replace blood lost through bleeding, as in surgery.

### Blood Products

Most blood banks increasingly separate out vital factors from whole blood so as to give only the needed factor to a patient. This policy has a three-fold benefit: (1) fewer donations of blood are necessary to meet the community's blood needs; (2) the individual is exposed to fewer elements that might precipitate a reaction; and (3) hepatitis, a viral disease transmitted by blood from an infected individual, is not transmitted by many blood products.

*Packed red blood cells* are red blood cells from

which the serum has been removed. They are used when hemoglobin is needed for its oxygen-carrying capacity. This may be the case in instances of severe anemia or slow blood loss in which the fluid was replaced by the body but red blood cell production could not keep up the body's needs.

*Platelets* are administered when the recipient would benefit from their ability to initiate the clotting process. One unit of platelets is the equivalent of those found in one unit of whole blood.

*Human serum albumin* is the protein albumin that is produced by the body. It is given when the body is not adequately manufacturing its own albumin supplies. It also serves as a volume expander because the protein molecules will not pass through the capillary walls and thus increase the colloidal osmotic pressure of the blood. Albumin is commonly administered in bottles of 50 to 100 ml.

*Plasma* is the fluid part of the blood after the red blood cells have been removed by centrifuge. Plasma will store for a prolonged period of time and provides clotting factors, proteins, and fluid volume. It may be used when whole blood is not available in emergency situations and when there is no lack of red blood cells but rather a decrease in fluid volume.

*Plasma protein fraction* is the part of the plasma left after fibrinogen and globulin have been removed. It may be used to provide proteins for colloidal osmotic pressure.

## Adverse Reactions to the Administration of Blood or Blood Products

### Potassium Excess

Blood that has been stored is subject to red blood cell breakdown. As these cells are broken down, their potassium is released into the plasma. Old blood may have a very high potassium level. Although not a problem for a person with adequate kidney function, this circumstance may cause problems for people with kidney disorders and those already having difficulties with potassium balance. The adverse symptoms presented are the same as those of any potassium excess. If such symptoms appear, the transfusion ought to be stopped until the physician decides on a course of action. It may then be restarted slowly.

### Hypocalcemia

In rare instances, very rapid administration of citrated blood may cause a calcium deficit due to the ability of the citrate to combine with the serum calcium. If blood is given no faster than one unit in thirty minutes, this will not be a problem. More rapid administration is indicated only in severe hemorrhage. The symptoms are the same as those of ordinary hypocalcemia (discussed on page 419). Treatment is to administer intravenous calcium compounds; the administration of blood may be continued.

### Circulatory Overload

The administration of whole blood to a person who has an adequate volume of blood may overload the circulatory system. Because the blood contains proteins and cells, the fluid cannot be moved into the interstitial spaces with ease and will thus accumulate, especially in the lungs. Circulatory overload is also a hazard if the patient has an existing cardiac problem; in such cases, packed red blood cells are usually administered. If circulatory overload occurs, the transfusion is slowed.

### Serum Hepatitis

Serum hepatitis is a viral disease transmitted from an individual blood donor to the recipient. In order to guard against serum hepatitis, a careful history must be taken before accepting blood from a donor. However, people who have had undiagnosed hepatitis may not be screened out, and donors who are paid for their blood may deliberately give false histories. The disease may appear at any time from six weeks to six months after the transfusion. Consult a medical-surgical text for information on symptoms and care. Hepatitis may be transmitted by whole blood, packed red cells, and plasma.

## Pyrogenic Reactions

Pyrogenic reactions, which are characterized by a fever, chills, and headache, are relatively common in people who receive blood. Attributable to sensitivity to white cells or platelets in the blood, pyrogenic reactions become increasingly common the more transfusions the individual receives and usually occur after at least 250 ml of blood or blood product has been administered. The pyrogenic reaction may also be a result of contamination of the blood or equipment. If the reaction is due to bacterial contamination, the symptoms are much more severe and may include nausea, vomiting, and diarrhea. A shock reaction may occur with gram-negative bacterial contamination. If the pyrogenic reaction is mild, aspirin may be ordered and the transfusion continued by the physician. If severe, the transfusion is stopped.

## Hemolytic Reaction

Hemolytic reaction, the most serious of all adverse transfusion reactions, is caused by incompatibility of types of red cells. In a hemolytic reaction, red blood cells are rapidly *hemolyzed* (broken down) and the reaction is due to the effects of these products on the body. This type of reaction usually occurs within the time it takes to administer the first 100 ml of blood but may occur more quickly. Symptoms include flank pain (from the red blood cell breakdown products precipitating in the kidney), dark urine (from the excretion of the hemolyzed red blood cells), constriction in the chest (from the precipitation of hemolyzed red blood cells in the lungs), rapid respirations and rapid heart rate (due to stress and lack of oxygen), fever, and chills. Later jaundice will set in if a large quantity of blood has hemolyzed. Death may result from damage to the renal tubules. It is crucial that the blood be stopped immediately when a hemolytic reaction is suspected.

## Allergic Reactions

Allergic reactions may include outbreaks of hives, itching, and flushing. Respiratory allergic response, with shortness of breath and broncho-spasm, is rare. Symptoms may occur after 125 ml have been infused or even after the entire transfusion is completed. Antihistamines are given, and if the reaction is mild the blood may be continued by the physician. Severe reactions require that the blood be stopped; in some cases adrenocorticosteroids may also be given.

## Nursing Responsibilities

The nurse is responsible for the safe administration of blood and blood products. Most facilities have established precise routines to maximize safety.

## Identification of Patient and Blood

The blood bank identifies the blood by the name and number of the donor as well as the type of blood (A, B, AB, O, and Rh negative or Rh positive). When the patient's blood is typed and cross-matched in the laboratory for compatibility, a form is filled out and attached to the blood, giving the patient's name and blood type and indicating the number of the blood unit that has been crossmatched. Usually two nurses double-check the unit of blood and the identification of the recipient to make sure that the correct blood is given to the correct patient. Check the policy in your facility.

## Setting Up the Intravenous Line

When blood is to be administered, the intravenous is started with a large-diameter needle (usually a size 19) that will accommodate the viscous fluid. It is the policy in most facilities to set up the intravenous with a Y-type administration set using normal saline (0.9 percent), which allows for maintenance of an open intravenous line if the blood must be discontinued or stopped temporarily. Saline is used because it is less likely than a dextrose solution to cause coagulation problems in the line. In the event that any fluid from the line backs up into the blood container, saline would not cause problems, but dextrose might precipitate some hemolysis (red blood cell breakdown). A filter is always used on blood to screen out any precipitate. Calcium-containing solutions might clot and clog the tubing upon contact with the blood.

## Checking the Blood

The blood itself should be examined to be sure that nothing untoward has happened to it. If clotting is visible in the bag, the blood should not be administered.

## Baseline Assessment

The patient's vital signs should be taken immediately before the transfusion is started so as to provide a baseline in case any reaction occurs.

## Temperature of Blood

Blood is kept very cold in storage. Transfusion should be started within thirty minutes after removal from the refrigerator to decrease the possibility of breakdown. If it is to be warmed before administration, a blood warmer should be used; using warm water is too inexact and may result in damage to protein and cells in the blood. Ideally, the blood should be completely transfused within two hours to guard against deterioration as the blood hangs at room temperature.

## Rate of Administration

The first 50 to 100 ml are given very slowly; continuous observation of the patient is highly desirable during this time to identify a hemolytic reaction immediately if it occurs. One unit (500 ml) should not be given in less than thirty minutes unless severe blood loss has occurred. Blood should never be allowed to hang for more than four hours.

## Ongoing Assessment

The patient should be checked at frequent intervals for problems with the transfusion itself and for symptoms of the various transfusion reactions.

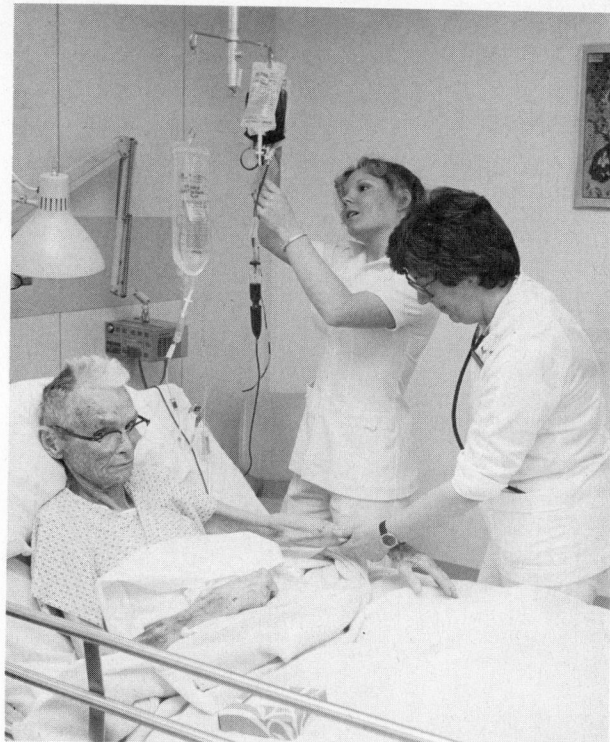

**Figure 24.21**
In most facilities, two nurses double-check the blood and the patient's identity before a transfusion is administered
(Russ Kinne/Danbury Hospital/Photo Researchers, Inc.)

The patient's subjective feelings should also be solicited. Many patients who experienced severe reactions have subsequently reported that the overt symptoms were preceded by feelings of anxiety and the sense that something bad was about to happen. Be careful, however, not to create anxiety.

## Response to Reaction

If a reaction occurs, it is usually appropriate to stop the transfusion, allow the saline to keep the infusion line open, and contact the physician. The physician might have been expecting a certain type of reaction and thus may have left orders for the transfusion to be continued at a slow rate and appropriate symptomatic treatment to be given. Under no circumstances should blood be discarded if a transfusion reaction is suspected. The laboratory will need the remaining blood for tests to determine the reason for the reaction.

# Conclusion

Because the circulatory system is very complex, circulatory assessment and intervention demand great depth of knowledge on the part of the nurse. The introductory material in this chapter should help you organize your thinking and actions. Alertness is crucial to identify impending problems before they become severe. The challenge is formidable.

## Care Study   A patient with electrolyte imbalance

Mrs. Eileen Merslake, R.N., the team leader, was at the desk when a nursing assistant approached her. "Mrs. Merslake, I just can't get Miss Stapleton to wake up enough to eat any lunch." Mrs. Merslake replied, "I'll go and check on her right away."

As Mrs. Merslake walked down the hall, she reviewed what she knew about Miss Stapleton, an eighty-two-year-old woman who lived independently in a large home. She had been admitted four days before with a diagnosis of congestive heart failure. Although Miss Stapleton had been very short of breath and fatigued upon admission, she had been completely alert and oriented. She had had severe fluid retention and had immediately been started on diuretics and medications for her heart. Mrs. Merslake remembered that the night nurse had commented in the morning report that Miss Stapleton had lost sixteen pounds in four days, her breathing was back to normal, and things were progressing well.

Mrs. Merslake found that it was almost impossible to rouse Miss Stapleton enough to speak. She seemed somewhat confused, could not grasp anything firmly, and was slumped in the armchair.

On the basis of all the information she had, Mrs. Merslake hypothesized that the patient might very well be suffering from a low potassium level.

The team leader was aware that she could ask for a blood chemistry to be run on a blood specimen that had already been drawn; the physician had ordered a fasting blood sugar measurement that morning. Mrs. Merslake placed a call to the doctor and asked the lab to run a potassium level. The lab called back with a report of a serum potassium level of 3.26 mEq/l. When the physician called back, she reported the patient's condition, reminding the physician of the medications being given, especially the diuretic, the fluid lost over the past four days, and the current laboratory report on potassium level.

The physician reduced Miss Stapleton's diuretic dosage by half and ordered an oral potassium supplement to be given immediately. Mrs. Merslake implemented these medical orders immediately. She also added this problem to the patient's nursing care plan and wrote nursing directives for observations to be made over the next forty-eight hours to evaluate the patient's response to the treatment.

## Study Terms

acid-base balance
acidity
acidosis
active transport
aldosterone
alkalinity
alkalosis
anion
antidiuretic hormone (ADH)
antigens
aorta
apex (of heart)
apical pulse
artery
ascites
atria
balanced solution
base (of heart)
base (pH)
blood pressure

bradycardia
buffer
capillary
cardiopulmonary resuscitation (CPR)
cation
central venous pressure (CVP)
circulatory overload
citrated
colloid
colloidal osmotic pressure (COP)
combining power
compensated
complete blood count (CBC)
cyanosis
Davenport Nomogram
diastolic
differential blood count

diffusion
edema
electrolyte
erythrocytes
external cardiac massage
extracellular fluid compartment
filtration
filtration pressure
fluid volume deficit
fluid volume excess
hematocrit
hemoglobin
hemolytic reaction
human serum albumin
hydrating solution
hypercalcemia
hyperkalemia
hypernatremia
hypertensive
hypertonic
hypocalcemia

hypokalemia
hyponatremia
hypotensive
hypotonic
interstitial fluid
intracellular fluid compartment
ion
isotonic
Korotkoff sound
leukocyte
mediastinum
membrane
metabolic acidosis
metabolic alkalosis
milliequivalent (mEq)
milliosmole (mOsm)
mouth-to-mouth resuscitation
orthopnea
osmolarity
osmosis
packed red blood cells

pallor
patency
pericardium
pH scale
pitting edema
plasma
platelets
postural hypotension
pulmonary edema
pulse
pulse deficit
pulse pressure
pulse rate
pulse rhythm
pulse strength
pyrogenic reaction

red blood cells (RBCs)
replacement solution
respiratory acidosis
respiratory alkalosis
serum hepatitis
systolic
tachycardia
tonicity
vein
ventricles
white blood cells
   (WBCs)
whole blood

## Learning Activities

1. Participate in a blood pressure screening clinic sponsored by an organization such as the Heart Association.

2. On a clinical unit, take and record the blood pressure of all patients. Using this list and the card index (Kardex), compare the blood pressures with the patients' ages and diagnoses. Talk with your instructor about how these relate.

3. Take your own pulse. Run in place or do some other physical activity for 5 minutes. Take your pulse again. Then take your pulse every 30 seconds and determine how quickly it returns to normal.

4. In your clinical group, discuss what occurred for each of you when doing Activity 3.

## Relevant Sections in
## Modules for Basic Nursing Skills

| Volume 1 | Module |
|---|---|
| Blood Pressure | 21 |
| Cardiopulmonary Resuscitation | 26 |

| Volume 2 | |
|---|---|
| Preparing and Maintaining Intravenous Infusions | 46 |
| Administering Intravenous Medications | 47 |
| Starting Intravenous Infusions | 48 |

## References

Anthony, C. P., and Kolthoff, N. J. *Textbook of Anatomy and Physiology*, 9th ed. St. Louis: C. V. Mosby, 1975.

Beaumont, E. "Product Survey: Blood Pressure Equipment." *Nursing '75* 5 (January 1975): 56–62.

Cohen, S. "Metabolic Acid-Base Disorders: Part 3, Clinical and Laboratory Findings." *American Journal of Nursing* 78 (March 1978): 1.

Gernert, C., and Swartz, S. "Pulmonary Artery Catheterization." *American Journal of Nursing* 73 (July 1973): 1182–1185.

*Guide to Fluid Therapy.* Deerfield, Ill.: Travenol Laboratories, 1973.

Hargest, T. S. "Start Your Count With Zero." *American Journal of Nursing* 74 (May 1974): 887–889.

Jarvis, C. M. "Vital Signs: How to Take Them More Accurately and Understand Them More Fully." *Nursing '76* 76 (April 1976): 31–37.

Jones, M. "Accuracy of Pulse Rate Counted for 15, 30, and 60 Seconds." Master's thesis, University of Washington, 1967.

Lee, C. A., *et al.* "Extracellular Volume Imbalance." *American Journal of Nursing* 74 (May 1974): 888.

Marcheondo, K. "CVP: The Whys and How of Central Venous Pressure Monitoring." *Nursing '74* 4 (January 1974): 21–24.

Metheny, N. M., and Snively, W. D. *The Nurses' Handbook of Fluid Balance,* 3rd ed. Philadelphia: J. B. Lippincott, 1979.

———. "Perioperative Fluids and Electrolytes." *American Journal of Nursing* 78 (May 1978): 840.

*Monitoring Fluids and Electrolytes Precisely.* Nursing '79 Skillbooks. Horsham, Pa.: Intermed Communications, 1979.

Shrake, Kevin. "The ABC's of ABG's." *Nursing '79* 9 (September 1979): 26–33.

Sparks, C. "Peripheral Pulses." *American Journal of Nursing* 75 (July 1975): 1132–1133.

"Standards for Cardio-Pulmonary Resuscitation (CPR) and Emergency Cardiac Care (ECC)." *Journal of the American Medical Association* 233 (August, 1980):32. Supplement.

Stright, P. A., and Soukup, S. M. "How to Hear It Right: Evaluating and Choosing a Stethoscope." *American Journal of Nursing* 77 (September 1977): 1477–1479.

Twombly, M. "The Shift Into Third Space." *Nursing '78* 8 (June 1978): 38.

# Chapter 25
# Neurological Function

## Objectives

After completing this chapter, you should be able to:

1. Briefly describe the four general parts of the nervous system.
2. Name two abnormal findings and two types of intervention for each of the eight areas of neurological assessment and intervention.
3. Discuss special nursing concerns in caring for the patient who is deaf or blind.
4. List special actions that must be added to routine care of the immobilized patient if the patient is also unconscious.
5. List the sequence of steps in emergency care of the patient undergoing a grand mal seizure.
6. Name the types of thermometers commonly in use.
7. Briefly discuss body temperature in relation to heat production and heat loss.
8. Discuss hypothermia and fever and the care of each.

## Outline

The nervous system is by far the most complex system of the body. Because of its complexity, we shall offer only brief descriptions of its anatomy and function, concentrating instead on assessment and intervention in neurological problems.

# The Nervous System

Anatomically, the nervous system can be subdivided into two large entities: the *central nervous system* (CNS) and the *peripheral nervous system* (PNS). The central nervous system is composed of the central organs for neurologic control—the brain and spinal cord—while the peripheral nervous system consists of all other structures and nerves. "The *brain* may be compared to a computer and its memory banks, the *spinal cord* to the conducting cable for the computer's input and output, and the *nerves* to a circuit supplying input information to the cable and transmitting the output to muscles and organs" (*New Columbia Encyclopedia*, 1975). See Figure 25.1.

## The Brain

The *brain*, the most vital and vulnerable of all the organs of the body, is encased in a bony structure called the *cranium*. The *cortex* of the brain is the thin outer gray-matter layer where reside awareness, cognition (thinking), and emotions. Other portions of the brain control and regulate vital functions, such as temperature, respiration, and heart action. The ability to move the body is controlled by the brain, as are the senses of sight, hearing, taste, touch, and smell.

## The Spinal Cord

The *spinal cord*, protected by the bony vertebrae that compose the spinal column, carries messages to and from the brain. It carries both *motor impulses*, having to do with movement, and *sensory impulses*, having to do with sensation.

## The Autonomic Nervous System

The *autonomic nervous system* is the involuntary part of our nervous system. We are not conscious of its functioning. Composed of *motor neurons* (nerve cells), it carries impulses from the central nervous system to the heart muscle and the smooth muscle of blood vessels and hollow organs, and also controls the secretions of glands.

The autonomic nervous system is further subdivided into two parts, the *sympathetic* and the *parasympathetic*. Distinguished only by function, the nerves of each part act in opposition to each other. For example, stimulation of the sympathetic branch increases the rate and strength of the heartbeat, while stimulation of the parasympathetic branch decreases both. Similarly, sympathetic stimulation of neurons to the stomach will decrease gastric secretions and parasympathetic stimulation will increase gastric secretions.

## Sensory Receptors

All over the body are millions of *sensory receptors*, which register sensations and elicit reflexes (involuntary responses to stimuli). Changes in the external and internal environment cause these receptors to "initiate the responses necessary for adjusting the body to these changes so as to maintain or restore homeostasis" (Anthony, 1978). See the discussion of homeostasis in Chapter 3. On a cold day, for example, the receptors in the skin register the sensation of coldness and send this message to the thalamus, a mass of gray matter in the inner portion of the brain, which interprets the sensation. By way of the motor neurons, a message is sent to the musculature and skin. The result is shivering, the body's attempt to generate heat.

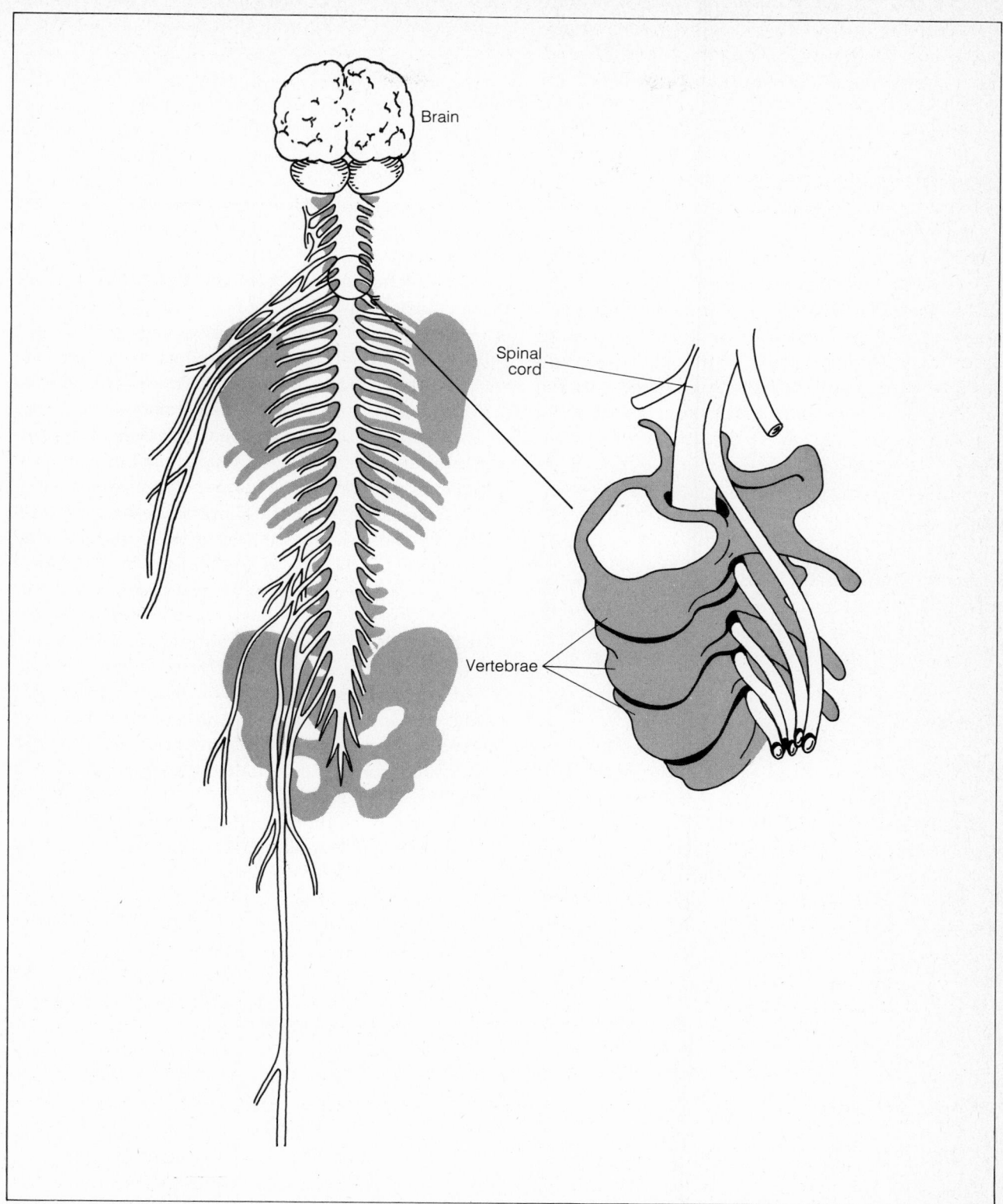

Brain

Spinal cord

Vertebrae

**Figure 25.1   The nervous system**

Reviewing the anatomy and physiology of the nervous system in an anatomy and physiology text will help you better understand the assessment, planning, intervention, and evaluation of the patient with neurological deficit.

# Common Neurological Problems

Let us examine the most common neurological deficits and the types of nursing intervention that are appropriate for each. In general, nursing actions for the patient with neurological problems have two purposes: to help the patient compensate for the loss or deficit and to provide safety for the patient.

## Mentation

*Mentation*, sometimes called "cognition," is the ability to think. Mentation includes memory, both recent and distant, and emotions. The normal person should be oriented and alert to the environment.

## Assessment

By means of a brief interview, the nurse can determine whether the patient is oriented on three points: person (who he or she is), place (where he or she is), and time (the general time of day, month, and year). It is important to verify how confused a patient is by testing for this information. For example, a patient may know his name and where he is but have no idea of the year; any variation is possible in a confused state. You must be cautious when gathering such information, for assertions that sound confused may not be so. For example, an elderly patient in an acute-care facility stated that she was dictating a book about Indians in Montana. Though she was severely handicapped and had come to the facility from a nursing home where she had resided for some time, she had indeed been writing such a book. Another patient stated that he had walked to a town 50 miles away the night before, when the nurses knew he had been in bed: this was clear evidence of confusion. When recording this information, the notation "Oriented x3" means that the patient is oriented in all three spheres.

The patient may have visual, auditory, or olfactory *hallucinations*, or perceptions of sights, sounds, or smells that are not present. *Illusions* are misinterpretations of real sights, sounds, or smells, such as perceiving a shadow on the wall as a cat. *Delusions* are faulty thinking patterns, exemplified by the patient who thinks he is the mayor of the city.

## Intervention

Patients who are confused or disoriented tend to make us uncomfortable; in our everyday lives, we expect people to react to us in rational ways. Nursing intervention should include neither arguing nor agreeing with confused perceptions. Identifying people in the immediate environment, naming the location and time, and explaining unfamiliar objects in the environment all help orient the patient. Your mode of orientation should depend on the specific areas of disorientation the patient displays. If the patient is not fearful, a gentle touch is a very effective way of communicating caring. Distraught and confused patients usually react positively to a quiet, confident attitude on the part of the nurse.

Some patients recognize and acknowledge their confusion and are quite upset by it. Telling such patients that you can appreciate how upsetting their confusion must be and assuring them that the confusion is due to their illness elicits a sense of relief in many. It is important to note that we are not considering the severely disturbed psychiatric patient here; the care of such patients requires special knowledge and training.

## Table 25.1
## Levels of Awareness

| Level | Behavior | Responsiveness |
|---|---|---|
| 1. Consciousness | Awake, alert, able to talk | Responsive to all verbal, visual, tactile, and auditory stimuli |
| 2. Lethargy or somnolence | Very sleepy or asleep; able to verbalize when awake | Can be awakened by and will respond appropriately to normal stimuli |
| 3. Stupor | Very sleepy, may fall asleep in the middle of a conversation; able to verbalize when awake | Can be aroused with concerted effort, which may have to be physical as well as verbal; constant input needed to stay awake |
| 4. Light coma or semicoma | No longer responsive to verbal stimuli, difficult to arouse; some spontaneous movement; restlessness in response to discomfort | Responsive to bright lights, light pin prick, discomfort, physical movement |
| 5. Deep coma | Totally unresponsive, many protective reflexes lost; if decerebrate, may emit high-pitched cry, assume opisthotonos position, exhibit disturbance of vital signs | May respond to severely painful stimuli |

## Levels of Awareness

*Levels of awareness* are associated with mentation, but there may be a considerable discrepancy. That is, a patient can be alert and interested in the surroundings, responsive to interpersonal relationships, and yet disoriented. For example, a patient may sit in the dayroom and play cards skillfully and animatedly, all the while recounting numerous telephone calls from the president requesting help with international affairs. Such a patient's level of awareness is considered normal, though he or she is obviously disoriented.

## Assessment

There are generally agreed to be five levels of awareness (see Table 25.1). At the *conscious* level, one is awake, alert, able to talk, and responsive to all appropriate verbal, visual, tactile, and auditory stimuli.

The second level of awareness is *lethargy* or *somnolence*. The person is sleepy and appears to be dozing much of the time. If genuinely asleep, the person can be awakened by normal stimuli and will respond appropriately. The lethargic person will not respond with enhanced awareness to such stimuli.

At the third level, *stupor*, the person is so sleepy that continual, concerted input is necessary to maintain wakefulness. The person's conversation may be confused or unclear.

At the fourth level of consciousness, *light coma* or *semicoma*, the patient no longer responds to verbal stimuli but may move spontaneously in response to physical stimuli. A light pin prick will elicit a reflex movement, and most of the body's reflexes are still present. The nurse may notice restlessness in response to discomfort such as hunger or wetness of the bed.

In *deep coma*, the fifth level, the patient is totally unresponsive to any stimuli except severe pain. There is no voluntary movement and many of the protective reflexes, such as gagging, blinking, and coughing, may be lost. The very seriously ill patient in deep coma may progress to a state of *decerebration*, which is partial or total interruption of the connection between the spinal tracts and the brain. The cerebellum has been isolated; thus, although vital function may continue, the person may have fluctuating vital signs. The patient often emits a high-pitched involuntary cry and may assume a backward, flexed, bridgelike position of the body called *opisthotonos* position.

## Intervention

As a patient becomes less alert, it is the function of the nurse to provide a safe environment—that is, to take precautions the patient would take on his or her own behalf, if able. Such measures include siderails, protection against exposure to dangerous temperatures, and many other actions that will be discussed throughout this chapter.

## Coordination

*Coordination*—the ability to move the extremities and body parts voluntarily in a balanced and effective manner—is disturbed in a variety of neurological conditions. Lack of coordination may be limited to a single extremity, such as an arm that moves randomly or fingers unable to grasp objects. It may also be generalized, as in the case of a person severely handicapped due to cerebral palsy.

## Assessment

Gross incoordination is often easily assessed by observing how the patient walks, which is known as *gait*. Is it steady and confident? Does the patient lurch? Does he or she reach out for the wall or furniture for support? Difficulty with gait is called *ataxia*. A more subtle sign might be difficulty locating the mouth with the toothbrush in oral self-care. *Tremors*—involuntary shaking of a body part, an extremity, or the head—sometimes contribute to the coordination problem. Tremors are most

common in the hands but may also afflict the knees and feet.

Difficulty with coordination has a variety of possible components, including lack of balance, dizziness, and impaired proprioception. *Proprioception* is the ability to discern the location of one's body parts. For example, people with disturbances of proprioception may not know the position of their feet if they close their eyes or are in the dark.

## Intervention

Although you can do little about the underlying causes of incoordination, you can help the patient accommodate. Caution the patient to ring for assistance when he or she wants to get out of bed or to ambulate. Encourage the patient to move slowly, and plan ahead on how you might help. Assistive devices, though designed primarily for the patient with weakness in the legs, can also provide security to the uncoordinated patient. A cane or even a walker steadies the gait. See Module 16, "Ambulation."

The patient whose hand coordination is impaired can use large-handled utensils and large mugs (see Figure 25.2). Always make sure hot liquids are kept at a safe distance so they cannot be spilled by involuntary movements. Smoking may have to be monitored for the sake of safety.

Some patients are embarrassed about their neurological deficits, referring to themselves as "walk-

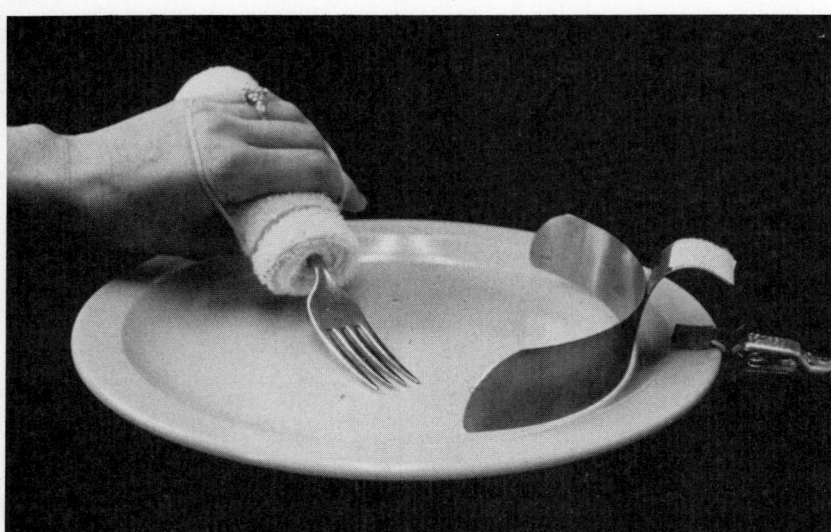

**Figure 25.2  Feeding utensil for the neurologically handicapped**
Florence E. Smith

ing like a drunk" or apologizing for their messiness at the table. You can help by offering encouragement, understanding, and a sense of humor.

## Muscular Weakness

Muscular weakness, which can afflict any of the skeletal muscles of the body, occurs because nerve innervation (stimulus) to a particular muscle or group of muscles has been partially interrupted. This condition, known as *paresis*, often accompanies incoordination. With decreased use, the muscle itself may *atrophy*, becoming smaller in bulk and size. Muscle weakness is not true paralysis.

### Assessment

Some muscle weakness can be assessed by observation. Does the patient drag one leg? Is there drooping of the eyelids (ptosis) or drooling at the mouth? Weakness can also be identified by means of simple testing. Ask the patient to grip both your hands and squeeze. Is the grip equal on both sides, allowing for handedness, or is one side much weaker than the other? You can test the shoulders and legs by asking the patient to push against your resistance.

### Intervention

The primary purpose of intervention is to maintain maximum muscle strength. This objective might be pursued by means of R.O.M. (range-of-motion) exercises, independent movement, and/or ambulation. See Module 14, "Range-of-Motion Exercises." Braces, canes, walkers, and crutches can facilitate movement and thus prevent unnecessary atrophy. Continue to offer the patient encouragement and realistic hope—not for complete return of function, perhaps, but for maintenance of whatever function is present.

## Sensation

The millions of sensory receptors all over the external surface of the body and in mucous mem-

brane are highly sensitive to changes in the environment. As we have described, these receptors send messages to the central nervous system, which stimulates a response or adjustment by way of the thalamus. If, for example, the fingers should touch a hot kettle, they are immediately drawn away.

Several diseases disturb sensory perception because they cause damage to the nerve endings. Among these diseases are diabetes, alcoholism, and multiple sclerosis. Because such disturbances follow the irregular distribution of nerves normal to the body, the affected areas are often uneven or patchy.

### Assessment

Disturbances in sensation most often afflict the extremities but may also involve the face or trunk. Asking the patient to describe the disorder is helpful in assessment. You should know the following terms. *Paresthesia* is distorted skin sensation, such as itching, tingling, crawling, or prickling. This term has also been used to describe a decrease in sensation, but a more accurate term for the latter is *hypesthesia*. *Hyperesthesia* is increased sensation. Decreased perception of pain is called *hypalgesia*; heightened perception of pain is *hyperalgesia*. In *astereognosis*, a less common sensory deficit, the patient cannot identify simple small objects by touch alone. For example, the patient may not be able to tell the difference between a safety pin and a quarter without looking.

Although the physician uses a variety of techniques to test sensory integrity, the best data may be the patient's subjective description.

### Intervention

Intervention for sensory loss focuses on protecting the area or extremity from injury and/or discomfort. A patient who cannot perceive high temperature or pain in a particular body part should not be exposed to heat or sharp objects of any kind. If an arm is involved, for example, injections should not be given there: a resulting reaction or inflammation could escape detection until much later due to decreased sensation.

## Paralysis

*Paralysis* is inability to move a body part voluntarily. The most common causes of paralysis are cerebral vascular accident (stroke) and trauma (injury). It is very important for nurses to understand that paralysis may or may not involve a disturbance in sensation. A paralyzed arm, for example, may have no sensation, normal levels of sensation, or hyperesthesia (increased sensation). Some patients experience pain in a paralyzed extremity.

*Hemiplegia* is paralysis of one side of the body. *Paraplegia* is paralysis of the lower part of the body. *Quadriplegia* is paralysis of all four extremities.

### Assessment

Paralysis is usually readily apparent. One side of the face may droop. The extremities may be flaccid and unable to move. Keep in mind that paralysis may not be complete. For example, the fingers may be capable of slight movement although the arm is paralyzed. The patient may be able to lift a paralyzed arm with the unaffected hand or to grasp a partially paralyzed leg and pull it forward.

### Intervention

Great care should be taken to protect a paralyzed part from injury. Never grasp and lift a patient under the axilla of a paralyzed arm since the shoulder could become dislocated (subluxation). If the patient is in a wheelchair, be sure that no part of the body is in a position to be caught. A foot can be twisted under the chair as it moves forward; fingers can become entangled in the wheel of the chair as it is moved. Patients can be positioned in bed on the paralyzed side if proper alignment is maintained with no twisting of or pressure on the extremities. Injections should be administered in the unaffected side for the same reasons as in cases of sensory deficit. Heat and sharp objects should be kept away from paralyzed body areas. Edema may occur if paralyzed extremities are allowed to hang in a lowered position for long periods. Slings can be used to keep the arms nearer the level of the heart, and footrests and footstools help keep feet in a less dependent position. Braces and walking devices may make ambulation possible. Muscle bulk can be maintained with regular R.O.M. exercises.

Paralysis distorts body image and is usually very difficult for the patient psychologically. Emphasizing the patient's strengths rather than weaknesses is a valuable aspect of nursing care.

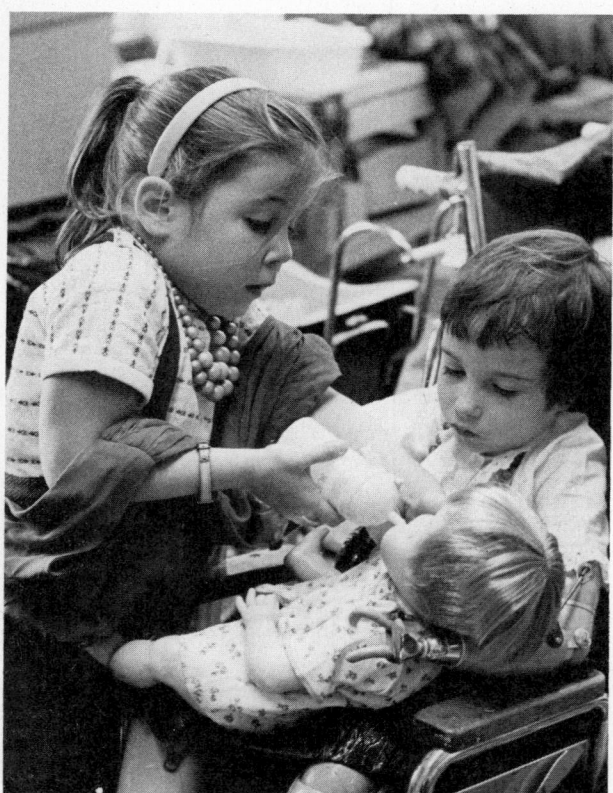

**Figure 25.3  Handicapped children having fun**
Hella Hamid/Photo Researchers, Inc.

### Dysphagia

*Dysphagia* is inability to swallow, usually due to partial paralysis of the esophagus. The patient with dysphagia may choke on fluids or food, aspirating the particles into the bronchi or lungs. The resulting irritation and partial obstruction can lead to an infection called aspiration pneumonia, a serious condition that can be fatal.

## Assessment

Careful assessment is called for when a patient reports any degree of difficulty swallowing. A sip of sterile water is an appropriate first step, since it will be less injurious than any other fluid if aspirated. Some patients can swallow solid substances easier than clear fluids, while others find thin liquids most acceptable. When testing, place the patient in high Fowler's position so that gravity flow can facilitate swallowing.

## Intervention

Choosing foods the patient can manage and positioning the patient in the sitting position both help swallowing. Encourage small bites and portions, and observe the patient carefully. If the patient is totally unable to take nutrients, a nasogastric or enteral tube may have to be passed for the purpose of feeding.

Fear of choking is likely to be prominent, and dysphagic patients need psychological support.

## Aphasia and Dysphasia

*Aphasia* literally means the absence of speech. The term is often used in practice to describe patients with disturbed speech, who should more accurately be called *dysphasic*.

Aphasia is a complicated phenomenon. It involves difficulty in using language, resulting from a disturbance in the speech center of the brain. *Sensory aphasia*, or receptive aphasia, is inability to receive and understand what others are saying. The person with *motor aphasia*, or expressive aphasia, is unable to form words. The severely disabled patient may have components of both conditions. Some patients can form certain words but use them inappropriately. Such a patient may, for example, recognize a television set but call it a chair. Some aphasic patients also lose the ability to recognize symbols and thus cannot interpret writing. They may or may not recognize photographs and other pictures. For example, the patient mentioned above may recognize a television set but not a picture of a television set.

## Table 25.2
## Neurological Assessment

| | Normal | Abnormal |
|---|---|---|
| **Mentation** | Alert, aware of surroundings; oriented to person, place, and time | Any disorientation, including confusion, hallucinations, illusions, or delusions |
| **Levels of awareness** | Alert and responsive to the environment | Any alteration in level of awareness; lethargy, stupor, semicoma, or deep coma |
| **Coordination** | Hand and finger movement and ambulation free of unsteadiness or tremor | Difficulty using hands or fingers, such as to hold objects; unsteady gait; tremor |
| **Muscular weakness** | Strong, equal grip; legs able to support weight; face symmetrical | Weak grip, difficulty elevating legs, drooping eyelids or drooling mouth |
| **Sensation** | Appropriately sensitive to all sensory stimulation | Distorted, increased, or decreased sensation, including pain |
| **Paralysis** | No evidence of paralysis; able to move all musculature normally | Unable to move one or more extremities or any other muscular area voluntarily |
| **Dysphagia** | Able to swallow solid foods, liquids, and saliva without difficulty | Unable to swallow solid food and/or liquids without choking |
| **Dysphasia** | Speaks clearly and understandably | Unable to speak and/or understand words; may be unable to interpret symbols. |

## Assessment

Because the patient may have a combination of any of the conditions described above, it is especially valuable for a speech therapist to make the assessment. Nursing intervention can then be tai-

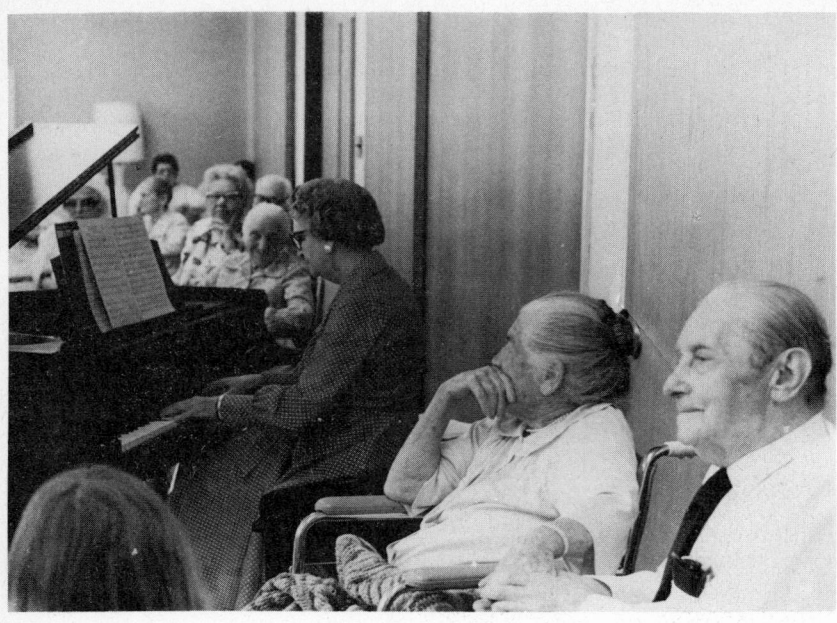

**Figure 25.4 Music therapy for aphasic patients**
Shirley Zeiberg/Taurus Photos

lored more closely to the patient's individual needs.

## Intervention

The patient who suddenly loses the ability to speak understandably becomes agitated, frustrated, and eventually very depressed over the inability to communicate. Such patients seem to respond well to a quiet, organized environment, devoid of confusion. Music can be very therapeutic, since it can be enjoyed without words. Most aphasic patients can hear normally, and shouting is not only unnecessary but upsetting. Unfortunately, some nurses assume that a patient who cannot speak also cannot hear.

Establishing some form of communication is essential to care. You should use whatever works best for the individual patient. If the patient understands simple words, use them; more complex sentences may only confuse the patient. Maintain eye contact and speak slowly and distinctly. If the patient understands symbols, you could make a simple symbol board with pictures of care items and other pertinent objects. If the patient can write, a magic slate or paper and pencil can provide for another type of communication.

The aphasic or dysphasic patient is often seen by a speech therapist for evaluation and treatment. If a patient of yours is in such a program, make it a point to become knowledgeable about the therapy. Consult with the therapist and find out how you can help the patient relearn speech.

## Special Senses

The special senses are hearing, vision, taste, smell, and touch. Loss of any of these senses is accompanied by a disturbance in body image. See Chapter 29, "Disturbances of Body Image Integrity." Loss of acuity in taste, smell, and touch can be

quite disturbing to patients; such a loss is often partial, however, and can be adjusted to gradually. This chapter will deal separately with deafness and blindness, which interfere so directly with the person's interaction with others and the environment. Sudden loss of hearing or sight can lead to deep depression, requiring the ultimate in sensitivity on the part of the nurse.

## Deafness

The patient may only have diminished hearing on one side. The older patient usually has hearing loss bilaterally (both sides), but one side will be better than the other. Hearing loss affects all ages, from the newborn (caused by congenital abnormality), through childhood (usually infections involving the ear) and on into later life (a result of nerve changes), when hearing loss occurs more frequently than blindness.

## Assessment

The patient is aware of such loss and will tell you often how you can be of assistance. "Could you please speak louder? I don't hear well," is a common response. The totally deaf patient may have learned to lip-read. Deafness may be accompanied by muteness, which is not the same thing as aphasia: completely deaf people who have never heard a human voice, including their own, have great difficulty learning speech, which ordinarily involves imitation of others' speech. Special teaching can enable many such people to acquire speech. Many deaf people communicate by means of *signing*—visual language that uses the positions of the hands and fingers to denote letters, words, and phrases.

## Intervention

There are several things to keep in mind when caring for a patient with a hearing deficit. When entering the patient's room, come into the patient's line of sight right away so he or she knows you are there and can identify you. If the patient has some hearing in one ear, stand on that side when speaking. With patients who lip-read, stand or sit directly in front of the patient and speak distinctly but normally. Electronic sound-amplification instruments enable some patients to hear better (see Figure 25.5). Write down important communications so they will not be misunderstood. Most large facilities have staff members who know signing and will be glad to help you communicate with the deaf. If there is no such person on staff, a call to the local organization for the deaf will locate a resource person. Sign lan-

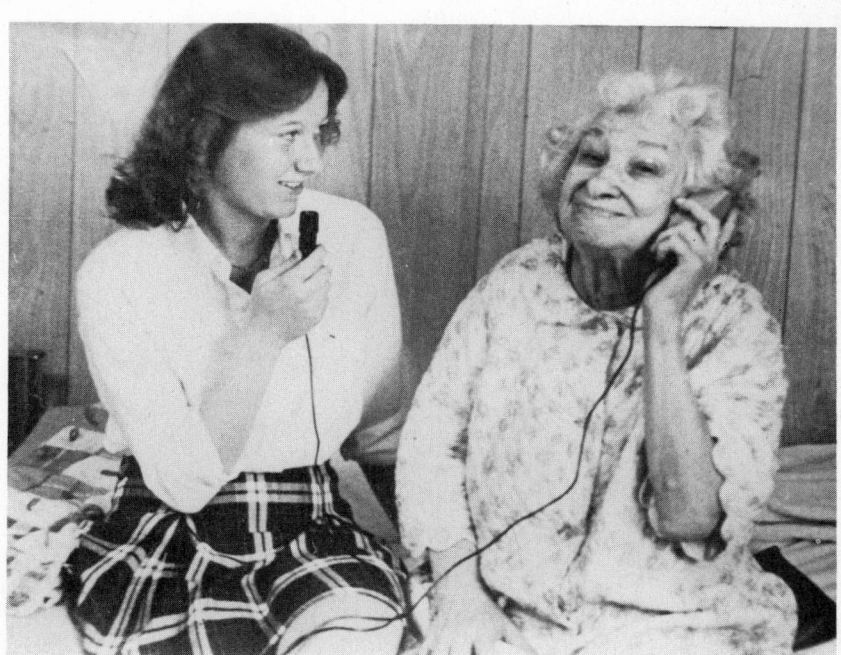

**Figure 25.5  A device used for sound amplification**
Photo courtesy of One to One Communications, Olathe, Kansas, and Eastern Kansas Register, Kansas City, Kansas

guages vary, and more than one method may be used in your area.

Safety is also a matter of particular concern since deaf people cannot hear alarms or verbal warnings. Fire alarm systems that employ bright lights instead of aural alarms are available for use in the home. There are also new but costly telephone systems equipped with a printed message device and a light in place of the ring.

## Blindness

No one who is sighted can truly understand what it means to lose one's sight—the familiar environment becomes unfamiliar and frightening, and one can no longer see the facial expressions of the people one loves. People who were born blind appear to function very well using their other senses to compensate. For those who have always relied on their sight, the adjustment to blindness can be extremely difficult.

Blindness may be total or partial. Some partially blind people retain their peripheral vision, which means they can see the area surrounding where they are gazing but not the center. Other patients lose their peripheral vision but retain central vision. Still others may be able to discern general shapes and light and dark areas but no details.

## Assessment

Visual assessment is performed by professionals with special training in the use of sophisticated instruments. Visually impaired patients can usually describe their disabilities and tell you how you can be of help.

## Intervention

Though the needs of sightless patients differ, there are several things you should always do when giving care to the blind. On entering the room, immediately identify yourself. This lets the patient know who is about and gives a sense of security. Most blind people welcome touch, and grasping the patient's hand or touching the shoulder is comforting. When an ambulatory blind patient is first admitted, orient him or her to the room by explaining where the furniture and bathroom facilities are located while at the same time helping the patient locate each object by touch. Do not rearrange the furniture, and arrange food items the same way on the tray at each meal. You might help the patient make selections from the menu, since it is usually printed.

Safety must be considered when a blind person is hospitalized. Hot liquids should be set safely

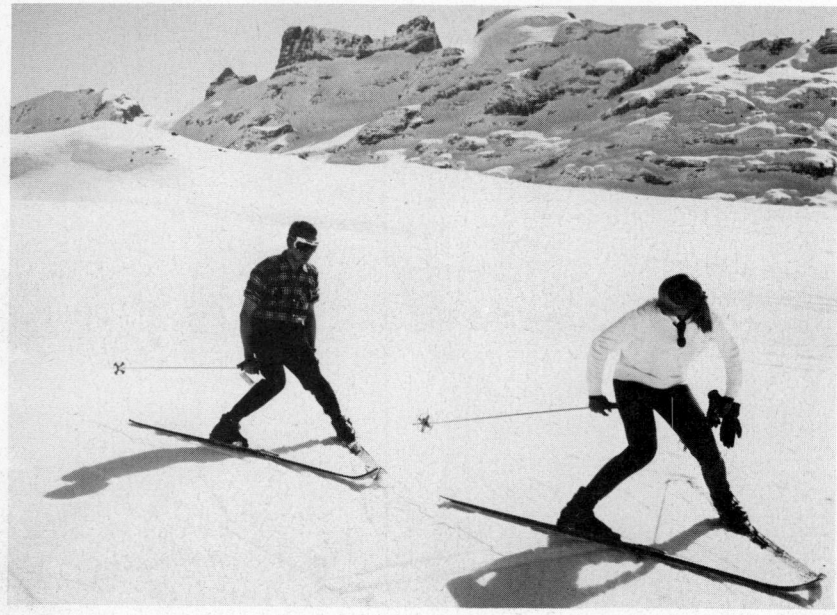

**Figure 25.6**
A blind skier enjoys the slopes with the help of a coach. (Lily Solmssen/Photo Researchers, Inc.)

aside until the patient is ready to drink them. Smoking may have to be monitored. Encourage the patient to ask for assistance when getting out of bed and ambulating.

The blind person is sensorially deprived. Music may be a valued diversion. If the patient reads Braille, many publications can be obtained. The Library of Congress has an excellent program for the sightless, providing the Bible, books, magazines, recipes, and instructional materials on tape or cassette free of charge; the tape and recording equipment is also provided at no cost. A blind person can also request that any material not already available be recorded on tape or record. Regional counseling services for the blind provide a variety of services, including special thermostats, dialing discs, and many other devices for use in the home.

The advent of blindness can be frightening and isolating. It is a time for family and friends to move close to the patient psychologically. The nurse can offer encouragement, caring, and support for the maintenance of maximum independence.

## The Patient With an Altered Level of Awareness

The somnolent, unconscious, or comatose patient requires special skills of assessment and intervention on the part of the nurse. The nurse must not only constantly assess the patient's level of awareness but also attempt to adjust to, supplement, and replace deficiencies that develop in any system of the body. Providing for safety is also essential.

### Assessment

As the patient's level of consciousness changes, you can determine what stimuli he or she responds to and what he or she is aware of. It is much more helpful to be specific than simply to use, for example, the word *stupor*, which may mean different things to different nurses and may prove insufficiently accurate.

Making the assessment as specific as possible renders changes in status more noticeable. For example, if a patient who did not previously appear aware of the lowering of a siderail begins to roll about when the rail is let down, this might indicate that the patient's level of awareness has risen and therefore might be regarded as a sign of improvement.

Specific testing is required, using various methods, to determine whether an unconscious patient's level of awareness is changing. One technique is to observe the patient for signs of awareness of nearby voices or noise. The patient may, for example, grimace or move about in bed. Calling the patient's name to see if he or she responds is referred to as *name-call* and charted as such. A bit more sophisticated is the *command*: instruct the patient to do something, such as to "move your left leg" or "squeeze my hand," and observe the response. The only requirement is to command something the patient is reasonably capable of carrying out. Neurologically, one step beyond response to a command is *verbalization*. Depending on the patient's visual acuity, you might ask what color the ceiling or a bright cup is.

Neurological signs or *neuro signs* are a set of brief tests of neurological status, usually performed to identify changes of status. Although there is some variation among facilities, neuro signs usually include (1) pulse, respiration, and blood pressure; (2) checking level of awareness; and (3) checking pupillary response to light (see Module 32, "Inspection, Palpation, Auscultation, and Percussion").

### Intervention

All the nursing actions directed toward care of the immobilized patient apply to the care of the unconscious patient (see Chapter 19). Most body systems, however, also require special attention. The critically ill unstable patient will probably be in the

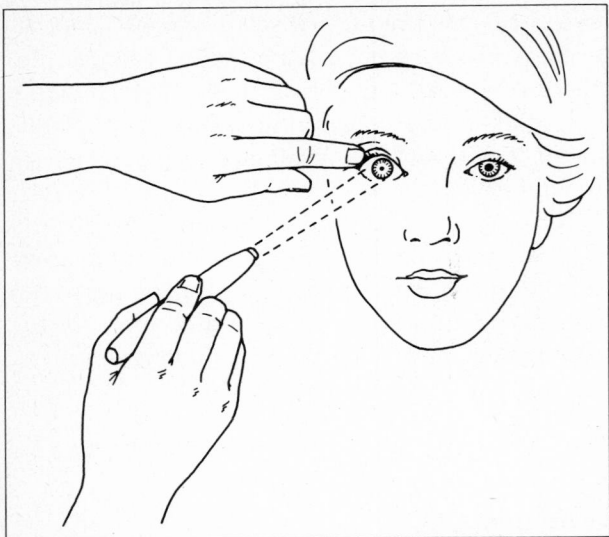

**Figure 25.7  Testing the pupillary reaction to light**
The light source is brought in from the side.

critical-care unit. As a nurse on a general unit or in a long-term care facility, however, you may care for a long-term comatose or unconscious patient.

Maintaining the patient's respiratory function is of primary importance. You must constantly assess for a patent (open) airway. Keep the patient's head to the side so that secretions can drain and, if vomiting should occur, vomitus will not be aspirated. Most unconscious patients can safely be placed in high position and turned from side to side, as well as placed prone, if done with utmost care. Change of position helps move secretions. The unconscious patient may have to be suctioned, since the cough reflex may be absent. If a tracheostomy has been performed, tracheostomy suctioning and care will be necessary (see Chapter 23, "Oxygenation," and Module 42, "Tracheostomy Suctioning and Care").

Oral care must be done carefully. Examine the mouth for loose teeth and be sure all equipment used is lint-free. Use oral-care equipment and solutions in such a way that the airway remains unobstructed at all times. Since unconscious patients frequently mouth-breathe, frequent oral care is called for.

Optimum nutrition provides the patient the best prospects for recovery. Since the patient cannot voluntarily ingest food, a nasogastric tube can be introduced for the instillation of tube feedings. Enteral feedings provide the patient a very nutritional solution through a small tube passed through the nose and directly into the jejunum. If the intestinal tract cannot absorb nutrients effectively, nutrition by hyperalimentation can be initiated (see Chapter 21).

Skin integrity and musculoskeletal maintenance are essential to keep the patient free of deformity. To some extent, circulation is always compromised in the comatose patient. Any pressure may cause the beginning of a pressure sore. Because the patient cannot report discomfort, you must be aware of positions that may cause undue pressure and change the patient's position completely at least every two hours. A nerve palsy (partial paralysis) could develop if a patient is allowed to lie on an arm or hand. Check every position change critically for body alignment. Use trochanter and hand rolls to prevent contracture (see Figure 25.8 and Module 12, "Moving the Patient in Bed and Positioning"). Frequent massage stimulates circulation and prevents skin breakdown. Monitor water temperatures closely to prevent burning. The use of heat lamps is discouraged for reasons of safety. Range-of-motion exercises are essential to maintain joint mobility in a patient who cannot move voluntarily.

Urinary incontinence is cared for by padding the bed and being conscientious about cleanliness. Some physicians regard use of the catheter as a safety threat because of the likelihood of infection; others may order a catheter to be inserted. Good perineal and catheter care help prevent infection. Monitoring output is crucial. To maintain bladder tone in a patient with a long-term catheter, a clamp-unclamp routine is sometimes used (see Chapter 22). This procedure is controversial since it is possible to forget to unclamp the catheter at the prescribed period (usually every two hours), causing damage to the bladder and/or sphincter. If this technique is used, a large sign should be placed over the bed to alert the nurse to adhere to the schedule.

Intestinal (bowel) incontinence also requires extreme cleanliness for esthetic reasons and to prevent infection.

All unconscious patients need ear care. Wax and foreign bodies should be removed in order to prevent inflammation. If the patient has suffered a head injury, inspect for the emission of blood or spinal fluid and report either to the physician immediately.

Eye care is needed to prevent permanent dam-

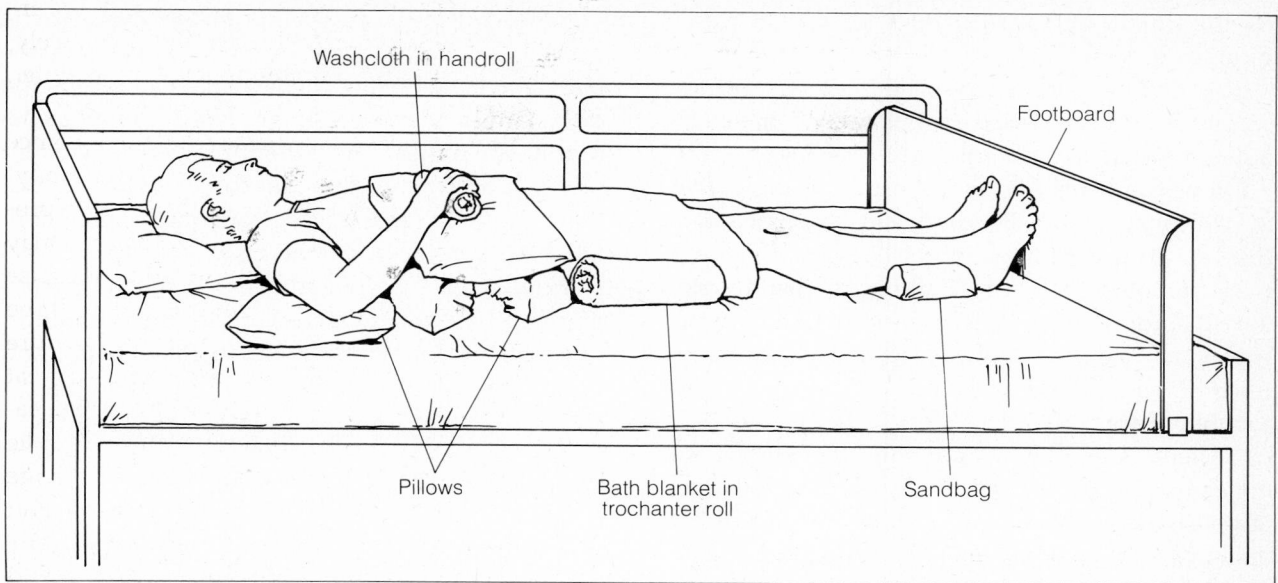

Washcloth in handroll

Footboard

Pillows

Bath blanket in
trochanter roll

Sandbag

**Figure 25.8  Positioning aids for the unconscious patient**

age. Contact lenses should be removed (for specific techniques, see Chapter 18, "Hygiene"). They should be carefully stored or given to the family along with other valuables. If the eyes of unconscious patients remain open, the corneas dry and ulceration can occur. The lids can be kept closed with eye patches; if patches are used, daily inspection is essential to detect any inflammation or infection. Sterile water can be administered as an eye wash. Eye drops are sometimes prescribed by the physician.

Patients in light coma can experience pain, which may be indicated by grimacing, restlessness, and/or moaning. Repositioning or adjustment of dressings, binders, or appliances may make the patient more comfortable. Pain medications should be used sparingly since they depress the central nervous system and may compromise respiration.

Sparks around oxygen, sharp objects, and unsafe temperatures are safety hazards to helpless patients. Siderails should always be raised when the patient is left alone, even for a few moments. Changes in level of awareness sometimes occur swiftly, and a quiet patient can become suddenly agitated and fall from bed.

Even comatose patients benefit from psychological care. Patients who appeared to be in deep coma have, upon recovery, reported hearing people and sounds. Hearing remains intact even when other senses are absent. The patient's level of awareness may be improved by the stimulation of familiar voices and sounds. Encourage the family and others close to the patient to visit and talk to the patient. Play music the patient has been known to enjoy. As you care for the patient, explain what you are going to do as if the patient were responsive. Converse with the patient. The nurse and others should remember not to say anything within earshot that could be disturbing or undermine the patient's dignity.

## The Patient With Seizures

A hospitalized patient who has never had a seizure may suddenly experience a convulsion. Or a patient who is known to be subject to seizures may be admitted for another cause. In any event, it is essential that nurses be knowledgeable about the care of a patient with a seizure. For information on the causes of seizures, refer to a medical-surgical text.

It is a myth that persons who have seizures are retarded. Some retarded individuals do have seizures, but seizures do not cause retardation. Convulsions can be caused by head injury, high fever in children, metabolic disorders, alcohol withdrawal, drug withdrawal, brain hemorrhage, and overwhelming infection. *Epilepsy,* a distinct seizure disorder, is generally well controlled with the use of new anticonvulsant drugs, and it is now uncommon to witness a seizure on the street or in a public place.

Society is finally abandoning the stigma on epilepsy. Until very recently, several states had laws that epileptics could not marry. There are epileptics in all walks of life, functioning completely normally. Nurses should encourage total social acceptance of people with seizure disorders.

## Types of Seizures

There are four types of seizures. *Simple partial seizures* involve only certain parts of the body. The person does not ordinarily lose consciousness. Movements may begin in a limited area, such as the upper arm, and proceed to other extremities. *Complex partial seizures* involve repetitious activities that appear purposeful. *Petit mal* or *absence seizures* are short lapses of awareness, during which the person does not usually fall to the ground. The seizure often consists of only a momentary interruption in activity or conversation, hardly noticeable to the observer. A *convulsive* or *grand mal seizure* is by far the most serious, since it involves unconsciousness.

## Phases of a Grand Mal Seizure

Grand mal seizures have several phases. It is important for nurses to be familiar with these phases so that we can describe them accurately. Accurate description is sometimes critical to diagnosis.

An *aura* is an awareness on the part of the patient that a seizure may occur. Auras vary: some people report only a feeling of apprehension; others see flashing lights or notice a numbness of the face. During the second phase, *relaxation*, the patient experiences subjective weakness before losing consciousness and falling to the ground. The *tonic* stage, which involves rigid stiffening of the body and clenching of the jaws, is followed by the *clonic* stage, characterized by jerking movements of the extremities. The patient may be incontinent of urine and may chew the tongue, causing lacerations. Most seizures last from one to three minutes and subside spontaneously. During the final *postictal* stage, movements cease and the person gradually regains awareness of the surroundings. The patient does not remember the seizure, and confusion and drowsiness may be present.

## Immediate Care of the Patient

The goal of care is the patient's safety. Thus it is important to know ahead of time what actions should be taken. Guidelines for care of the seizure victim follow:

1. Establish an open airway and prevent injury to the tongue. If the teeth are already clenched, do not try to pry the mouth open; doing so may loosen teeth. If the mouth can be easily opened, place something soft between the teeth to keep the tongue from being chewed. A clean handkerchief or gauze, twisted like a rope, is best. Avoid plastic objects or even tongue depressors, which have been known to be shattered or chewed and to obstruct the patient's airway.
2. Place something soft under the patient's head to absorb the impact of its backward thrust onto a hard surface. A pillow or coat serves the purpose. Pad or lower siderails.
3. Turn the patient's head to one side to prevent secretions and vomitus from being aspirated.
4. Loosen the patient's clothing so breathing is not restricted.
5. Never attempt to restrain the patient. Dislocations and fractures have resulted from this practice. Instead, remove potentially injurious objects.
6. Stay with and reassure the patient throughout the episode.
7. When the postictal stage begins, turn the patient on one side and allow to rest.

## Seizure Observations

Although we now have very sophisticated instruments, such as the *CAT (computerized axial tomo-*

*gram) scanner*, capable of definitive diagnosis of the patient with seizures, observation and accurate reporting of the seizure remain important. The factors that need to be noted are listed below. Because you may have to make your observations while giving care, it is important to know what observations to make.

1. Did the patient convey the aura by crying out or speaking?
2. When did the patient fall to the ground?
3. How soon did the clonic phase begin?
4. In which limb did clonus first appear?
5. Were all the extremities subsequently involved?
6. How tightly was the mouth clenched?
7. Was the patient incontinent?
8. When did clonus subside?
9. What injuries did you note in inspecting the patient?
10. Was the patient confused postictally?
11. On regaining awareness, what subjective feelings did the patient recall having preceded the seizure?
12. What were the patient's vital signs during the rest period following the seizure?

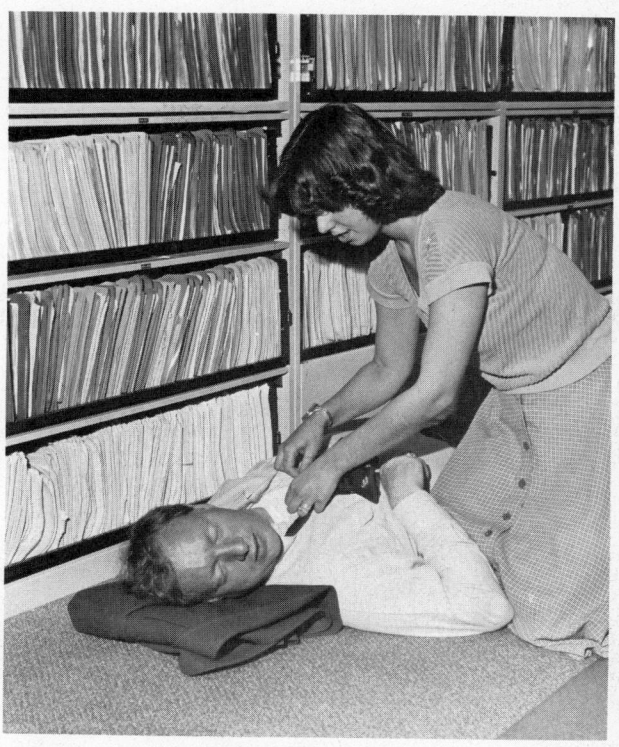

**Figure 25.9   Helping the victim of a grand mal seizure**
Russ Kinne/Danbury Hospital/Photo Researchers, Inc.

## Health Teaching

Health teaching can contribute significantly to the well-being of a patient with a seizure disorder. Conscientiously taking the prescribed anticonvulsant medication is usually the most important preventive measure. If the patient is in the hospital for surgery or another condition that renders the patient N.P.O. (nothing by mouth), be sure the physician is aware of the patient's seizure history so a decision can be made about continuing the drug regimen. The medications may be given by injection.

Maintaining a regular life style, good nutrition, and regular meals is important for people with seizure disorders. Because sleep patterns should not be disturbed, shift work is usually inappropriate. Avoiding stress and staying active are both advisable.

# Body Temperature

Body temperature is regulated by the hypothalamus in the brain, which balances heat production and heat loss. The human body's temperature must be maintained within very narrow limits for the optimal functioning of its various physiological processes. The normal temperature range is only 3.5–4.0°F (6–7°C), from 97°F (36.1°C) to 100.4°F (38°C). The "normal" body temperature is considered to be 98.6°F (37°C) when measured orally. Axillary temperature (temperature measured under the arm) is normally 1°F (.6°C) lower, and rectal temperature is 1°F (.6°C) higher. Some researchers believe, however, that imprecise measuring techniques account for these differences.

Because it is subject to a twenty-four-hour cycle

called its *circadian rhythm*, body temperature is highest from 4:00 to 8:00 p.m. and lowest in the early hours of the morning. Women also experience a temperature-change cycle associated with the menstrual cycle: the body temperature increases 0.5–1°F at the time of ovulation and decreases again at the time of menstruation.

"Normal" temperature varies among individuals. The elderly often have relatively low normal temperatures, which is probably a function of their slower metabolisms. Infants' and young children's normal temperatures may be a full degree higher than adults'. For this reason, a single temperature reading provides only very general information unless it is considered in light of other data on the patient.

## Measuring Temperature

In the United States, body temperature is usually measured in degrees Fahrenheit, but hospitals are increasingly adopting the Celsius (sometimes called centigrade) scale. Though Fahrenheit measurements are more familiar, Celsius measurements are more readily used in combination with other measurements, such as when calculations of calorie or fluid requirements must be made.

The most common instrument for temperature measurement is the glass thermometer containing mercury (see Figure 25.10). Although careful attention is paid to quality control in their manufacture, some thermometers do exhibit errors in calibration or other aspects of manufacture. Whenever an extremely low or extremely high temperature reading is made on a glass thermometer, therefore, the temperature should be rechecked with a different thermometer.

To obtain an accurate measurement, the glass thermometer must be correctly positioned. For an oral temperature reading, it must be under the tongue, touching the tissue, with the lips closed. A rectal thermometer's bulb must be inserted 1 inch beyond the internal sphincter. The bulb of the axillary thermometer should be placed against dry skin of the axilla itself, not against the upper arm and chest.

The length of time a thermometer is left in place may be the greatest contributory factor to errors in measurement. Oral thermometers must be in place ten minutes for children and eight minutes for adults to ensure accurate readings. Only three minutes are required to obtain a maximum reading from a rectal thermometer. An axillary thermometer should be left in place ten minutes.

Although smoking two minutes before insertion of an oral thermometer does not significantly raise mouth temperature, the mouth temperature is lowered by drinking ice water and does not return to normal until five minutes later. There appears to be no significant change in oral temperature when a nasal oxygen catheter or nasogastric tube is in use. Therefore, rectal temperatures appear to be necessary only for persons who mouth-breathe and thus cannot keep their lips tightly closed.

Another instrument for measuring temperature is the electronic thermometer, which provides a much more rapid and accurate reading than does a glass thermometer. Its use also eliminates the hazards of broken glass and escaping mercury, and, because the probe covers are disposable, makes cleaning and sterilizing unnecessary. Furthermore, it is not necessary with some models for the patient to hold the mouth closed, because the reading is taken directly over a small artery under the tongue. However, these instruments are both very expensive and easily damaged if dropped or handled roughly. The method of use is specific to each brand, but, in general, a temperature-sensi-

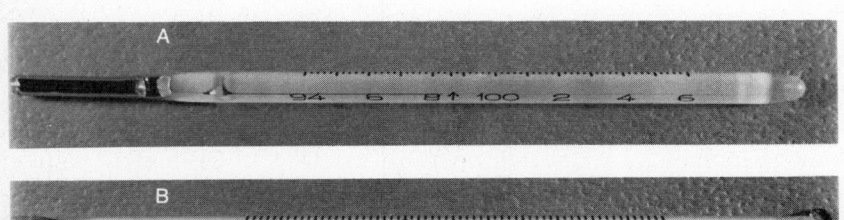

**Figure 25.10 Oral and rectal thermometers**
*A:* Oral thermometer; *B:* rectal thermometer. (Courtesy Ivan Ellis)

tive probe is attached to an energy source and a measuring device. The temperature appears as lighted numerals or is indicated on a dial. Duration of use and placement are specified by the manufacturer. Various procedures for measuring temperature are described in Module 20, "Temperature, Pulse, and Respiration."

## Heat Production

Heat is produced by metabolism and is therefore a by-product of all activities and processes within the body. The *specific dynamic action* of foods is the energy expended in the process of digestion and absorption. Because heat is always produced in this process, eating can produce an almost immediate increase in feelings of warmth. Muscular activity also produces considerable heat. Shivering is involuntary muscular activity that has the effect of increasing the body temperature. Infections and inflammations increase tissue metabolism and thus increase tissue heat.

## Heat Loss

Heat is lost through four processes: radiation, conduction, convection, and evaporation. *Radiation*, the loss of heat to another object without contact, occurs constantly. *Conduction* is loss of heat through direct contact with another object. *Convection* is heat transfer caused by moving air, which carries heat away from the body surface to be replaced by cooler air. *Evaporation* also has a cooling effect because the conversion of liquid to a gas requires heat energy. Evaporation of moisture occurs constantly from the surface cells, and more extensively through the secretion of perspiration from glands beneath the skin.

Heat loss is increased by the dilation of peripheral vessels, which transfers heat from the body core to the surface where heat loss can occur more readily. Increased perspiration also hastens heat loss by providing for more evaporation. The process of heat loss can be enhanced by using fans or a breeze to increase convection or by applying moisture to the body to bring about evaporative cooling. An automatic cooling blanket increases conduction of heat from the body by circulating cool water through tubing within the blanket.

Such a blanket is usually equipped with a rectal thermometer and a means of regulating the temperature of the blanket.

Heat loss is minimized by the contraction of muscles in the hair follicles, causing "goose pimples," which in turn raise hairs on the body surface to provide an insulating layer and decrease convection. This process is most effective in individuals with large amounts of body hair. Vasoconstriction on the body surface decreases all forms of heat loss and preserves the heat of the body core. Adding layers of clothing or blankets decreases radiation and conduction and also reduces convection losses by preventing air movement next to the skin. Because the blood vessels of the head do not constrict in response to cold, covering the head is particularly effective in preserving body heat.

## Hypothermia

When the body loses more heat than it can produce, a condition known as *hypothermia* occurs. Its initial symptoms are loss of judgment, confusion, and uncontrollable shivering. After a brief period this massive effort to generate body heat may exhaust the body's energy reserves. The body is then no longer able to maintain heat-producing activity, and temperature continues to drop until death ensues.

Hypothermia may occur accidentally due to exposure. Air temperatures need not be below freezing to cause fatal hypothermia. Winds that greatly increase convection cause "wind chill," whose effect is the same as that of a much lower temperature without wind. Getting wet can contribute to hypothermia by greatly increasing heat loss through evaporation and by providing a medium for conduction of heat away from the body. The combination of wetness and wind can cause hypothermia even when the air temperature is above 50°F. Treatment consists of providing hot drinks, food, and an external source of heat such as a fire or another person's body. Simply providing covering will not restore body heat because the body has lost the ability to produce its own heat.

In the hospital, the patient undergoing hypothermia is gradually warmed in conjunction with close monitoring of all vital systems. If the condition is severe, peritoneal dialysis is performed, using warmed solution (see Chapter 22).

Hypothermia may also be purposefully induced to facilitate the performance of certain types of surgery. Because metabolism is slowed, tissues can be deprived of blood supply for a certain period of time without sustaining permanent damage. This technique has been particularly useful in certain heart and brain surgeries. The patient is anesthetized and given medications to prevent the body from exerting its heat-producing abilities, and the body temperature is then lowered to the desired level by means of hypothermia blankets and drugs. In the past, ice-water baths were used. When the surgery has been completed, the patient is either rewarmed with heating pads or allowed to recover his or her own heat-producing abilities. The body temperature must be closely monitored during the entire process to ensure that it does not fall too low. Care must also be taken to see that, upon return to normal, the body's heat-regulating mechanisms function correctly.

## Fever

Fever, or *pyrexia*, is defined as a body temperature 1°F (0.6°C) or more higher than normal. Fever occurs when the body sets its temperature-regulating mechanism higher than usual because of infection, the presence of a toxin, or a disease of the endocrine or central nervous system. Because the body both increases heat production and initiates measures to prevent heat loss until the new temperature is attained, a fever is often preceded by "chilling." Shivering is thus a heat-producing mechanism. Withholding blankets and other aids to comfort will not prevent the development of a fever; it will simply increase the cost in energy of reaching the temperature level set by the hypothalamus.

Various terms are used to characterize fevers. In a *remittent* fever, the temperature is always elevated but may rise and fall considerably. An *intermittent* fever is one in which the temperature rises each day but returns to normal sometime during each twenty-four-hour period. A *constant* fever is one in which the temperature remains elevated at a constant level.

A high temperature is not always harmful. It is now recognized that some slight rises in temperature help the body to combat infections by increasing metabolic rates and providing a less favorable climate for some disease organisms. Often, however, the temperature rises so high that the body's energy stores are depleted and the temperature interferes with tissue functioning. For example, high temperatures may interfere with the functioning of the central nervous system and induce confusion, hallucinations, and even convulsions. Infants and children are especially susceptible to these effects.

## Assessment

A person with a fever commonly has flushed, dry skin that feels warm or even hot to the touch. The eyes lose their luster. The person may report feeling listless and weak and may complain of headache. Although the need for food is great because of the high metabolic rate, lack of appetite and even nausea may be present. "Fever blisters" on the lips are caused by the herpes simplex virus, which may set in due to the weakened resistance of the body. The effect of elevated temperature on the central nervous system tends to cause irritability and anxiety. The body may lose quantities of water through perspiration, resulting in symptoms of dehydration.

If all patients' temperatures are taken daily to screen for fevers, doing so in the late afternoon or early evening, such as at 6:00 p.m., will be most likely to reveal low or intermittent fevers. The temperatures of patients with infections, those at particular risk of infection (new surgical patients, new mothers), and those whose temperature-regulating mechanisms might not be functioning (the brain-injured, young infants) are often measured every four hours.

Whenever a patient has "chills" or appears to have a fever, the temperature should be taken as part of a complete assessment. Although healthcare facilities adopt policies on the frequency of temperature-taking, such policies are not intended to substitute for individual decision making. You should not hesitate to perform this task more frequently if necessary. While a temperature is rising, and again when steps have been taken to reduce it, you may check the temperature every fifteen to thirty minutes.

## Intervention

The physician must be notified of a fever so that it may be diagnosed and appropriate medical treatment ordered. If an infection is thought to be the cause of the fever, it may be necessary to culture wound drainage and to take steps to prevent the spread of infection to others (see Chapter 11).

In addition to medications or special baths the physician may order, many independent nursing actions can be taken for the patient with a fever. Comfort is a primary need. The skin may be dry and characterized by excessive salt deposits due to perspiration. Frequent bathing followed by the application of a lotion will promote a feeling of well-being and preserve the integrity of the skin. Because the skin of a feverish person is often very sensitive, bedding should be kept smooth and tight and should be changed as needed. Care should be taken to avoid bright lights and direct sunlight, to which the eyes may be sensitive. A cool, moist cloth placed over the forehead and eyes will often be welcome. Petroleum jelly or another lubricant will prevent cracked or dry lips. The patient will be most comfortable if the hair is arranged off the forehead and neck.

Providing adequate nutrition can be very challenging. Liquids are of primary concern in order to prevent dehydration. Frequent offerings of cool liquids, especially slightly tart drinks such as fruit juice, may be welcome. Foods ought to be light and simple. The prostration and weakness brought about by the fever may necessitate feeding the patient; otherwise the patient may fail to eat simply because the effort is too great.

Temperatures above 114.8°F (46°C) are not compatible with life, and tissue damage may begin to occur at 105°F (40°C). In order to maintain a margin of safety, then, measures to combat fever are usually undertaken when the temperature reaches 101°F (38.4°C). Measures to lower body temperature include antipyretic medications such as aspirin and acetominophen; cooling baths of tepid water, ice water, or alcohol; the use of fans; and special cooling or hypothermic blankets. There is some controversy over the use of the various kinds of baths. All are cooling, but alcohol causes excessive dryness of the skin and ice water causes profound vasoconstriction in the skin. Both are extremely uncomfortable for the patient. For these reasons, tepid baths may be preferred. In life-threatening situations, enemas of cold water—or even ice water—may be used to bring about rapid cooling of the body core. When a fever recedes, it is said to have "broken." Profuse sweating occurs as the body resets its temperature at a normal level.

## Charting Neurological Function

Charting information about neurological function accurately is every bit as important as recording any vital sign. You should use the same terms employed by the other members of the health-care team. The value of the nurse's assessment, description, and charting of neurological data cannot be overestimated. Such assessment can, in many cases, indicate whether or not a particular treatment is successful and can guide revisions in the nursing and medical care of the patient.

## Conclusion

Caring for the patient with a neurological deficit can be one of the most challenging and rewarding experiences nursing has to offer. The nurse can directly influence the consequences of recovery by maintaining the patient's highest possible level of function. In giving care, the nurse assumes the role of the patient's advocate, speaking, hearing, feeling, and caring for the patient who may not be able to do so independently for some time, if at all. Neurological nursing requires the highest level of physical, psychological, and social skill.

## Care Study   A deaf boy

Kevin had been deaf since birth. An outgoing, happy black youngster of four, he seemed to bounce into the room with his mother for his evening admission prior to a tonsillectomy scheduled for the early morning. Although Kevin had not yet learned words, he had some ability to read lips. It was obvious that he was able to indicate yes or no—usually no!—by means of a vigorous shake of the head. His mother stayed to give the nursing interview and for the collection of a urine specimen and other routine preoperative matters. A set of picture cards kept on the pediatric unit to illustrate routine care allowed Kevin to point to various items that might be needed, such as a water glass, urinal, or tissues. This would be a type of game, yet meet care needs. But how to prepare Kevin psychologically for the surgery?

Jim Kistler, R.N., called the operating room. Did the surgical nurse have any ideas? "I'll be right up," replied Tina Renfrow, R.N., who soon appeared with a book in hand. The title was *Hey, I'm Having My Tonsils Out Tomorrow.* Mr. Kistler was delighted with the book, as he knew Kevin would be. Although there was a caption under each brightly colored picture, the pictures conveyed everything. A small boy on a stretcher was hugged by

mother and waved goodbye to her as she sat down to await his return. The faces were cheerful. The surgeon wore a mask but revealed his face before surgery to allay fear in the child. The young patient was shown after surgery with an obviously sore throat but surrounded by his caring parents and a nurse.

"Just what I needed," said Mr. Kistler. Carrying the book and a surgical mask for Kevin to try on, he disappeared into Kevin's room.

An hour later, Mr. Kistler had the feeling Kevin was perhaps as well prepared for surgery as a hearing child would be. He then pointed to his back and cavorted like a frisky horse. "Climb on," he said, and Kevin excitedly did so. Mr. Kistler "rode" Kevin to the operating-room door. Tina Renfrow greeted them at the door, held up a mask to indicate she was part of the surgical team, and hugged Kevin. Mr. Kistler took Kevin back to his room. He removed the water pitcher, since Kevin was to have nothing by mouth until morning. Kevin tugged at Mr. Kistler's sleeve and pointed vigorously at a picture in the book. Mr. Kistler laughed. The picture showed a nurse emptying a water pitcher.

## Study Terms

aphasia
astereognosis
ataxia
atrophy
aura
autonomic nervous
  system
awareness
CAT scanner
central nervous system
  (CNS)
circadian rhythm
clonic
coma
command
conduction
consciousness
constant fever
convection
coordination
cortex

cranium
decerebration
delusion
dysphagia
dysphasia
epilepsy
evaporation
fever
gait
grand mal seizure
hallucinations
heat loss
hemiplegia
hypalgesia
hyperalgesia
hyperesthesia
hypesthesia
hypothermia
illusion
intermittent fever
lethargy

levels of awareness
mentation
motor aphasia
motor impulses
motor neurons
name-call
neuro signs
olfactory
opisthotonos position
palsy
paralysis
paraplegia
parasympathetic
  nervous system
paresis
paresthesia
partial seizure
peripheral nervous
  system (PNS)
petit mal seizure
postictal
proprioception

pyrexia
quadriplegia
radiation
relaxation
remittent fever
seizure
semicoma
sensory aphasia
sensory impulses
sensory receptors
signing
somnolence
special senses
stupor
symmetrical
sympathetic nervous
  system
tactile
tonic
tremors
verbalization

## Learning Activities

**1.** Take your own temperature every 2 to 4 hours for 2 days. Graph your temperature. Determine your circadian rhythm. When is your temperature highest? lowest? What is your average temperature?

**2.** Obtain and review a checklist or flow sheet used for recording neurological signs in your facility.

**3.** Contact a chapter of the Epilepsy Association and find out what programs are offered in your community for people with seizure disorders.

## Relevant Sections in
## Modules for Basic Nursing Skills

| Volume 1 | Module |
|---|---|
| Moving the Patient in Bed and Positioning | 12 |
| Range-of-Motion Exercises | 14 |
| Ambulation | 16 |
| Temperature, Pulse, and Respiration | 20 |

| Volume 2 | |
|---|---|
| Inspection, Palpation, Auscultation, and Percussion | 32 |

## References

Amacher, Nancy J. "Touch Is a Way of Caring and a Way of Communicating with an Aphasic Patient." *American Journal of Nursing* 73 (May 1973): 852–854.

Anderson, C. A. "Making the Right Moves in Discharge Planning: Home or Nursing Home?" *American Journal of Nursing* 79 (August 1979): 1448–1449.

Anthony, Catherine Parker, and Kolthoff, Norma Jane. *Textbook of Anatomy and Physiology,* 9th ed. St. Louis: C. V. Mosby, 1975.

Bangs, Cameron; Hamlet, Murray P.; and Miller, William J., Jr. "Help for the Victim of Hypothermia." *Patient Care* (15 December 1977): 46–56.

Blainey, C. G. "Site Selection in Taking Body Temperature." *American Journal of Nursing* 74 (October 1974): 1859–1861.

Bumbalo, J. J., *et al.* "The Self-Help Phenomenon." *American Journal of Nursing* 73 (September 1973): 1588–1596.

Felder, L. "Neurogenic Bladder Dysfunction." *Journal of Neurosurgical Nursing* 11 (June, 1979): 94–104.

Geary, Ruth Patton. "Journey Into Fog." *American Journal of Nursing* 78 (February 1978): 246–248.

Gedrose, Judith. "Prevention and Treatment of Hypothermia and Frostbite." *Nursing '80* (February 1980): 34–36.

Hazzard, M. E., and Scheuerman, M. "Family System Therapy." *Nursing '76* (July 1976): 22–23.

Holmes, J. E. "The Physical Therapist and Team Care." *Nursing Outlook* 20 (March 1972): 182–184.

Hunko, Veronica. "Numidia Looked Like a Model— But She Wasn't a Model Patient." *Nursing '78* 8 (December 1978): 51–52.

Jones, Cathy. "Glasgow Coma Scale." *American Journal of Nursing* 79 (September 1979): 1551–1553.

Krieger, Dolores. "Therapeutic Touch: The Imprimatur of Nursing." *American Journal of Nursing* 75 (May 1975): 784–787.

McAllister, B. "Liberation Time for the Handicapped." *RN* 39 (March 1976): 57–60.

McVan, B., ed. "What the Nose Knows." *Nursing '77* 7 (April 1977): 46–49.

Moorat, D. S. "The Cost of Taking Temperatures." *Nursing Times* 72 (20 May 1976): 767–770.

Moss, B. K. "Hearing Loss—the Invisible Handicap." *Patient Care* 13 (15 September 1979): 124–125.

*The New Columbia Encyclopedia,* 4th ed. New York: Columbia University Press, 1975.

Nichols, G. A.; Kucha, D. H.; and Mahoney, R. P. "Rectal Thermometer Placement Times for Febrile Adults." *Nursing Research* (January/February 1972): 76–77.

Perron, Denise M. "Deprived of Sound." *American Journal of Nursing* (June 1974): 1057–1059.

# Part Seven

## Major Challenges in Patient Care

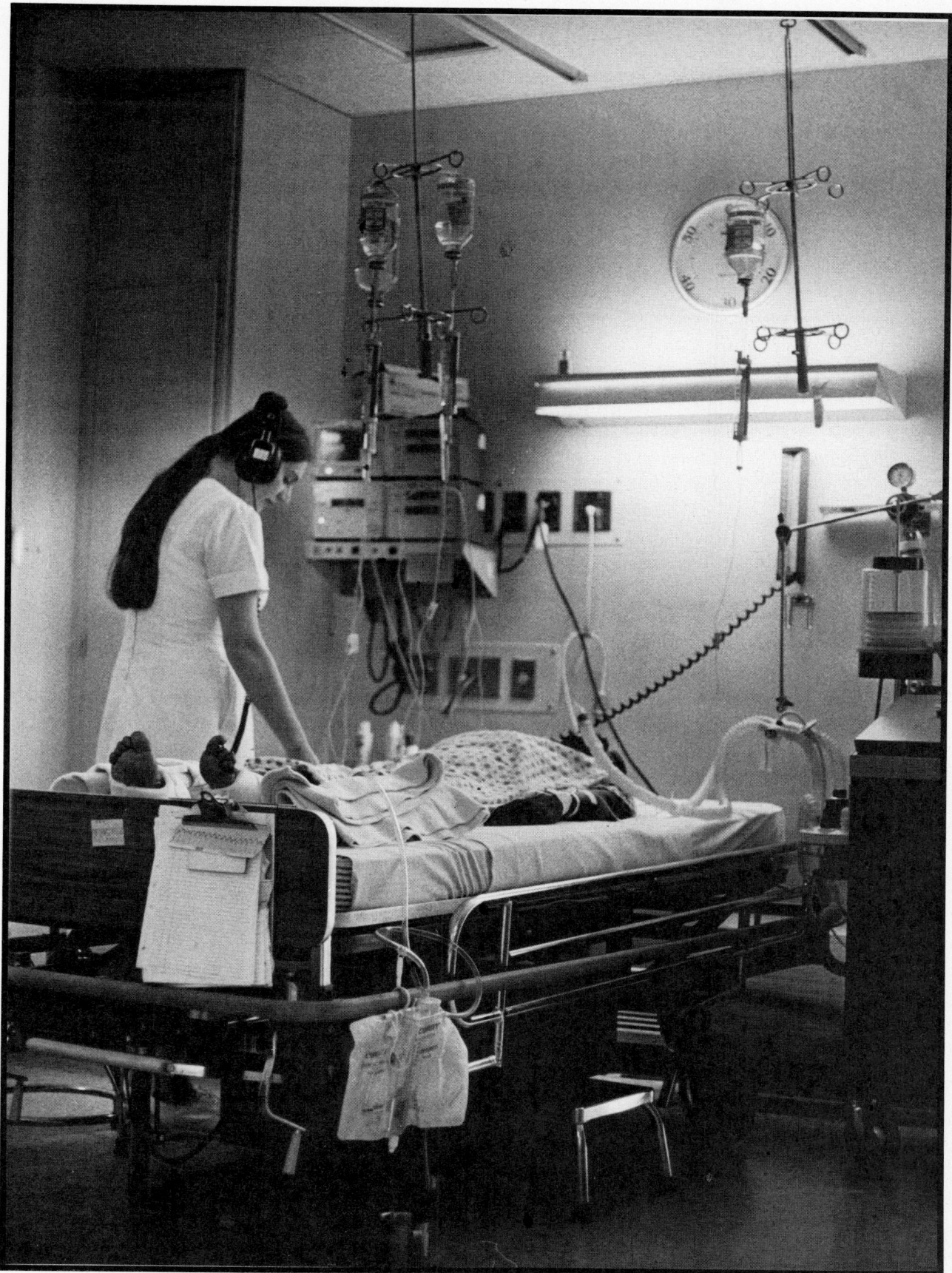

# Chapter 26

# Pain

## Objectives

After completing this chapter, you should be able to:

1. Explain, in your own words, the purpose of pain.
2. Discuss the three routes the pain impulse may travel after reaching the spinal cord.
3. List the physiologic responses to pain.
4. Discuss the various other ways people respond to pain.
5. List data to be gathered when assessing for pain.
6. List five major categories of nursing intervention to relieve pain and give examples of specific actions in each category.
7. Discuss differences in approach to treatment of chronic pain and terminal pain.

## Outline

Pain is an essentially lonely experience. It cannot be shared, and words are inadequate to explain the feeling to someone else. Pain can crowd out the rest of the world, making itself the center and focus of consciousness. Pain is frequently what prompts a person to seek medical care and often continues to be the person's primary concern during treatment. What is pain? What is its purpose? What causes it? What can be done to alleviate pain? Answers to these questions are highly important for nurses.

## The Nature of Pain

Pain is a warning system. It lets us know when something is wrong and thus alerts us to protect ourselves from injury or to care for an injury that has already occurred. Some individuals' pain perception is decreased or lacking due to disease or a congenital defect; they are at risk of unnoticed injuries, such as burns from an excessively hot heating pad. Lack of ability to perceive pain might also lead to neglect of an injury and thus to infection and further tissue damage.

### Receiving the Pain Stimulus

*Free nerve endings,* which are pain receptors, pervade all tissue but are most prevalent in skin and surface tissues. Receptor nerve endings, for touch and temperature, also appear to be able to transmit pain impulses when they are excessively stimulated. Thus pain may be caused by a variety of stimuli, including some that have chemical, mechanical, and thermal sources.

*Ischemia* (lack of adequate blood supply to tissues) may, in some instances, cause very severe pain in the affected part. *Excessive stretching* of tissues is a source of much visceral or internal pain, such as when the bowel is overstretched or the bladder excessively distended.

*Neurogenic pain* is pain that arises from damaged or injured nerves or nerve roots. Such pain may accompany crushing injury, infection, inflammation, or scarring. Due to the effect on the nerve itself, neurogenic pain may continue long after the initial damaging agent has disappeared.

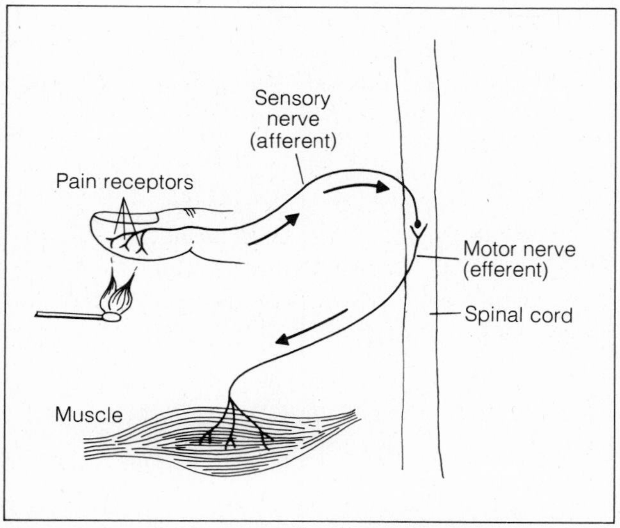

### Pathways for Pain Impulses

When sensory nerves are aroused by a painful stimulus, three processes occur. First, a *reflex* withdraws the body part from the stimulus. The pain impulse travels along the sensory nerve (afferent nerve) to the spinal cord and is transmitted directly to a motor nerve (efferent nerve) (see Figure 26.1).

Second, the impulse travels up the spinal cord to the brain stem, where the *autonomic nervous system* is activated. *Cutaneous (superficial) pain* usually stimulates the sympathetic division of the autonomic nervous system, which results in increased respiratory rate, increased heart rate, and high blood pressure. *Visceral (internal) pain* may cause the parasympathetic division of the autonomic nervous system to be stimulated, which increases

**Figure 26.1  First pathway for pain impulses: The simple reflex arc**

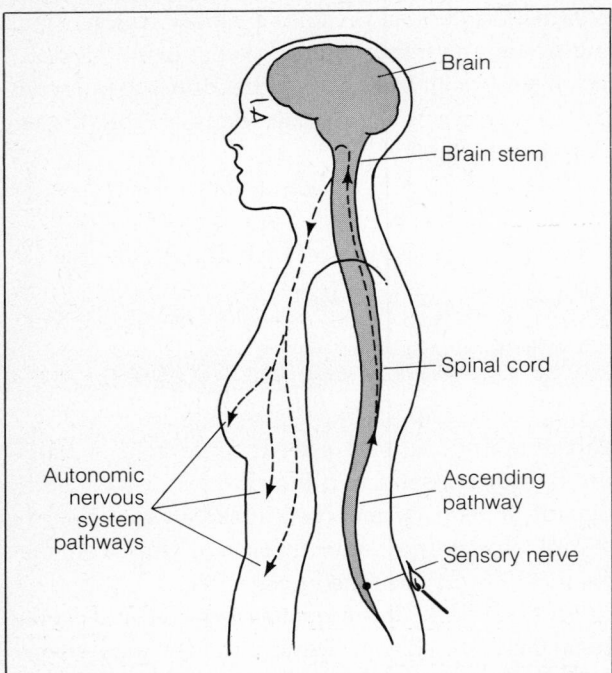

**Figure 26.2  Second pathway for pain impulses**

the impulses to be spread to adjacent nerve fibers, which transmit the pain impulse as if it originated at their point of origin.

## The Gate-Control Theory of Pain

Melzack and Wall (1965) have proposed that the spinal cord, where the transmission of impulses from sensory fibers to ascending fibers occurs, is characterized by a complex mechanism they call "gate control." According to this theory, pain-inhibiting impulses travel down the spinal cord constantly. Therefore, pain impulses must be sufficient to overcome these pain-inhibiting impulses if they are to travel upward to the brain and be perceived. Theorists suggest that disturbances in this mechanism may be responsible for cases of constant pain with no observable cause. If the inhibiting impulses are lacking, there may be a constant upward flow of minor impulses that are perceived as pain. Though neither proven nor disproven, this theory has been valuable in enhancing our understanding of chronic pain.

blood flow to internal organs and decreases respiratory rate, pulse, and blood pressure (see Figure 26.2).

Other autonomic responses to pain are increased perspiration; tearing of the eyes; dilation of the pupils; increased blood flow to the brain, which increases alertness and causes restlessness; and changes in gastrointestinal function, resulting in nausea and even vomiting.

Third, after reaching the brain, the pain impulse moves through the *thalamus*, where the pain is perceived (recognized as pain), to the *cortex*, where the perception is registered and interpreted and appropriate action is determined. It is in the cortex that the location of the pain is identified (see Figure 26.3).

On occasion, pain may be perceived by the patient as occurring elsewhere than its actual location. This phenomenon, called *referred pain*, occurs most frequently in the internal organs, where there are fewer pain receptors because larger areas are served by the same pathway. A familiar example is the heart attack that manifests itself as pain radiating down the left arm. The severity of the pain and the strength of the impulses cause

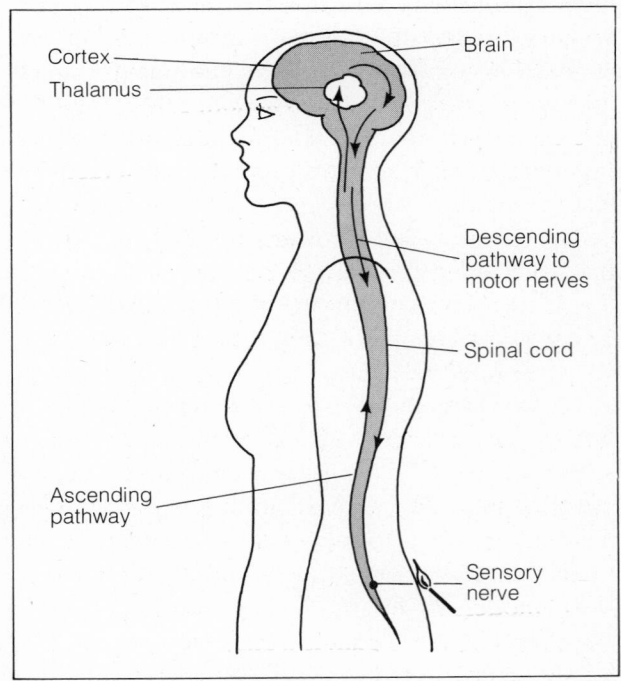

**Figure 26.3  Third pathway for pain impulses**

## Phantom Pain

*Phantom pain* is pain perceived in a body part that is no longer present, such as an amputated leg. This phenomenon does not seem to result from stimulation of the sensory nerves, since surgery to sever nerves at the spinal level has not always relieved such pain. Phantom pain is not well understood, and research into its cause is continuing. Application of the gate-control theory to this problem suggests the possibility that the pain impulses originate higher in the spinal pathways, at some point where the gate-control mechanism has failed, or in the brain itself. It is important to recognize that phantom pain is not imaginary; the person truly experiences pain.

Phantom pain is initially treated with medication as an acute pain that is expected to be self-limiting. In most instances phantom pains gradually subside and do not recur. When phantom pain persists, it is treated as a chronic long-term problem (see page 470).

# Responses to Pain

## Physiological Reactions

The intensity of the basic physiological reaction to pain initiated by the autonomic nervous system varies greatly in response to the intensity of the pain. Reactions may range from mild, in which the heart rate and respirations increase only slightly, to massive, in which a state of shock ensues and the person loses consciousness. That people can learn to alter basic autonomic responses to pain is apparent in certain Native American cultures that accorded recognition to individuals able to endure great pain with no visible reaction. Hindu mystics also develop the same ability for religious reasons. It generally takes a long time and considerable effort to achieve such control.

The *pain threshold* is the amount of painful stimulation needed for pain to be perceived. Experiments have shown that the pain threshold is fairly uniform in all people. Pain reaction, however, varies dramatically.

Other reactions to pain are determined by the interpretation of the cerebral cortex. A given sensation of pain is compared with other experiences of pain and defined as "sharp," "aching," "cramping," or whatever term is appropriate. Its intensity is classified in light of prior experience as mild, moderate, or severe. It is important to remember that, since pain is a subjective experience, its intensity is rated subjectively. In other words, you cannot classify the intensity of someone else's pain. Although you may become highly knowledgeable about the levels of pain that usually accompany given conditions or procedures, the individual's pain is unique. Researchers have developed external means of measuring pain, but they are still experimental.

The cortex also notes the location of pain, its original source, whether it *radiates* (appears to spread from its source), and whether position changes or movements ease or increase it.

Interpretations of the type, intensity, and location of the pain are then integrated with feelings about pain, prior experiences of pain, cultural and social attitudes toward pain, ideas about the origin or purpose of this particular pain, and current emotional and physiological status to produce a reaction to the pain.

Reaction to pain may be very different, if it has been experienced before, and the person knows exactly what to do about it, than if the pain is entirely unfamiliar. For example, a person who suffers chronic sinus headaches may have a whole regimen of pain-relieving measures, including medications prescribed by a physician, and will thus react very differently to sinus pain than to unfamiliar pain of equal intensity in the abdomen.

## Cultural Responses

Different cultures are characterized by very different patterns of response to pain. The passive or nonresponsive attitude of members of certain Native American tribes in the face of the most extreme pain has become legendary. This attitude, manifested in many cultures throughout history, has been named for the Stoics of ancient Greece. *Stoicism*, then, is one way of responding to pain.

Other cultures encourage *expressive responses*, both verbal and nonverbal; to keep one's feelings hidden is considered inappropriate. Such expression may take the form of talking, moaning, praying, or cursing. That verbal and nonverbal expressions of pain are not necessarily congruent with the intensity of the pain stimulus is understood and accepted among people of the same cultural background.

The mainstream of American culture tends to lean toward the stoic attitude. It is considered good and brave not to express pain and, conversely, weak and bad to do so. However, such acquired responses are not so potent that autonomic responses to pain are inhibited.

As a nurse, you must carefully examine your own attitudes toward pain in order to guard against value judgments of another person's response to pain. If you feel that pain should be expressed and encourage the characteristically stoic individual to do so, the patient may feel demeaned and lose some self-esteem. If, on the other hand, you try to induce an expressive person to withhold such feelings, you may be seen as rejecting his or her needs.

Recognizing the cultural values of the patient is also necessary when you are planning intervention. In the case of a patient who is stoic, you may need to base intervention on nonverbal cues, since the pain may be greater than the patient's statements indicate. You also need to be very alert to nonverbal cues in the case of the expressive person, because intervention based only on verbal statements might be inappropriate to the actual degree of pain experienced.

## Psychological Responses

Because it indicates that something is wrong and interrupts normal life patterns, pain arouses anxiety in many individuals. Anxiety may be manifested in a variety of ways, depending on its severity (see Chapter 15). The severity of the anxiety is not necessarily a function of the severity of the pain. Pre-existing anxiety often greatly accentuates reactions to pain.

Other emotions may also be evoked by pain. Some people feel guilt because they have previously learned to equate pain with punishment; they often perceive severe pain as punishment for wrongdoing, and children in pain tend to do the same. For some people, pain may be a means of relating to others in such a way as to elicit their attention and concern. For them, pain is rewarding.

In some situations, pain may be seen as a means to an end. A woman in childbirth may see the pain of labor as worthwhile because it results in the birth of a much-desired child. Adherents of certain religious beliefs see pain as earning merit or favor from God.

When pain seems useless or undeserved, the reaction to it may be anger or increased tension and anxiety. This reaction may characterize the woman delivering an unwanted child or the person who has a body part removed. Such feelings tend generally to exaggerate both the perceived intensity of pain and reaction to pain.

# Assessing the Patient's Pain

## Observations

As in all other nursing situations, the first task is to assess the patient with regard to pain. Respiration, pulse, skin color, wincing, restlessness, and inability to sleep are important indications of the patient's physical response to pain. The patient's muscles may be tensed, the brow may be furrowed, and a position that relieves stress on the painful part may be maintained. The person

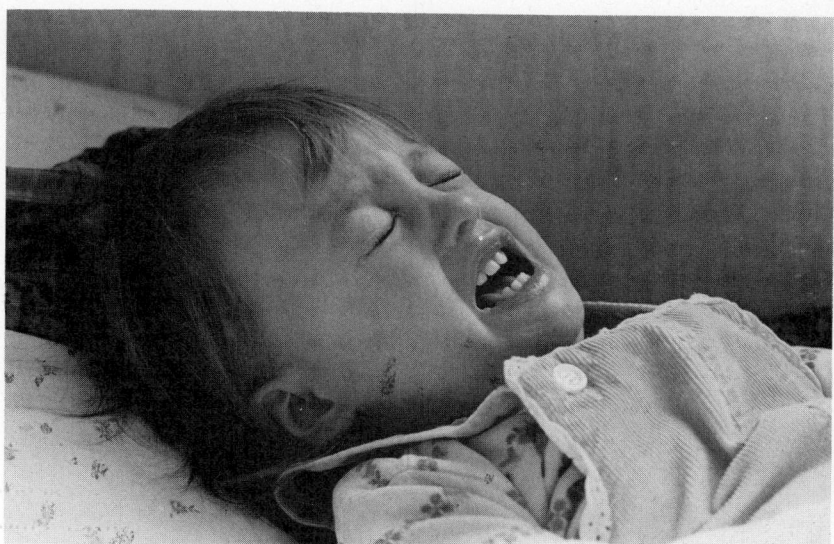

**Figure 26.4**
Nonverbal cues may indicate the presence of pain. (Sam Sweezy/Stock, Boston)

may move slowly and carefully in order to protect the painful site, or may resist moving at all. Such nonverbal cues may be the only evidence of pain in the child or the person unable to communicate.

## Interviewing

It is essential to try to elicit the patient's subjective sensations and description of the pain since pain is so personal and subjective in nature. You will need information on the *location, severity* (or intensity), and *quality* (sharp, dull, throbbing, or whatever) of the pain. (See Exhibit 26.1 for a list of terms commonly used to describe pain.) Severity may be estimated by asking the patient to identify the level on a scale of zero to ten, with zero being no pain and ten equaling the worst pain ever felt by the patient. Related factors, such as *when the* pain began, *changes* since it began (increasing, decreasing, radiating), and *measures* previously successful in combating it are also important. Factors that might have *precipitated* the pain or might be *related* to it are also significant. Remember that not all questions are appropriate to ask every patient. For example, a person who has just had surgery and complains of severe pain should be asked where the pain is located to make sure it is the expected postsurgical pain. If so, it is not necessary to ask further about precipitating factors and related events; they are self-evident. In such an

Exhibit 26.1
**Terms Used to Describe Pain**

| | |
|---|---|
| Aching | Intractable |
| Burning | Knifelike |
| Cramping | Lancinating |
| Crushing | Pinching |
| Cutting | Pounding |
| Dartlike | Radiating |
| Dull | Tearing |
| Electriclike | Throbbing |
| Gnawing | Sharp |
| Heavy | Shocklike |

instance, you should proceed rapidly to intervention in order to relieve the pain.

Some individuals express themselves better than others with regard to pain. Because pain is a subjective sensation, words are often inadequate to describe it. For some, the effort of talking about the pain they are experiencing is too great for their physical and emotional strength; such individuals should not be pressed to do so. Children may not have large enough vocabularies to describe their pain or may use words in their own ways. For example, one four-year-old repeatedly told the nurse she had a headache. This was duly noted on the chart. Only when a more perceptive nurse asked the child to "point to the hurt" was it discovered that the pain was in the abdomen. The child called any kind of pain a "headache."

## Integrating Background Knowledge

Information gathered by means of observation and interview must be integrated with information on the patient's sociocultural background and current medical status. A complaint of severe, sharp abdominal pain is interpreted differently if the patient has just had abdominal surgery than if the patient is newly admitted to the hospital and has not previously complained of such pain.

## Relieving the Patient's Pain

After a thorough assessment, plans for nursing intervention are formulated. Such intervention can take many forms, depending on such factors as the origin and severity of the pain, the patient's response to it, and medical orders regarding drugs, activity, and the like.

One of the most helpful ways to approach intervention is to consider the various aspects of the experience of pain and to decide at which point intervention is possible. Intervention may be aimed at (1) eliminating the source or stimulus of pain, (2) preventing the pain receptors from reacting, (3) interrupting the impulse somewhere along the pathway, (4) decreasing perception of pain, or (5) altering the patient's interpretation of and response to the pain. An approach that aims at more than one aspect of the pain simultaneously may be more effective than intervention directed at only a single aspect.

### Eliminating the Source of Pain

Eliminating its cause is certainly the most long-lasting and effective means of dealing with pain. Such actions as removing open safety pins, changing wet bedding, and smoothing wrinkled sheets are all aimed at eliminating the source of pain. For the postsurgical patient who has gas pains, helping expel the gas by administering return-flow enemas or encouraging movement to increase peristalsis is the most effective approach. The nurse who automatically thinks "medication" when a patient says "I hurt!" is doing the patient an injustice.

Complex or inaccessible sources of pain are more problematic, and may not be subject to nursing intervention. The surgeon must remove painful calluses on the feet or a gall bladder filled with stones to provide long-term relief of pain.

Certain drugs may, by reducing inflammation and swelling of a body part, reduce or eliminate the pain caused by those conditions. When severe muscle spasms are the cause of pain, muscle relaxant drugs will help. Massage can also relieve muscle spasms, especially in the neck and back. When pain is caused by ischemia (lack of blood supply to a body part), measures to increase blood flow may reduce pain. Intervention to remove the source of the pain is the best long-term response to pain and the preferred method of intervention. However, it is not always possible.

### Protecting Pain Receptors From Stimuli

It is sometimes possible to protect the receptors from the source of pain. Examples are putting petroleum jelly on excoriated buttocks to protect the skin from urine and putting a cloth over the eyes to protect them from light. The patient with trigeminal neuralgia, a disorder of the fifth cranial nerve, may use a silk scarf to protect the overly sensitive nerve from air movement that might stimulate it. There is evidence that aspirin may exert some of its effect by decreasing the sensitivity of pain receptors. Ointments containing topical anesthetic agents are also used, notably in products for hemorrhoids and sunburn, to decrease the pain receptors' ability to function.

## Interrupting the Pathways for Pain

Interruption of the pathways for pain is usually a physician's responsibility, though nurses performing in expanded roles are also acting in this capacity. A local anesthetic may be injected at a point along the nerve pathway to interrupt the transmission of pain impulses. Injections are most commonly done just proximal to the origin of the pain (as in dental work) or close to the spine. Spinal anesthesia—the injection of drug agents into the spinal canal to provide total blockage of the pathway—allows surgery to be performed.

Pain pathways in the spinal thalamic tracts (a group of nerves in the spinal cord) may be interrupted surgically in certain cases of long-term intractable pain. This procedure, called a *chordotomy*, cannot be guaranteed successful because of anatomic variations in the spinal cord but has been immeasurably helpful in certain cases.

The *dorsal column stimulator* (D.C.S.) is an electric stimulation device recently developed for use in the control of intractable pain. The device is surgically implanted along the spinal column. When activated, it provides an electrical stimulation, felt as a buzzing sensation, which can interrupt a pain impulse and prevent pain perception. The person can activate the D.C.S. when pain sets in, thus stopping the pain. It is expected that use of the dorsal column stimulator will increase as more information becomes available about its effectiveness.

A *transcutaneous nerve stimulator* (T.C.S. or T.N.S.) functions in the same manner as a dorsal column stimulator through electrodes attached temporarily to the skin. Some peripheral nerve stimulators are being implanted into the tissue to avoid the constant skin irritation that characterizes the T.C.S.

## Decreasing the Perception of Pain

### Analgesic Administration

Any drug, narcotic or nonnarcotic, that decreases pain perception is termed an *analgesic*. Pain is perceived in the thalamus and then transmitted to the cortex. Narcotics given before pain occurs or be-

fore it becomes severe block pain perception. Thus relief is more effective if medication is given before pain becomes severe. When a painful experience is anticipated, a narcotic given beforehand can prevent the perception of severe pain.

Nonnarcotic analgesics act in a variety of ways. Most, like narcotic analgesics, act to block pain perception; the anti-inflammatory effects of some may also help to eliminate the cause of the pain.

*Addiction* is a complex physiologic and psychologic dependence on a substance, giving rise to characteristic physical and psychologic problems when the substance is withdrawn. Concern about addiction to narcotic analgesics sometimes prevents nurses from using these drugs effectively. Available evidence indicates that addiction is extremely rare among those who are experiencing severe pain. It also seems to show that the chance of addiction is reduced if the person in pain is not required to demonstrate excessive reaction to pain in order to receive such medication. Thus, the person with short-term acute pain (such as a new surgical patient) does not become addicted when given narcotics regularly during the acute postoperative period. The person with severe pain of a terminal nature, such as in terminal cancer, is less likely to become addicted or to need increasing amounts of medication when pain medication is given on a regular schedule and pain relief can be depended on. Absence of anxiety about pain and absence of fear that relief will be withheld seem to be key factors in preventing addiction.

### Hypnosis

Pain is relieved by *hypnosis* for the duration of the hypnotic trance, and pain relief may last due to the effect of posthypnotic suggestion on pain perception. Though used in some health-care settings, hypnosis is not yet a common method of pain relief. The person using hypnosis must be trained in all aspects of its use.

### Acupuncture

*Acupuncture*, which has been practiced as a medical art in the Orient for hundreds of years, is receiving increasing attention from medical researchers. In acupuncture, long slender needles are inserted into specific points on the body. These needles may be twirled, heated, or attached to a mild electrical current. The effect is to provide anesthesia to a given body part. Interestingly, the part anesthetized is not necessarily in close proximity to the entry point of the needle. For example, a point near the base of the thumb may be used to relieve pain in a tooth. Many kinds of surgery are performed in China using only acupuncture to prevent pain, and the process has also been used to treat different types of long-term pain. Understanding of acupuncture is still limited, and there are many theories about how it works. Its use is experimental in this country.

## Distraction

By preoccupying the attention, distractions can prevent pain from being perceived. If a person with a headache becomes engrossed in a hobby, for example, the head pain may recede from awareness, only to return when the distraction ceases. Pain is not perceived because all cerebral cortex activity is focused elsewhere, and impulses from the thalamus are blocked. When concentration decreases, impulses will be transmitted to the cortex and pain will be noticed. This mechanism is most effective in cases of relatively mild pain. However, if concentration is extreme enough, even severe pain may not be perceived until the attention disperses. For example, a football player may not realize he is injured until after an important play is completed. Thus you can sometimes help a person in pain by engaging him or her in an engrossing activity. This approach will not necessarily minimize perception of very severe pain that is already present but may serve to increase such a patient's comfort. Visitors, a television program, a book, or anything else the patient is interested in can be an effective distraction. You need to be careful not to convey the idea that pain from which a person can be distracted is trivial; the importance or strength of the distractor is the primary factor.

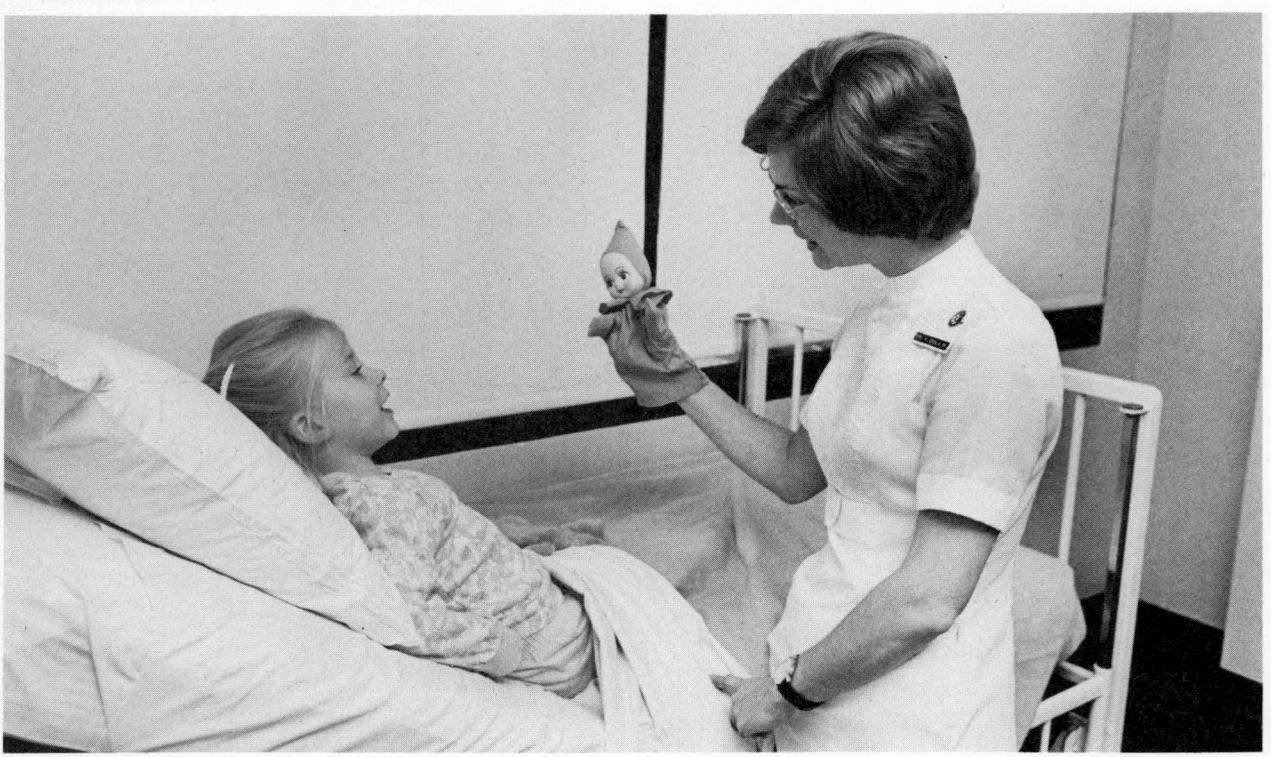

**Figure 26.5**
Diversion may decrease pain perception. (Dan Bernstein)

## Modifying the Interpretation of Pain

### Narcotic Administration

Pain interpretation may be modified by many factors. In the hospital, the most common agents are, again, the narcotic analgesics. A narcotic given before pain becomes severe may block perception of pain; the same narcotic given after pain has become severe acts to modify interpretation. The patient may even say that the pain is still present but no longer matters. The patient may appear less anxious and able to rest or relate to others, and physiological responses to pain may disappear.

### Interpersonal Relating

Pain interpretation may also be modified beneficially by an interpersonal process involving the nurse and the patient (see Chapter 12). For example, a person who interprets pain as punishment can be helped to examine and deal with such feelings. This process may in turn decrease anxiety about pain, reduce physiologic response to pain, and change the patient's interpretation of the severity of pain. Other interpretations of pain may be dealt with in the same manner.

### Comfort Measures

Interpretation of pain may also be influenced by comforting measures that counteract the pain impulses. Bathing to remove excess perspiration, combing the hair, or providing a backrub that is soothing to the skin may help decrease the severity of the pain. It is important to find out what the individual regards as soothing, since people vary greatly in their choice of comforts.

### The Placebo Effect

A *placebo* is an inert substance administered in place of a pharmacologically active drug. It is considered effective when it has the effect that might be expected from the drug for which it substitutes. Though the effectiveness of placebos is not clearly

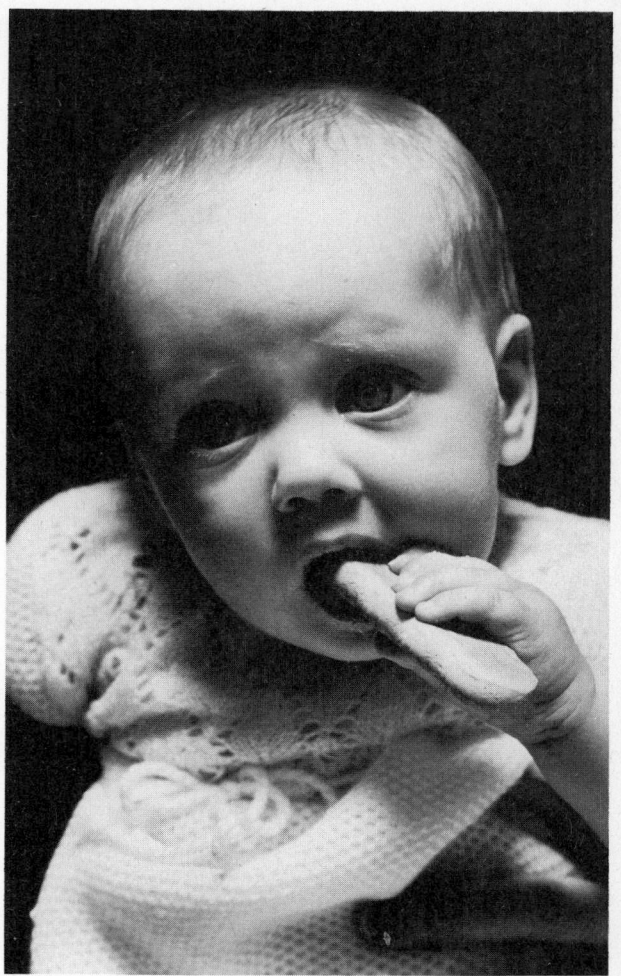

**Figure 26.6**
A teething baby is experiencing pain. (Russ Kinne/Photo Researchers, Inc.)

understood, we do know that *all* medication is subject to a *placebo effect*—that is, the effect may be greater than the drug itself accounts for. This phenomenon appears to be related to the atmosphere of trust and confidence in which the drug is given. You will find that medications for pain are more effective if you accompany them with explanations of their effectiveness and an attitude of certainty that they will indeed help to relieve the patient's pain.

Occasionally a physician may order an inert substance, usually normal saline for an injection or flavored syrup administered orally, instead of a narcotic in response to a patient's request for pain medication. This approach raises many ethical questions. The patient does have the right to know what treatments are being used, and dishonesty with the patient is considered unethical. On the other hand, if you tell the patient a placebo has been prescribed, it may not work. The purpose of giving a placebo is usually to guard against or treat drug dependence associated with pain relief measures or to determine whether the pain has an organic cause. Pain whose origin is psychological rather than organic is likely to respond more fully to a placebo.

Every nurse must make an individual decision, on the basis of conscience, with regard to each individual case in which a placebo is ordered. When you have made your decision, you can act on it by giving the placebo or by asking not to participate in that aspect of care. Whatever your choice, you should also support the rights of other health-care workers to make contrary ethical choices.

In some settings, the patient is informed in advance that a placebo may be used at some point in treatment but that he or she will not be so notified at the time the placebo is administered. The patient is then asked to consent to this mode of treatment. Placebos also prove effective in these circumstances, which eliminate the ethical problem.

## Helping the Person With Chronic Pain

Chronic pain is pain that persists for weeks, months, or even years. The condition responsible for the pain may be one for which there is currently no means of correction, such as severe arthritis, or there may be no visible cause. Narcotic analgesics are not advisable in such cases because they can become addicting. This kind of chronic pain may threaten one's occupation, undermine interpersonal relationships, and destroy the fabric of life.

To modify reactions to such pain, a variety of methods have been used. Behavior modification techniques that reward non–pain-oriented behavior and ignore pain-oriented behavior are meeting with some success. This approach assumes not that the pain is not real but that it is the person's response to pain that disrupts his or her life.

Such techniques are not to be used lightly, since they can change a person psychologically as surely as surgery does so physically. The patient must be informed about the situation and consulted about the treatment plan and must give informed consent such as would be required for surgery. Success with these techniques depends on a total health-team approach.

Another approach is to reduce pain medication gradually while encouraging the person to remain active and involved. Use of a liquid pain medication composed of a syrup and an undisclosed amount of drug allows for the amount of the syrup to remain the same while the drug content is gradually reduced. This approach helps prevent psychological reactions to the withdrawal of the drug.

Surgery is an alternative method of pain relief in cases of chronic pain. Though such surgery does not alter motor function, it may adversely affect other sensory perception. The resulting inability to perceive harmful heat and cold may create safety problems. Surgery for pain relief is not always successful.

The various nerve stimulators, such as the T.C.S. or T.N.S., have had their greatest success in treating chronic pain. The stimulator may at first be used continuously; gradually the duration of use is reduced, and eventually the stimulator is turned on only as needed. The final step is to stop using the stimulator altogether. In cases in which use of the stimulator is a permanent necessity, implanted electrodes are used in preference to those that must be attached to the skin. Skin electrodes must be removed for short periods of time daily, the skin cleaned and checked for irritation, and the electrodes replaced in a slightly different location.

# Helping the Person With Terminal Pain

Pain related to a terminal illness, usually called *terminal pain,* requires a different approach to pain management. During the early stages of the illness, through surgeries and treatment, pain may be managed much the same as it is for any other patient. When the disease is far advanced and there is no expectation of cure, the approach changes.

The patient is encouraged to become an active participant in managing pain. Many drugs used to control pain may cause drowsiness and diminished ability to relate to others or perform tasks. Only the patient can decide whether pain relief or alertness is more desirable. Often patients are encouraged to characterize the intensity of pain on a scale of 1 to 5 or 1 to 10, and many patients become quite adept at doing so. Because terminal pain is not necessarily uniform, nor always progressively worse, this assessment technique can lead to more individualized treatment.

In order to minimize discomfort and promote independence, oral medications are used as long as possible. The use of *pain cocktails*—mixtures of drugs in alcohol, water, and flavoring syrup—is becoming quite common. The drugs in such a mixture usually include a narcotic analgesic and phenothiazine. Cocaine may be added for its mood-elevating effects, although some authorities recommend against doing so. Sometimes other drugs are added. You may hear of *Brompton's mixture,* a mixture with a heroin base used in England. Some facilities in the United States use a mixture they call *modified Brompton's,* or simply *pain mixture,* which substitutes another narcotic (often methadone or morphine) for the heroin. Phenothiazine is included to counteract the nausea sometimes induced by oral morphine and for its tranquilizing effect; the alcohol helps prevent the growth of microorganisms in the syrupy base.

Medication is given on a regular schedule, not on a p.r.n. (whenever necessary) basis. This approach is used because the pain is always present, and allowing pain to increase substantially before giving the next dose would be counterproductive. The patient may be allowed to increase or decrease the dose in light of the severity of the pain and the desirability of being alert and active.

Using this approach, most patients can be kept relatively pain-free and free of symptoms of drug dependence. Though some physiologic drug dependence may be present, it is of minimal concern since there is no expectation that the person can be free of the need for drugs. Because the mixtures are given orally, the patient is saved the prospect of repeated injections.

This approach can work only with a person who is conscious and able to take oral fluids. If severe nausea and vomiting are present, those conditions must be controlled before an oral pain mixture can be given.

At least one leading authority, Richard Twycross, opposes the use of mixtures, on the grounds

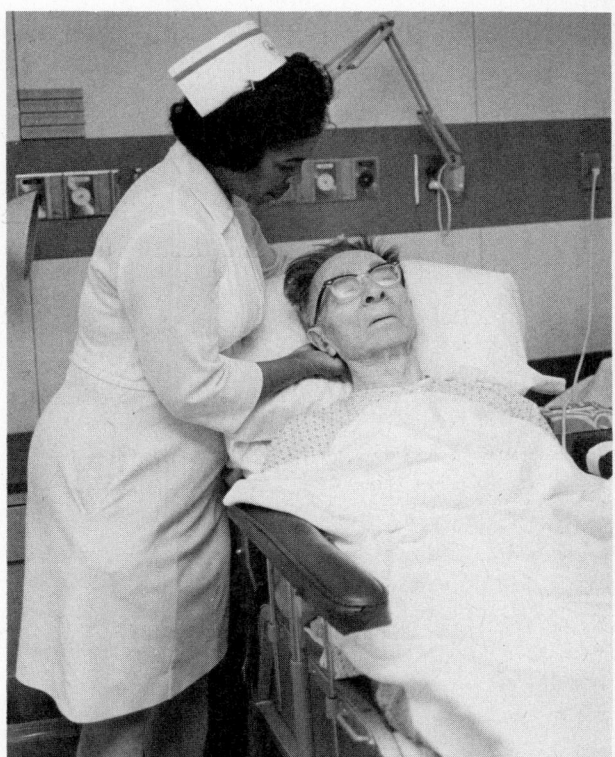

**Figure 26.7**
The nurse has much to offer the patient with terminal pain. (Russ Kinne/Danbury Hospital/Photo Researchers, Inc.)

that they make it harder to adjust dosages of individual drugs. He suggests, instead, that each individual drug be given separately. Twycross also recommends that the medication schedule never be adjusted but that the dosage be adjusted as needed to achieve the desired level of pain relief. Basic to his approach is the selection of a single drug for pain relief. This drug would be given every four hours around the clock, even waking the patient if necessary. Additional drugs (tranquilizers, antiemetics, mood elevators, and the like) can be given as needed on separate schedules. He also strongly recommends the addition of aspirin to the regimen when bone pain is present.

Of course, the patient with terminal pain also needs all the other skilled care the nurse is able to provide. Medications must not be viewed as lessening the patient's need for personalized care. Whether it is a simple physical act, such as straightening wrinkled bedclothes, or the immeasureable value of the presence of another human being, the nurse has much to offer the patient with terminal pain.

## Evaluating Pain-Relief Measures

The result of nursing intervention to relieve pain must be evaluated at each point. The most effective way to evaluate pain relief is to ask the patient whether the pain has diminished. Be specific in your questions. Often the pain will still be present but of less intensity; activity may again be possible, and the patient may feel less distressed by the pain.

Another important way to evaluate pain relief is to observe the patient's behavior. If you identified the presence of pain by assessing nonverbal behavior, look to see if that behavior has changed. Is the facial expression more relaxed? Is the body less tense? Is the patient willing to move about?

In order to evaluate the effectiveness of a medication accurately, you need to know its expected effect and the time needed for it to work. For example, an injected narcotic might begin to take effect in ten minutes and reach its maximum effect within half an hour. An oral medication, on the other hand, might not begin to work for twenty to thirty minutes.

If the initial efforts at pain relief do not prove adequate, additional steps may need to be taken to make the patient more comfortable. If you conclude that the medication ordered is not effective, it may be necessary to consult with the physician. Whatever the situation, the patient will benefit from the knowledge that you care about his or her pain and are actively working to alleviate it.

## Conclusion

Pain is a complex phenomenon. In planning intervention for the relief of pain, you will find it useful to consider the various aspects of the total pain experience and to try to intervene as early as possible. Intervention is often more effective if it is multifaceted and aimed at more than one component of the pain.

Although medications to relieve pain are an important tool, they are by no means the only way of dealing with pain. The effective nurse carefully assesses the patient and brings to bear measures specially selected in light of the individual and nature of the problem.

## Care Study   A patient in pain

Jeff Brown, a student nurse, is assigned on Friday to care for Mr. Ralph Jarvis, who had a cholecystectomy (gall-bladder removal) on Tuesday morning. Mr. Brown is standing at the nursing station, checking the card index (Kardex), when the orderly walks up and says, "Mr. Jarvis needs a shot for pain."

Mr. Brown goes to Mr. Jarvis's room to make an assessment before planning intervention. He enters the room, introduces himself and explains his role, and then asks Mr. Jarvis to describe his pain. Mr. Jarvis says, "It's sharp and all across here," indicating his lower abdomen. Mr. Brown thinks about the surgery, the length of time since the surgery, and the patient's description of the pain, and then says, "Mr. Jarvis, it sounds to me as if you

may be having gas pains, which is usual this length of time after surgery, and the location of your pain indicates the same thing. Your doctor has ordered a 'return-flow enema' to relieve gas." Mr. Brown then explains the procedure. "I'll give you one right now and we'll see if it helps."

Mr. Brown performs the enema, and a large amount of gas is returned. After the procedure is over, he asks Mr. Jarvis how he feels. Mr. Jarvis replies, "Wow, that did the trick—I feel pretty good. I don't think I need that shot now."

Mr. Brown returns to the nursing station to record the entire process on Mr. Jarvis's chart.

## Study Terms

acupuncture
addiction
analgesia
anesthesia
ascending fibers
autonomic responses
behavior modification
Brompton's mixture (modified Brompton's mixture)
chordotomy
cutaneous (superficial) pain
dorsal column stimulator (D.C.S.)
expressive responses
"gate-control" theory
hypnosis
ischemia
neurogenic pain

pain cocktail (pain mixture)
pain impulse
pain interpretation
pain perception
pain reaction
pain receptor
pain response
pain threshold
phantom pain
placebo
radiating pain
referred pain
spinal anesthesia
stoicism
terminal pain
transcutaneous nerve stimulator (T.C.S. or T.N.S.)
visceral (internal) pain

## Learning Activities

1.  Recall an occasion when you experienced pain. List words to describe that pain.
2.  In a group meeting, take the words listed in Activity 1 and discuss their meaning to each per-

son in the group. Do the words have different meanings to different individuals?
3.  Write a brief paper on different cultural groups' attitudes toward pain.
4.  Prepare a case study of a patient with pain. Include your assessment, planning, implementation, and evaluation.

## References

Armstrong, M. E. "Acupuncture." *American Journal of Nursing* 72 (September 1972): 1582–1588.

Bellars, K. "You Have Pain? I Think This Will Help." *American Journal of Nursing* 70 (October 1970): 2143–2145.

Capp, L. A. "The Spectrum of Suffering." *American Journal of Nursing* 74 (March 1974): 491–495.

Goloskov, J. "Use of the Dorsal Column Stimulator." *American Journal of Nursing* 74 (March 1974): 506–507.

Janzen, E. "Relief of Pain: Prerequisite to the Care and Comfort of the Dying." *Nursing Forum* 13 (January 1974): 48–51.

Johnson, J. "Sensory and Distress Components of Pain." *Nursing Research* 23 (May–June 1974): 203–209.

Lauer, J. W. "Hypnosis in the Relief of Pain." *Medical Clinics of North America* 52 (January 1968): 217.

McCaffrey, M. "Intelligent Approach to Intractable Pain." *Nursing '73* 3 (November 1973): 26–32. Care study.

————. "Patients in Pain." *Nursing '73* 3 (June 1973): 41–50. Pictorial.

McCaffrey, M., and Moss, F. "Nursing Intervention for Bodily Pain." *American Journal of Nursing* 67 (June 1967): 1224–1227.

McLachlan, E. "Recognizing Pain." *American Journal of Nursing* 74 (March 1974): 496–497.

Melzack, R., and Wall, P. "Pain Mechanisms: A New Theory." *Science* 150 (November 1965): 970–979.

Pain. Part 1, Basic Concepts and Assessment. *American Journal of Nursing* 66 (May 1966): 1085–1108. Part 2, Rationale for Intervention. *American Journal of Nursing* 66 (June 1966): 1345–1368.

Schultz, N. V. "How Children Perceive Pain." *Nursing Outlook* 19 (1971): 670–673.

Siegele, D. S. "The Gate Control Theory." *American Journal of Nursing* 74 (March 1974): 498–502.

Turnbull, F. "Pain and Suffering in Cancer." *Canadian Nurse* 67 (August 1971): 28–30.

Wiley, L., ed. "Intractable Pain: How Nursing Care Can Help." *Nursing '74* 4 (September 1974): 54–59.

# Chapter 27
# Loss

## Objectives

After completing this chapter, you should be able to:

1. Briefly discuss the importance of hope, the family, the team approach, and support for care providers in care of the terminally ill.
2. Name the six stages of dying and give an example of how each might affect care.
3. Describe the physical, social, and psychological factors in care of the terminally ill.
4. Identify the special needs of children who are dying.
5. Discuss how euthanasia poses a dilemma for the nurse.
6. Describe nursing actions at the time of death that may help prepare the family for grieving.
7. Name the four stages of grief Engel has identified.
8. Compare normal and abnormal grief.
9. Specify ways the nurse can help survivors.
10. Briefly discuss the hospice approach to care of the terminally ill.

## Outline

Death is the ultimate and loneliest experience all human beings face. We are the only species aware of our own mortality, and this knowledge may bring not only loneliness and helplessness but also outright fear of annihilation. However, even these feelings can be accompanied by growth—a growth in perceptiveness leading to a feeling of relative contentment and acceptance. It is to these ends that we as nurses must direct our actions.

Asked why they have chosen nursing as a profession, most student nurses quickly and understandably reply that they wish to help people get well. We are a recovery-oriented society. Medicine is designed to cure, or at least to prolong life. Only recently has this stance begun to become less rigid. The subject of death and dying is being explored honestly, with the result that guidelines are being developed for those who interact with dying people and their families.

## Society and Death

In primitive societies, death was accepted as the natural conclusion to life. Death occurred daily in the life of the village, to animals and humans alike, usually within full view of members of the community. Observance of the loss was in direct proportion to the value of the deceased to the tribe: a young hunter or prestigious leader elicited an outpouring of grief not paralleled by grief for the elderly or even children. Except for those wounded on hunting expeditions or in accidents and worthy of salvage, dying people who could no longer feed themselves were rarely helped to eat; instead they were allowed to die.

In contemporary society, death is no longer visible, except on television and in the movies. Though it is not unusual to read about the death of thousands in a natural disaster as we sit comfortably in our living rooms, many people live their entire lives without viewing a dead person. Thus death is often depersonalized in our culture. That is, death is perceived as something abstract that happens only to others, and even thinking about it can be largely avoided.

## Who Is Dying?

The capacity of modern technology to prolong life far beyond the natural course of disease makes the classification of patients as dying less clear-cut than it once was. A troubling situation nurses frequently face is preparing psychologically for the impending loss of the patient and then watching him or her live on indefinitely, sometimes in pain and hopelessness, with the help of life-sustaining devices. Families face the same painful situations. Equally disturbing are patients who might be expected to respond to life-saving medical measures but who die suddenly when such measures are not forthcoming. And there are those with life-threatening conditions whom the nurse does not classify as dying but who are experiencing the same feelings and reactions as those close to death. In summary, the nurse must interact with each seriously ill patient by sharing his or her fears and cares and simultaneously living with uncertainty as to the patient's prognosis. This is a difficult task.

# Concepts Basic to Care

Before addressing specific aspects of care of the terminally ill, let us examine certain concepts basic to such care. Care planning should offer the patient *realistic hope* by providing for attainable short-term goals. Inclusion of the *family* as well as the patient in decision making is paramount. A *team effort* provides the best comprehensive care of the patient but sometimes proves difficult for professionals to whom this concept is unfamiliar. All team members should work together as colleagues, and no one member of the team should exercise control all the time. Lastly, *emotional support for care providers* allows them to discharge their feelings and recharge their energies so they can continue to offer the best of care.

## Realistic Hope

Of all human needs, perhaps none is more important than hope. Patients hope that their illnesses will be brief or their surgery successful. Disabled people hope for maintenance of function and mobility. Nurses share these hopes with their patients.

For terminal patients and their families, hope for long-term survival may not be realistic, but this does not mean that hope is lost. There are other things to hope for, such as a brief return home, a talk with a long-estranged loved one, a walk unaided to the dayroom, or a pain-free period of time with friends and family. Hope is contagious, as is hopelessness. If, as a care provider, you lose all hope, so do the patient and the family. Nurses are in the fortunate position of being able to turn hope into action; thus hope can be as sustaining as our nursing skill and creativity allow for. Maintaining the quality of the patient's life is the ultimate hope in nursing the terminally ill.

## The Family

The dying patient is losing family as well as everything and everyone he or she has ever loved. The family members in turn are losing one of themselves. As in any crisis, the members of a dying person's family relate to one another intensely. Because the impending loss is upsetting and may evoke old grievances, family disruption can occur. More commonly, families draw closer together and old grievances are forgotten in the immediacy of losing a family member. A caring nurse can facilitate communication among family members.

From the family, the patient needs affirmation of his or her importance to them and to be treated, until the last, as a contributing member of the group. The patient needs the family to share a review of what life has meant, considering both good times and bad. We shall consider this process, called a *life review*, in more detail later. The patient needs to grieve along with the family. And, finally, the patient needs to be assured that although his or her death will change the family in a significant way, the family will cope by continuing to share the loss.

## Team Effort

The most effective way of caring for terminally ill patients and their families is by making available to them an interdisciplinary team. Such teams, which are being used increasingly in the hospital setting and in home-care situations, usually consist of a physician, nurses, social workers, and a chaplain. There may also be a need for the services of other professionals, such as an occupational therapist, physical therapist, dietitian, or speech therapist. The needs of the patient and the family are by no means confined to medical and nursing needs but may also be of a social or spiritual nature. The patient and family are integral parts of the team and should play the foremost role in making decisions involving fundamental values and the circumstances surrounding death.

## Support for Care Providers

Until recently, little thought was given to the physical and emotional toll on those who care for

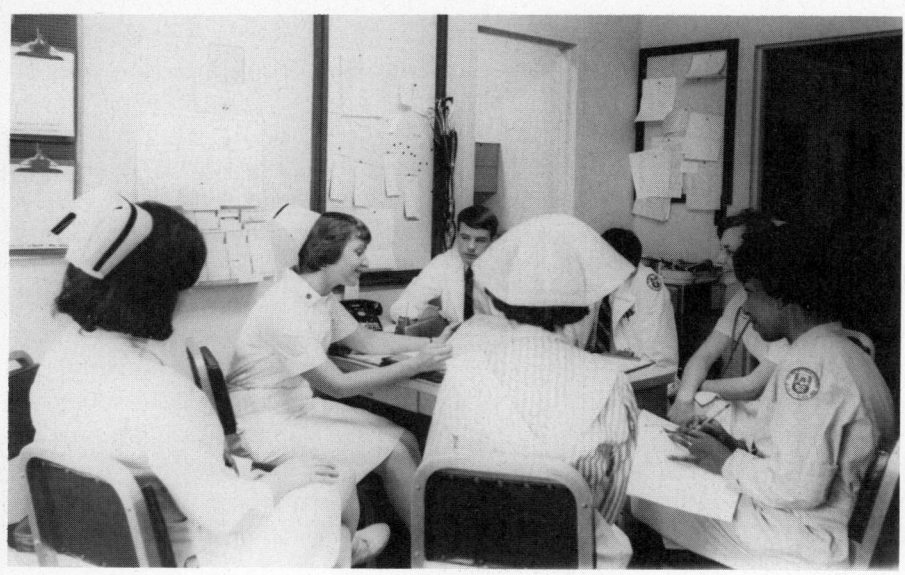

**Figure 27.1 An interdisciplinary team sharing thoughts and feelings**
Elizabeth Wilcox

the terminally ill. Now that care of the terminally ill has become a specialty within the practice of nursing, the *burnout* syndrome has been identified (Storlie, 1979). Burnout occurs because nurses are sensitive people who feel the loss of their patients deeply. This is as it should be. However, the experience of repeated losses can give rise to such signs of stress as fatigue, irritability, and insomnia. Some nurses have reported disruption of personal relationships.

In some facilities, nurses caring for dying patients regularly meet with a psychiatrist as a group to explore their feelings. On a more informal basis, staff nurses provide mutual support by recognizing each others' feelings and encouraging the sharing of loss with one another. Research is continuing on burnout among nurses who are repeatedly subject to high stress, including loss, in their work. Ways are being sought to minimize this syndrome among nurses and other professionals.

Though you may not, in practice, care exclusively for terminally ill patients, it is always important to recognize that feelings are healthy and to develop methods of coping with emotional stress. Taking time for pursuits you enjoy and talking with a peer or close friend (taking care to maintain confidentiality) are essential. As you share your feelings, you will develop a greater understanding of yourself and your personal philosophy about death.

## Stages of Dying

In the late sixties, Dr. Elisabeth Kübler-Ross identified five stages of dying, which are helpful as guidelines when caring for the terminally ill. These are stages of denial, anger, bargaining, depression, and acceptance. There is sometimes a sixth stage, disengagement. Not only the patient but also the family and care providers experience these stages, though not necessarily simultaneously. For example, at the same time the patient is sharing feelings about dying with the nurse in an open and realistic way, the family may be talking about taking the patient on a trip "as soon as she gets well."

Nurses—as observers, sharers, helpers, and supporters in the dying experience—must understand that not all patients pass sequentially through the various stages or experience every stage. It is not uncommon for a dying person to revert from apparent acceptance back into a state of depression. Bargaining may punctuate the dying process, only to be replaced by depression or anger. The family and members of the health team may in a sense accompany the patient through the stages of dying, sharing many of the patient's feelings.

Because each of these stages is a mechanism for coping, premature intervention is unwise. Only if the patient's outlook is interfering with necessary aspects of care and treatment, or if it is disrupting the family, should intervention take place. Any such intervention should be undertaken by a skilled person who can point out an alternative outlook and behavior. The patient should have the right to die in his or her own way. The uniqueness of the individual patient, in dying as well as in living, is an absolute principle in nursing care.

## Denial

During the stage of denial, the individual is consciously or unconsciously denying that something of serious consequence is occurring. This stage is that of "No, not me!" Denial usually lasts a relatively short time, primarily because events make the truth apparent and denial no longer possible. During this stage the patient may "doctor shop," request the repetition of certain tests, or flatly state that the test results are someone else's. Within cer-

tain limits, denial should not be contradicted but allowed to subside slowly as the patient gradually adjusts to the upsetting news.

## Anger

No other stage is as difficult for nurses to deal with as anger. This is the "Why me?" stage. It seems blatantly unfair to the patient that he or she has been "chosen" to die while so many others remain healthy. The feeling of anger becomes almost intolerable at times, and the health-care team may bear the brunt of it. The family is sometimes reprieved because the family's love makes such outpourings unacceptable to the patient. The physician may also escape anger, as the one person who may be able to help and whom the patient does not dare to alienate; sometimes, however, the physician is the target of anger.

In any case, the patient's anger is often focused on the nurse, taking the form of excessive demands or complaints about care. The nurse may be made very uncomfortable by feeling angry in return and regretting that the person will not recover so an appropriate response can be made. By marshaling your communication skills, firmness, and kindness, you can tell the patient you understand that he or she is seriously ill and angry about the consequent restrictions and that you would

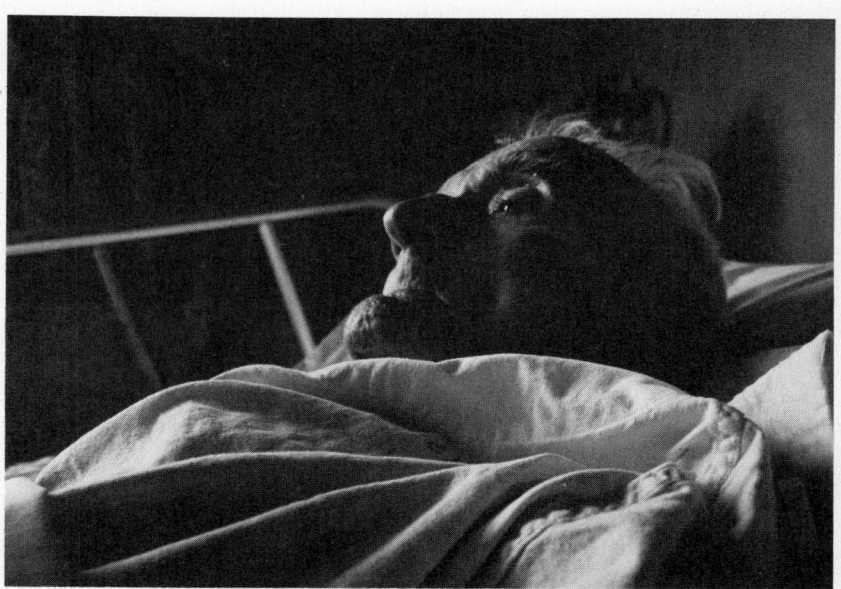

**Figure 27.2**
Death is the ultimate and loneliest experience all human beings face. (Frank Siteman/Stock, Boston)

like to provide the very best care. However, you can say, some limitations must be set so both your goals can be accomplished. Such a confrontation is not disconcerting to the patient, and at times a patient will express relief at being treated as a person who can still elicit feelings in others. "Clearing the air," in such instances, is very therapeutic.

## Bargaining

The third stage, bargaining, may be quite short, intermittent, or not overt. Often the patient bargains for time: "If I can only make it until my son's graduation. . . ." Occasionally a patient will say, "If only I were a better person. . . ." Bargaining is an attempt to postpone and can be helpful to the patient.

## Depression

When bargaining fails to delay the course of the illness or bring about a cure, impending death becomes a reality that can no longer be avoided psychologically. The sense of losing one's life, family, and total earthly environment is often accompanied by feelings of deep depression and profound sadness. To do your own "grief work" but remain close to the patient is a notable nursing achievement. Crying during this stage denotes awareness, and it is therefore inappropriate for the nurse and/or family to admonish the patient not to cry. The stage of depression may be lengthy

and in some patients does not lift. Ideally, the patient will pass through this stage to acceptance.

## Acceptance

Acceptance should not be confused with resignation (Kübler-Ross, 1969). It can be a time of contentment, a final sharing with close friends and family, and a conclusion of unfinished business. It is hoped by all that the pain is controlled and the struggle, which can be very exhausting, is almost over. The patient's circle of interest narrows, and attention is given only to events and people close to the patient. The family may need particular support during this period, for they may not have reached comparable acceptance of the loss.

## Disengagement

The period of acceptance, the final stage described by Dr. Kübler-Ross, is sometimes followed by a sixth stage that might be called disengagement. One frequently sees this phenomenon shortly before death occurs. The dying person may become very quiet, even withdrawn, but not necessarily sad. He or she wants to see only intimates or no one at all, is apathetic, and appears aware that the end is very near. A dying teenager said to his father, "Take the radio home, Dad, I won't be needing it anymore," and died within a few hours. The dying person has, in fact, passed beyond acceptance and said his or her goodbyes.

# Needs of the Terminally Ill Patient

The needs of the terminally ill are many. For purposes of planning, we shall address in turn the three major categories of needs—physical, social, and psychological—with the understanding that they overlap and have impact on one another and that each is as important as the others. Not all patients have needs in all three areas, but assessments must be made in each to ensure total care of the patient.

## Physical Needs

The physical changes that may accompany serious illness can understandably be very alarming to the patient and the family. The systems of the body are not functioning as they should. Deterioration means that death is approaching. The patient's body image is also changing, and accommodation to these changes is very difficult; sometimes patients refuse to look in mirrors or are reluctant to have visitors. Some patients strive to compensate with mental competence for physical deterioration. Reassurance that the person remains valuable and attractive is essential. The following physical problems are common among dying patients.

## Pain Management

Although no attempt is made to assign priorities to physical problems, pain management must come first in assessment and treatment. Without good management, pain influences and interrupts all aspects of a relationship. As a dying woman put it, "Pain consumes you." Chronic pain is different from other pain in that it has no beginning and no end. Management of chronic terminal pain and the use of pain mixtures are discussed in Chapter 26.

Pain has different meanings for different individuals. It may mean that the disease is progressing, that "things are getting worse." That death is impending is an understandable interpretation, and occasionally a welcome one, if the illness has been long and painful. But pain is ordinarily unwelcome to the dying, destroying hope and draining the individual of energy that could be used to relate to family and friends. About 40 percent of dying patients experience severe pain during the course of their illnesses. One study shows that the pain can be adequately controlled in 95 percent of these patients (Lamerton, 1973).

Just as one's previous experiences with death affect one's dying, past experiences with pain affect response to pain. For example, a patient who has experienced only infrequent moderate pain, which has been satisfactorily controlled, is unlikely to be very fearful that pain will get out of control. On the other hand, the patient who has had severe uncontrolled pain fears it and lacks trust that it can be controlled.

Managing the pain of the terminally ill is a very important component of care planning. Drug addiction is uncommon in the terminal patient suffering severe pain, and large dosages of drugs are tolerated without bringing about psychological or physiological dependence. The patient should be given liberal amounts of pain medications so as to be made as comfortable as possible until death.

Tranquilizers are often prescribed in conjunction with narcotics, primarily to relieve anxiety.

Medication should be administered before the pain becomes intense and more difficult to control. Oral pain medications are given to terminal patients routinely, "by the clock."

The objective of pain control is to anticipate and eliminate pain and to erase the memory of it. Pain is controlled best if the medication is given every four hours, even throughout the night. If the dosage proves inadequate, it should be increased, rather than shortening the time intervals (Twycross, 1979). No dying person should ever have to ask to have pain relieved. Almost all patients can remain on oral preparations until twenty-four to forty-eight hours before death and can be kept relatively pain-free with proper management. The pain of dying is very real, directly related to the pathology of its cause, and aggravated by anxiety. It must never be treated lightly. Pain management also involves finding time to listen and to allow the patient to talk freely about his or her fears.

## Nausea

Nausea may have a variety of causes. Systemic reactions and local pathology can both cause nausea and vomiting. Nausea is also a common side effect of treatment, such as chemotherapy (the use of drugs to combat cancer) and irradiation.

Several measures may be used to counteract nausea. Foods of the patient's choice should be offered in small amounts and at frequent intervals. Antiemetic drugs, such as the prochlorperazine group (Compazine, Marezine), can be given approximately thirty minutes before chemotherapy or irradiation treatments to prevent the onset of nausea. Cannabis (marijuana), though controversial, is being accepted in some medical circles for treating nausea in terminal patients and for reducing intraocular pressure in patients suffering from glaucoma; its antiemetic effects are impressive (Andrysiak, 1979). Rest, quiet, and diversion are also helpful in treating nausea.

## Edema and Skin Changes

In the later stages of disease, most patients experience some skin change and/or edema. If the liver or pancreas is involved, the skin may take on a yellowish tinge and the patient is said to be jaundiced. This color change appears first in the sclera (white portion) of the eyes and then becomes more generalized. If itching is a problem for the jaundiced patient, special drugs can be administered along with soothing baths. *Edema*, the presence of fluid in the interstitial tissues, may be detected first in the upper buttocks and later in the lower extremities, particularly the ankles. If edema becomes generalized in the later stages of illness, the nurse must remember that the tissues cannot readily absorb medications by injection. The patient with edema may prefer longsleeved garments for the sake of appearance. For females, light makeup often elevates mood by improving appearance.

## Distention

Abdominal distention, which may be a final symptom of terminal disease, is particularly distressing for the patient since it causes bloating and can also interfere with breathing and eating. Distention may be caused by gas, large amounts of feces due to intestinal immobility, free-floating fluid in the abdominal cavity (ascites), or tumor mass. Regardless of the cause, conservative nursing measures are often helpful. These include positioning the patient high in the bed and encouraging ambulation. If the cause is gas, a nasogastric tube may afford some relief, and the use of suppositories may bring about defecation. If the cause of the distention is fluid in the abdominal cavity, some physicians choose to perform a paracentesis (introducing a large needle into the abdomen to withdraw the fluid) to make the patient more comfortable. Paracentesis is at best only a temporary measure since the fluid usually reaccumulates; it also depletes the patient of needed protein, which is a major constituent of the fluid.

## Constipation

All the drugs used to control chronic terminal pain cause some degree of constipation. If the dosage is high, the constipation may be profound and impaction is not uncommon (see Chapter 22).

Such nursing actions as increasing fluid intake and roughage in the diet and promoting ambulation and exercise are all very helpful. If, for medical reasons, the patient cannot pursue these actions, constipation can become a serious problem. The patient feels both psychologically and physically unwell, since regular elimination is a component of our concept of wellness.

You may have to resort to the use of suppositories and enemas to relieve the constipated patient. Laxatives are often prescribed as a preventive measure along with drugs for pain.

## Intestinal Obstruction

Obstruction, which may occur in cases of abdominal or pelvic tumor, makes the patient unable to eat or drink without pain and cramping. If the obstruction occurs early in the illness, surgical intervention is usually undertaken. The physician bypasses the obstruction or, if possible, removes the tumor mass that is occluding the passage. If the patient's physical condition contraindicates surgical intervention, a nasogastric tube is sometimes used to relieve the gas and distention caused by the obstruction. If the obstruction occurs very late in the disease process, near death, a treatment being used with increasing frequency in the United States is to give the patient diphenoxylate hydrochloride (Lomotil), a drug that stops motility of the bowel. The patient becomes comfortable and can take small amounts of fluids, and the nasogastric tube may be avoided.

## Respiratory Secretions

Some dying patients develop a buildup of respiratory secretions, which produces in the final hours of life what has been called a "death rattle." This phenomenon can be more disturbing to the family than to the patient. Oxygen is sometimes given but usually has little effect since respiratory exchange may be compromised. However, this measure too may comfort the family.

Suctioning can increase secretions because of irritation and should be used prudently. An increasingly common treatment is to administer large dosages of atropine (as much as 1 mg), a drug that dries secretions, during the final hours.

The pulse may increase and the face become mildly flushed, but these effects are harmless.

## Social Needs

Most patients who discover they have a disease from which they will not recover, experience some degree of social isolation. A primary reason for this isolation is that some healthy people feel uncomfortable and threatened by contact with people they know are dying. The feeling "It could be me" is disturbing, and we may feel uncertain about what to say or how to act. This behavior is unfortunate, since it occurs precisely when the patient most needs closeness to family and friends.

In the hospital, dying patients are often placed far from the nursing station in an unconscious attempt to minimize contact. Time studies have shown that nurses spend less time in the rooms of dying patients than in those of patients who will recover (Glaser and Strauss, 1968).

The degree of isolation a terminal patient experiences largely depends on his or her pre-illness life style. If the patient has always been outgoing and enjoyed strong support from family and friends, such support usually continues. For a patient who has been a quiet, private person, isolation can be profound. Sometimes the reverse is true: a popular, outgoing patient may frighten off social contacts, while an introspective person may know better how to cope with loneliness and isolation. The nurse may become close to the patient when others find closeness too painful, and the nurse's caring can alleviate the patient's feelings of being totally alone.

## Psychological Needs

### Independence

Some people find dependence—reliance on someone else to meet most of their needs—very depressing. As nurses, we should try to maximize the independence of dying patients by encouraging them to make decisions about care and to participate in their own care. For example, the patient should decide how far he or she is able to walk and whether or not a visit to the local library is feasible. Too often the family, in an effort to protect the patient from stress, excludes him or her from family decisions. Such behavior is a disservice to the patient.

## Productivity

In conjunction with the need for independence, terminal patients also need to feel productive and should be encouraged to continue their jobs as long as possible. One dying woman continued to fold letters soliciting funds for a charitable organization until shortly before she died. An elderly man reported to the occupational therapy department in his wheelchair each morning to work on a doll house for his granddaughter; three days after gluing on the chimney, he peacefully died. Nurses should appreciate the need for productivity since it is the essence of nursing care.

## Communication

What should the patient be told? Whether or not to tell the patient the extent and prognosis of the illness is up to the physician. Interviews with dying people reveal that most know they are dying. The kindest and most reasonable approach on the part of the physician is to reveal whatever the patient wants and is willing to know, which varies from patient to patient. Nurses often find themselves in the uncomfortable position of not knowing exactly what the patient and family have been told. It is appropriate to ask the attending physician what information has been shared with the patient and the family. Experience in interacting with dying people will enable you to discern how much the patient knows or is willing to know about the diagnosis.

Professionals are sometimes uncomfortable talking with the dying. One social worker wrote, "I know he wanted to talk to me. . . . The patient knew and I knew, but as he saw my desperate attempts to escape, he took pity on me and kept to himself what he wanted to share with another human being. And so he died and did not bother me" (Kübler-Ross and Warshaw, 1978).

Nurses often express the fear that, if the patient asks a direct question, they "won't know what to

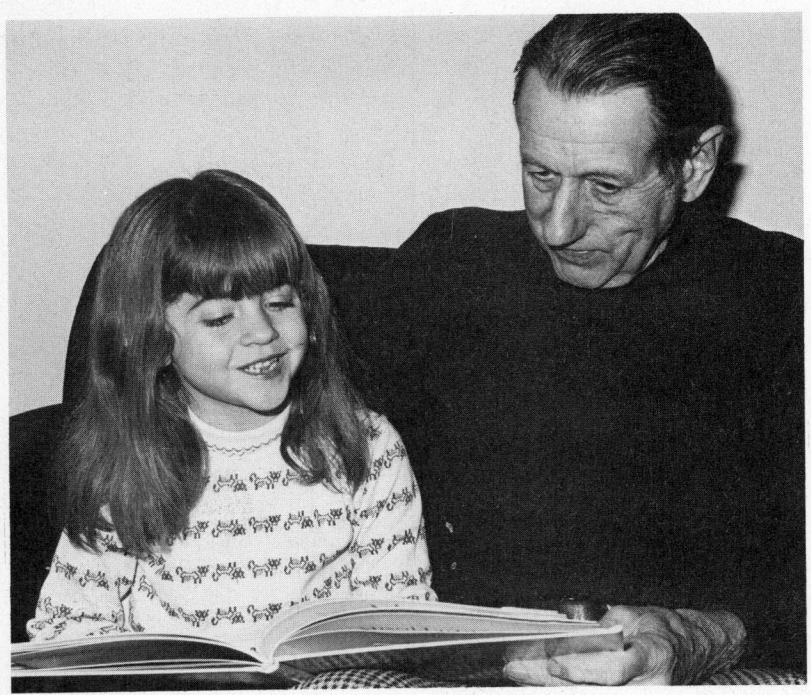

**Figure 27.3 Enjoying the last days of life**
Lester V. Bergman & Assoc., Inc.

say.'' Such direct questions are fairly infrequent. Although each case is unique, certain guidelines for communicating with the dying can be offered.

Probably the most valuable thing the nurse can do is to plan sufficient time to sit with the patient and listen undisturbed. It has been all too common for nurses to enter the patient's room only to perform a task and then leave immediately after completing it, fearful that the patient will confront them about the illness. Keep in mind that, even with very critical patients, you do not know whether or when they will die. Thus it is very risky, for your own peace of mind as well as the patient's, to make rigid predictions. It is far better, if the occasion arises, to let the patient know you understand that he or she is seriously ill. Nurses are often so concerned about *giving* information that they fail to simply *listen* to the patient, which is the essence of therapeutic interaction with the dying. Patients really do not expect their care givers to have the answers to their philosophical questions, but they do appreciate someone who will explore the profound ''whys'' with them.

Losing a loved one is a heart-wrenching experience for the family and can be nearly unbearable in cases of extended terminal illness when the goodbyes seem never-ending. If the family is unable to communicate or be ''in touch'' with the dying person, the consequence can be true isolation.

Long after the patient accepts and wants to talk about dying, the family may deny it. Family members may talk endlessly about the patient coming home. Or they may keep all conversation superficial, saying nothing that is meaningful to the patient. Visits become shorter. One young mother always brought her young children, who naturally became bored and rambunctious, necessitating her early departure from the bedside of her dying mother. An even more extreme example was the mother of an eight-year-old boy dying of leukemia. The boy was asking for his mother and several phone calls were made, all unsuccessful. Finally she said sadly, ''Don't you understand? I simply *can't* come.'' With the support of the nurse, many families are able to maintain contact with their loved one, finding out for themselves that patients do not talk about dying at great length but only want to communicate their feelings on occasion to those who mean the most to them.

## Strengths Instead of Weaknesses

All too often nurses focus on the patient's weaknesses, since they are the source of the patient's problems. However understandable, such an emphasis can be detrimental to the spirits of the dying patient. Every person retains many strengths until the final hours of life, and emphasizing those strengths is essential. If, for example, the patient expresses sadness and discouragement about no longer being able to drive a car, we can reflect with him about his ability to take short walks and enjoy outings. It is important not to deny or trivialize a patient's statements in our efforts to emphasize the positive. One patient, too weak to write letters to close friends, was able to use a tape recorder to send caring messages; it was the nurse who suggested doing so and procured the recorder and tapes. When writing a care plan for a terminally ill patient, the nurse is encouraged to maximize strengths in this way.

### Life Review

Every dying patient grieves for loss of self. As part of the grieving process, most feel a need to review their lives. The family too may feel a need to reflect on the past with the patient. They may look at photographs together. This process appears to be a way of "letting go," giving meaning to death, and making certain one will be remembered.

Because the nurse is likely to have known the patient only a short time and to be an objective listener, the patient may find the nurse a particularly valuable participant in life. The reviewing process is also valuable for the nurse, who thus gets to know the patient more fully. The process of life review tends to have the beneficial effect of eliciting *anticipatory grief*, or grieving before the actual death.

### Planning Death Rites

The patient may or may not feel a need to participate in planning his or her funeral or memorial service. Many patients express a real need to do so as a completion or resolution of their own grieving. Making such plans is a clear expression of acceptance on the part of the patient. One woman, a mountain climber, planned a memorial service consisting solely of beautiful music accompanied by slides of the patient, smiling, at the summit of a mountain. Her family and friends found this personal remembrance extremely moving. You may be fortunate enough to be asked by the patient to participate in these plans, such as by contacting a member of the clergy or close friends.

## The Death of a Child

Children die of many causes: congenital defects, injury, suicide, cancer, and other diseases of the major systems of the body. It is painful to contemplate children dying, and it takes a very special nursing team to provide the support the child and the family need. Though it is beyond the scope of this chapter to deal in depth with a child's death, some observations are in order.

A child's conception of death depends on how old he or she is. A very young child has not developed a concept of death as we understand it but is aware of being ill and of the threat of separation from those who love him or her. This separation anxiety is the focus of sensitive care of young children who are dying.

Every effort should be made to include the family in planning and providing care and to encourage them to be with the child as much as possible. Urge family members to share this commitment so that the child's brothers and sisters are not neglected. Indeed, the other children should be made welcome in the hospital so they too can better understand the illness and eventual loss.

At about age eight or nine, the child begins to understand the finality of death. A dying child of this age or older may exhibit anger, regression, withdrawal, anxiety, and sadness. Children who have learned to associate being hurt or punished with being bad may harbor feelings of guilt; this response is particularly characteristic of young

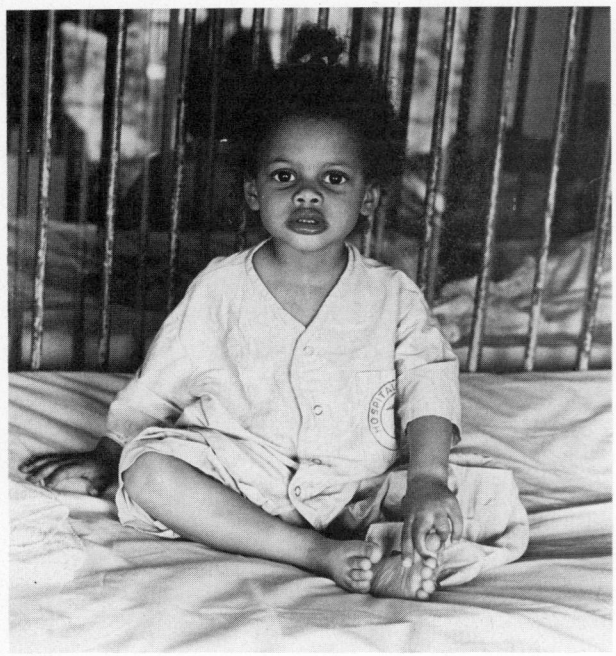

children. Letting the child talk out these feelings with a trusted staff member is very helpful. It must be emphasized to the child that being sick is not a punishment for bad behavior and that family and friends recognize that the child is good. As with adults, realistic hope should never be taken away. Peers, teachers, and friends of the family may also need support from the nursing staff. Because it is hard to know what to say under such difficult circumstances, the families of terminally ill children can be inadvertently isolated.

Children, including teenagers, who have the support of a loving family and a sensitive, caring team, approach death with amazing openness, honesty, and acceptance. Nothing is so sad, yet so inspiring.

**Figure 27.4**
Children often face death with openness and honesty.
(Anna Kaufman Moon/Stock, Boston)

## Euthanasia

No current ethical issue except abortion is of more immediate concern to nurses than *euthanasia*, which means "peaceful death." There are two kinds of euthanasia: active (positive), which is the use of toxic substances or other methods to end life; and passive (negative), which is the withdrawal of or decision not to use extraordinary means to prolong life. Active euthanasia is legally murder. Public sentiment, as well as that of the medical community, appears to be growing in support of

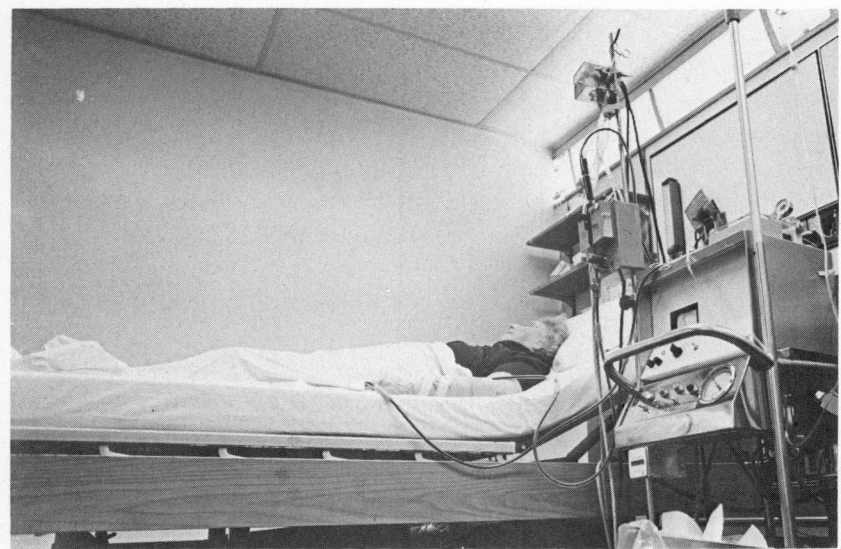

**Figure 27.5 Modern technology can prolong life.**
Frank Siteman/Stock, Boston

negative euthanasia, which is, in fact, practiced. Local medical societies, the Catholic Church, and many other religious denominations have spoken out against the dehumanization brought about by the use of extraordinary means when there is no reasonable hope of recovery. This issue relates directly to that of "death with dignity." In our recovery-oriented zeal, do we on occasion deprive dying patients of their dignity? This is a searching question for nurses, and far too complicated an issue for absolute answers to suffice. Among the questions that must be answered are: What are extraordinary means? What do the physician, family, and patient see as appropriate? Nurses must be true to themselves. No nurse should participate in any decision or practice he or she considers ethically unacceptable.

Several states have enacted natural-death acts. These laws, whose titles vary from state to state, allow a person, before illness or disability sets in, to declare their wishes with regard to the use of heroic or extraordinary measures in the event they are determined to be incapable of recovery and are deteriorating. There continues to be legal and medical controversy over such legislation.

## The Death Event

However long-expected and emotionally prepared-for, the actual death of the patient may be difficult to accept. Whether the moment of death is sad but memorable or painful and distressing is, to some degree, influenced by your care as a nurse.

Some people close to the dying patient are likely to feel a deep need to be present at the moment of death. Their presence allows for a decisive, final letting-go and for the beginning of a new phase of grief that will eventually be resolved. Every effort should be made by the nursing staff to honor these wishes. Families frequently say that they have been very comforted by a nurse who talked with them about the death and stayed with them during the final moments. Because most people in our society have not witnessed a death and thus feel some fear, the nurse can explain what it might be like: that death usually comes quietly and that the patient is often unresponsive and pain-free but probably able to hear. Everyone should be aware that the dying person's hearing may be intact and that they should speak with respect and say only what would be appropriate for the person to hear.

The children of the family should also be allowed, if the family wishes, to share the natural end of life. Their presence should depend, of course, on their prior preparation as well as their relationship to the dying person.

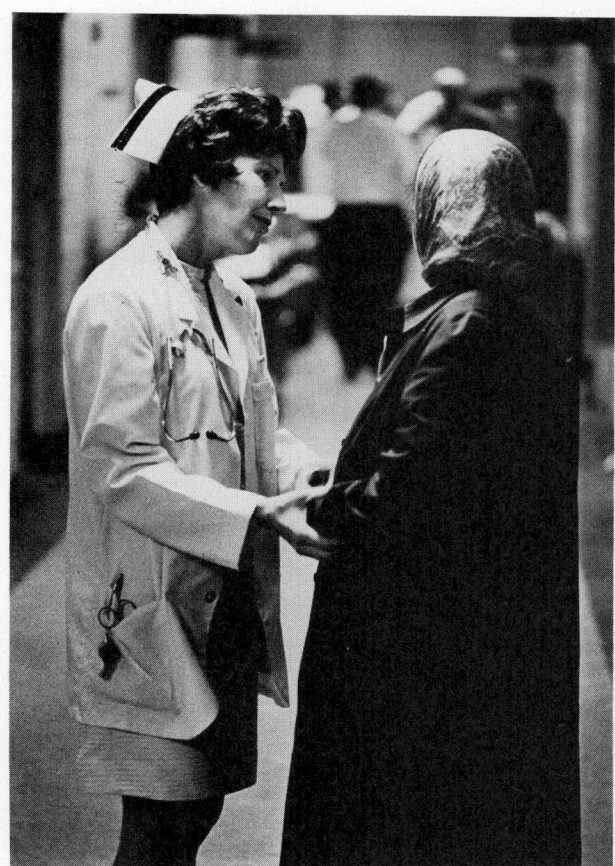

**Figure 27.6**
Family members need nursing support at the time of death. (Cary Wolinsky/Stock, Boston)

Viewing the body in the care setting is becoming more widespread as a way of helping families through the grieving process. After caring for the body, the nurse may want to join the family and others in visiting or sitting with the body.

Confrontation with the body is a healthy part of the grieving process. It sharpens the reality of death. Some families, however, prefer to view the body later at a funeral home or not at all. Nurses should respect the rights and wishes of all those involved.

The health-care team grieves together with the family and others who were close to the patient. Crying denotes awareness of the loss. Nurses and physicians often weep with the family.

## Death Care

*Death care*, the cleansing and preparation of the body after death, may be as simple or as detailed as the hospital requires. It is best to check the procedure of the facility where you practice. After the patient is pronounced dead by the physician, usual practice is that all equipment is discontinued, clean dressings are applied, teeth and eyeglasses are sent with the body, and valuables are signed for and given to the nearest relative. It is a nursing responsibility to see that the body leaves the unit properly and with dignity. For a description of the tasks and procedures involved in caring for the body, consult Module 17, "Postmortem Care."

## The Grief of the Survivors

Life is, among other things, a series of losses: loss of a prize in school, loss of a desired position in one's working life, loss of a relationship due to divorce, and so on. Again, how one has coped with previous losses largely determines how one copes with the loss of a beloved person.

That loss can also foster creative energies is attested to by the Taj Mahal, built as a memorial to a dead wife, and Igor Stravinsky's lovely Symphonies for Wind Instruments, composed to commemorate the death of the composer Debussy. Finding some meaning in loss can diminish the pain. Though survivorship is difficult, many experience a new surge of inner strength.

## The Stages of Grief

Grief is not exclusive to death. It is a healthy response to other losses as well. This is an important point for nurses. The elderly stroke patient with a flaccid and useless arm grieves. The woman who loses a breast to cancer grieves. Hospitalized children separated from their parents grieve. The man who is losing his sight grieves. The relationship between loss and body image is discussed in Chapter 29.

The stages of grief are not very different from the stages of dying, since in dying we grieve for ourselves. A number of writers have described the stages of grief, most in fairly similar terms. Engel (1964) outlined four stages: shock and disbelief, developing awareness, restitution, and resolution.

## Shock and Disbelief

Shock can accompany expected death as well as sudden death. Nurses are sometimes surprised when a family that has long expected a loved one to die expresses disbelief at the time of the death. We should understand that this is a normal stage of grief. Sometimes people have to disbelieve before they can believe. This stage may recur days later, when a family member may say, "I still can't believe this actually happened." Quiet support is needed during this period.

## Developing Awareness

The unconscious mind, functioning protectively, allows painful reality to enter consciousness gradually. This mechanism explains why some people do not cry until some time after a death. As aware-

ness becomes more complete, the survivors often feel fear, abandonment, or deep depression. Such depression is a painful but normal reaction and should not be treated lightly. This is a time to touch and be close to the survivor. The nurse should convey understanding that this is a very difficult and sad time. Reassurances that "tomorrow will be better" ring hollow and are unhelpful. Letting the survivors share their feelings of rejection and depression and move through these feelings is of real value.

## Restitution

*Restitution* is recognition of the death. Formal observance of the death may take the form of a funeral or memorial service, or a simple gathering of friends and family to share memories of the deceased. Some form of restitution is important to complete the grieving process. Death counselors report that families that abstain from any type of gathering, thereby denying themselves and others an opportunity to focus on the loss, do not come to resolution as soon or as smoothly as families that grieve more openly.

## Resolution

*Resolution* is sometimes referred to as *replacement*. This term is by no means intended to suggest that

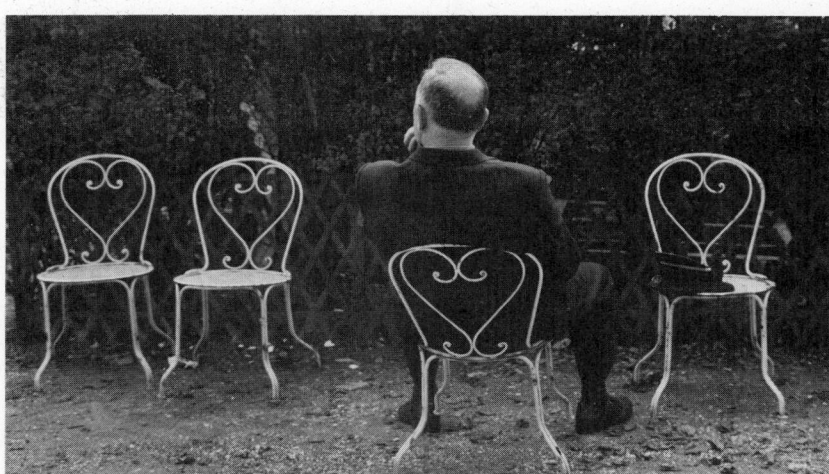

**Figure 27.7**
Replacement is often difficult for the elderly. (Gabor Demjen/Stock, Boston)

the loved one can be replaced. Its meaning is that the survivors need to find replacements, different from what has been lost, in their lives. For example, a large number of widowed people return to school; some remarry, and others make career changes. Parkes writes of an aspect of resolution called "the search," during which the survivor seeks out the deceased. Repetitive dreams of the deceased may occur, or the survivor may suddenly see someone who resembles the dead person and fleetingly but piercingly hope that he or she is still alive.

Resolution is most difficult for the elderly. Although steps such as remarriage or entering an educational program are certainly possible, many elderly people do not view these as options. A large proportion of elderly have spent forty or fifty years in a traditional marriage in which the woman did not work outside the home and the man did not perform routine household tasks. The death of one partner thus requires an enormous adjustment to the loss. Also, the restitution process may be hampered by real or perceived limitations on the elderly person's options: remarriage or returning to school, for example, may not be desired or feasible. The literature on widowhood reports that the death rate of surviving spouses within six to twelve months of the death is higher than that of the same age group in the general population. Nurses who recognize the particular dilemma of the elderly survivor can help provide the special support and counseling that may be needed.

## Recognizing Normal and Abnormal Grief

Nurses usually spend more time with the family and friends of the terminal patient than do other members of the care team. This proximity represents an opportunity to assess grieving. Though guidance for the person experiencing abnormal grief is the province of a trained counselor, assessment by the nurse can be of considerable value. To assess appropriately, you should be familiar with normal and abnormal grief reactions.

### Normal Grief

Hofling and Leininger (1960) compare the experience of normal grief to a ship that has lost its anchor in a heavy sea. The grieving person must put aside other things for a time and attempt to right the floundering ship. A substitute anchor is found and the sea also calms. It is not unusual for much of the grieving process to occur even before the patient is biologically dead. The end of the relationship, due to coma or disengagement, may trigger the grief mechanism. During the period of bereavement, the nurse may note the survivor acting more dependent, taking on symptoms or manner-

isms of the deceased, needing to talk about the deceased, and gradually refocusing attention on reality. Such phrases as "the way he would have wanted me to be" and "carrying on for her" are commonplace. All these are normal reactions to grief. It may be said that grieving has taken place satisfactorily when the survivor can remember the deceased comfortably, recalling both the pleasures and the disappointments of the relationship.

### Abnormal Grief

It is important to recognize incomplete or abnormal coping in order to be able to provide help or possibly to refer the person to a grief counselor. Extreme exaggerations of the normal grief process, such as dependence to the point of nonfunctioning, persistent symptoms or mannerisms of the deceased, and constant dreams or even hallucinations of the deceased, all constitute unsuccessful coping and may indicate a need for help. Disturbances of the digestive tract, insomnia, heavy sighing, pacing, and unresponsiveness to others are other signs to watch for.

# Caring for Survivors

In addition to the actions we have already mentioned, there are other measures nurses can take to help the survivors of a loss.

## Informing the Survivors

If the family was not present at the time of death and has not yet been informed by the physician, the nurse can help prepare for news of the loss. The environment in which word is received should not be amid the general confusion of the unit; a quiet room, chapel, or comfortably furnished conference room may be suitable. It is helpful to arrange for coffee and comfortable chairs for all. You may ask a member of the clergy to be present if you know this to be the wish of the family.

It is best if all family members are present so that news of the death can be given to all at the same time, preventing possible misinterpretation and allowing for family members to comfort and support one another.

## Cultural and Religious Factors

The religious and cultural background of the family must be taken into consideration: different religions and cultures grieve in different ways, and comfort to the family should be foremost in the mind of the nurse (see Chapter 5).

## Responding to Anger

Grieving family members occasionally express anger at the nursing staff and physician. The nurse should recognize that such accusations are usually expressions of guilt and grief and should be treated as such; they should not be taken personally. It is more helpful to the family for the nurse not to accept misplaced or unjustified anger. This can be conveyed by saying something like, "I can understand your angry feelings, since this must be a very difficult time for you." A reply such as this very often elicits an apology and tears.

## Supporting Constructive Changes

During the grieving period, the survivor may make a frantic attempt to regain control of life by means of hasty decisions, such as selling a beloved home, and may turn to the nurse for counsel. The nurse can be most helpful by trying to refocus the survivor's thoughts on the everyday changes that must take place rather than major ones that might be regretted later. Major decisions should be delayed. Realistic and constructive adaptive changes in the lives of the survivors should be supported, but it is not up to the nurse to suggest such changes.

## Touch

Perhaps the most meaningful gesture the nurse can offer a survivor is touch. At a time when words seem inadequate, a steady arm, a gentle hand, or a meaningful hug expresses care and shared feelings.

# Hospice

To many people in our country, the word *hospice* is becoming a familiar term. It represents a philosophy of care and a system for delivering care to the terminally ill and their families.

Hospices offer both inpatient and outpatient care of the terminally ill. Their origins can be traced to small shelters for the injured, ill, and infirm established along the routes of the Crusades, and hospices are still widespread throughout Great Britain and Europe. The hospice movement has spread to the United States and Canada, where several hundred active and ambitious hospice programs are in varying stages of development.

## The Philosophy of Hospice Care*

In general, the foremost goals of hospice care are to foster and support patients' rights to self-determination and control over the last stages of their lives and to assist patients and families before death occurs and to provide follow-up care for the family during bereavement. Many hospices also provide support and education for those involved in terminal care, including professionals, family members, and friends.

## The National Hospice Organization (NHO)

In an effort to coordinate the development of hospices in the United States, the National Hospice Organization was established in 1978; its central office is near the nation's capital in Vienna, Virginia. According to the NHO bylaws, the organization has four main purposes:

1. To promote the principles and concept of hospice care for the terminally ill and their families
2. To act as a clearinghouse for the dissemination of information and ideas to groups and individuals dedicated to the hospice concept
3. To develop and promote educational projects for professionals and the public focusing on the concepts of hospice care
4. To oversee legislation relevant to hospice development.

Inherent in the general goals of the organization is a commitment toward establishing and promoting standards for high-quality care.

*Based on Hospice of Seattle.

## The Interdisciplinary Hospice Team

Hospice care is provided by an interdisciplinary team composed of physicians, nurses, social workers, chaplains, volunteers, and professionals in related disciplines. Trained volunteers are an essential element of hospice care, and their importance cannot be overemphasized. Volunteers perform in a variety of roles, offering patients recreation and companionship and sometimes performing tasks and errands patients cannot accomplish by themselves. One objective of the team is to maintain the patient at home as long as the patient and family wish. To accomplish this requires the availability of a support team twenty-four-hours a day; the members of the team are on call on a rotating basis. The patient and the family together are considered the unit of care. Whether the patient is in a hospital, a hospice, or at home, communication among the team, the patient, and family is never interrupted. Expert symptom management is central to hospice care.

## Care Options

Hospice programs offer alternative types of care and care settings, and many models have been developed. Some offer home care as well as inpatient care. Some hospices have special clinics where outpatients, their families, and the staff can share concerns. Some programs are developing day-care services, which provide a full day of physical, occupational, recreational, and medical management, as needed, as well as nutritional advice and other services. Some hospices with inpatient units offer respite care, which is short-term inpatient care designed to provide special attention to a patient's specific needs or a rest for the family members who have been caring for the patient at home.

## Bereavement Counseling

A unique aspect of hospice care is the provision of bereavement counseling from the time of the team's first encounter with the patient and family until one year or more after the death. Bereavement contacts continue until a level of satisfactory resolution has taken place.

Hospice care provides the nurse opportunities for a broadly expanded role. It requires special training, often given by hospice organizations. Assessing and assigning priorities to care is very different from traditional nursing. Emphasizing the quality of life, rather than cure, requires some adaptations of what we have learned. For example, rather than carefully describing chest sounds, the hospice nurse focuses on what the patient sees as a problem and how it is affecting his or her life.

Hospice care allows the nurse to develop and apply new skills in bereavement counseling and understanding of family dynamics. The nurse also grows through the experience of loss, learning the wider meaning of care, growing close to families, and developing the inner strength to terminate that relationship when it is no longer needed and to move to new experiences.

## Conclusion

Nursing the dying, while certainly sad, is not without its satisfactions. A long-term relationship with a dying person can be deeply meaningful for the nurse. Each patient dies in his or her own way, and some dying patients are examples of human beings at their finest. The dying person who talks less about dying than about living can be a rare and treasured experience for the nurse.

Care of the dying and the management of grief have rightfully come into prominence during the last few years. If we could choose, children and adults would never die in our care, but death is a sober fact of nursing practice. No one needs our skills, caring, and gentleness more than those whose lives are about to end.

## Care Study   Managing death through a team effort

Tom Simmons was only thirty-six, too young to die, thought Peg Johnson, R.N., as she reviewed the physician's orders and prepared to write the nursing care plan for tomorrow's team conference. Tom was a new admission. She read over the nursing interview and began.

Physically, pain was the priority problem and the reason for admission. Tom's pain medication was not providing adequate pain relief. Tom was irritable and demanding with his wife Sue, who was close to tears most of the time.

Socially, Tom had been at home, dealing not only with the pain, which kept him from sleeping, but also with boredom. He had been an engineer in a busy computer design firm and had had lots of friends, but calls and visits from these friends over the last seven months had diminished to the point of nonexistence.

Tom's mother visited daily, however, trying to "cheer him up" and talking about how the entire family would go up to the island next summer. "Doesn't she know I'm not going to have another summer!" Tom would yell after his mother left. Sue would rush from the room in tears.

Psychologically, Tom's boredom was increasing, along with his concern over his two sons, ages eight and eleven. Tom usually saw the boys only on Sundays, since his mother had taken them to stay with her until "Tom feels better." Although Sue did not like this arrangement, she acquiesced rather than make an issue of it. The school principal reported acting-out behavior problems on the part of the older boy, which had not existed before his father's illness. The younger boy was acting withdrawn.

The following morning, Mark Vatalie, a social worker, took a chair from the lounge and joined the others: Dr. Phil Bennett; Peg Johnson; Joan Seward, R.N.; Ken Tratner, the hospital chaplain, and Dick Brown, the hospital pharmacist. Peg presented her care plan assessment data and the discussion began. Over an hour later, the plan was complete and the team was anxious to start.

Peg would be the primary-care nurse, relating directly to Tom's changing needs. Joan would provide backup and play a special advocacy role with Sue. Mark would consult with the teachers at school. Ken would introduce himself to the family, be available for any religious needs they might have, and consult with a family pastor if indicated. Dr. Bennett, after consultation with Dick on the best pain management, would coordinate the team and evaluate progress.

The next month entailed hard work and yet considerable satisfaction. Much of the intervention went much more smoothly than the team had anticipated. After trying various combinations of agents, a pain mixture was devised that almost totally controlled Tom's pain. He re-corded the levels of pain he was experiencing on a paper-and-pencil evaluation scale, and the dosages of administration were altered accordingly. This process gave Tom a feeling of control over what was happening to him.

With the control of his pain, Tom became much more communicative and able to express deep feelings of guilt over leaving Sue with the boys. Ventilating these feelings with Peg released much of his anger, and visits with Sue took on a new ease and meaning for them both.

Joan and Sue began to spend coffee breaks together, and Sue soon released her pent-up anger toward her mother-in-law. Joan and Sue decided it was time for the boys to be at home and to begin visiting their father, who would not be with them much longer. Tom's mother was a capable and well-meaning woman who wanted to help but could not accept the death she knew was approaching. Joan asked Tom's mother to join them for a coffee break and suggested that if she had some free time while at the hospital, the unit was badly in need of volunteer help to shop and write letters for other patients. Sue then said she was feeling alone with Tom in the hospital and that if the boys came home and Tom's mother could help with dinner two nights a week, she would appreciate it. Tom's mother turned to Sue with tears in her eyes "Oh, it's so good to have you ask me to do something. It's so hard to lose a son, you know." Sue gently put her arms around Tom's mother and said how good it felt.

Mark met twice a week with the boys' teachers and also spent considerable time with the boys, both separately and together. He drove them to soccer on Saturdays, after which they had a good talk over hamburgers and went to the hospital to see Tom. Mark and the teachers decided not to discuss the changes in their behavior with the boys but simply be available and supportive. Apparently as a result of the changes in Tom and Sue, and their new relationship with Mark, the boys' behavior in school began to improve; though behavior changes were still apparent, they seemed to Mark a natural response to the home crisis.

Tom left the hospital four weeks after his admission. Home care nursing services were provided. Peg thought a great deal about Tom and Sue, and the team often asked her what she had heard. Two weeks after discharge, Sue called Peg to invite her to a small gathering to celebrate Tom's thirty-seventh birthday. Sue had invited a few friends and wives from the office, "and they're coming!" she said excitedly. It was a quiet, good time. Peg loved the evening, so different from the first day on the unit.

Tom died peacefully six weeks later at home with his family and Peg nearby.

## Study Terms

| | |
|---|---|
| acceptance | hope |
| anger | hospice |
| anticipatory grief | isolation |
| bargaining | independence |
| burnout | interdisciplinary team |
| communication | life review |
| death care | productivity |
| denial | replacement |
| depression | resignation |
| developing awareness | resolution |
| disbelief | restitution |
| disengagement | strengths |
| edema | |
| euthanasia | |
|    active (positive) | |
|    passive (negative) | |

## Learning Activities

**1.** Read a book about death and dying and report on it to your class. Check your selection of a book with your instructor first.

**2.** Using references, write a five- to eight-page paper on one of the following topics. If another topic seems more appropriate or compelling, check with your instructor.

   Communicating with the Dying Patient
   Supporting the Family of the Dying Patient
   Hope in Relation to Dying
   Dying with Dignity
   I Have Just Been Told I Have a Fatal Disease
   My Personal Views About Death (or What
      Dying Means to Me)

**3.** Talk with a person in your community whose job or profession involves confrontations with death.

## References

Andrysiak, Theresa; Carroll, RoseMary; and Ungerleider, J. Thomas. "Marijuana for the Oncology Patient." *American Journal of Nursing* 79 (August 1979): 1396–1398.

Brantner, John. "Positive Approaches to Dying." *Death Education* 1 (Fall 1977): 293–304.

Butler, Robert N. "The Need for Quality Hospice Care." *Death Education* 3 (Fall 1979): 215–225.

Engel, G. L. "Grief and Grieving." *American Journal of Nursing* 64 (September 1964): 93–98.

Fulton, Robert, ed. *Death and Dying: Challenge and Change*. Reading, Mass.: Addison-Wesley, 1978.

Glaser, B., and Strauss, A. L. *Awareness of Dying*. Chicago: Aldine, 1965.

Goffnett, Carol. "Your Patient's Dying—Now What?" *Nursing '79* 9 (November 1979): 26–33.

Griffin, J. G. "Family Decision: A Crucial Factor in Terminating Life." *American Journal of Nursing* 75 (May 1975): 794–796.

Hofling, C. K., and Leininger, M. M. *Basic Psychiatric Concepts of Nursing*. Philadelphia: J. B. Lippincott, 1960.

Kavanaugh, R. E. "Helping Patients Who Are Facing Death." *Nursing '74* 4 (May 1974): 35–42.

Kobrzycki, P. "Living with Dying at Home." *American Journal of Nursing '75* (August 1975): 1312–1313.

Kopel, Kenneth, and Mock, Lou Ann. "The Use of Group Sessions for the Emotional Support of Families of Terminal Patients." *Death Education* (Winter 1978): 409–421.

Kübler-Ross, Elisabeth. *On Death and Dying*. New York: Macmillan, 1969.

Kübler-Ross, Elisabeth, and Warshaw, Mal. *To Live Until We Say Goodbye*. Englewood Cliffs, N.J.: Prentice-Hall, 1978.

LaCasse, C. M. "A Dying Adolescent." *American Journal of Nursing* 75 (March 1975): 433–434.

Lamerton, Richard. *Care of the Dying*. London: Priory Press, 1973.

Lester, D., et al. "Attitudes of Nursing Students and Nursing Faculty Toward Death." *Nursing Research* (January 1974): 50–53.

Lewis, C. S. *A Grief Observed*. New York: Seabury Press, 1973.

Markel, William M., and Simon, Virginia. *The Hospice Concept*. American Cancer Society, 1978.

Nowlis, Elizabeth Ann. "Odyssey to Mare Street: Lessons Learned at St. Joseph's Hospice." In *Current Perspectives in Oncologic Nursing*, Volume II, pp. 132–138. St. Louis: C. V. Mosby, 1978.

Paula, Sister. "The Work of the Hospice." *Nursing Times* 75 (April 1979): 667–669.

Reiner, E. E. "Helping the Survivors of Expected Death." *Nursing '75* 7 (March 1975): 60–65.

Robbins, T. *Even Cowgirls Get the Blues*. Boston: Houghton Mifflin, 1976.

Shubin, S. "Burnout: The Professional Hazard You Face in Nursing." *Nursing '78* 8 (July 1978): 22–27.

Stoddard, Sandol. *The Hospice Movement*. New York: Random House, 1978.

Stoller, Eleanor Palo. "Effect of Experience on Nurses' Responses to Dying and Death in the Hospital Setting." *Nursing Research* (January/February 1980): 35–38.

Storlie, Frances J. "Burnout: The Elaboration of a Concept." *American Journal of Nursing* 79 (December 1979): 2108–2111.

————."Caring for a Patient Who Wants to Die: Should You Let Her?" *Nursing '80* 10 (February 1980): 50–53.

Twycross, R. G. "Overview of Analgesia." In *Advances in Pain Research and Therapy*. New York: Raven Press, 1979.

Ufema, J. K. "Dare to Care for the Dying." *American Journal of Nursing* 76 (January 1976): 88–90.

Wald, Florence S., and Wald, Zelda Foster and Henry J. "The Hospice Movement as a Health Care Reform." *Nursing Outlook* 28 (March 1980): 173–178.

Wertenbaker, Lael T. *The Death of a Man*. New York: Random House, 1957.

Whitman, H. H., and Lukes, S. J. "Behavior Modification for Terminally Ill Patients." *American Journal of Nursing* 75 (January 1975): 98–101.

Williams, J. G. "Understanding the Feelings of the Dying." *Nursing '76* 6 (March 1976): 52–56.

Zopf, D. "The Dying Patient: Meeting His Needs May Be Easier Than You Think." *Nursing '75* 5 (March 1975): 16–18.

# Chapter 28

# Sensory Disturbance

## Objectives

After completing this chapter, you should be able to:

1. Define sensory deprivation and sensory overload.
2. Identify situations that might predispose to sensory disturbance.
3. Assess for sensory deprivation and sensory overload, taking into consideration the condition, environment, and symptoms of the patient.

4. Describe nursing intervention in both sensory deprivation and sensory overload.
5. Evaluate the effectiveness of prevention and intervention in cases of sensory disturbance.
6. Identify people other than patients who are at risk of sensory disturbance.

## Outline

497

For many years, nursing assessment of patients' problems focused virtually exclusively on physical needs. It gradually became apparent that psychological needs must be assessed as well. Only very recently, however, have nurses seen the necessity of assessing for disturbances related to sensory input.

When we speak of *sensory input*, we are talking about all the messages and impressions transmitted to the brain by any of the five senses. Sights, sounds, tastes, odors, and the sensations of temperature and texture all constitute what we call *input*. During our waking hours, thousands of these stimuli are registered in one's consciousness, where they are not only received but also interpreted and sometimes acted on. These messages are received in a repetitive, "rapid-fire" manner, though we perceive them in a smooth-flowing pattern. For example, a symphony is actually a series of sounds—high and low, short and prolonged—all bombarding the ear. Without appropriate sensory input, we can become disoriented and out of touch with reality and lose our ability to interact with those around us.

## Sensory Level

The optimum level of sensory input to which we can respond appropriately at any given time may be influenced by several factors: the meaningfulness of the stimuli; our interpretation of the input in light of our past experiences, knowledge, and attitudes; and the presence of other stressors, such as illness or fatigue. All affect the reception of input.

One's optimum level of sensory input is very changeable. Suppose you are spending the evening studying. The input you are receiving is mostly visual, from books and papers, accompanied by some tactile input from the texture of the paper and the shape of the pencil. At such a time, relatively low input is appropriate; higher input would make you uncomfortable and interfere with your concentration. The next day you attend a football game, where you experience very high sensory input; the colorful uniforms, the roar of the crowd, a marching band, and the smells of popcorn and hotdogs all combine to make for a multitude of stimuli. Human beings enjoy and need variations in sensory input. We tend in general to cope better if high-input periods are followed by lower levels of input.

## Sensory Disturbances

### Sensory Deprivation

*Sensory deprivation* results from a lower level of sensory input than the individual needs for optimal functioning. Studies show that normal people experimentally subjected to sensory input as low as possible experience irritability, inability to think clearly, perceptual distortion, and changes in brain-wave pattern (Bexton, Heron, and Scott, 1954). That such symptoms occurred even though the subjects were aware of participating in an experiment on sensory deprivation suggests that sensorially deprived persons have little control over their reactions.

The first symptoms may be irritability and childish responses. If sensory disturbance becomes severe enough, lack of clarity in thought and illusions can occur. *Illusions* are false interpretations of visible objects. An example is a rounded vase of fluffy pussywillows that the patient sees as a bird with a large feathery tail. If sensory disturbance becomes extreme, actual *hallucinations* can develop. A patient who hallucinates sees sights and/or hears sounds that are not actually there. A thorough assessment of the patient and the situation is necessary to determine whether sensory deprivation or sensory overload is responsible for hallucinations.

## Sensory Overload

*Sensory overload* occurs when an individual receives more sensory stimuli during a given period than can be tolerated. It is usually a combination of stimuli, such as auditory, visual, and tactile (touch), that overtaxes the patient's sensory receiving mechanism. A persistent barrage of input produces symptoms similar to those of sensory deprivation.

## Assessing for Sensory Disturbance

In assessing a patient for sensory deprivation or overload, you should know something about the sensory level to which the patient is most accustomed and accommodates best. A busy, outgoing, aggressive businessman who is suddenly placed on strict bedrest in a private room may develop sensory deprivation fairly rapidly. Conversely, a nursing-home resident who is transferred to the hospital could develop sensory overload because of a sudden rise in the level of input.

Patients in hospitals are in a "captive" environment in the sense that they typically have little control over the quantity of input they receive. Because the study of sensory input is relatively new, many patients and health-care workers are unaware that certain feelings and symptoms are attributable to sensory disturbances, and not directly to the disease process.

Assessment for potential or existing problems of sensory disturbance consists of studying (1) the *condition* of the patient, (2) the *environment* in which the patient is placed, and (3) whether or not the patient is experiencing any of the *symptoms* we have mentioned. The nurse sees such symptoms manifested in the behavior of the patient. Assessment is especially important when the patient is immobilized or less responsive than usual psychologically because such patients are often unable to give clear cues as to the source of their discomfort.

Each patient must be assessed as an individual. Irritability and unclear thought do not necessarily mean that a patient is sensorially disturbed. The same symptoms may be caused by such other conditions as generalized infection, electrolyte imbalance, drug intoxication, or the illness itself. Keeping in mind the patient's diagnosis will thus make your assessment more accurate and complete.

## Patients at High Risk of Sensory Disturbance

### Identifying Sensory Deprivation

Some patients are more susceptible than others to sensory deprivation. Using one or more of the three parameters—condition, environment, and symptoms (behavior)—consider several categories of patients for whom you might care. Patients residing in chronic-care facilities, who are in bed much of the time and may have roommates who are unable to communicate, infrequent visitors, and contacts with the staff only when care is given, commonly suffer sensory deprivation. Pri-

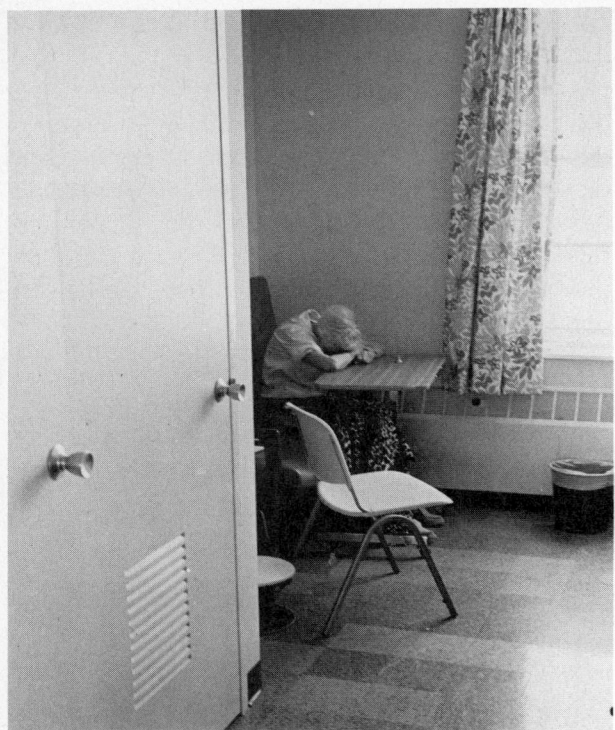

**Figure 28.1 A patient at high risk of sensory deprivation**
Stephen J. Potter/Stock, Boston

experience sensory deprivation because coronary-care units are designed to provide low sensory input in order to allow for complete rest. Sensory deprivation can also afflict any patient who has suffered partial or total loss of sight or hearing. The wearing of eye patches after eye surgery can contribute to sensory deprivation, as can immobilization.

Patients with mild sensory deprivation often complain simply that they are bored. At this early stage, you can prevent further disturbance by supplying additional input, such as reading material, music, or visitors.

After less than three hours of lying in the recumbent position, patients can begin to exhibit signs of sensory deprivation (Downs, 1974). The recumbent position distorts visual images and auditory perception and forces the patient to adapt to a new spatial environment.

Because of new understanding of sensory deprivation, hospital rooms are becoming more colorful and visually stimulating. However, many rooms in institutions remain plain and dull, painted white or tan and sparsely furnished. Such a setting offers the patient little visual input.

vate rooms, intended to provide for rest in an undisturbed environment, may unwittingly promote deprivation of the senses.

When a fragile older adult with diminishing senses appears listless and withdrawn, the cause may be insufficient sensory input. Efforts to engage the remaining senses can bring about a remarkable reversal in attitude and behavior, making the person more outgoing and contented.

Particularly susceptible to sensory deprivation are patients in isolation. Patients may be isolated for various medical reasons and with different degrees of stringency (see Chapter 11). It appears that sensory deprivation is directly related to the degree of isolation imposed. As a case in point, when you care for a patient in protective isolation for leukemia or burns, you usually wear a gown, a cap over your hair, a mask, gloves, and cloth boots over your shoes. The room is often sparsely furnished in order to diminish the likelihood of the spread of bacteria. We rely greatly on visual impressions of the people with whom we interact, and to see only people's eyes can be very disconcerting.

Patients who have suffered heart attacks often

## Identifying Sensory Overload

Assessment for sensory overload employs the same parameters as does assessment for sensory deprivation: condition, environment, and symptoms. Is the patient's condition such that he or she needs constant surveillance by sophisticated medical equipment and personnel? This situation makes for a multiplicity of stimuli within a small area and can be a clue to sensory overload.

A hospital unit, which is quite different in appearance, routine, and pace from a private home, can bombard the patient with unfamiliar input. The patient awakened for the measurement of vital signs, disturbed for morning care, and subjected to many tests and procedures will commonly exhibit irritability. Patients who are quite ill fare worse. The insertion of tubes or catheters and frequent injections represent additional input, as well as causing discomfort. Touch, which is very valuable to the patient suffering from sensory deprivation, can arouse anxiety in the patient with an overload of stimuli. Constant touching, turning, and testing may raise anxiety to the level of panic.

# Intervention in Sensory Disturbance

Nursing actions in response to sensory disturbance are twofold: prevention and intervention. Preventing problems from arising is a primary aim of all nursing action, and it is far preferable to prevent sensory disturbance than to intervene once it has occurred. If the patient's condition and/or environment seem to be a potential cause of sensory disturbance, the nurse may be able to modify one or the other. It is usually easier to change the environment than it is to alter the patient's condition. For example, you might be able to push the immobilized patient, bed and all, to an environment that provides a more satisfactory level of input, if only for a brief time. The bedridden patient with low sensory input could be transferred in bed to an occupational therapy session. And the patient who is experiencing too much input might be moved to a quiet area. Intervention to alleviate an existing disturbance uses similar tactics. The physician may allow the patient on strict bedrest to get up once a day, which would increase input. If the sensorily overloaded patient's condition permits, the physician might order the discontinuation of monitoring equipment.

## Intervening in Sensory Deprivation

Studies show that the input provided to relieve sensory deprivation must be meaningful to the patient. For example, music the patient enjoys stimulates the senses, while incidental noise in the hallway has no meaning for the patient and may be not only annoying but also ineffective in relieving symptoms. Only stimuli that are received and interpreted to serve some purpose for the individual represent effective input.

It may be that the hallucinations experienced by some persons suffering extreme deprivation are functional in that they provide input. That is, the creation of hallucinatory images compensates for lack of real input in the environment. When input is increased, hallucinations usually disappear.

The most meaningful input experienced by human beings is personal contact with others. The few people who have dared lone voyages across the ocean have reported severe sensory deprivation and hallucinations, despite the abundance of sensory input provided by the sea, changing weather, and wildlife. They attributed this phenomenon to loss of human contact, a hypothesis that has important implications for nurses. Every member of the health-care team has meaning for the patient in that each helps plan and provide care. It is frequently the nurse who spends the most time with the patient and thus has the best opportunities to offer the patient meaningful input. Family and friends are equally important. Personal contact has the advantage of providing input in various modalities: the nurse presents a

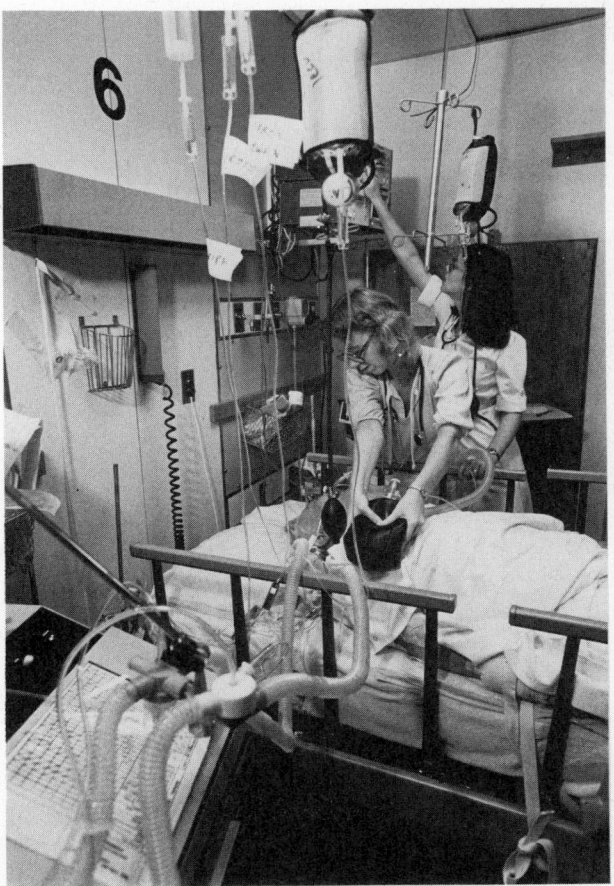

**Figure 28.2   A patient at high risk of sensory overload**
Daniel Bernstein

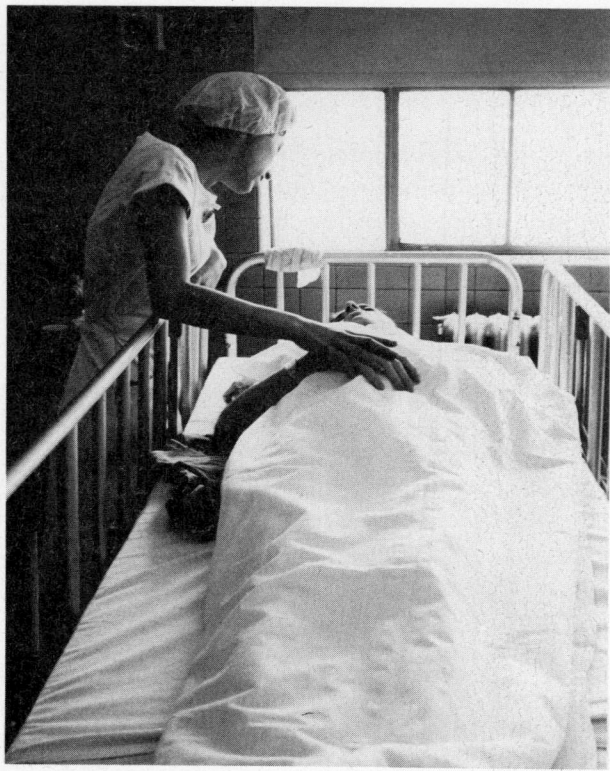

**Figure 28.3**
Touch is therapeutic sensory input. (Herb Levart/Photo Researchers, Inc.)

visual image, provides auditory input by speaking, and may touch the patient as well.

The significance of touch cannot be overemphasized. The earliest meaningful input in our lives is touch: long before the infant can focus on objects or interpret sounds, stroking and fondling quiet cries and produce a sense of contentment. Touch continues to be an important part of our lives. For the patient in the hospital, touch is a means of orientation to the environment, reassurance in stressful situations, and an expression of caring. In adulthood, some people use touch more expressively and more spontaneously than others. Though you may initially have to make a conscious effort to use touch, it soon becomes automatic to touch a patient's hand or shoulder while speaking. It is unusual for a patient to show any objection to this practice. In fact, most find touch a warm, pleasant experience. However, there are always exceptions, so it is essential to be perceptive and use touch with discretion.

Another effective source of input is the radio or television. Television has the advantage of being visual as well as auditory. If the patient is unable to do so, you should choose music or a program suitable for the patient. The family may be of help here. For example, a soul-rock radio station is inappropriate for a seventy-six-year-old patient but suitable for a teenager.

Taste is another source of input. If you are selecting a menu for a patient who is unable to do so, you might choose foods characterized by a variety of tastes and consistencies. Taste can be particularly meaningful if a special treat is prepared and brought from home by a family member. An example is a teenager of Italian descent who had been badly injured. After several weeks in a coma, he regained consciousness and was beginning to

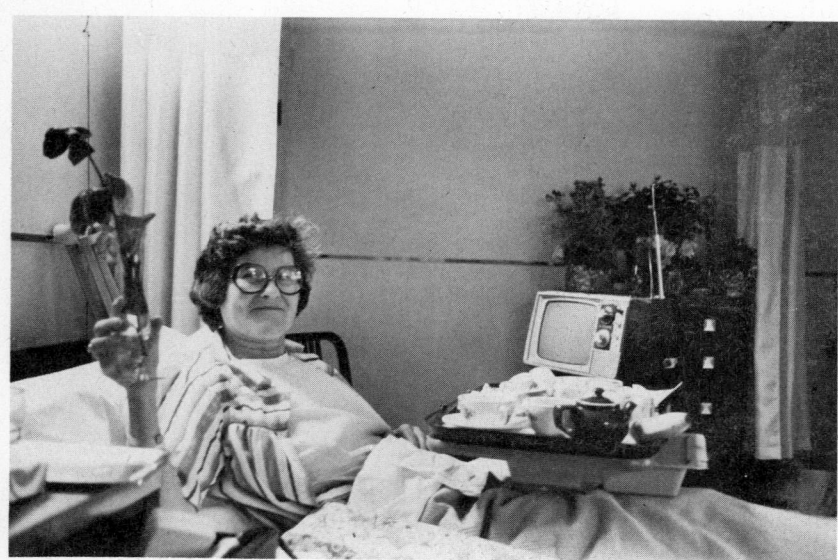

**Figure 28.4**
Nonpersonal stimuli can help a patient with sensory deprivation. (Carol Palmer)

feed himself. His sister brought in a small hot dish of homemade spaghetti, and with the initial spoonful he grinned broadly for the first time since his accident.

Olfactory stimulation (smell) should not be overlooked. A friend brought a teenage patient a small box of incense—an odor the patient associated with home. You might apply mildly scented skin lotions, deodorants, aftershave lotions, or colognes to the patient after a bath. And you might yourself wear a very light fragrance. Again, use discretion: some colognes may cause nausea in particularly sensitive persons.

## Intervening in Sensory Overload

After making an assessment, you can devise a plan for preventing or relieving sensory overload. It is a sound first step to make a careful nursing care plan, taking into consideration sources and levels of sensory input. Some of these sources might be eliminated, and input might be timed more satisfactorily. For example, you could plan to perform several procedures at once, allowing the patient periods of low input between periods of care. Input simultaneous with but unrelated to medical procedures can be therapeutic and relieve anxiety. Soft music for limited periods of time has proven effective.

## Communicating With the Health-Care Team

Communicating with others on the health-care team is essential when intervening in sensory disturbance. The plan should be written in accordance with the nursing process, including data, assessment, and actions. Other members of the team can then participate in implementing it. For ex-

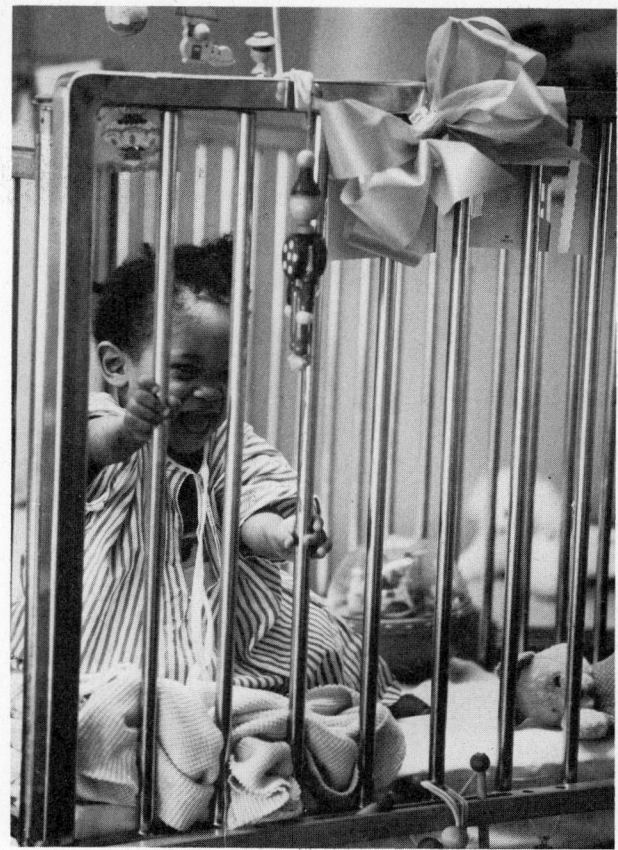

**Figure 28.5**
Toys and mobiles are appropriate for the sensory-deprived child. (Elizabeth Wilcox)

ample, in the case of a patient with sensory overload, the drawing of a blood sample by a laboratory technician may be deliberately scheduled to coincide with nursing care, after which the plan could provide for the patient to have quiet and low input.

Evaluation involves checking for the presence and intensity of symptoms. If symptoms have diminished or disappeared, intervention is successful. What is effective with one patient, however, may not work with another. Individualization is a necessity.

## Occupations Prone to Sensory Disturbance

Sensory disturbances do not happen exclusively to patients in the hospital. The person who is not in the hospital can, by changing the environment or moving elsewhere, adjust sensory input to meet his or her needs. If while studying you want to increase input, you need only turn on the phonograph and continue to work. If the phone begins to ring repeatedly, the family or others return home, or street noises become obtrusive, you may gather up your books and papers and take refuge in the local library, where the environment is more subdued and input is decreased. However, some people whose professions do not allow them to adjust their environments may suffer from sensory disturbance. Night-duty nurses, astronauts in spaceships, miners, and people who work in windowless rooms have all been reported to suffer from the effects of sensory deprivation due to mo-notony and lack of sensory stimuli. Control-tower operators in busy airports have experienced sensory overload due to the input produced by incoming and outgoing aircraft, monitoring equipment, and radio interchange with pilots.

Nurses who work in particularly busy and stressful areas of the hospital, such as the emergency room and intensive care, often feel the effects of sensory overload, notably irritability and undue fatigue. A quiet period at home reading or a walk usually alleviates these symptoms.

## Conclusion

Sensory disturbance in patients has only recently been recognized as a problem. The irritability and confusion it elicits is upsetting not only to the patient but also to the family and staff as well. With basic knowledge of sensory disturbance, assessment is not difficult. And once the problem is properly identified, nursing intervention is remarkably effective. Because sensory disturbance is a problem that calls for creativity and imagination, formulating a solution can offer a high degree of satisfaction.

## Care Study    A patient with sensory deprivation

Tim is a twenty-one-year-old college student who suffered extensive injury to the right side of his head in an explosion. After several weeks in a coma, he gradually regained awareness but remained confused much of the time. More time has passed and the confusion continues. An assessment is undertaken.

Though the surgical site is healing well, Tim has a large defect (depression) on the right side of his head—an area where part of the skull has been removed, leaving only the skin as a covering for the brain tissue. The physician has ordered the patient turned only to his left side and back to protect the area from pressure. Tim's left arm and leg are paralyzed, and he cannot turn himself. Because of the injury to the brain, he cannot see to his left with either eye. This, then, is the condition of the patient.

As for Tim's environment, the head of his bed is against the left wall of the room as the nurse enters, so that he faces a wall. The combination of this arrangement and the limitations of Tim's vision means that Tim can see only the ceiling and a part of the upper wall. The room itself is sparsely furnished. Symptoms of confusion are present: Tim thinks he is in his dormitory room and carries on long conversations with friends who are not present.

It is decided to offer Tim a variety of stimuli. A friend brings in a radio and tells the nurse the kind of music Tim likes. The radio is left on for measured periods of time and then turned off, in order to avoid monotony of input. Extension cords for electrical equipment allow for the bed to be moved to the right wall, and Tim to face the open doorway to the hall. His body position is changed frequently. Brightly colored travel posters, obtained free-of-charge from a local travel agency, are taped to the wall within Tim's line of vision. (Tim traveled all over the world with his widowed father, who was in the military before his accident.) The posters recall to Tim many of the places he has visited, and he tells the nurse some of his experiences. Initially placed high on the wall near the ceiling, the posters are gradually lowered as Tim becomes able to view objects at a more normal level. Since Tim has always been interested in aquatic diving, a friend buys him *Diving* magazine, and friends and staff take turns reading passages to him when time permits. A small amount of his favorite shaving lotion is applied after morning care.

Tim's mental status gradually clears as input is increased. He begins to talk more and soon becomes active in his own care and enthusiastic about recovering and continuing his college studies. He states later that he remembers the silence of his room and the blankness of its white walls. He talks about the frightening images he saw and his relief when familiar sights and sounds were introduced into his environment.

## Care Study   A patient with sensory overload

Maria Palmucci, a thirty-eight-year-old woman of Italian descent, is admitted to the acute-care unit of the hospital with severe cardiopulmonary problems. Her room is designed for intensive care, the glass on the upper half of the wall contiguous to the hallway permitting close observation by the nursing staff. The room itself is a clutter of equipment, mostly electrical. Lights blink and sounds emanate from the appliances constantly. Oxygen and suction equipment bubble and gurgle. The ceiling lights are left on night and day to allow the nursing and medical staffs to perform tests, treatments, and procedures. Vital signs are taken hourly, oxygen and intravenous fluids are under constant scrutiny, and the patient is turned frequently. Mrs. Palmucci is becoming increasingly apprehensive.

The condition of the patient is such that almost constant attention and touching are required. Tubes and catheters add to the general confusion experienced by the patient. The environment inflicts a high level of visual, auditory, and tactile input on a continuing basis. A heart-monitoring machine is equipped with an alarm that rings loudly in response to even moderate movement on the part of the patient, as well as to heart irregularity. Mrs. Palmucci's symptoms are apparent in her behavior. Apprehension is fast escalating into panic. Mrs. Palmucci grasps the sheets until her knuckles are white. She hyperventilates (takes rapid, deep breaths) and her eyes appear frightened. At times she pulls at her gown and violently shakes her head. Though it is believed that the loss of REM sleep (see Chapter 20) exaggerates her state of mind, the primary problem is sensory overload.

The nursing care plan is reviewed in assessing the patient's condition and environment. All unnecessary equipment is removed from the room. The ceiling lights are dimmed for long periods of time, leaving only a small, dim wall light. When the nurse is in the room, the shade on the large hallway window is pulled to shut out the sight of busy traffic up and down the hall. The door is kept closed to diminish sound. The heart-monitoring alarm is moved by the hospital's mechanical department so that it rings only at the nurse's station and does not continue to distress the patient. Suction equipment is turned off when not in use. The nurse plans for care to be provided at a few set times so that the patient will not receive constant stimuli. Soft music is played in the unit for short periods of time. The nurse sets aside time to hold Mrs. Palmucci's hand in silence.

Within a very short time, Mrs. Palmucci grows quieter and her breathing becomes more regular and efficient. With the improvement in breathing, her cardiac status also improves. The look of fear on her face disappears and her muscles relax.

## Study Terms

hallucinations

illusions

olfactory

sensory deprivation

sensory input

sensory level

sensory overload

tactile

## Learning Activities

1. Lie down alone in a quiet, darkened room for ten minutes. Then describe the state of each of your senses and the amount of input received by each.

2. If you can, enter an environment with a high input level and again describe each of your five senses.

3. Select a patient whom you consider to have a comfortable balance of input. What factors make this so?

4. Select a patient whom you consider to be suffering from sensory disturbance. What do you see as causative factors?

## References

Bexton, W. H.; Heron, W.; and Scott, T. H. "Effects of Decreased Variation in the Sensory Environment." *Canadian Journal of Psychology* 8 (June 1954): 70.

Black, Sister Kathleen. "Social Isolation and the Nursing Process." *Nursing Clinics of North America* 8 (December 1973): 575–586.

Bolin, R. H. "Sensory Deprivation: An Overview." *Nursing Forum* 13 (March 1974): 240–258.

Cameron, C.; Kessler, J.; Kramer, W.; and Warren, K. "When Sensory Deprivation Occurs." *The Canadian Nurse* 68 (November 1972): 32–34.

Chodil, J., and Williams, W. "The Concept of Sensory Deprivation." *Nursing Clinics of North America* 5 (May 1970): 544–548.

Dolan, M. "A Return to Laughter—and Tears." *Nursing '76* 6 (November 1976): 43.

Downs, F. S. "Bed Rest and Sensory Disturbance." *American Journal of Nursing* 74 (March 1974): 434–438.

Ellis, R. "Unusual Sensory and Thought Disturbances After Cardiac Surgery." *American Journal of Nursing* 72 (November 1972): 2021–2024.

Hahn, J., and Burns, K. R. "Mrs. Richards, A Rabbit and Remotivation." *American Journal of Nursing* 73 (February 1973): 302–305.

Heron, W. "The Pathology of Boredom." In *Altered States of Awareness*. San Francisco: W. H. Freeman, 1971.

Kratz, C. R. "Sensory Deprivation in the Elderly." *Nursing Times* 75 (February 22, 1979): 330–332.

McCorkle, Ruth. "Effects of Touch on Seriously Ill Patients." *Nursing Research* 23 (March/April 1974): 125–132.

Thomson, L. R. "Sensory Deprivation: A Personal Experience." *American Journal of Nursing* 73 (February 1973): 266–268.

Woods, Nancy Fugate. "Noise Stimuli in the Acute Care Area." *Nursing Research* (March/April 1974): 144–149.

# Chapter 29

# Disturbances of Body Image Integrity

*Body image* was defined in Chapter 15 as a multi-dimensional view of one's body that takes into account its appearance, kinesthetic feedback, sensory feedback, and internal feelings. Appearance is the actual look of one's body seen directly and in a mirror. Kinesthetic feedback is the perceived location of one's body in relation to its surroundings and the relationship of body parts to one another. Sensory feedback is perception of the external environment. Internal feelings include the full range of psychological-emotional responses to one's own body and appearance.

An individual whose body image is accurate and flexible, changing as the individual changes, and who feels comfortable with his or her body is said to have *body image integrity.* Such integrity can be disturbed if the individual persists in viewing his or her body in a way that is no longer realistic.

Illness frequently causes changes in the body. Because these changes are usually undesirable and often happen suddenly, disturbances in body image integrity are commonplace among ill people. As a nurse, you will need skill in (1) identifying situations in which body image integrity may be threatened, (2) assessing the patient's response to such a situation, and (3) intervening to prevent a disturbance or to help restore body image integrity if a disturbance occurs.

## The Development of Body Image

Body image changes throughout one's life as the body changes and as one's understanding of and feelings about the body change. Body image changes and develops throughout life according to a pattern, which roughly corresponds to the patterns of other aspects of development (review Chapter 4 on the life cycle).

### Infancy

The infant is born without a body image. In the womb the infant and the environment are one, and the self is not perceived as a separate entity. The processes that lead to the development of the adult self-image begin at birth.

The infant responds to the internal stimuli of pain and hunger and does not at first distinguish between them. Gradually the infant begins to identify those feelings of discomfort that are relieved by food and to distinguish them from other feelings. The same process occurs with regard to all internal stimuli, and as a result the infant learns to trust his or her body and develops an understanding of its signals.

External stimuli also help infants to identify their own bodies. Little babies sometimes cause themselves pain by biting their own toes, since they cannot distinguish the boundaries between the self and the nonself. The touch of those who care for the infant is central to the process of learning to differentiate self from nonself.

### The Toddler (One to Three)

The toddler can distinguish self from nonself, has learned to trust feelings (one hopes), and begins to ascribe value to body parts. Some parts are seen as important, some as pretty, and some perhaps as unmentionable. These values are largely acquired from the people who are significant to the child and from the direct experience of pleasure or pain derived from body parts. The toddler typically perceives the limits of the body as more encompassing than does the adult. For example, feces, urine, fingernails, and hair are considered parts of the body, and their disappearance may be upsetting.

### Early Childhood (Three to Six)

Along with physical stature, the young child's body image is also changing. The child no longer feels like a baby and may ascribe this term to a younger sibling. Children of this age may see themselves as "little adults," the boy pretending to act "like Daddy" and the girl imitating the activities of her mother.

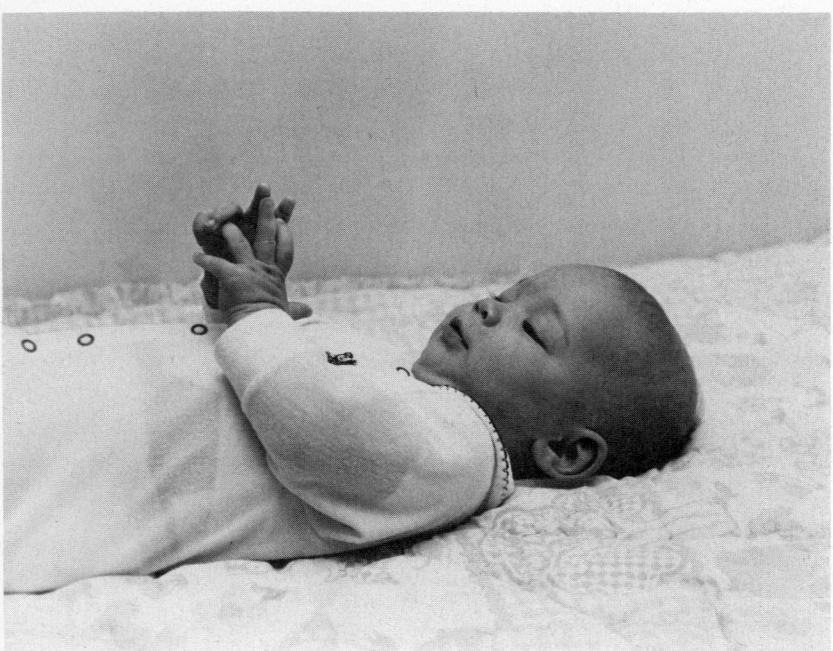

**Figure 29.1**
An infant must learn the limits of his or her own body. (Russ Kinne/Photo Researchers, Inc.)

## Middle Childhood (Six to Twelve)

By the time children reach school age, they have become highly aware of others' bodies and begun to make close comparisons between themselves and others. The child may be acutely aware of differences that are not even noted by the adult. Although the child has already begun to learn about the body's functioning at the beginning of this stage, real understanding is not achieved until age nine or older. Before then, the child's ideas are often inaccurate and may be very confused. Both boys and girls of this age group may seek out magazines and books that include pictures of the human body.

## Adolescence (Twelve to Eighteen)

The adolescent undergoes many physical changes, both overt and internal, as discussed in Chapter 4. Plenty of physical activity and exercise can help teenagers become more comfortable with their changing bodies.

The changes associated with sexual development give rise to an intense awareness of and preoccupation with one's body. Adolescents often compare themselves with others, exhibit concern about whether or not they are normal, and exhibit exaggerated modesty. They may spend prolonged periods in front of the mirror and express profound dissatisfaction with their appearance. It is common for adolescents to feel very unsatisfied with a particular facial feature—often the nose, which becomes more pronounced as adult features begin to emerge. Acne (pimples and other blemishes), which varies from mild and intermittent to severe and scarring, may cause particular distress. Adolescents with severe acne often withdraw from social contacts.

Adolescents are often confused by their sexual feelings and may control them poorly. There is considerable pressure on American adolescents to act on their sexual feelings. Those who do not do so, for whatever reasons, may wonder whether they are normal in sexual feelings and function. Menstruation, seminal emissions, and erections at inopportune times can make the adolescent feel that his or her body has become unreliable and a cause for anxiety.

## Young Adulthood (Eighteen to Forty)

The body image of the young adult is deeply influenced by prevailing standards of beauty and

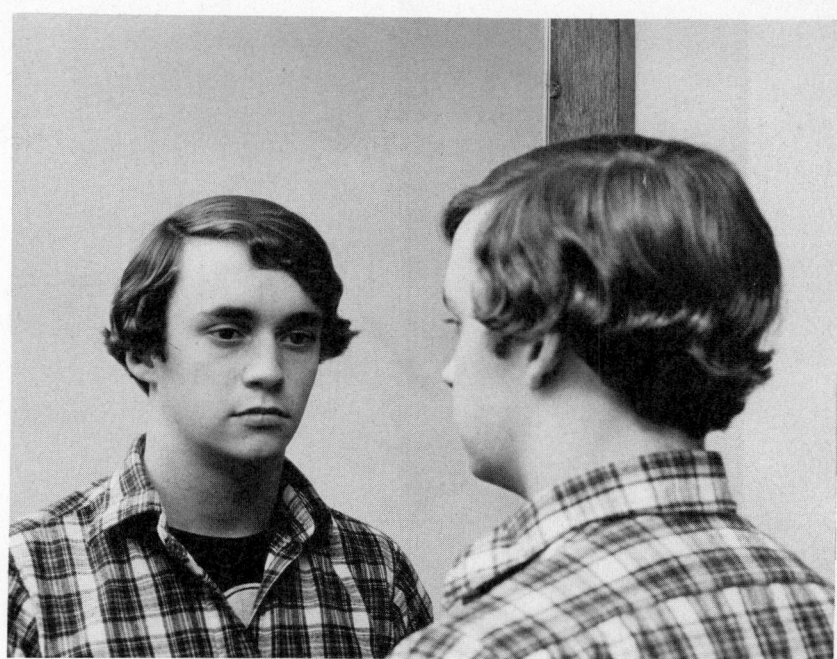

**Figure 29.2**
The adolescent may spend time gazing into the mirror. (Russ Kinne/Photo Researchers, Inc.)

value judgments about the body. Efforts to discern character on the basis of appearance have a dubious but very long history: the belief that people with beady eyes are untrustworthy, for example, originated centuries ago. More recently, psychological studies of body types have been undertaken in an effort to legitimize such "folk wisdom," but they have not succeeded in demonstrating a correlation between body and personal characteristics. Stereotyping is nevertheless very common. (Health-care workers who try not to respond to patients stereotypically sometimes forget that patients may respond to them, in turn, on the basis of stereotypes. Ideally, any health-care worker would be equally acceptable to a patient, but reassignments must be made if the patient's response to care is affected by his or her attitude to the provider of that care.)

In Western cultures, and especially in the United States, the young, beautiful body is idealized. For women, the standard is a very slim figure and conformity to a rather narrow definition of beauty. The spectrum of what is considered handsome in men is broader: for example, the older man with a slightly portly figure and graying hair may be seen as "distinguished." However, height is often equated with leadership ability in men, and studies have shown that the short man may be handicapped in job advancement.

Women seem to have clearer and more accurate images of their bodies than do men (Murray, 1972). They are more acutely aware of physical changes, especially those that affect the face, than men. Women also tend more to equate body with self; men tend to be less specific in their views of their own bodies and to relate self more to accomplishment and position in life. The women's movement and related phenomena may bring about a convergence of men's and women's attitudes toward their bodies.

## The Middle Years (Forty to Sixty-five)

Because of the physical changes occurring in the middle years (discussed in Chapter 4), the body image may become more negative. The body may be perceived as less attractive, less able, and less valuable. The extent of these negative feelings is based on the individual's personality and how satisfactory life has been to this point. Many middle adults see the changes as evidence of maturity and experience and are therefore comfortable with the changes. Today, many middle adults conscientiously work to "keep in shape," thereby avoiding the decreased function that comes from inactivity. Most middle adults adjust gradually to the changes occurring with some feelings of regret for passing youth and some positive feelings about the values inherent in maturity.

## The Later Years (Over Sixty-five)

The older adult is frequently faced with chronic illness as well as with diminished function and change in appearance. Sensory deficits are common in the older adult and these may lessen the ability to participate in social functions and to enjoy such hobbies as music and reading. Decreased strength and increased fatigue may lessen the ability to be a productive worker. These are all distressing to the older adult and may lead to feelings of worthlessness and despair over lost abilities. Or, the older adult may make realistic adaptations to decreased function and accept these changes, becoming a secure person able to relate to others and positive in outlook.

# Common Problems With Body Image Integrity

In order to identify situations that may threaten body image integrity, you must pay close attention to both the situation and the individual.

## Failure of Normal Development

Children are prone to interrupted body image development during illness, due to having missed normal situations and interactions that contribute to development. The child may thus emerge from the illness having made no gains in psychological development. For example, an infant needs appropriate tactile input if he or she is to learn to distinguish the body from the environment; touch is provided by cuddling, feeding, bathing, and playing with the infant. Insufficient touch retards development. An infant deprived of enough touch due to illness may still be exploring his or her own body when he or she should be ready to begin exploring the environment. The infant also needs to learn to identify feelings, such as hunger, that occur in the body. To do so, the infant must feel the discomfort, express it, be fed, and feel satisfaction. If fed according to a schedule without regard to the body's responses, the infant will not learn about them.

The toddler needs from others an accepting attitude toward touching various body parts, without labeling some body parts good and others bad. Such simple procedures as shaving a body part before surgery can upset a toddler, who considers hair part of the body and does not necessarily recognize it as expendable. The toddler may view an intravenous tube infused to the arm as part of the body and may need help understanding both its placement and its removal.

School-age children need contact with peers and reassurance that they are normal and acceptable. Lacking such support, they can be expected to suffer self-doubt and become withdrawn.

In summary, the individual needs appropriate input at each stage of development in order to develop body image integrity.

## Changes in External Body Appearance

Disturbances in body image integrity can also be caused by changes in external body appearance. The person who experiences formation of a scar, hair loss from chemotherapy, loss of a limb, or a colostomy (surgery to open the colon through the abdominal wall) will probably need some support and assistance to maintain body image integrity.

In order to participate fully in life, one must accept such changes and incorporate them into one's self-image. The difficulty of doing so is a function of the individual's developmental level, previous life experiences, and previous body image. For example, a facial scar may be readily incorporated into the body image, and even worn as a badge of pride, by a young man who fences

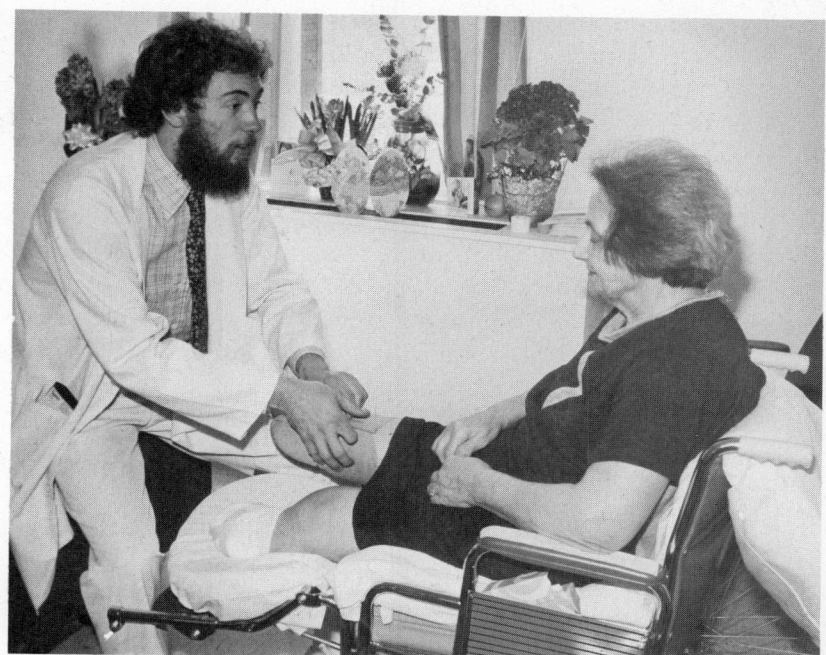

**Figure 29.3**
A change in body structure may be accompanied by a disturbance of body image. (Russ Kinne/Danbury Hospital/Photo Researchers, Inc.)

as a hobby. The same scar on a teenage girl might elicit severe depression and cause her to withdraw from normal social life.

## Changes in Body Function

Body image integrity can also be affected by changes in the body's functioning. Examples are a lung disease that limits physical activity, a stomach problem that requires dietary changes, and medications whose side effects include diminished alertness. The body does not respond as it previously did and may be less acceptable. Some individuals deny such changes and jeopardize their health by failing to follow prescriptions for activity and diet. Others find the change so overwhelming that they feel life is no longer meaningful.

# Patients' Responses to Problems With Body Image Integrity

A change in the body evokes responses similar to those observed in a dying person, who is coping with the total loss of self (see Chapter 27).

## Shock, Disbelief, and Denial

At first the patient may exhibit *shock, disbelief,* and *denial.* For a while, denial may actually be helpful: the patient whose energy is invested in coping with the physical problems of healing may not have adequate resources for simultaneous psychological changes. But if denial persists for a long time and interferes with the patient's ability to participate in his or her own care, skilled psychiatric help may be needed.

## Anger

As the reality of the change is acknowledged, the patient may express *anger,* more often at the world in general than at someone in particular. Such anger is characterized by a "Why me?" attitude. On occasion, anger may be directed at the most accessible targets, the nurse and the family. Although such anger is not really personal, it is often difficult to make this distinction, and families may need to talk to someone who understands what they are feeling. If you are the target of anger, you too may need someone with whom to discuss your feelings if you are to continue to function effectively with the patient. It is important that you not reject the patient at this time. Though rejecting of others, the patient needs their acceptance in order to move toward self-acceptance.

## Bargaining

Bargaining is less common in body image disturbance than in other types of loss and impending loss. On occasion, a person might engage in bargaining for a period of time. However, a person with a new colostomy might say, for example, "If I am very careful about how I take care of myself, maybe the doctor will be able to operate and put everything back to normal." Though such bargaining is unrealistic, it needs to be accepted in light of the patient's feelings at the time.

## Depression

Anger and bargaining may be followed by severe *depression* as the patient grieves for what was and might have been. Attempts to cheer up a depressed patient are inappropriate. Instead, such a patient needs the constant concerned care and presence of others, even when he or she is rejecting of others. Sitting with the patient in silence, with no expectation of response, may be especially helpful. Touch and other nonverbal communication are particularly important.

## Acceptance

Gradually, the person develops *acceptance* of the new body image. Integrity is restored, and energy can be focused on rehabilitation and/or returning to the mainstream of life. Therapeutic interaction—to help the patient think about the entire experience, verbalize it, and give it meaning—is most effective at this time.

Health-care workers sometimes make the mistake of expecting this entire process to be accomplished very rapidly. Time is needed: time with others and time alone. Trying to hurry a person in the development of a new body image may only impede progress.

## Assessing for Problems of Body Image Integrity

### Developmental Level

When you have identified a situation in which body image integrity may be disturbed, you will need to make a thorough assessment of the individual patient. First, consider the patient's developmental level. What might be his or her primary needs and concerns? How are those needs and concerns related to the current situation? Is the patient, for example, a young adult just beginning to develop interdependent relationships with the opposite sex? If so, changes perceived as diminishing sexual attractiveness or sexual ability may

be especially upsetting. The removal of a uterus is likely to be less upsetting to a woman past childbearing age than to an eighteen-year-old who has never had a child.

### Occupation and Life Style

Another area of concern is the person's occupation or role. A singer's throat is important to her, while a telephone lineman may consider his legs much more significant. The person whose occupation is sedentary will be less threatened by an illness that necessitates being sedentary than will someone whose previous job involved considerable physical activity. A businesswoman who considers it necessary to entertain frequently may be excessively upset by an ulcer that requires a special diet.

## Cultural Expectations

Cultural expectations may greatly affect a person's response to a body change. Because of Western society's definition of beauty in women, a woman who loses a great deal of weight might not be too upset; a man who associates large size with masculinity might find weight loss of greater concern.

## Strengths and Weaknesses

As you assess the patient, consider his or her strengths and weaknesses. What assets will the person be able to bring to bear on the crisis? Some people have developed strength by confronting previous crises successfully. Others have the support of strong religious beliefs. Always try to meet the family or significant others in the patient's life and to assess their strengths. Some family members may be very helpful, while others also need assistance in dealing with the crisis. Each individual has some strengths that can be built on.

Some individuals do not have supportive families and friends. Some are undergoing other major crises in addition to body changes. Problems such as these will need to be considered when you plan for care of the patient.

## Behavioral Response

Identifying the particular stage the person is experiencing in the process of re-establishing body image integrity will help you to respond in the most helpful way. What are the patient's behavior patterns? Observe for activity level, pacing the floor, chain-smoking, and other signs of anxiety. The person may refuse to discuss the change or, alternatively, become completely absorbed with it to the exclusion of all other topics. Neither is a healthy response. What are the patient's facial expressions? Muscles may be tense and the lips tightly drawn if the person is upset and anxious. The entire face may droop if depression is severe. Does the person's reaction seem appropriate to the situation? For example, laughing and joking about the loss of a leg indicate a serious problem. Such a loss is a major disability and requires considerable adaptation. Denial of the seriousness of the disability is a barrier to rehabilitation.

## Individual Perception

Always keep in mind that it is the person's own perception of the seriousness of the change that most profoundly affects his or her response. To determine how the individual sees the change, and how he or she feels about it, an interview is essential. One colostomy patient may express fear that he will be unacceptable to others; another individual recovering from the same surgery may express relief that the colostomy will allow for participation in social events previously impossible due to chronic pain and diarrhea.

# Intervening in Problems of Body Image Integrity

There are many ways you can help the patient maintain body image integrity. Most are valuable in prevention as well as in dealing with an existing problem. Planning ahead for the maintenance of body image integrity may prevent the patient from experiencing severe difficulties.

## Therapeutic Environment

A *therapeutic environment* that helps the patient accept the change can be provided by promoting cleanliness, enhancing the patient's personal appearance, and performing other tasks that demonstrate respect. Providing privacy and preserving modesty are also important. These considerations are sometimes overlooked in the case of children, but they too respond to recognition of their personal modesty.

## Emphasizing Strengths

Emphasizing unimpaired abilities and assets and putting no undue stress on the disability may help the person accept the change. Help the patient look for his or her own strengths.

By avoiding an exclusive focus on one part of the body, you may help the patient retain a broad perspective on the self. If, on the other hand, everyone who contacts the patient is interested only in his or her bowel function, the patient too will focus on that alone. When appropriate, remind the patient of previous occasions when he or she has coped successfully with stress and of the family and friends available for support.

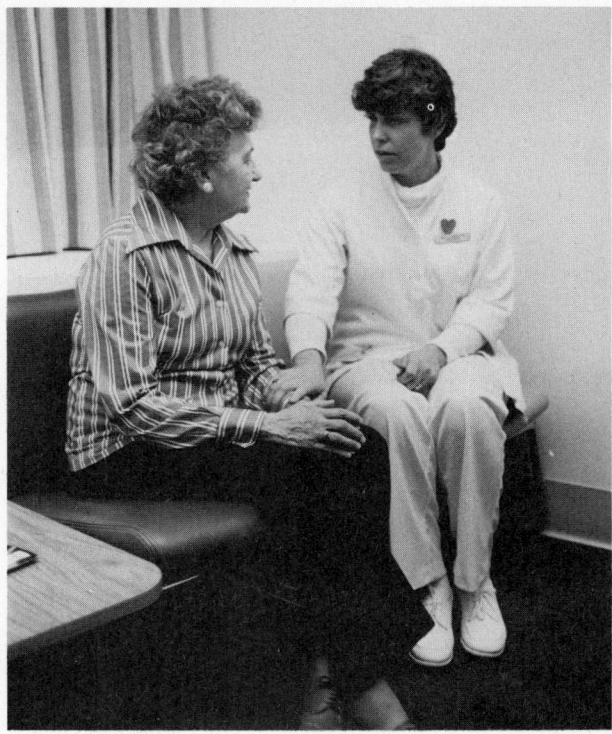

**Figure 29.5**
Preparing the family for what they will encounter helps them be supportive to the patient. (Russ Kinne/Danbury Hospital/Photo Researchers, Inc.)

## Perceptual Feedback

Such *perceptual feedback* as touching a scar or the stump of an amputated arm can provide valuable sensory input. Encouraging active movement of a changed part, such as an arm affected by a stroke, will provide for *kinesthetic feedback*. When active movement is not possible, passive movement (movement whose energy is provided by another person) is helpful. *Visual feedback* by means of mirrors allows the patient to face reality and not be overwhelmed by imaginings that exaggerate reality. Feedback must be appropriate to the individual's level of development.

## Verbal Feedback

*Verbal feedback* on the movements being performed is valuable in establishing understanding of the body's new feelings. For example, while exercising a patient's leg, you may state, "Now I

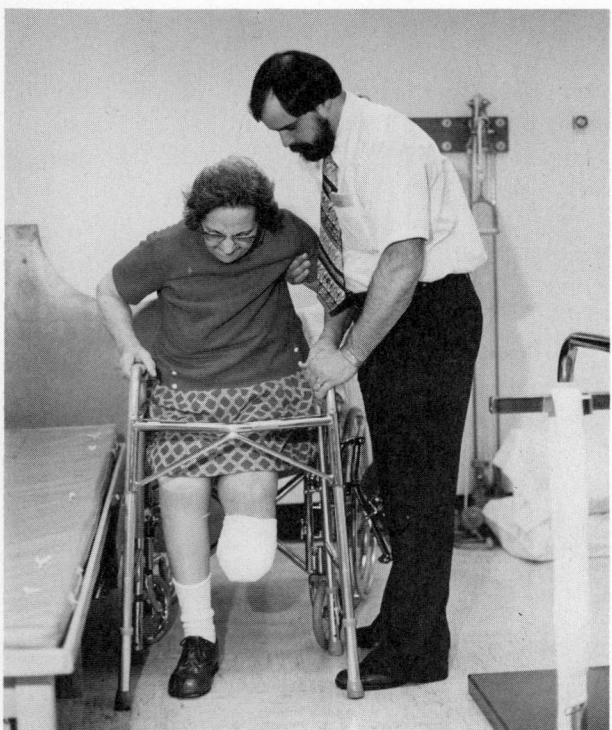

**Figure 29.4**
Perceptual feedback helps a patient cope with a body-image disturbance. (Russ Kinne/Danbury Hospital/Photo Researchers, Inc.)

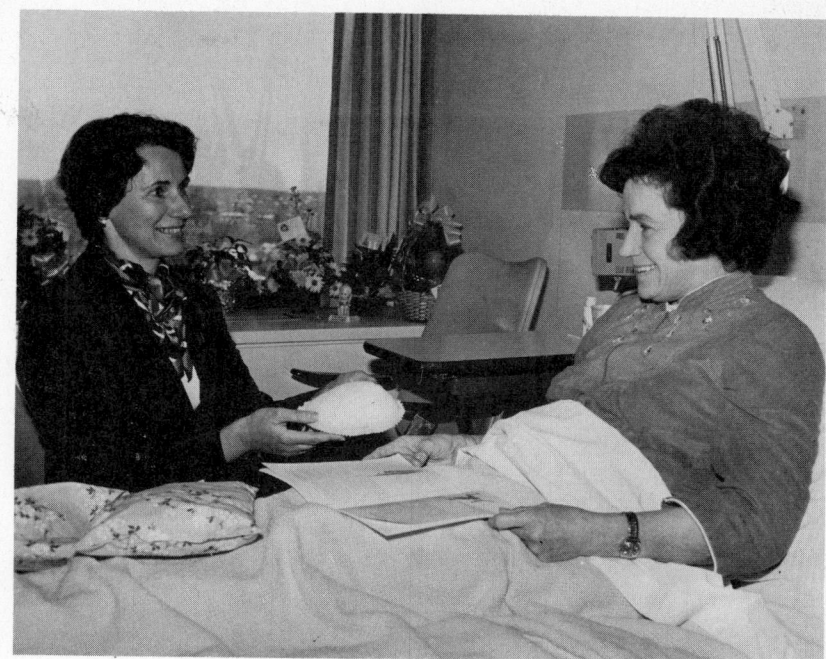

**Figure 29.6**
A Reach to Recovery volunteer demonstrates a breast prosthesis to a mastectomy patient. (Russ Kinne/Danbury Hospital/Photo Researchers, Inc.)

am bending your knee. Now I am straightening it out.''

## Helping Family and Friends to Be Supportive

The patient, family, and friends may deal more effectively with a profound change if they are adequately prepared before actually confronting it. It may thus be beneficial to describe the expected changes to the family in advance so they can maintain composure and provide support to the patient when they first view the change. You may also counsel family and friends to help them understand the stages the patient may go through. Sometimes they may benefit from explanation of the value of feedback and a therapeutic environment.

## Health Teaching for the Patient

There is a fine line between adequate preparation of the patient and frightening disclosures he or she is not ready for. The individual's response must be your guide in making such decisions. For example, a young woman refused to look at her colostomy for days after the surgery and would not consider learning to care for it herself. A nurse, assessing the situation, learned that the patient was envisioning a "horrible black mess" and explained that the colostomy is a rosy-pink mucous membrane approximately 2 inches in diameter. The patient then looked at her colostomy, found it was not as bad as she had expected, and began learning self-care.

Explanations of changes in functioning should be at a level of sophistication appropriate to the patient. Such explanations should note possible changes in feeling and the effects that treatments and medications will have on functioning. Mistaken ideas often add greatly to the patient's fears and burdens.

## Therapeutic Interaction

Finally, the nurse may be able to help the person understand what he or she is feeling. The techniques of interpersonal communication (see Chapter 12) are valuable in this endeavor. The purpose of such interaction is to help the patient explore personal feelings and make independent decisions about self-care, future plans, and methods of coping with the change.

# Conclusion

Body image is a complex phenomenon encompassing all the ways a person perceives his or her own body. The development of body image is a lifelong process characterized by constant shift and change. Although patterns of body image development are identifiable, each person must be considered as an individual.

Body image integrity is essential to optimal functioning. Because illness causes myriad changes in the body and requires adaptation of the body image, the nurse must develop skill at identifying threats to body image, assessing for disturbances of body image integrity, intervening to prevent problems, and helping resolve existing problems.

## Care Study    A patient with a disturbance of body image integrity

Eleanor Jacal, a student in a Fundamentals of Nursing course, is assigned Mrs. Katherine Meindl, age forty-eight, who had a left radical mastectomy three days ago. In preparing to care for this patient, Eleanor notes the following:

1. A radical mastectomy involves removal of a large amount of chest and axillary tissue, as well as the breast itself. The resulting scar is quite large. There may be some weakness and difficulty of movement in the arm on the operated side because of the role chest muscles play in arm movement.

2. A radical mastectomy is usually performed for a malignancy of the breast and there is likely to be considerable concern about the potential spread of malignancy.

3. Although radical mastectomy is extensive surgery, by the fourth postoperative day it is usual for the patient to be ambulating and beginning self-care.

4. Movement of the arm on the operated side is usually ordered by the surgeon, and exercises are usually started in the postoperative period.

5. It is usual for the mastectomy patient to be upset about this change in body structure. She often feels a loss of femininity and concern over the response of significant family members, especially her sexual partner. Depression is common.

In making her plans, Eleanor anticipates spending a lot of time with Mrs. Meindl, who will probably be sad and need support.

When Eleanor enters Mrs. Meindl's room the next morning, she is surprised to see a woman in a beautiful bed jacket, hair perfectly arranged and makeup expertly applied, though it is only 7:30 a.m. Mrs. Meindl greets her with a smile and says, "I'm sure having a student will be fun. Of course, I'm not really a sick patient, so you won't have much to do." This is not at all the response Eleanor expected. She wonders if Mrs. Meindl is just an exceptionally well-adjusted woman.

When the surgeon arrives to change the dressings, Mrs. Meindl says "You do what you must—I'm really not interested. Eleanor and I will just continue our chat." Mrs. Meindl looks the other way and ignores the surgeon's comments throughout the dressing change.

Later, when Eleanor is discussing with Mrs. Meindl her plans after leaving the hospital, the patient states that she expects to begin her old activities immediately. "You see, my daughter will be coming home from college for vacation. She doesn't know I've had surgery. I don't want her to know that she has only half a mother."

The staff nurse visits during the morning to say, "Mrs. Meindl, often women who have had a mastectomy wonder about the various kinds of 'falsies' available. There is an organization called Reach to Recovery made up of women who have had mastectomies. A member of that group would be glad to visit and would be able to discuss this with you." "No!!" Mrs. Meindl almost shouts. "I—I mean, no, thank you. I'm not interested," she continues, in a calmer tone of voice.

As Eleanor is preparing to report off to the team leader at noon, she reviews her assessment data.

1. Mrs. M. appeared cheerful and outgoing on first contact.

2. She refused to look at the surgical incision or to listen to the surgeon's discussion of the surgery.

3. Mrs. M.'s plans are to take up her former activities without a recuperative period. This is not realistic.

4. She has kept the operation a secret from a college-age daughter.

5. She had called herself "half a mother."

6. Mrs. M. appeared upset when a "Reach to Recovery" visitor was suggested.

Eleanor decides that Mrs. Meindl has a problem of body image integrity, on the grounds that she is not discussing or showing evidence of facing the physical change in any way and that her emotional response to the problem appears to be interfering with her ability to be realistic about her care.

Since Eleanor will not be caring for Mrs. Meindl during the rest of her hospital stay, she decides to report her findings to the team leader. The team leader says, "I've been concerned about Mrs. Meindl. Her cheerfulness is too good to be true. After all, any surgery is serious and her attitude doesn't seem very realistic. I appreciate the specific information you've been able to give me. I do agree with your analysis of the problem. During our team conference this afternoon, we can bring this problem to the attention of the entire team and develop a plan for helping Mrs. Meindl."

The student nurse has researched background information, collected data on the patient, and analyzed the data, determining that a problem exists. In considering a plan of action, she recognizes her own limitations and reports her concerns to someone with the skill and opportunity to act. The process of assisting Mrs. Meindl with her problem is begun.

## Study Terms

acceptance
anger
body image
body image integrity
denial
depression
disbelief
feedback
kinesthetic feedback

perceptual feedback
stimuli
  external
  internal
  therapeutic
    environment
verbal feedback
visual feedback

## Learning Activities

**1.** List as many of your own physical characteristics as you can. Consider your appearance, sensations, and kinesthetic sense.

**2.** Review the patients on a hospital unit, possibly during morning report. List those you consider prone to a disturbance in body image integrity.

**3.** For a patient in the clinical area whom you have identified as suffering from a disturbance of body image integrity, outline the appropriate nursing process. Include assessment, goal, plan for intervention, and evaluation.

## References

Blaesing, S., and Brockhaus, J. "The Development of Body Image in the Child." *Nursing Clinics of North America* 7 (December 1972): 597–607.

Bucy, N.; Unruh, I.; and McFadden, G. A. "Lead Your Maimed Patient Back to Independence." *RN* 40 (June 1977): 29–33.

Compton, C. Y. "War Injury: Identity Crisis for Young Men." *Nursing Clinics of North America* 8 (March 1973): 53–66.

Corbeil, M. "The Nursing Process for a Patient With a Body Image Disturbance." *Nursing Clinics of North America* 6 (March 1971): 155–163.

Craft, C. A. "Body Image and Obesity." *Nursing Clinics of North America* 7 (December 1972): 677.

Dempsey, M. O. "The Development of Body Image in the Adolescent." *Nursing Clinics of North America* 7 (December 1972): 609–615.

Fujita, M. "The Impact of Illness or Surgery on the Body Image of a Child." *Nursing Clinics of North America* 7 (December 1972): 641.

Gallagher, A. M. "Body Image Changes in the Patient With a Colostomy." *Nursing Clinics of North America* 7 (December 1972): 669–676.

Hill, S. "The Child With Ambiguous Genitalia." *American Journal of Nursing* 77 (May 1977): 810–814.

Leonard, B. J. "Body Image Changes in Chronic Illness." *Nursing Clinics of North America* 7 (December 1972): 687–695.

Loxley, A. K. "The Emotional Toll of Crippling Deformity." *American Journal of Nursing* 72 (1972): 1839–1840.

McCloskey, J. C. "How to Make the Most of Body Image Theory in Nursing Practice." *Nursing '76* 6 (May 1976): 68–72.

Miles, M. S. "Body Integrity Fears in the Toddler." *Nursing Clinics of North America* 4 (March 1969): 39–51.

Murray, R. L. "Body Image Development in Adulthood." *Nursing Clinics of North America* 7 (December 1972): 651–660.

———. "Principles of Nursing Intervention for the Adult Patient With Body Image Changes." *Nursing Clinics of North America* 7 (December 1972): 697–707.

Nev, C. "Coping With Newly Diagnosed Blindness." *American Journal of Nursing* 75 (1975): 2161–2163.

Riddle, I. "Nursing Intervention to Promote Body Image Integrity in Children." *Nursing Clinics of North America* 7 (December 1972): 651–661.

Smith, C. A. "Body Image Changes After Myocardial Infarction." *Nursing Clinics of North America* 7 (December 1972): 663.

Tierney, E. A. "Accepting Disfigurement When Death Is the Alternative." *American Journal of Nursing* 75 (December 1975): 2149–2150.

# Chapter 30
# The Fragile Older Adult

## Objectives

After completing this chapter, you should be able to:

1. Describe the physical changes that take place in the various body systems with aging.
2. Discuss the psychosocial needs of the older adult with regard to life style, retirement, finances, housing, and loss.
3. Name three organizations for the elderly.
4. Enumerate the purposes of organizations that provide for the aging population.
5. List the types and characteristics of long-term care settings available to older patients.
6. Discuss institutionalization, communication, confusion, and safety with reference to the patient in the long-term care setting.
7. Explain how you might help meet patient needs specific to long-term care.

## Outline

There are more elderly people in the United States today than ever before: one out of every ten Americans is over sixty-five. This phenomenon is attributable to a dramatic increase in life expectancy. At the turn of the century, one could expect to live an average of forty-five years; at present, the average person lives into the late seventies. Many more people are living into their eighties, nineties, and beyond. Since living longer increases one's chances of disease and illness, older people are seeking health care and being admitted to acute- and chronic-care facilities with growing frequency. Forty percent of physicians' office visits are accounted for by the elderly, and they also occupy 33 percent of hospital beds in the United States (Aiken, 1978). This phenomenon has obvious implications for nurses. Schools of nursing are recognizing the importance of providing student nurses clinical experience in caring for geriatric (aging) patients. The skills of caring for the aging patient are essentially the same skills the nurse offers every patient, adapted to the physical changes and limitations that may accompany aging. In addition, special attention must be given to the psychological needs of the older person. Although the student nurse may not wish to pursue a career in geriatric nursing, knowledge of older patients and their needs is essential; contact with older persons is inherent in nursing. Even in pediatrics, you may find that an older family member greatly influences the decisions and eventual recovery of a young patient.

Two terms with which you should be familiar are *geriatrics*, the specialty in health care dealing with the aged patient, and *gerontology*, the study of the aging process, including the illnesses and diseases of old age. Nurses can specialize in both these areas.

## What Is Aging?

Though there are many theories of aging, no one knows precisely why some people age more rapidly than others. Hans Selye and others have postulated that each person has an individual "aging clock" whose rate depends on inherited adaptive energies. Selye further suggests that one's degree of ability to cope with stress is a central factor in aging. In other words, aging is seen by Selye and others as a function of life stress and the degree to which one can successfully resolve or adapt to stressors.

Another theory of aging postulates that the autoimmune system of the body, which protects us from disease and combats injury by producing antibodies and hormones that have a homeostatic action, becomes less responsive with age, allowing structural deterioration and diseases to increase in occurrence.

According to the complicated cross-linkage theory, aging is accompanied by an increase in accidental crossings-over or linkages between the intracellular and extracellular molecules, resulting in a stiffening of all of the connective tissues of the body. This phenomenon is accompanied, it is suggested, by a realignment of DNA particles, an essential component of all living cells.

Easier to grasp is the "wear-and-tear" theory, according to which all plant and animal life is subject to wearing out after a certain period of time.

No single theory of aging has been proven; aging may possibly be attributable to a combination of factors. We can, however, say with certainty that aging, like all human experiences, is individual. Consider for a moment the eighty-three-year-old retired attorney, hospitalized for minor surgery, who sits up at night studying the new math, because, as he says, "It's so exciting. There's so much to know." At the other end of the spectrum is the sixty-eight-year-old woman lying impassive in a nursing-home bed, staring blankly at a rain-spattered window. Why do people age so differently? We can only speculate that variations depend on such factors as the patient's heredity, previous mental attitudes, health, and nutritional status, as well as the support of the family. Other factors, known and unknown, affect different individuals. Theories about the causes of aging are not germane here; it is important only that we remember that aging is a natural process.

## The Needs of the Fragile Older Adult

By no means are all older people fragile: for example, only 6–7 percent of people over the age of sixty-five live in chronic-care facilities. Nevertheless, our older patients are often frail and vulnerable to injury, stress, and complications of illness.

The fragile older adult, like the healthy, vigorous adult, has numerous needs and problems. For purposes of assessment, let us look in turn at the physical and psychosocial ramifications of aging, keeping in mind that they overlap.

## Physical Changes

The body of a young person makes the adaptations necessary to maintain homeostasis rather quickly. The elderly, due to cellular and tissue changes, respond or adapt more slowly to physiological and emotional stresses and thus have more difficulty maintaining a state of balance. As nurses, we can help the older patient to make needed adaptations. This ought, in fact, to be the focus of care.

Because diminishing physical strength is readily obvious, we often tend to mistakenly identify this aspect of a person as representative of the total being. This tendency leads us astray, since many older adults who are fragile physically remain strong and viable otherwise. Nevertheless, changes unavoidably occur in the body as one ages.

Though people do not all experience the same bodily changes with aging, patterns can be discerned. The assessment process will be facilitated by familiarity with the potential effects of aging on the systems of the body.

### Cardiovascular

Cardiovascular conditions are the leading cause of death among the elderly. Changes in the cardio-

vascular system are complex. The most generalized complication that arises in the elderly is *arteriosclerosis*, a thickening of the middle wall of blood vessels that narrows the opening through which the blood flows. A more severe form of vascular compromise occurs with *atherosclerosis*, an additional thickening of the inner wall of arteries caused by the presence of deposits. This condition, which makes the vessels even more rigid and narrows the *lumen* (the interior of the vessels), affects every system of the body by diminishing the supply of blood to all organs.

The heart muscle itself is less efficient due to decreased blood supply, and a weaker beat often described as "thready" results. In conjunction with degenerative changes in the vessels supplying the heart muscle, the valves of the heart itself do not close as tightly as they once did. What are the consequences of all this for the patient? The blood pressure rises due to the increased force with which an unchanged volume of blood is pushed through a smaller lumen in the vessels. Because circulation is slow, the patient feels cold. Standing for a long period of time pools blood in the lower extremities and may cause dizziness. Lying on the extremities causes tingling and can disturb rest. The muscles stiffen, the muscles of respiration are no longer as vigorous, and over-

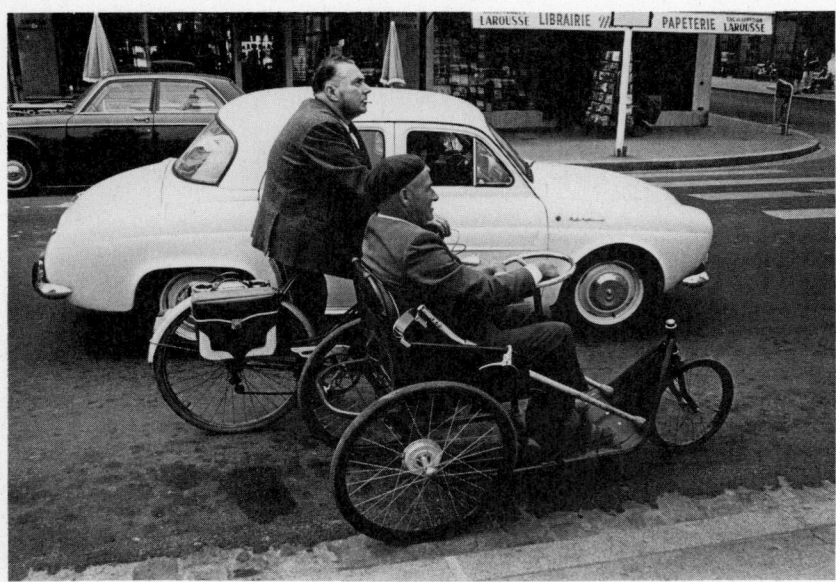

**Figure 30.1   Out on an errand**
Harry Wilks/Stock, Boston

exertion can quickly exhaust the individual. The kidneys also receive less blood supply and are less productive than before. Drugs are excreted more slowly and can build up in the body, necessitating close observation for drug effects. The patient may be prescribed special drugs to facilitate functioning of the cardiovascular system, perhaps for the rest of his or her life.

## Respiratory

The respiratory system is affected by changes in the musculoskeletal system. Bone and muscle changes decrease actual chest size. There are also fewer alveoli, and those present become larger and less elastic. The older person breathes slightly faster than the younger person in order to compensate for these changes. More important than actual chest size is decreased ability to cough. The collection of secretions that are not *expectorated* (spit out) is often a source of infection. Encouraging patients, especially those who are bed-ridden, to cough and deep-breathe can help ward off respiratory complications.

## Musculoskeletal

Musculoskeletal changes due to aging affect the joints, long bones, and muscles and can be very troublesome. Many people become more seden-

tary as they grow older and may change position less frequently. It has been shown that the active, healthy person need not lose more than 30–40 percent of muscle tone and strength through aging. However, lack of exercise and improper diet often cause older people to lose a much greater proportion of their muscle tone. Weak muscles enhance the danger of broken bones, since they cannot provide adequate support. A moderate exercise program and a good diet adequate in protein will help the patient maintain muscle strength.

Bones often undergo degenerative changes with aging. The most common condition is *osteoporosis*, a metabolic failure to replace bone tissue, which leads to thin, porous bones that fracture easily. Although this condition occurs primarily in older women, due to the reduction of estrogens, it also afflicts men. Symptoms include low back pain, weakness, stooped posture, and a tendency to fracture bones. It is hoped that hormonal supplement therapy after menopause will greatly lessen the incidence of osteoporosis in older women, and early data appear to support this hypothesis. In general, the diet should contain adequate calcium, protein, and vitamin D. Excess calcium in the diet will not prevent osteoporosis because it is a metabolic problem.

The nurse must take extra precautions to protect a patient with osteoporosis against accidents that could lead to the breakage of bones. If osteoporosis is severe, even grasping the long bones to turn the bed patient can result in a fracture. Ambulatory patients most often suffer fractures of the neck of the femur and the trochanter. It has been speculated that in many cases of hip fracture, the hip fractures spontaneously and causes the fall, rather than the reverse.

Most geriatric patients have some degree of osteoarthritis, which is assumed to be caused by the wearing of joint cartilage until the underlying bone is exposed. This situation in turn causes pain and immobility, and sometimes swelling, of the joint. Almost every person over the age of forty has some osteoarthritis in the cervical spine or neck, which may be asymptomatic until later in life when joints of the extremities also become involved. Treatment of arthritis consists of moderate exercise to maintain mobility, medications for inflammation and pain, and special therapies such as heat. When caring for the person with arthritis, a gentle touch is needed. The patient may be able to tell you how he or she moves most easily. Remember that the patient may be in constant pain.

*Gout* is a systemic illness whose most common symptom is swollen and inflamed joints. In addition to medication, the patient is often ordered to consume 3000–4000 ml of fluid a day. Seeing to a fluid intake this high may take ingenuity on your part: a variety of juices and beverages and an intake schedule designed with the patient's help are both beneficial.

## Urinary

The urinary system may also be affected by the aging process. The vessels and renal arteries narrow and the filtering process is less efficient. However, the volume of urine produced in a day remains relatively stable throughout life. Studies show that bladder capacity lessens as one ages, necessitating that the bladder be emptied more frequently. Getting up at night to urinate is common but interrupts the patient's rest. The sphincter, because it is muscular, loses some of its elasticity, and urine leakage can occur in both males and females. This is understandably disturbing to the patient, and a solution is not easy. The male can wear a device that consists of a penile covering, much like a condom catheter, connected to a leg bag. Females may wear a light padding to protect against accidents. Corrective surgery is sometimes indicated. Muscular deterioration can also

prevent the bladder from emptying completely, encouraging the growth of bacteria. Susceptibility to infections and the formation of stones (calculi) are common results.

## Genital

The female's ability to produce children ends at menopause. The male's ability to produce sperm persists throughout life, though their number diminishes. Thus the male can procreate well into his eighth decade. There is little reason, physically, for libido (sexual desire) to wane in later life on the part of either sex. Frequency of intercourse may decrease and it may take longer to reach orgasm, but libido remains. The unavailability of a sexual partner is the most common reason for cessation of sexual activity (Masters and Johnson, 1977).

Estrogen deficiency in the female may cause thinning of the vaginal walls and decreased lubrication. Vaginal creams are available to alleviate this problem. Use of supplemental estrogens is currently being discouraged because of a possible link to cancer, but women should be encouraged to consult with their physician about their own particular situation.

## Gastrointestinal

The gastrointestinal tract probably causes the elderly more distress than any other system of the body. Foods once easily digested can in the later years cause gastric or intestinal discomfort. Actually, the digestive system undergoes far less change than do other systems of the body. There is some decrease in the digestive juices and some reduction in the ability of the gall bladder to secrete bile. Much of the problem appears to be due to inadequate chewing of food because of ill-fitting dentures or poor teeth, inappropriate food choices, and emotional upset. Constipation in the elderly results largely from early and continued use of laxatives. Constipation is much more frequent than diarrhea. With old age and its accompanying muscular changes, the bowel becomes less responsive and laxatives less efficient. You may have considerable difficulty convincing the older patient of the

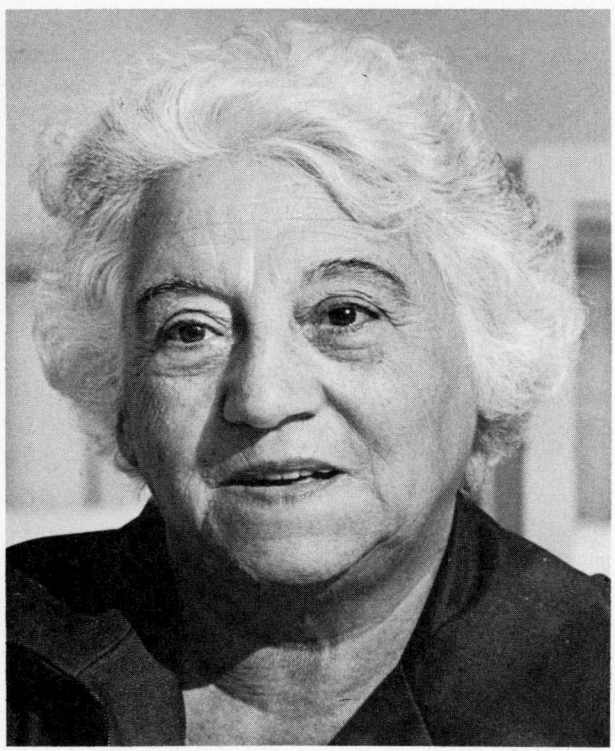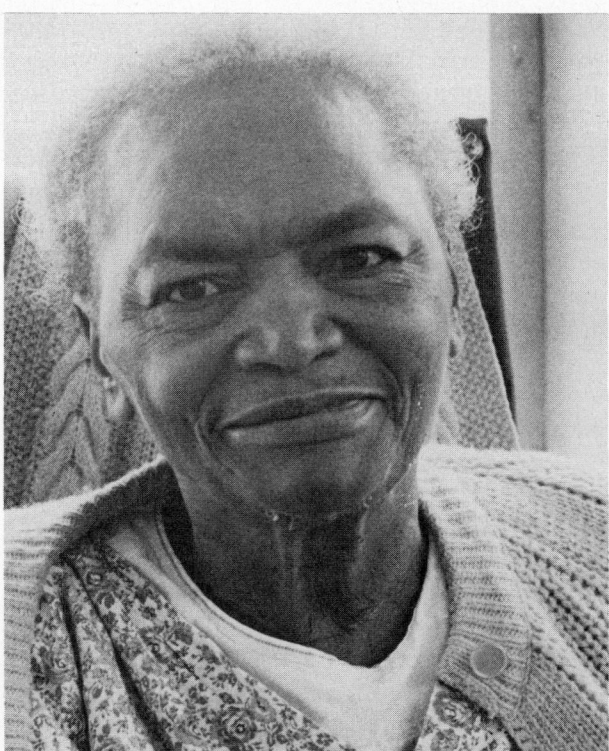

**Figure 30.2**
Changes in the hair and skin accompany aging. (*Left:* Ellis Herwig/Stock, Boston; *right:* John Goodman)

need to increase fluid intake, include roughage in the diet, and exercise, though all contribute to healthy bowel functioning. It is often impossible to eliminate the use of laxatives once they have become a habit.

## Skin

The integument (skin) undergoes profound changes with aging. Wrinkling, though present to a degree even in children, is an overt sign of aging. Research tells us that smoking, poor diet, and exposure to sun and weather hasten wrinkling. Thus it can to some degree be prevented, but a person who already has extensive wrinkling has little recourse except cosmetic surgery, seldom undertaken by the elderly.

Because skin becomes thin and dry as it ages, it is helpful to add oils directly to the bath water and to apply palliative oils or lotions sparingly to the skin immediately after the bath. Alcohol, often used in conjunction with rubs, should be avoided because of its drying effect on skin. Lotion is the better choice. Patients need not be bathed daily,

since bathing is drying to the skin. Many older patients are used to bathing only once a week and become upset at what they consider undue emphasis on cleanliness. Use care when placing an identification armband on the wrist of an elderly patient. An overly snug band can cause an abrasion, as can a tight watchband. Rubbing on sheets, lying on wrinkled bedding, and striking a siderail can also cause skin damage to the elderly. The slightest redness may be the forerunner of a difficult-to-heal decubitus ulcer or bedsore.

## Hair

The hair grays or whitens with age. Hair texture may also change, becoming curlier or straighter.

*Alopecia,* the loss of hair, is another common result of aging. Not only scalp hair but also hair in the axilla and genital area and general body hair becomes sparse. Baldness, though more common in the older male, also occurs in females. In women, baldness of the scalp is often patchy. It has been suggested that excessive shampooing, tight hats, and the practice of setting the hair tightly all promote balding, but evidence is not conclusive. Much male baldness is genetic and cannot be prevented. Baldness is important only as it affects the patient's body image. The use of a hairpiece should not be discouraged if it is beneficial to the patient's self-concept.

## The Five Senses

The five senses—seeing, hearing, smelling, tasting, and touching—diminish to some extent with age. It is thought that these alterations occur because of degeneration of nerves, vascular irregularities, and/or local tissue changes. In some patients such diminishment is almost undiscernible; in others it is rather profound. While it may be obvious that a patient is partially blind or hard-of-hearing, you may overlook decreased sensitivity of taste, smell, and touch. When the patient has suffered a significant loss in one or more senses, a degree of sensory deprivation can result (see Chapter 28), which can in turn cause psychological depression. Patients are sometimes defensive about a loss of hearing or sight, and some frankly deny it. The nurse with ingenuity can frequently channel a patient's interest toward the use of a compensatory sense. For example, the elderly patient who was an avid reader and television viewer until loss of vision made both impossible could make use of "talking book" records available through public libraries and organizations for the blind. Books with very large print are also available from libraries, and some newspapers print large-type editions. The mentally agile older person may want to learn a new skill, such as Braille. Specific nursing interventions for people suffering sensory impairment are suggested in Chapters 25 and 28; some modifications may be appropriate for the elderly.

## Vision

The pupils of elderly people's eyes become smaller, admitting less light to the retina. Because one result is difficulty seeing in the dark, the use of a nightlight may be helpful. Older patients can distinguish bright colors more easily than dark ones, so the use of red, orange, yellow, and pink may enhance vision. Speaking as you enter the room, identifying yourself, and expressing caring through touch are all helpful when tending a patient with diminished vision.

There is a high incidence of glaucoma in the elderly. *Glaucoma,* a condition characterized by increased intraocular pressure, is controlled by the frequent and uninterrupted use of eye medications administered in drops. If a patient with glaucoma is admitted to your unit, be sure that the eye medications are available, the physician writes an order for their use, and they are given conscientiously. If the patient wears contact lenses or glasses, make sure they are properly cared for and that the patient is assisted in their use if necessary.

## Hearing

Loss of hearing is far more common among the elderly than loss of sight. It has been estimated that one out of four people over age sixty has a degree of hearing loss sufficient to be characterized "medically deaf." Among the several causes of deafness are disturbances of the auditory nerve or cerebral cortex and changes in the structure of the ear itself. A hearing aid is not helpful in all cases, and an examination by a specialist can determine whether or not such a device would improve hearing.

In assessment, it is not enough to observe that a patient has a hearing loss. Determine which ear is least affected, and, when speaking, face the patient and position yourself nearer that side. Sitting or standing at eye level is also helpful since visual cues and lip-reading help the patient understand what you are saying. Because hearing loss is often more severe in the higher voice range, lowering your voice slightly also facilitates communication. Speaking clearly and distinctly is important because an elderly person may process information somewhat more slowly than the young. Never shout at the deaf; shouting may be interpreted as a hostile outburst.

## Taste

Although it does not usually pose a serious problem, diminishment of the sense of taste may cause a patient to lose interest in food and thus become malnourished. Older patients frequently remark that food "just doesn't taste as good as it once did." Dentures can interfere with the perception of both taste and texture. Tastes in food appear to change with age: one patient will crave sweets; another, who has always been fond of sweet foods, finds them no longer appealing. Diets planned with color and consistency in mind enhance appetite and are no more expensive to prepare than bland, colorless diets.

## Smell

The ability to smell also diminishes with age. Some older people use fragrances excessively due to a loss of olfactory acuity. Because smell is a major factor in appetite, *anorexia* (loss of appetite) is in part attributable to olfactory impairment. Inability to smell smoke in time to flee from a fire could affect the safety of the elderly person.

## Touch

Although testing has shown that the sense of touch diminishes somewhat with age, this process rarely interferes with the individual's life. Men as well as women enjoy crafts such as needlepoint, knitting, and weaving. Difficulty working with fine yarns and patterns is often attributable to both visual loss and impairment of touch. The best solution is for the patient to use bulky knits or larger patterns. The primary problem posed by impairment of touch is the possibility of injury from sharp or hot objects. Such accidents might be prevented by avoiding hot-water bottles and heating pads and by wearing shoes at all times to protect the feet. A deficit in touch could also cause a person to overlook an injury and thus to go without care. Older people should be encouraged to examine the extremities daily for signs of injury.

## Metabolism

Decrease in metabolism results in lower body temperature. Heat is also lost because of decreased muscle bulk and underlying adipose (fat) tissue in the extremities and, in the case of very thin people, the trunk. Elderly people should not be exposed to very cool temperatures because of their difficulty in maintaining body temperature. On the other hand, an excessively warm environment can also be a problem due to decreased ability to perspire, which cools the body. Moderate temperatures and adequate clothing are appropriate.

## Central Nervous System

Although brain mass (weight) diminishes in later life and cerebrovascular changes may result in decreased blood flow to the brain, a direct link between these conditions and reasoning and thinking has not been established. Brain function is known to depend on many factors. The physiological changes described above, as well as motivation and stimulation, are factors that may affect the ability to think and learn. Older people tend to learn more slowly than the young but can learn as well. The synapses (connections) of the spinal column with the peripheral nerves may lengthen, slowing reaction time. For this reason, precautions should be taken in the operation of motor vehicles and machinery.

Though the word *senile* technically means nothing more than the state of being old, it is now commonly used with reference to mental deterioration and thus has offensive connotations for many people. Lately, however, the term has come into use in diagnosis and appears on the charts of many older patients. In the context of diagnosis, senility means a state of physiological and psychological deterioration with age. At best, it is a broad and ill-defined term. Though no one knows whether the state of senility is reversible, a study undertaken several years ago sheds some light on the question. Five nursing-home patients who had been classified as senile were organized into a sharing group by the nurses. They met daily and talked about their past experiences and skills. At first, talk was minimal, but as time went on, these patients renewed their interest in life, began caring for themselves again, and improved physically. One wonders, then, whether these people were truly senile. If so, can the state of senility be reversed? Far different, in any event, is the 107-year-old woman who exhibits little in the way of mental faculties, does not respond to sensory input, and completely lacks reasoning power. Has her body outlived her brain?

The National Institutes of Health recently stated,

"Senility is not an inevitable consequence of growing old; in fact, it is not even a disease. . . . Rather, 'senility' is a word commonly used to describe a large number of causes, many of which respond to prompt and effective treatment." Unfortunately, less money was spent in 1975 for medical research on aging than on any other medical field. A vigorous investigation of the causes of senility does not appear to be in the offing at this time.

## Psychosocial Needs

The attitudes of society impose many problems on the elderly. Social restrictions may bring on more significant psychological problems than does the aging process itself. On the other hand, our society is beginning to take increasing responsibility for responding to such problems and initiating programs to help meet the needs of the aging.

Chapter 4 examined Erikson's description of late adulthood as characterized by conflict between integrity and despair. Similarly, Robert Havighurst assigns to late maturity development tasks whose purpose is to maintain integrity. He defines successful coping with late maturity as adjusting to decreasing physical and psychological health, adjusting to retirement and reduced income, establishing appropriate living arrangements, adjusting to the death of a spouse or others of significance, establishing an explicit relationship with one's age group, and meeting social and civic obligations. Fulfillment of these developmental tasks would lead, finally, to acceptance of one's own death.

### Stable Life Style

Only in the last few years has adjustment to life changes been investigated in any depth (see Chapter 15). Life change may be internal, such as illness, or external, such as changes in relationships or employment or social status. According to Dudley and Welke, "Too much life change over a short period of time initiates illness, and the greater amount of life change, the more serious the illness" (1977). Statistics appear to bear out this hypothesis. In general, adjustment to life change is more difficult for the elderly since their life styles and relationships are of longer standing.

Within a very brief time span, the older person may find it necessary to adjust to retirement, decreased income, relocation, and disruption of relationships due to loss of contact or even the death of a spouse or beloved friend.

### Retirement

Traditionally, retirement age was fixed at sixty-five, regardless of whether or not the individual was able and wanted to continue working. Fortunately, this practice is changing; some places of employment allow the age of retirement to be extended to seventy if doing so is mutually desirable. The people who look forward to retirement are usually those with long-standing interests in hobbies and other leisure activities. People who have devoted themselves wholeheartedly to their jobs may find that retirement brings on feelings of worthlessness and depression. The adjustment for the retiree's spouse can be equally traumatic. Both may find it unnatural for the worker to be around the house all day with little to do, and conflicts

---

Exhibit 30.1
**Havighurst's Developmental Tasks for Later Maturity**

**1.** Adjusting to decreasing physical and psychological health.
**2.** Adjusting to retirement.
**3.** Adjusting to reduced income.
**4.** Establishing appropriate living arrangements.
**5.** Adjustment to the death of a spouse or others.
**6.** Establishing an explicit relationship with one's age group.
**7.** Meeting social and civic obligations.

---

can result. Preparation for retirement helps to alleviate these problems.

Dr. Carl Eisdorfer of the University of Washington suggests that in our younger years we purposely exercise more than one of our senses or abilities in leisure activities in order to guard against the loss of such outlets in later life. For example a person who always enjoyed classical music, and spent time collecting fine recordings and attending concerts, may react with depression and despair to the loss of hearing in later life. Despair might also afflict the outdoor-oriented hiker and backpacker who suffers a stroke and can no longer walk. The elderly who pursue skills and hobbies using two or more modalities are better able to compensate for the loss of one.

Retirement often disrupts established social patterns and may require the making of new friends. Ideally, these new contacts include people of all ages. Many older people make younger friends by attending classes on college campuses or in the community. City dwellers sometimes have an ad-

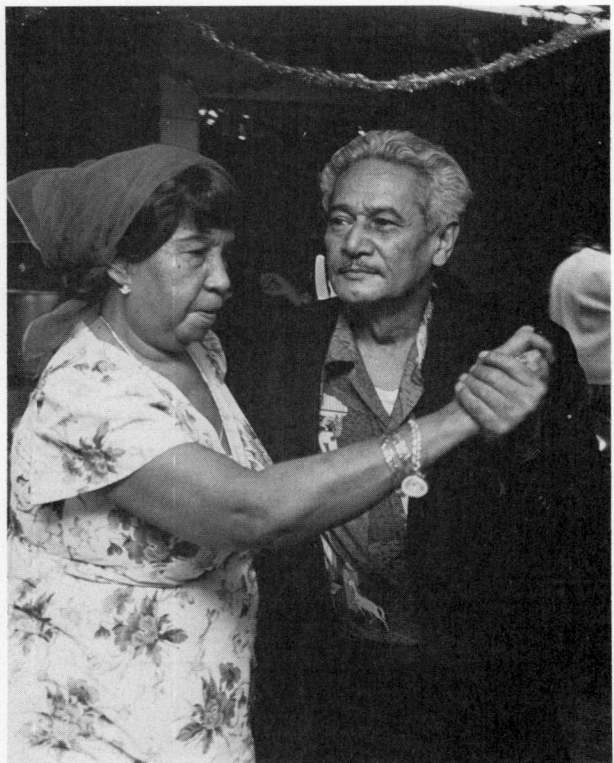

**Figure 30.3**
Older adults find enjoyment and companionship in social events. (Eric Kroll/Taurus Photos)

vantage over the rural elderly in that they have access to more opportunities for community participation. Many cities' daily newspapers list educational, recreational, and social events for the elderly. In any location, however, the elderly can be isolated and alone.

## Finances

Diminished income can be another burden of retirement. Sixteen percent of the elderly have incomes below the official poverty level; in this group, blacks outnumber whites two to one (U.S. Census Bureau, 1973). Although this figure is appalling in itself, many more older people live just above the poverty level.

What are the causes of financial distress on the part of the elderly? First, though most have accumulated retirement income through the federal Social Security program, these funds alone have proven inadequate to meet the high cost of living today. Second, because employment savings plans were uncommon until relatively recently, the individual worker had to look ahead independently to secure his or her financial future. Third, money put aside years ago has been severely devalued by inflation. Furthermore, people are living longer, and any savings they have accumulated must thus last longer. And some elderly people who suffered illnesses or injuries before Medicare and Medicaid were established sustained financial losses they have never recovered.

Living on a fixed income has penalized many older citizens. Increased Social Security payments and subsidies for high fuel costs have helped but not kept pace with spiraling price increases resulting from inflation.

Lack of money also affects the diets of older people, for whom adequate nutrition should be a priority. Because food costs have risen so steeply in the last few years, elderly people spend approximately one-third of their incomes on food. The older population has been found to have a high incidence of chronic malnutrition, due largely to food costs, the difficulties of shopping, longstanding poor eating habits, and poor meal planning. Eating alone also undermines appetite and proper eating. Sharing a meal occasionally with a friend or neighbor helps somewhat to alleviate this

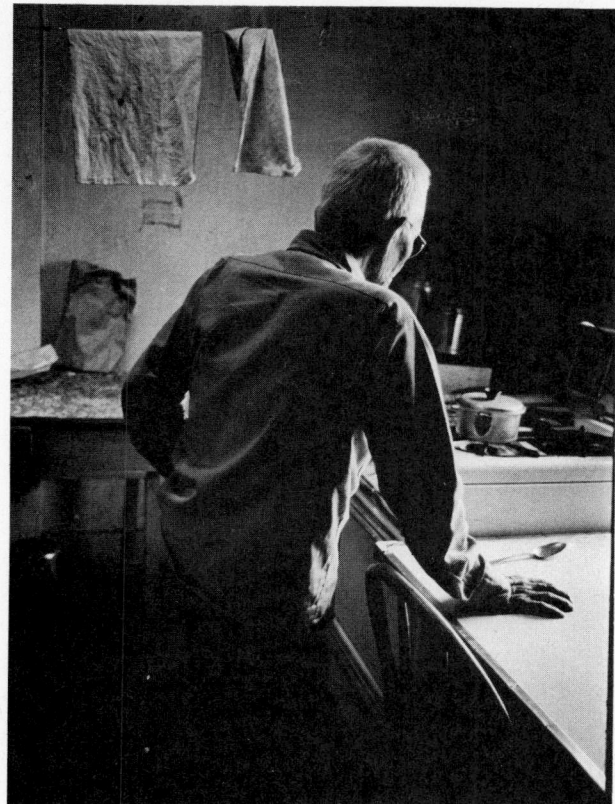

**Figure 30.4**
Lonely meals may contribute to poor nutrition. (James Mot-low/Jerobaam)

homes and form their own retirement communities, while others must accommodate themselves to small furnished or unfurnished rooms with minimal cooking facilities. The U.S. Department of Housing and Urban Development (HUD) has subsidized a limited number of low and moderately priced public housing units, but the waiting lists for such accommodations are very long.

Housing for the elderly should be located in an area with easy access to transportation, shopping, and social contacts. Pets should be permitted since they can be a great comfort to those who live alone. Homes must be in good repair to prevent injury. Ramps can be easily constructed to facilitate wheelchairs. A number of elderly people may need occasional help from housework agencies to maintain the cleanliness of their homes.

## Loss of Others

Adjustment to the loss of a lifelong spouse or friend is particularly hard for the elderly. The loss

problem. Federal food stamps and community centers that provide one well-balanced meal each day both represent attempts to solve nutritional problems of the elderly. Also, programs such as Meals-on-Wheels deliver inexpensive, well-balanced frozen meals to the elderly and disabled.

## Housing

Housing for the elderly is a problem of considerable magnitude. Many who have lived in the inner city for years no longer find their neighborhoods desirable—or even safe. Deteriorating neighborhoods, theft, and street violence have placed undue stress on older citizens and forced them to seek out less threatening environments. Finding adequate housing on a low fixed income is not easy. Large homes with high maintenance costs must often be traded for smaller, less expensive houses. Some elderly people purchase mobile

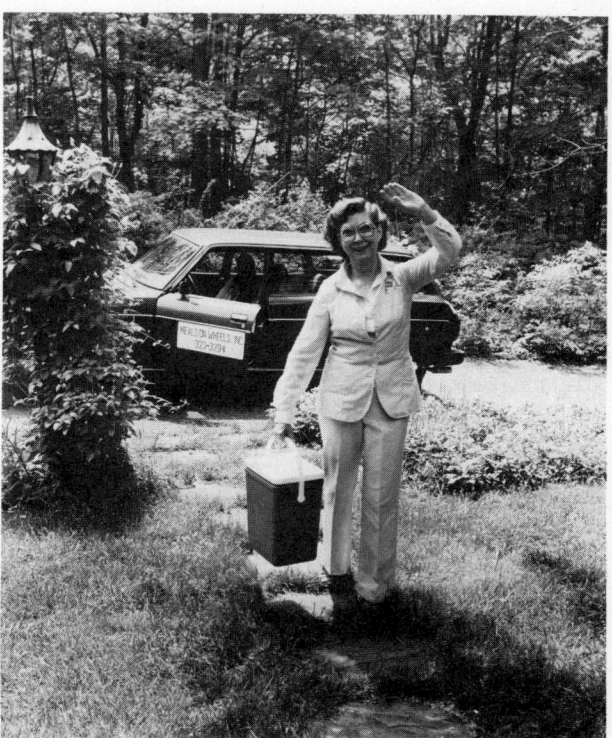

**Figure 30.5**
Community services may help the elderly maintain independence. (Russ Kinne/Photo Researchers, Inc.)

is made more acute by limited diversions and the difficulty of finding a new companion (see Chapter 27). Such losses may even necessitate a new living arrangement. Many researchers have cited the high incidence of mortality among surviving partners after the death of a spouse. The will to live is a strong factor in survival; the mutual dependence of many older couples, though inspiring to observe, can be devastating to the survivor. The family of a bereaved older person can facilitate the process of emotional reinvestment by offering love and care and by encouraging independent decision making on the part of the bereaved person. Rapidly relocating the survivor and taking over the making of necessary decisions only intensifies the depth of his or her depression and feelings of bereavement.

## Organizations for the Elderly

The realization that older citizens can, with proper organization, influence economic change and promote consumer rights has brought into being a number of organizations geared to the interests of the elderly. By the late 1970s, about six million older Americans were active in such organizations, twenty-four times as many as during the previous decade (Aiken, 1978).

In addition to those groups devoted to political change, there are many more informal groups that stress social interaction. Dues are usually no more than token. Retired and elderly people who live in rural areas should be encouraged to start such groups in their area. Younger people can be helpful by supporting the efforts of these organizations and by such contributions as volunteering to transport aging citizens to voting polls. Exhibit 30.2 lists a few of the larger organizations and agencies, both federal and private, devoted to the interests of the elderly. Each state also has its own organizations with which you should become familiar.

## The Healthy Older Adult

As nurses, we may develop a tendency to assume that most elderly people are fragile or infirm, since the elderly people we care for all have health problems. We should constantly remind ourselves that most older people remain vital and active until death. Many of our most distinguished political leaders are chronologically old; artists in their later years have produced some of our finest music, paintings, poetry, and prose. And we too are aging.

## Long-Term Care

With increased longevity, elderly people are more likely eventually to become unable to meet all of their own physical and psychological needs. This process may necessitate a change in living arrangements, ranging from minimal supervision to total skilled care.

Many older citizens get along well in their own homes; moving to an apartment setting has allowed others to continue to live independently. Some cities have telephone services that check on older people daily to assess their welfare.

## Reasons for Long-Term Care

There are many reasons why an older person might need some type of long-term care: diminishing senses, such as loss of sight or hearing; a physically limiting disability, such as paralysis of one or more extremities following a stroke; or cognitive and psychological factors, such as memory loss and confusion.

Extended families used to be quite common—that is, grandparents were an integral part of the family and often lived with their children long before disability required them to do so. However, the prevailing family structure has changed, and caring for an elderly person within the home setting is no longer so common. The mobility of the modern family would in many cases require the older relative to relocate, perhaps repeatedly, which is a particularly difficult and psychologically hazardous life change. Because people who require long-term care may be very old, their children may also be getting along in years and thus physically unable to take on the demanding task of caring for their parents. Frequently both husband and wife work outside the home, making continuity of care impossible. Family disruption due to divorce may preclude a home environment conducive to care. Another obstacle is the high cost of housing, which makes it difficult to afford extra space for the older person.

## Settings for Long-Term Care

There are several types of settings for long-term care of the elderly, some of which are still quite rare. Some people who live independently in a house or apartment are able to maintain themselves with some outside help and/or a supportive effort by family members and neighbors.

### Shared Living

In several parts of the country with large elderly populations, it is becoming increasingly common

Exhibit 30.2
**Organizations for the Elderly**

**Private**
American Association of Retired Persons (AARP)
1909 K Street, N.W.
Washington, D.C. 20006

American Geriatrics Society
10 Columbus Circle
New York, New York 10019

Gray Panthers
3700 Chestnut Street
Philadelphia, Pennsylvania 19104

National Alliance of Senior Citizens (NASC)
Box 40031
Washington, D.C. 20016

National Caucus on the Black Aged (NCBA)
1730 M Street, N.W.
Washington, D.C. 20006

**Federal**
Administration on Aging
Social and Rehabilitation Service
U.S. Department of Health, Education and Welfare
300 C Street, N.W.
Washington, D.C. 20201

National Institute on Aging
National Institutes of Health
U.S. Department of Health, Education and Welfare
9000 Rockville Pike
Bethesda, Maryland 20014

Office of Long-Term Care
Public Health Service
U.S. Department of Health, Education and Welfare
5600 Fishers Lane
Rockville, Maryland 20852

for older people to choose to live together, often in the home of one member of the group. Sharing expenses and responsibilities in this way allows some people to remain independent longer than they otherwise would.

## Retirement Apartments

Retirement apartments provide for privacy within a community. For such an arrangement to be suitable, the older person must be able to perform all ordinary activities of daily living, including preparation of meals. In some such facilities, limited household help is available. Many also sponsor social activities.

## Retirement Homes

Retirement homes have also become popular. Each resident has his or her own room and bath, and sometimes a small kitchenette. Served meals are available for people who cannot prepare their own. Some homes provide all meals; others offer only one or two meals. Still others require payment for all meals. Some retirement homes provide household services, though residents take care of their own personal needs. Emergency medical services are usually available.

## Minimal-Care Centers

Minimal-care centers offer primarily supervisory care, such as helping residents maintain hygiene and supervising medications. They are appropriate for people who do not need a great deal of help fulfilling their needs but who cannot manage totally alone.

## Total-Care Centers

Nursing homes exist to meet the needs of elderly people who need skilled nursing care for physical or psychological reasons. Though some such facilities are called convalescent centers, most of their residents are the fragile elderly who will stay on until death. The quality of care in nursing homes varies from excellent to poor. Complex economic issues, particularly involving public funding, have fed national controversy over the nursing-home industry and the ways government and the private sector can best serve the aging. The answers are not easy.

# Concerns in Long-Term Care

## Institutionalization

Relocation to a chronic-care institution on a long-term basis can permanently disrupt a person's equilibrium. Many recent studies have found elevated mortality rates among recent arrivals to long-term care facilities, especially when the move was not voluntary. Entering long-term care can be a tremendous blow to one's self-concept: "I have always prided myself on being independent and now everyone tells me what to do and when. They are always doing things for me." Treating the person with respect and recognition of individuality, capitalizing on strengths, and allowing for personal decision making can help offset this reaction.

If familial, social, and cultural ties are severed, further identity problems may emerge. Institutionalized individuals may begin to see themselves in an unfavorable light, internalizing a poor self-concept and diminished self-esteem: "People are now seeing me as a debilitated person—a patient." Care providers should try to help the new arrival to reinstate former relationships and should make an effort to provide familiar or new social and cultural opportunities. Because separation from a loved pet can also be traumatic, some facilities allow pets to visit in specified areas.

If care intensifies, further diminishing independence, the message that "you are ill and incapable of doing as you wish" can further erode the person's self-concept. Constant reinforcement of the patient's value as a person should be offered with sincerity and respect.

Compliance, another consequence of institutionalization, is often welcomed by a hard-working staff but may increase the patient's despair. Total compliance, even with nonpriority routines like hygiene, may not be healthy since it promotes dependence.

As assimilation into the institutional environment proceeds, identity may continue to deteriorate until withdrawal is complete and the resident sees himself or herself as "just one of the others," a passive recipient of procedures, medications, and hygiene, waiting out the remainder of life (see Table 30.1).

It is important to stress that many long-term

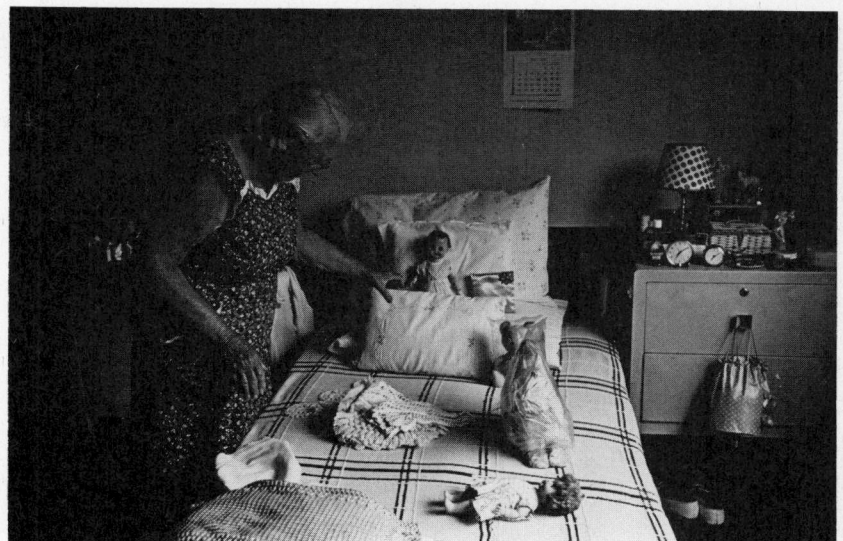

**Figure 30.6 Memorabilia help provide a sense of being in familiar surroundings for the chronic-care patient.** Lucy Fleeson/Stock, Boston

care facilities offer personalized and sensitive care. Many provide a wide range of crafts, classes, and social activities and encourage residents to maintain interest in the wider community. Inclusion of the family in the care program is a high priority in a number of facilities.

## Communicating Effectively

In communicating with the elderly, it is beneficial to speak of the past, the present, and the future.

The past is familiar, the present keeps thinking current, and the future—even the near future—suggests hope. Some nurses complain that care of the elderly is time-consuming because older patients seem to talk endlessly. "It's hard to get away," they complain. Remember that such patients are lonely and cherish the nurse's presence for even a short time. If the nurse visits the patient frequently when care is not needed, communication will be improved.

Overly familiar communication can undermine a potentially good relationship with an elderly pa-

Table 30.1
**Stages in the Development of Institutionalization**

| Stages of development | Symptoms | Prognosis |
|---|---|---|
| Stage of uncertainty | Loss of identity | Readily reversible |
| Deprived of cultural and social reinforcement | Looks for success and adaptation; hypersuggestible | |
| Doubts about physical and mental condition | Questioning; faltering | |
| Feels relieved of responsibility because he or she is receiving message: "Something is wrong with you" | Less interest in personal care; resents being treated as incompetent | Therapy is increasingly difficult |
| Compliant but still feels more competent than other residents | | |
| Loss of contact with family and friends | Fewer letters and visits; socially awkward | |
| Identifies self with others in institution | Complete psychosocial degradation | Not readily reversible |

Adapted from Maurice E. Linden, "You Won't Believe It." Paper presented at State of Delaware Governors' Conference on Aging, 1967. Mimeograph copy available from New Jersey Department of Community Affairs, Division on Aging, Trenton, N.J. 08601.

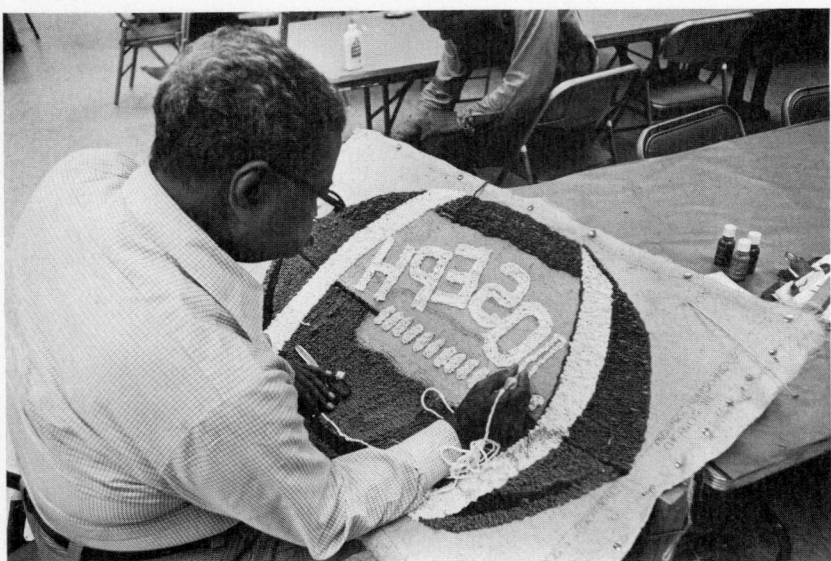

**Figure 30.7**
Learning new skills gives meaning to life. (Stephanie Dinkins/Photo Researchers, Inc.)

tient. Most older patients were raised with much more social formality than is usual now. First names were not used casually. It is best, then, to address the older patient by his or her last name until the patient requests that you do otherwise. Though hospitals are becoming increasingly informal, and many nurses and patients are on a first-name basis, it is prudent to show respect to the older person in this way. Another unfortunate commonplace practice is "talking down" to the elderly as if they were children. Terms such as "honey" and "dear" may be interpreted as degrading by the patient. The inclusive "let's do that" is also inappropriate, for it intrudes on the dignity of the patient and suggests dependence.

## Coping With Confusion

For a variety of reasons, including the anxiety of relocation, confusion is not uncommon in the geriatric patient. Often the patient recognizes his or her confusion and is frightened by it. Such a situation is not easily remedied, but there are things you can do to help. An older patient who is able to be of service in some manner will benefit from feeling needed. One older woman became much less confused and depressed when she was asked to help fold linen. Another patient wrote a letter for a fellow patient who could not write. A creative

approach in developing the nursing care plan can do a great deal to alleviate confusion.

Intervention is essential for the confused older patient because confusion often increases if nothing is done about it. If the patient is confused about the time and place, informing the patient where he or she is and what time it is, including the day and month, is helpful. You might ask the family to bring a large-faced clock and a large-print calendar as aids to orientation. Sometimes confusion is only evident at night. A nightlight and side-rails give the patient a feeling of security and enhance safety. Any necessary changes in routine should be undertaken slowly, since confused patients adapt poorly to sudden change. Another helpful technique is to make out a daily schedule, in large print, which allows the patient to keep track of the day's plan and to know what to expect at a given hour. Unrealistic plans and behavior should not be supported by the nurse. For example, if a patient tells you that he is going on a picnic and the snowy weather obviously makes such a plan impossible, it is not a kindness to agree. Simply point out that, although picnics are great fun on warm sunny days, the weather is poor and no plans for such a picnic have been made. Then, to minimize the patient's disappointment, offer an enjoyable substitute.

It is poor practice to tell an elderly patient you will do something or be back at a specified time and not to follow through. Such a practice not only confuses the patient but also rapidly destroys trust. Specifying a time is good but only if it is adhered to. Five minutes may seem like twenty to the inactive patient. Thus it is wise when you inform the patient that you will return in five minutes to suggest that he or she watch the clock. This practice calls on the patient's sense of time and enhances confidence that you will return as promised. These suggestions may seem like little things, but they are valuable to the aged.

## Safety

Accidental injury or trauma sustained by the older patient is a particularly serious problem. The older patient heals slowly and may develop pneumonia due to immobilization during recovery. Safety demands that you constantly observe the patient and the environment for potential hazards.

In a state of confusion, overzealous independence, or night disorientation, the patient may try to get out of bed unaided. In many institutions it is mandatory for the siderails of every patient over sixty-five to be placed in the upright position at night, unless a waiver has been signed by the patient or the family. If the nurse describes this practice to the patient as a form of protection and not a punitive action, the patient will usually accept it. However, some patients will attempt to crawl over the rail, intensifying the danger. Soft wrist

restraints or a vest restraint may then have to be applied. The call bell or button must always be placed so that even the restrained patient may call for help. The most restless patient becomes much quieter if he or she understands that the nurse can be summoned at will.

Falls are of special concern for the elderly. Well-fitted hard-soled leather shoes are safest for older people. Bedroom slippers are often slippery, tend to fit poorly, and give inadequate support; tennis shoes "catch" because of the rubber sole covering and do not provide enough support. Spills can be dangerous for both patients and nurses and should be wiped up immediately. Loose floor tiles, throw rugs, and small items such as bobby pins on the floor may all imperil the patient. Furniture should not obstruct passageways. Showers and tubs can also be dangerous; a bath towel placed on the bottom of the tub provides for better footing. Handrails on bathroom walls also offer support to the unsteady person. Good lighting is essential for safety in all areas.

Other hazards include electrical appliances with worn cords or connections, which may cause a shock or start a fire. Smoking is distinctly dangerous, and many facilities have rules controlling it. Smoking in bed, dangerous for anyone, is particularly so for the older person whose reflexes may be impaired. The patient's safety is imperative, and perpetual vigilance by care providers is indispensable.

# Personal Attitudes Toward the Older Adult

As a student, you will probably spend several weeks in a nursing-home setting caring for the older or geriatric patient. Even if not, you will surely care for many aging patients in the hospital setting. Basic care will always focus on psychosocial needs, communication, and safety, with adaptations to meet the needs of the individual patient. Before beginning such an experience, it is helpful to examine your own attitudes toward the elderly. How quickly and how well you relate to the older patient depends largely on past experi-

ences with elderly people. A nurse whose elderly aunt or grandparent has been cantankerous or disruptive to the family might find it harder to be empathic and close to an elderly patient than would a nurse who has had a cherished relationship with an older relative.

One must guard against stereotyping the aged. Often a patient's age elicits an unfortunate response before he or she even arrives, a response expressed in such remarks as, "Oh, but she's ninety-one. What are we supposed to do?" It sometimes appears that the limitations age imposes on good recovery promote lack of interest on the part of the nurse.

"Since attitudes influence behavior, it is essential for nurses to develop positive attitudes toward aging and the care of the aged" (La Monica, 1979). As nurses, we can restore respect and dignity to the aging. Your older patient has been a child, a teenager, perhaps a student. Your older patient has loved, had friends, taught others, acquired wisdom and skills. Your older patient has feelings much like your own. By caring, you can provide your patient what you would want and need in the same circumstances, meaningful human contact.

## Conclusion

The growing number of elderly people, and their vulnerability to health problems, makes it more essential than ever for nurses to gain skill in the care of the fragile older adult. Research has opened new vistas by suggesting that the mental deficiencies and physical disabilities that often accompany aging can be minimized and sometimes reversed. Our skills must keep pace with new knowledge on aging; this is an exciting challenge for the nurse.

Developing an understanding attitude toward the aged enhances interaction and effectiveness. Nursing leadership can help by supporting new programs for the aging that will benefit all people, not just those in our care.

## Care Study   The value of occupational therapy

Nursing student Susan Tapp suddenly realized how sad she felt. In the past three weeks, while practicing in a nursing home, she had grown very fond of Mrs. Aldrich, a ninety-one-year-old patient. She had not known either of her grandmothers, who had both died when she was a baby. She realized now how nice it would have been to have had a grandmother like Mrs. Aldrich.

Mrs. Aldrich was a quiet, gentle lady who missed her only grandson and his family, who lived in California, and particularly her only great-grandson, Mike. The holidays had just ended, and they were not planning to visit until summer. Mrs. Aldrich talked a great deal about the arthritis in her hands that kept her from doing any fine handiwork. The diminished strength of her legs kept her wheelchair-bound most of the day, which seemed to increase her depression. "I feel so worthless, no good to anybody," she had remarked one day. Ms. Tapp had read the Bible with Mrs. Aldrich at her request and taken her to the activities room, but Mrs. Aldrich had shown little interest in participating, saying, "There is nothing for me to do there."

Ms. Tapp looked back over her assessment. Mrs. Aldrich certainly had strengths. She liked to work with her hands and was alert and communicative. She had a family who cared for her, though they were far away. Mrs. Aldrich needed a short-term goal, perhaps something to do, and also a way of communicating with her family, particularly Mike. Ms. Tapp decided to work further on her plan that evening. Perhaps she'd think of something.

As she hurried down the hallway to her car, Ms. Tapp glanced into the ceramics room. A friend of Mrs. Aldrich, along with several other women and a man, were making clay mugs. A plan began to form in Ms. Tapp's mind: a mug for Mike!

The following day, she could hardly wait to start on her plan. She told Mrs. Aldrich about the ceramics room, which they then visited together. She showed Mrs. Aldrich how easy and how much fun it was to mold the clay and set up a schedule so that she could accompany Mrs. Aldrich to the ceramics class twice a week.

The following weeks were spent sharing the creation of a loving gift for Mike. The gray clay was rounded and formed, mainly by Mrs. Aldrich. Then came the drying period and the selection of a deep blue glaze. When the mug emerged from the kiln, all agreed that it was beautiful. Ms. Tapp and Mrs. Aldrich celebrated with coffee. Mrs. Aldrich reacted with enthusiasm when Ms. Tapp suggested making the mug unmistakably Mike's by painting his name on it. With Ms. Tapp's encouragement, Mrs. Aldrich lettered MIKE around the side in white paint.

Ms. Tapp and Mrs. Aldrich gave the mug a special place in her room to await Mike's next visit. Ms. Tapp promised to return for the presentation to meet Mike and the family.

Seven weeks later, Ms. Tapp thought back over her experience. Mrs. Aldrich had changed in several ways. She had become more talkative about matters other than her problems. She seemed more optimistic and, best of all, she had decided to continue going to the ceramics classes. "I hope she doesn't stop when I leave," thought Ms. Tapp.

That afternoon after her clinical experience ended, Ms. Tapp ran into her friend Ginny Colbert. "Ginny, aren't you going to be at Meadowdale next quarter?" Ginny Colbert shook her head affirmatively. "Well, I'd really like to have coffee with you soon and tell you about a patient of mine you could help." "Sure, Susan, let's do that."

## Study Terms

| | |
|---|---|
| alopecia | glaucoma |
| anorexia | gout |
| arteriosclerosis | life change |
| atherosclerosis | lumen |
| expectorate | osteoarthritis |
| fragile | osteoporosis |
| geriatrics | senile |
| gerontology | |

## Learning Activities

1. Talk with an older person who is in good health.
2. Talk with a hospitalized older patient.
3. Compare the concerns and/or problems of the two people with whom you talked in Activities 1 and 2.
4. Visit a community resource designed to help the elderly.
5. While caring for an elderly patient in the clinical area, write a nursing care plan emphasizing matters affected by aging.

## References

Aiken, Lewis. *Later Life.* Philadelphia: W. B. Saunders, 1978.

Cahill, J. B., and Smith, D. "Considerate Care of the Elderly: Little Things Mean a Lot." *Nursing '75* 5 (September 1975): 38–39.

Combs, K. L. "Preventive Care in the Elderly," Part III. *American Journal of Nursing* 78 (August 1978): 1339–1341.

Costello, M. K. "Sex, Intimacy and Aging." *American Journal of Nursing* 75 (August 1975): 1330–1332.

Diekelmann, N. "Pre-retirement Counselling," Part II. *American Journal of Nursing* 78 (August 1978): 1337–1338.

Dresen, S. E. "Autonomy: A Continuing Developmental Task," Part V. *American Journal of Nursing* 78 (August 1978): 1344–1346.

Gotz, B. E., *et al.* "Drugs and the Elderly," Part VI. *American Journal of Nursing* 78 (August 1978): 1347–1351.

Griggs, W. "Sex and the Elderly," Part VII. *American Journal of Nursing* 78 (August 1978): 1352–1354.

Harris, Diana K., and Cole, William E. *Sociology of Aging.* Boston: Houghton Mifflin, 1980.

Havighurst, Robert J. *Developmental Tasks and Education,* 2nd ed. 1952.

Hirschfeld, M. J. "The Cognitively Impaired Older Adult." *American Journal of Nursing* 76 (December 1976): 1981–1984.

Hogstel, M. O. "Staying Well While Growing Old: How Do The Elderly View Their World?" Part I. *American Journal of Nursing* 78 (August 1978): 1334–1336.

Kastenbaum, Robert. *Growing Old: Years of Fulfillment.* New York: Harper & Row, 1979.

Kalish, Richard A., and Reynolds, David K. "The Role of Age in Death." *Death Education* 1 (Summer 1977): 205–227.

La Monica, Elaine L. "The Nurse and the Aging Client: Positive Attitude Formation." *Nurse Educator* 4 (December 1979): 23–26.

Lore, A. "Supporting the Hospitalized Elderly Person." *American Journal of Nursing* 79 (March 1979): 496–499.

Markson, E. W. "Readjustment to Time in Old Age." *Nursing Digest* 2 (February 1974): 32–39.

Malasanos, Lois, *et al. Health Assessment.* St. Louis: C. V. Mosby, 1977.

Masters, W. H., and Johnson, V. E. "Sex After Sixty-Five." *Saturday Evening Post* (February 1977): 48–52.

Meissner, Judith E. "Assessing a Geriatric Patient's Need for Institutionalized Care." *Nursing '80* 10 (March 1980): 86–87.

"Mortality, Morbidity and Voluntary Change of Residence by Older People." Paper read at the Annual Meeting of the American Psychological Association, 2 September 1967, in Washington, D.C.

Patrick, M. "Little Things Mean a Lot in Geriatric Rehabilitation." *Nursing '73* 3 (August 1973): 7–9.

Pugsley, J. R., and Kolb, P. "Jane and Sara Were Old and Helpless." *Nursing '75* 5 (April 1975): 10–12.

Putnam, P. A. "Orienting the Young to Old Age." *Nursing Outlook* 22 (August 1974): 519–521.

Robinson, K. D. "Therapeutic Interaction: A Means of Crisis Intervention With Newly Institutionalized Elderly Persons." *Nursing Clinics of North America* 9 (March 1974): 89–96.

Thralow, J., and Watson, G. "Remotivation for Geriatric Patients Using Elementary School Students." *Nursing Digest* 3 (July/August 1975): 48–49.

Tyberg, Delores A. "Creating an Intermediate Care Facility." *American Journal of Nursing* 79 (July 1979): 1237–1239.

Uhler, D. M. "Common Skin Changes in the Elderly," Part IV. *American Journal of Nursing* 78 (August 1978): 1342–1344.

Vlack, J. E. "When a Nursing Home Is the Best Choice." *American Journal of Nursing* 79 (August 1979): 1450–1451.

Wilhite, M. J., *et al.* "Changes in Nursing Students' Stereotypic Attitudes Toward Old People." *Nursing Research* 25 (November/December 1976): 430-432.

# Appendix A

## Common Abbreviations

| Abbreviation | Latin Meaning | English Meaning |
|---|---|---|
| @ | | at |
| abd. | | abdomen |
| a.c. | ante cibum | before meals |
| A.D.L. | | activities of daily living |
| ad lib. | ad libitum | at will |
| ax. | | axillary |
| b.i.d. | bis in die | twice a day |
| B.M. | | bowel movement |
| B.P. | | blood pressure |
| B.R.P. | | bathroom privileges |
| c̄ | cum | with |
| cap. | | capsule |
| c/o | | complains of |
| D.O.A. | | dead on arrival |
| et | et | and |
| Frax., Fx. | | fractional, fracture |
| gtt. | gutta | drop |
| h. | hora | hour |
| H/P | | history and physical |
| h.s. | hora somni | hour of sleep (bedtime) |
| I.M. | | intramuscular |
| I.V. | | intravenous |
| K.V.O. | | keep vein open (with intravenous infusion) |
| L.L.Q. | | left lower quadrant (of abdomen) |
| L.U.Q. | | left upper quadrant (of abdomen) |
| N.P.O. | non per ora | nothing by mouth |
| n.r. | non repetatur | not to be repeated |
| "o" | | orally |
| o.d. | omne die | every day |
| O.D. | oculus dexter | right eye |
| O.S. | oculus sinister | left eye |
| O.T. | | occupational therapy |
| O.U. | oculi uterque | each eye |
| p.c. | post cibum | after meals |
| p.o. | per ora | by mouth |
| p.r.n. | pro re nata | when needed |
| P.T. | | physical therapy |
| q.s. | quantum sufficiat | sufficient quantity |
| q.d. | quaque die | each day |

| Abbreviation | Latin Meaning | English Meaning |
| --- | --- | --- |
| q.h. | quaque hora | every hour |
| q.2h. | | every two hours |
| q.3h., etc. | | every three hours, etc. |
| q.i.d. | quater in die | four times a day |
| q.o.d. | quaque alto die | every other day |
| R.L.Q. | | right lower quadrant (of abdomen) |
| R.O.M. | | range of motion |
| R.U.Q. | | right upper quadrant (of abdomen) |
| s̄ | sine | without |
| s.o.b. | | short of breath |
| s.o.s. | si opus sit | if necessary |
| spec. | | specimen |
| stat. | statim | immediately |
| sub q. | | subcutaneous |
| tab. | | tablet |
| t.i.d. | ter in dies | three times a day |
| T.K.O. | | to keep open (intravenous infusion) |
| T.L.C. | | tender loving care |
| T.P.R. | | temperature, pulse, and respiration |
| U.A. | | urine analysis |
| ung. | unguent | ointment |

# Appendix B

## Abbreviations of Medical Conditions

| | |
|---|---|
| A.R.D.S. | adult respiratory distress syndrome |
| A.K. Amp. | above-knee amputation |
| A.S.C.V.D. | arteriosclerotic cardiovascular disease |
| A.S.H.D. | arteriosclerotic heart disease |
| B.E. | bacterial endocarditis |
| B.K. Amp. | below-knee amputation |
| B.P.H. | benign prostatic hypertrophy |
| Ca. | cancer (carcinoma) |
| C.F. | cystic fibrosis |
| C.H.D. | coronary heart disease |
| C.H.F. | congestive heart failure |
| C.O.P.D. | chronic obstructive pulmonary disease |
| C.V.A. | cerebral vascular accident |
| D.&C. | dilation and curettage (of uterus) |
| D.I.C. | disseminated intravascular coagulation |
| D.T.'s | delerium tremens |
| F.U.O. | fever of undetermined origin |
| G.B. | gall bladder |
| G.C. | gonococcal infection |
| H.C.V.D. | hypertensive cardiovascular disease |
| L.T.B. | laryngo-tracheobronchitis |
| M.I. | myocardial infarction, mitral insufficiency |
| M.S. | multiple sclerosis |
| P.A.P. | primary atypical pneumonia |
| P.I.D. | pelvic inflammatory disease |
| P.V.D. | peripheral vascular disease |
| R.D.S. | respiratory distress syndrome |
| R.F. | rheumatic fever |
| R.H.D. | rheumatic heart disease |
| S.B.E. | subacute bacterial endocarditis |
| S.I.D.S. | sudden infant death syndrome |
| T.&A. | tonsillectomy and adenoidectomy |
| T.B. or T.B.C. | tuberculosis |
| T.I.A. | transient ischemic attacks |
| T.U.R.B. | transurethral resection of the bladder |
| T.U.R.P. | transurethral resection of the prostate |
| U.R.I. | upper respiratory infection |
| U.T.I. | urinary tract infection |

# Appendix C

## Combining Forms

The combining form may appear at the beginning, within, or at the end of a term. By identifying the meaning of each combining form contained in a word, it is possible to discern the meaning of the word. A dash preceding the form indicates that it is most commonly a suffix (appearing at the end of a term); a dash following the form indicates that it is most commonly a prefix (appearing at the beginning of a term).

| Form | Meaning |
|------|---------|
| a-, an- | without |
| ab- | away from |
| ad- | to, toward |
| adeno- | gland |
| -algia | pain |
| ambi- | on two sides |
| angio- | vessel |
| ano- | anus |
| ante- | before, forward |
| arterio- | artery |
| arthro- | joint |
| bis- | two |
| broncho- | bronchus |
| cardi-, cardio- | heart |
| -cele | hernia, tumor, protrusion |
| -centesis | puncture |
| cepha-, cephalo- | head |
| cerebro- | cerebrum of brain |
| cervico- | neck |
| chole- | bile |
| cholecysto- | gall bladder |
| chondro- | cartilage |
| circum- | around |
| cranio- | head |
| cysto- | sac, cyst, bladder (most often urinary bladder) |
| -cyte | cell |
| derm- | skin |
| dys- | abnormal, painful |
| -ectasis | expansion, dilation |
| -ectomy | excision |
| -emia | blood |
| encephalo- | brain |
| endo- | within, inner layer |

| Form | Meaning |
|------|---------|
| entero- | intestines |
| ex- | out, out of, away from |
| exo- | outside, outer layer |
| gastro- | stomach |
| hem-, hema-, hemo-, hemato- | blood |
| hemi- | half |
| hepato- | liver |
| histo- | tissue |
| hyper- | excessive |
| hypo- | low, lesser |
| hystero- | uterus |
| -iasis | condition, formation of, presence of |
| ileo- | ileum (part of small intestine) |
| ilio- | ilium (part of pelvic bones) |
| intra- | within |
| -itis | inflammation of |
| laparo- | loin, flank, abdomen |
| laryngo- | larynx |
| latero- | side |
| lympho- | lymph |
| -lysis | dissolution, breaking down |
| macro- | large |
| mal- | bad, poor |
| -malacia | softening |
| masto- | breast |
| medio- | middle |
| -megaly | enlargement |
| meningo- | meninges |
| micro- | small, microscopic |
| mono- | single |
| myelo- | bone marrow, spinal cord |
| myo- | muscle |
| naso- | nose |
| neo- | new |
| nephro- | kidney |
| neuro- | nerve |
| non- | not |
| oculo- | eye |
| odonto- | tooth |
| -oma | tumor |
| oophoro- | ovary |
| ophthalmo- | eye |
| orchio-, orchido- | testes |
| oro- | mouth |
| -orrhaphy | suture/repair of |
| os- | bone, mouth |
| -osis | condition, disease, increase |

| Form | Meaning |
|------|---------|
| osteo- | bone |
| -ostomy | artificially created opening into an organ |
| oto- | ear |
| -otomy | incision into |
| ovario- | ovary |
| para- | beside, along with |
| -pathy | disease |
| -penia | deficiency, decrease |
| peri- | around |
| -pexy | suspension, fixation |
| pharyngo- | pharynx |
| phlebo- | vein |
| -plasty | surgical correction, plastic repair of |
| -plegia | paralysis |
| pneumo- | lungs, breath |
| post- | after |
| pro- | in front of, before |
| procto- | rectum |
| pseudo- | false |
| -ptosis | falling, drooping |
| pyo- | pus |
| retro- | behind |
| rhino- | nose |
| salpingo- | Fallopian tube |
| sclero- | hard |
| -spasm | involuntary contraction |
| spleno- | spleen |
| sterno- | sternum |
| super-, supra- | above, more than |
| teno- | tendon |
| thoraco- | thorax, chest |
| thyro- | thyroid |
| tracheo- | trachea |
| trans- | across, throughout |
| urethro- | urethra |
| uro- | urine, urinary |
| utero- | uterus |
| vaso- | blood vessel |
| veno- | vein |

# Appendix D

## Table of Equivalencies

1. Metric doses and apothecaries' equivalents

### Liquid

| Metric | Approximate apothecaries' equivalents |
|---|---|
| 1,000 ml | 1 quart |
| 500 ml | 1 pint |
| 250 ml | 8 fluidounces |
| 30 ml | 1 fluidounce |
| 15 ml | 4 fluidrams |
| 5 ml | 1 fluidram |
| 1 ml | 15 minims |
| 0.06 ml | 1 minim |

### Solid

| | |
|---|---|
| 30 gm | 1 ounce |
| 15 gm | 4 drams |
| 4 gm | 60 grains (1 dram) |
| 1 gm | 15 grains |
| 0.5 gm | 7½ grains |
| 60 mg | 1 grain |
| 30 mg | ½ grain |
| 15 mg | ¼ grain |
| 10 mg | ⅙ grain |
| 8 mg | ⅛ grain |
| 1 mg | 1/60 grain |
| 0.6 mg | 1/100 grain |
| 0.4 mg | 1/150 grain |
| 0.3 mg | 1/200 grain |
| 0.2 mg | 1/300 grain |
| 0.1 mg | 1/600 grain |

2. Approximate household measures

| | | |
|---|---|---|
| 1 teaspoonful | 1 fl dr | 4–5 ml |
| 1 tablespoonful | ½ fl oz | 15 or 16 ml |
| 1 jigger | 1½ fl oz | 45 ml |
| 1 cup | 8 fl oz | 240 ml |

3. Prescription abbreviations

| | |
|---|---|
| gr | grain or grains |
| gtt* | drops |
| ʒ | dram |
| ℥ | ounce |
| aa | equal parts |
| ss | one half |
| cc** | cubic centimeter |
| gm | gram |
| mg | milligram |
| mcg | microgram |
| ml | milliliter |
| mEq | milliequivalent |
| ℳ | minim |

*Gutta(e)
**Although technically not exactly equivalent, ml and cc are often used interchangeably.

# Appendix E

## Special Visual Examinations (Endoscopy)

Hollow organs that open to the body's exterior surface are examined by means of a hollow tube and a light. These "scopes" are of two basic types: the rigid and the fiberoptic. The rigid scope is a metal or plastic tube, and the passageway into the organ must be straightened to allow entry of the tube. The light allows the inside of the organ to be visually inspected. It is also possible to insert a special instrument to take a specimen of tissue. This procedure is called a *biopsy*. The fiberoptic scope is a flexible tube containing a bundle of fibers that reflect light. These fibers are so perfectly aligned that the image at the bottom of the tube is seen clearly at the top. Fiberoptic scopes can conform to the shape of the passage or organ and can thus be inserted into areas of the body not accessible to metal scopes. They cause less discomfort than do rigid scopes and also have attached instruments to take tissue samples.

| | Organ Studied | Preparation | Special Nursing Concerns |
|---|---|---|---|
| Bronchoscopy | Bronchi and (with fiberoptic scope) lung segments | NPO and sedatives. If general anesthesia, routine preop. If local, special explanation of procedure. Dentures out. | If performed with local anesthesia, do not give fluids or food until gag reflex returns. Complications to watch for include bleeding due to tissue trauma, laryngospasm, and respiratory distress. Also, in any procedure that uses a local anesthetic, watch for allergic reaction. |
| Colonoscopy | Entire large bowel (with fiberoptic scope) | Measures to cleanse bowel completely begun evening before and completed morning of test. | Bleeding due to trauma |
| Cystoscopy | Bladder | Same as for bronchoscopy. | Urinary tract irritation from scope. Possible infection. Encourage fluids. |
| Esophagoscopy | Esophagus | Same as for bronchoscopy. | If performed with local anesthesia, do not give fluids or food until gag reflex returns. |
| Gastroscopy | Stomach (with fiberoptic scope) | Same as for bronchoscopy. | Same as for esophagoscopy |
| Laryngoscopy | Larynx | If general anesthesia, routine preop. If local, special explanation of procedure. | If performed with local anesthesia, do not give fluids or food until gag reflex returns. Complications to watch for include bleeding due to tissue trauma and laryngospasm. |

|  | Organ Studied | Preparation | Special Nursing Concerns |
|---|---|---|---|
| Proctoscopy | Rectum | Measures to cleanse bowel completely begun evening before and completed morning of test. | Bleeding due to trauma |
| Sigmoidoscopy | Sigmoid colon and rectum | Same as for proctoscopy | Same as for proctoscopy |

# Appendix F

# X-Ray Examinations

X rays produce a negative-type film that shows images of the outlines of various structures whose different densities allow varying amounts of radiation to penetrate through to the film.

Most x rays are simple images of body parts; examples are x rays of the chest and of the extremities to check for fractures. The view or patient position is usually designated by the physician.

Some organs do not appear on routine x rays because they are not sufficiently dense to block any radiation. In these cases *contrast studies* are performed: a contrast material (radio-opaque substance) is introduced into the organ so that a clear outline of it can be seen on the x ray. The functioning of an organ can sometimes be studied by taking a series of x rays as the contrast material moves through the organ. Intravenous "dyes" (contrast materials) are potent and can cause severe allergic reactions.

| | Organ Studied | Preparation | Method | Special Nursing Concerns |
|---|---|---|---|---|
| Angiogram | Blood vessels. Usually used to examine a system of veins and arteries within an organ. | Usually NPO. Sometimes surgical prep of site. | Catheter is threaded into artery (often the femoral), and contrast medium is injected under pressure into the organ's vascular system. | Allergic reaction to contrast medium. Bleeding from puncture site. Thrombus formation. |
| Arteriogram | Arteries (but often used as a synonym for angiogram) | Same as for angiogram | Same as for angiogram | Same as for angiogram |
| Barium Enema (Lower Bowel) | Large intestine | Measures to cleanse bowel completely begun evening before and completed morning of test. | Barium is given as enema. Large plug is inserted in rectum to prevent loss of barium. | Barium causes severe constipation or even obstruction, if not removed by means of enemas or laxatives. |
| Bronchogram | Bronchi | NPO. Routine preop. General anesthesia usual. Dentures out. | Contrast medium is inserted through bronchoscope, then suctioned out. | Same as for bronchoscopy. Also irritation from contrast medium causes increased secretions. Retained contrast medium may cause pneumonia. |

| | Organ Studied | Preparation | Method | Special Nursing Concerns |
|---|---|---|---|---|
| Cystogram | Bladder | None usual | Patient is catheterized and contrast medium inserted through catheter. | Encourage fluids to prevent infection. |
| Cholecystogram (Gall Bladder Series) | Gall bladder | NPO. Fat-free meal evening before. Oral contrast pills evening before as directed. | Material excreted in bile is given in pill form. X rays are taken to determine whether gall bladder contains the material. Then a fatty liquid is given, and further x rays are taken to observe function of gall bladder. May give contrast medium IV just before test. | Pills often cause nausea and vomiting. Vomiting of pills makes test invalid. Burning on urination as contrast medium is excreted. |
| Cholangiogram | Bile ducts | NPO. Preparation for surgery. Usually done during gall bladder surgery. | Contrast medium is injected into bile ducts themselves. | None usual |
| Intravenous Pyelogram (IVP) | Kidney, ureters, and bladder | NPO. Measures to cleanse bowel completely evening before test. | Contrast medium is injected intravenously and excreted by kidneys. A series of x rays made of entire urinary tract. | Contrast medium can cause urinary irritation. Encourage fluids. |
| Myelogram | Spinal canal | NPO. Sedative given. Usually not general anesthesia. | Lumbar puncture is done, some spinal fluid removed, and contrast medium injected into canal. Patient is positioned on tilt table, which is tilted to allow contrast medium to flow to desired level. | Same as for lumbar puncture. (See Appendix J.) Allergic reactions to dye. |
| Pneumo-encephalogram | Ventricles of brain | NPO. Sedative given. Full: 100 cc of air, general anesthesia. Limited: 10–15 cc air, local anesthesia. | Lumbar puncture is done, some spinal fluid removed, and air inserted. Air rises to ventricles when patient is placed in upright position. | Headache until air is absorbed. Pain medications are given. Quiet and darkened room and flat bedrest are usually helpful. |

|  | Organ Studied | Preparation | Method | Special Nursing Concerns |
|---|---|---|---|---|
| Retrograde Pyelogram | Kidney | NPO. Laxatives to clear bowel. | Cystoscopy is performed. Ureteral catheters are inserted, films taken of catheters, and contrast medium is then injected into renal pelvis for films. | Same as for cystoscopy |
| Upper G.I. | Esophagus, stomach, duodenum | NPO after midnight | Barium is swallowed. Films are taken as material fills upper gastrointestinal system. | Same as for barium enema |
| Ventriculogram | Ventricles of brain | Complete surgical preparation as for neurosurgery. | Burr holes are drilled in skull and cannula is inserted to inject contrast medium into ventricles. | Complete postop. care for a neuro patient. (See a medical-surgical textbook.) |

# Appendix G

## Measurement and Recording of Electrical Impulses

Some organs of the body undergo changes in electrical potential in the process of functioning. These changes in electrical potential can be of significance in evaluating the functioning of the organ.

| | Organ Studied | Preparation | Method | Special Nursing Concerns |
|---|---|---|---|---|
| Electrocardiogram (EKG or ECG) | Heart | None usual | Electrodes are secured to the chest wall with electrode paste and tape or suction cups. Other electrodes are attached to the extremities. The machine then records the electrical activity of the heart. | None |
| Electroencephalogram (EEG) | Brain | None usual | Electrodes are attached to the scalp with small needles or paste. The patient is at rest in a darkened room, and may be asked to deep-breathe (hyperventilation) or watch a flashing light (photic stimulation) at certain times. | None |
| Electromyogram (EMG) | Muscles | None usual | Electrodes are attached to the muscles tested with small needles or paste and the electrical impulses are recorded. | None |

# Appendix H

## Miscellaneous Tests of Specific Body Functions

A great many tests have been devised to examine the functioning of body processes. Those listed here are only a few of the more common tests.

| | Purpose | Preparation | Method |
|---|---|---|---|
| Basal Metabolism Rate (BMR) | To test the rate at which the body uses oxygen at complete rest (not sleep) in order to measure metabolic rate | NPO. Test performed first thing in the morning. No activity allowed preceding test. | The nose is clamped; the patient breathes through a mouthpiece so that oxygen consumption can be measured. |
| Gastric Analysis | To measure the stomach's production of gastric juices | NPO | A nasogastric tube is inserted into the stomach. All gastric contents are aspirated and saved over a period of time. Samples are taken at specified time intervals according to laboratory procedure. |
| Glucose Tolerance Test (GTT) | To measure the ability of the body to metabolize a glucose "load" | NPO | A fasting urine sample is obtained, and a blood sample is drawn for a fasting blood sugar test. Then a solution containing a known amount of glucose is drunk by the patient. At intervals specified by the laboratory, urine samples are taken and blood samples are drawn (usually by the laboratory technician). |
| Indirect Gastric Analysis (Tubeless Gastric Analysis "Diagnex Blue," "Azurea") | To measure the production of gastric acid by determining the rate at which the dye material is absorbed and excreted | NPO | Dye material is given as directed by the manufacturer. Urine is saved for 24 hours and sent to the laboratory for analysis. Urine will continue to be blue for several days after the test. |

# Appendix I

## Tests Using Radioactive Materials

In these tests, small amounts of radioactive substances are injected or ingested into the body and a scanning device that registers the presence of radioactive particles is used to determine their distribution. Some substances are simply circulated in the blood stream to allow circulatory pathways, and changes or interruptions in those pathways, to be seen. In other tests, differential rates at which the radioactive substance is absorbed by different tissues allow rates of activity, types of tissue, and ability to function to be determined. The amounts of radiation are so small that they pose no hazard to personnel or patient. However, caution must be used in considering such a test for a pregnant person.

|  | Organ Studied | Preparation | Method |
|---|---|---|---|
| Brain Scan | Brain | None | Material is injected IV and the scanner is used to trace the circulatory pattern of the brain. Because some tissues will absorb more of the material, abnormal tissue can be located. |
| $I^{131}$ Uptake | Thyroid gland | NPO before test. Meals are resumed after taking iodine preparation. | An oral solution containing this radioactive isotope of iodine is given. The thyroid is scanned to determine its rate of metabolism of the iodine 24 hours after the $I^{131}$ is ingested. |
| Liver Scan | Liver | None | Material is injected IV and the scanner is used over the liver. Areas of obstruction result in increased uptake of the material. |
| Lung Scan | Lung | None | Material is injected IV and scan films are taken of the lungs. Circulatory patterns are apparent and diseased areas often show up as blocks in circulation on the scan. |

# Appendix J

## Tests Involving Introduction of a Large Needle into an Organ or Body Cavity

These tests are all performed by a physician with the careful sterile technique appropriate to minor surgical procedures. Because of the size of the needle, a local anesthetic is administered. If the patient is especially anxious, some sedation may be given before the procedure is begun.

| | Purpose | Method | Special Nursing Concerns |
|---|---|---|---|
| Abdominal Paracentesis | To remove fluid that has accumulated in the peritoneal cavity | With the patient in a sitting position, the needle is inserted through the abdominal wall. A 3-way stopcock, syringe, and tubing may be attached to the needle to allow aspiration of the fluid. | The patient should void first. Shock may occur during the procedure. (See a medical-surgical text.) The wound must be dressed afterwards. Be alert to the amount of fluid removed. |
| Bone Marrow Biopsy | To obtain a sample of bone marrow tissue to examine its production of blood components | The patient is lying down. The sternum or the iliac crest is commonly punctured. | The procedure may be very upsetting to the patient. Some pain is felt when the bone is entered, and the aspiration of tissue may be painful. The sound of bone penetration may be upsetting. Afterwards, pressure is applied for 5 minutes to prevent bleeding. |
| Lumbar Puncture | To puncture the spinal subarachnoid space to remove a sample of fluid for study or to inject dye for a contrast x ray | The patient lies on side in a flexed (bowed) position to allow access to the lower spine. During the procedure, a measurement of spinal fluid pressure is made. | Afterwards the patient is kept flat for a time. The prone position is preferred to allow "welling" of the puncture site, preventing further loss of fluid. Fluids are encouraged to facilitate replacement of spinal fluid. Headache occurs infrequently as a complication. |
| Thoracentesis | To puncture the pleural space to remove fluid or allow for the insertion of chest tubes | With the patient usually sitting up and leaning over a table, the puncture is made in the lower posterior chest to remove fluid and in the upper anterior chest to remove air. | Possible respiratory distress and pain during aspiration |

# Glossary

**acceptance** Affirmation of a belief in a situation or state.

**accommodation** (1) A term used by Piaget to describe the needed adjustment in thinking to understand old and new information. (2) The second stage in the life of a group when individuals adjust their own behavior in order to work more effectively with others.

**acid–base balance** The balance of the acidity and alkalinity of the body fluids for optimum homeostasis.

**acidity** The property of giving off hydrogen ions; the quality of being acidic is measured at less than 7.0 on the pH scale.

**acidosis** A disturbance of the acid–base balance resulting in the accumulation of acids in the body; a serum pH of less than 7.35.

**active assistive exercise** Movement that is partially accomplished by oneself and assisted by another.

**active exercise** Voluntary movement of a body part resulting from muscular contraction and relaxation.

**active transport** An energy-consuming process for moving substances across a cell wall against the concentration gradient.

**activities of daily living (ADL)** Those tasks necessary to meeting personal basic needs.

**acupuncture** A technique for relieving pain or providing regional anesthesia by inserting needles into specific points in the body.

**acute care** Health care for a condition that requires treatment of a fairly intensive nature for a limited time span.

**acute illness** Illness that is usually of rapid onset, requires short-term treatment, and resolves itself with no apparent residual.

**active participation** Personal involvement in doing a task or activity.

**adaptive forces** Any forces, internal or external, that tend to maintain or restore homeostasis.

**adaptive response** A response by a person that tends to restore homeostasis.

**addiction** Dependence on a substance for daily functioning in which illness results from withdrawal of the substance.

**adolescent** A person in the age group from twelve to eighteen.

Selected definitions in this glossary are from *The American Heritage Dictionary of the English Language,* © 1980 by Houghton Mifflin Company. Reprinted by permission from *The American Heritage Dictionary of the English Language.*

**adrenals** A pair of small endocrine glands each of which is located on the top of each kidney. Each adrenal is composed of a center called the medulla and an exterior layer called the cortex. Each portion functions as a separate endocrine gland.

**adventitious sounds** Abnormal sounds, as in the lungs.

**aerobic** Designating bacteria that live only in the presence of free oxygen.

**aesthetic needs** In Maslow's hierarchy, the top needs' level that relates to the need for beauty and artistic endeavor.

**affective** Designating the type of learning that relates to attitudes and values.

**aggregate** A number of people found in one place considered collectively and who have no common goal.

**agnostic** An individual who neither accepts nor rejects the existence of God or a higher being.

**agreeing-disagreeing** A blocking response when used in regard to feelings.

**aids to decision making** Facilitating responses that assist another person to plan a course of action.

**airborne** Designating a route of transmission whereby pathogens are transmitted via dust particles in the air.

**alarm reaction** The first stage of Selye's General Adaptation Syndrome (G.A.S.).

**albuminuria** The abnormal finding of protein in the urine.

**aldosterone** An adrenocorticosteroid hormone that causes salt and water to be reabsorbed and potassium to be excreted by the kidney tubules.

**alignment** The position of body parts in relationship to one another.

**alkalinity** The property of being basic; measured as greater than 7.0 on the pH scale.

**alkalosis** A disturbance of the acid–base balance resulting in an accumulation of bases in the body; a serum pH greater than 7.45.

**allergy** An abnormal body hypersensitivity to a specific antigen that is ordinarily harmless.

**alopecia** Loss of hair; baldness.

**alveoli** Small pouches of thin, single-layered membrane in the lungs where the exchange of gases occurs.

**ambulation** Walking.

**amulet** An object worn as a charm against evil or injury.

**anaerobic** Designating pathogens that grow best in an oxygen-free atmosphere.

**anal stage** Freud's psychosexual stage from the age of two to three when the anal and urethral areas provide sensual satisfaction.

**analgesia** Absence of pain sensation.

**androgens** Male hormones.

**anesthesia** Loss of all sensation.

**anger** A feeling of extreme displeasure toward someone or something.

**anion** An ion with a negative charge.

**ankylosed** Designating a joint in which the bones are fused to make it immovable.

**Anointing the Sick** A sacrament or ceremony found in several Christian groups in which prayers are said and oil touched to the ill person.

**anorexia** Lack of appetite or interest in food.

**antibiotics** Drugs that are effective in inhibiting the growth of or destroying bacteria.

**antibody** A protein, having a specific structure, produced by the body that interacts with a specific antigen to destroy or inactivate it.

**anticipatory grief** Feelings of grief that occur when it is perceived that a loss may be imminent.

**antidepressives** Agents that decrease feelings of depression.

**antidiuretic hormone (ADH)** A hormone secreted by the posterior pituitary that causes the kidneys to reabsorb water independently of solids.

**antiemetic** A substance that prevents and/or controls nausea and vomiting.

**antifungal** Designating agents that inhibit the growth of or destroy fungi.

**antigen** Any substance that can cause the body to form an antibody.

**antihistamines** A group of drugs that depress the action of histamine in the body, which results in decreased secretions and decreased swelling of mucous membranes.

**antihypertensive** Tending to counteract high blood pressure.

**antimicrobial** Capable of suppressing the growth of microorganisms.

**antiseptic** Capable of inhibiting the growth of microorganisms.

**anuria** Total absence of formation of urine by the kidneys; suppression.

**anxiety** A subjective experience of apprehension initiated by a threat to oneself, whether physical, mental, emotional, or spiritual.

**apex of heart** The lower, more pointed end of the heart.

**aphasia** Inability to use language caused by brain dysfunction.

**apical pulse** The heart rate as counted by listening to the heart over its apex.

**apnea** Absence of respiration.

**appetite** A subjective desire for or interest in food.

**approving-disapproving** Blocking responses when used in relationship to feelings.

**approximated** Describing edges of an incision that are touching.

**arteriosclerosis** Thickening and hardening of the inner and middle wall of vessels, thus narrowing the opening through which blood flows.

**artificial tears** A neutral, sterile solution used to lubricate the eyes.

**ascending fibers** Those nerves in the spinal cord that transmit impulses up to the brain.

**ascites** The accumulation of excess fluid in the peritoneal cavity.

**asepsis** Absence of all disease-producing microorganisms.

**aseptic conscience** In the practice of nursing, feeling an obligation to be the strictest and most rigid judge of whether or not technique has been broken.

**asexual** Lacking sexual awareness.

**Asians** A large, diverse group consisting of Japanese, Chinese, Filipinos, Koreans, and South East Asians.

**assault** A threat to do bodily harm.

**assessment** The first step of the nursing process, which includes collecting data and making a nursing diagnosis.

**assimilation** Piaget's term for the process by which information is absorbed.

**associate degree program** A college level education of approximately two years in length that awards an associate degree.

**astereognosis** The inability to identify, without looking, small objects by touch.

**asynchrony** Disproportionate growth, although normal for early childhood.

**ataxia** Difficulty with gait or walking.

**atelectasis** The collapse of portions of the lung due to lack of air in the alveoli; often the consequence of secretions blocking the airways and absorption of air distal to the plug.

**atheist** An individual who believes that there is no God or higher being.

**atherosclerosis** A condition in which plaques of a cholesterol-based material are deposited in the interior of the arteries.

**atony** Lack of muscle tone.

**atrophy** The condition of becoming smaller in bulk or size such as the wasting or deterioration of a body part.

**audiovisual aids** Objects or methods to provide visual and auditory information for learning.

**audit** A method of evaluating by checking what care was provided and comparing it to a previously established standard for care.

**aura** A warning sign or an awareness to a person that a seizure may occur.

**authoritarian** Autocratic.

**autoclaving** A process of steaming under pressure for a period of time in order to destroy microorganisms.

**autocratic** A style of leadership in which decision making and authority are located in the leader.

**autogenic training** A set of exercises designed to help one focus on physical sensations, shut out psychosocial stressors, and induce the relaxation response.

**autonomic nervous system** The involuntary part of the nervous system that sends and receives impulses from the heart muscle, smooth muscles, blood vessels, and hollow organs; it also controls the secretions of glands.

**autonomy** Erikson's task of the toddler; becoming important to self and developing assertiveness.

**autonomic responses** Involuntary body responses controlled by the autonomic nervous system.

**baccalaureate program** A college-level education, approximately four years in length, that awards a bachelor's degree.

**bacteria** One-celled microorganisms, the most numerous of all pathogens.

**bactericidal** Referring to agents that kill all bacteria, pathogens and nonpathogens alike.

**bacteriuria** The presence of bacteria in the urine.

**balanced solution** An intravenous electrolyte solution that provides water, calories, and electrolytes in concentrations commonly found in the body.

**Baptism** A sacrament of Christian churches in which water is used and prayers are said to receive the individual into the Christian faith.

**bargaining** Negotiating for a change in circumstances in return for changes in behavior or feelings.

**barrier** (1) A boundary or limit. (2) A technique for limiting the spread of microorganisms.

**barrio** A Spanish-speaking community within a larger community.

**base of support** A foundation that supports the body weight.

**Basic Four** A simplified way of planning meals to include all essential nutrients in adequate amounts. The four groups are bread, meat, milk, and fruits and vegetables.

**basic life skills** The abilities needed to manage one's time, finances, and interpersonal relationships.

**battery** Touching or harming a person without consent.

**behavior** The actions of an individual.

**behavior modification** An approach to changing conduct by using manipulation of the environment, especially by manipulating the consequence of the conduct.

**belittling** A blocking response in which a person's feelings or problems are categorized as not major or less than those of others.

**bereavement** Grief or mourning.

**bias** Adverse judgments or opinions without knowledge or facts; prejudice.

**bioethics** A field of study dealing with questions of right and wrong that relate to human life.

**biofeedback** A mechanical means of providing information on specific body processes.

**Biots' respirations** Similar to Cheyne-Stokes except that the respirations between the periods of apnea appear normal. (See *Cheyne-Stokes respirations*.)

**bisexual** Sexual feelings toward members of both sexes.

**Black English** A variation of English having certain words, phrases, and sentence structure that are special to some blacks.

**blocking responses** Responses that tend to inhibit another person from sharing thoughts and feelings.

**blood gases** The gas components of the blood, primarily oxygen and carbon dioxide.

**body image** A multidimensional view of one's body that takes into account its appearance, kinesthetic feedback, sensory feedback, and internal feelings.

**body image integrity** An accurate body image that

changes as the individual changes and with which the individual feels comfortable.

**body mechanics** The analysis of the action of forces on the body parts during activity.

**bradycardia** An abnormally slow heart rate, usually defined as below 60 beats per minute in the adult.

**bradypnea** Slow respirations, usually below 16 per minute in the adult.

**bridging** A method of supporting the body parts on pillows so that areas where pressure usually occurs are bridged between the pillows.

**Brompton's mixture** An oral solution of heroin, cocaine, an antiemetic, and other needed drugs in an alcohol-based syrup used in England for terminal pain. Modified Brompton's is a mixture similar to Brompton's but with morphine or methadone substituted for the heroin.

*Brujas* Persons capable of causing illness or discomfort among the Hispanics.

**Buddhism** A religion based on the teachings of Siddhartha Gautama Buddha who lived in India about 500 B.C.

**buffer** A substance that can combine with either a strong acid or a strong base and bring them closer to a neutral pH of 7.0.

**"burn out"** Symptoms of emotional, social, and physical exhaustion due to the stress of the role of the care provider.

**calculi** Stones.

**calorie counting** A method of planning a reducing diet by keeping a record of the calories contained in food and planning menus that stay within a specific calorie range.

**carbohydrate** A compound of carbon, hydrogen, and water used for energy by the body.

**carbohydrate counting** A method of planning a reducing diet in which only the grams of carbohydrate are monitored and limited.

**carcinogenic** Cancer-causing.

**cardiopulmonary resuscitation (CPR)** A combination of rescue breathing and external cardiac massage.

**caries** The decay of bone or teeth.

**carrier** An infected person without signs or symptoms but capable of transmitting a disease to another.

**casts** Small dish-shaped, hardened mucus particles formed in the renal tubules and discarded in the urine.

**CAT scanner** Computerized axial tomogram scanner, a noninvasive instrument for discerning abnormalities of the brain and other body tissues.

**catheterization** The process of inserting a catheter, most commonly used in reference to inserting a catheter into the bladder.

**cation** A positively charged ion.

**center of gravity** A point in an object or person at which gravitational pull functions as if the entire weight of the object or person were at that single point.

**centering** A part of Piaget's preoperational stage; the inability to see a complete situation; seeing only those aspects pertaining to the moment.

**central nervous system** The division of the nervous system pertaining to central neurologic control, the brain and spinal cord.

**central venous pressure** The pressure of the blood in the vena cava and right atrium; normally 5–10 cm of water.

**Century tub** A brand name for a device that, with the use of a hydraulic lift, places a person secured in a plastic chair into a whirlpool tub for bathing.

**cephalocaudal** Relating to the neuromuscular motor development from the head downward to the feet, evident from birth to two years.

**certification** A process of obtaining a credential attesting to ability in a specialized field.

**challenging** A blocking response in which a person's statements of concerns or feelings are questioned.

**chaplain** A member of the clergy who has a specific relationship with or is employed by the health-care facility to assist in meeting the spiritual needs of the patients, families, and staff.

**chemical theory of sleep** The theory that sleep is brought on by increased carbon dioxide levels in the blood.

**Cheyne-Stokes respirations** Respirations gradually tapering off to the point of cessation. After a period of apnea, the respirations gradually return to become deep and rapid.

**Chicano** A Mexican-American.

**chordotomy** A surgical procedure that severs afferent pain nerves.

**chronic illness** Illness that persists; statistically identified as persisting for three months or more.

**chronic obstructive pulmonary disease (C.O.P.D.)** A group of respiratory diseases in which there is obstruction to airflow and therefore difficulty in breathing.

**circadian rhythm** The approximately twenty-four-hour cyclic pattern of rest and activity in humans.

**citrated blood** Blood to which citrate has been added to prevent clotting during storage.

**clean technique** A technique designed to decrease the number of pathogens on persons or objects.

**clergy** Individuals who have fulfilled the requirements to become full-time, paid workers for their religious groups.

**clichés** Routine social phrases or responses that tend to block depth of communication.

**climax** Sexual orgasm.

**clonic** Pertaining to the stage of a seizure during which jerking movements of the extremities occur.

**cognition** Rational thinking processes or knowledge.

**cognitive learning** The type of learning that relates to knowledge.

**cohesion** A mutual attraction that holds a group together.

**colloid** A large molecule substance that cannot pass through a semipermeable membrane.

**colloidal osmotic pressure** The osmotic pressure created by the presence of colloids on one side of a semipermeable membrane that tends to cause water to move through the membrane to the colloids.

**colostomy** A surgically devised opening directly from the large intestine to the abdominal wall.

**coma** A level of awareness in which a person no longer responds to external stimuli except, in some cases, to painful stimuli.

**common law** The broad area of common knowledge, customary procedure, and judicial decisions upon which a current legal decision may be made.

**communication** The process by which one person makes thoughts, feelings, and concerns known to another.

**compensated** Designating an acid-base state in which the pH is within the normal range due to adjustments in electrolytes and buffers.

**compensation** Emphasis on a trait or traits to make up for perceived deficiencies of the self.

**complete blood count (CBC)** A measurement that establishes the values of a variety of components of the blood, usually including red blood count, white blood count, hemoglobin, and hematocrit.

**concrete operational** Piaget's cognitive stage of seven to eleven years of age during which a person can understand the physical environment in relation to technology.

**conduction** The transfer of nerve impulses by neurons.

**confidentiality** The protection of the patient's privacy through careful use of both written and oral communication.

**conjoint therapy** The treatment of a couple by a male and female therapist.

**consciousness** The state of being awake, alert, and able to communicate.

**consensus** A decision reached by general agreement by all group members.

**consent** A decision to accept an offered plan of care.

**considering consequences** A facilitating response in which a person is helped to look realistically at the potential result of a particular course of action.

**constant fever** One in which the temperature remains elevated at a uniform level.

**contaminated** Having been in contact with microorganisms.

**content** The topics discussed, decisions made, and actions taken by a group.

**continuing education** Learning programs undertaken after graduation from a basic program to maintain or expand competence.

**contraception** Prevention of impregnation.

**contracture** A shortening of a muscle that causes distortion or deformity of a joint.

**contraindications** Indications that a certain plan of treatment is inadvisable.

**convection** Heat transfer caused by moving air that carries heat away from the body surface and that will be replaced by cooler air.

**conventional** Kohlberg's level of moral development that incorporates the need to please or be accepted by others.

**conversion** The development of a physical illness or disability to substitute for a psychological problem.

**coordination** (1) The ability to voluntarily move the extremities and body parts in a balanced and effective manner. (2) Facilitating the functioning of the health-care team to provide better care.

**coping mechanisms** Any action that assists an individual in tolerating a stressor and relieving unpleasant feelings.

**cornea** The central, clear convex surface of the eye over the pupil and iris.

**cortex** Thin, outer layer of the brain.

**cough reflex** The involuntary reflex that protects a person from foreign bodies lodging in the respiratory tract.

**cranium** The portion of the skull that encloses the brain.

**credé** Manually exerting pressure on the bladder to force out urine.

**credential** A written evidence of one's qualifications.

**crisis** A situation in which previous methods of coping are no longer useful and which threatens to overwhelm the individual.

**criteria** Specific standards upon which an evaluative judgment may be based.

*Curanderos* Folk healers of the Hispanic culture who derive their powers from God.

**cutaneous pain (superficial)** Discomfort occurring in surface tissue.

**cyanosis** A bluish discoloration of the skin due to oxygen deficiency.

**dangling** Sitting on the side of the bed with the feet and lower legs hanging off the edge.

**data base** Information gathered about a patient and used to establish a plan of care.

**data collection** A part of the first step in the nursing process; gathering information.

**death care** The cleansing and preparation of the body after death.

**decerebration** Deep coma progressing to total or partial interruption of the connection of the spinal cord tracts to the brain.

**deciduous teeth** Temporary teeth.

**decubitus ulcer** An open sore or lesion of superficial tissue caused by pressure.

**defending** A blocking response in which one person opposes another by defending against critical statements made.

**defense mechanisms** Largely unconscious behaviors that serve to relieve feelings of anxiety and tension.

**dehydration** A condition in which there has been an undue loss of body water.

**delusion** Faulty thinking pattern inconsistent with reality.

**demanding an explanation** A blocking response in which a reason for feeling and behavior is strongly requested.

**democratic** Pertaining to the form of rule in which decisions are made by all group members.

**denial** An unconscious refusal to recognize a happening or circumstance.

**dentures** Artificial teeth.

**dependency** The inability to function satisfactorily without the aid of another.

**dependent functioning** Working under the direction of another individual.

**deposition** A legal testimony given in written form.

**depression** A state of being in low spirits, feeling dejected, and often without hope.

**dermis** The inner, thicker layer of the skin.

**despair** Erikson's unsuccessful outcome of the later years; to feel useless and lose hope.

**developing awareness** Gradually recognizing reality and the changes related to it.

**developmental crisis** A crisis arising out of the changes that occur within the life cycle.

**diagnostic test** A procedure designed to provide information that will aid in the identification of a disease process.

**dialysis** A procedure for replicating kidney function.

**diet order** The physician's prescription for diet; *content*: the kinds of foods to be eaten; *form*: whether the daily intake is to be in three meals, six meals, three meals plus snacks, or any other pattern; *texture*: whether the food is pureed, chopped, or regular.

**dietary history** A complete record of the eating patterns, likes, and dislikes of an individual.

**diffusion** The movement of particles from their area of greater concentration to their area of lesser concentration.

**diploma program** A basic education of approximately three years in length, associated with a hospital, that awards a diploma upon completion.

**direct-care audit** Evaluation of care through checking the actual care given.

**direct contact** The direct transmission of pathogens from one surface to another when the surfaces touch.

**disadvantaged** Designating those in our society who do not have quality of life socially or economically.

**disbelief** Refusal to believe.

**discharge planner** An individual with the responsibility for planning for care of the patient after discharge from the facility.

**discrimination** Taking actions directed by bias, prejudice, or stereotyping.

**disengagement** A natural withdrawal from the environment.

**disinfectants** Agents that destroy pathogens.

**displacement** Focusing feelings related to one person or situation on another.

**dissolution stage** The final stage in the life of a group during which the group is ended.

**distress** A level of stress within the body great enough to disturb homeostasis.

**diuretic** A drug that increases the production of urine.

**dorsal column stimulator** A battery-powered electrical device with an electrode surgically placed at the spinal nerves that produces electrical stimulation, thus interfering with pain impulses; used for intractable chronic pain.

**dosage** A specified quantity of a therapeutic agent, prescribed to be taken at one time or at stated intervals.

**double-bagging** A procedure performed by two persons for disposing of contaminated linens or objects by placing the inner or contaminated bag inside an outer or clean bag.

**doubt** Erikson's unsuccessful outcome of the toddler; to be uncertain and to distrust others.

**douche** A stream of water applied to a part or a cavity of the body for cleaning or medicinal purposes, most frequently the vagina.

**droplet** A means of transmission of pathogens by the moisture of a sneeze or cough.

**dyspareunia** Painful intercourse.

**dysphagia** Difficulty in swallowing.

**dysphasia** Difficulty in using language.

**dyspnea** Difficulty or pain when breathing.

**dysuria** Difficulty or pain on urination.


**Eastern Orthodoxy** A Christian religion based in Eastern European and Mideastern countries and professing a specific body of beliefs.

**edema** An excessive accumulation of serous fluid in the tissues.

**egocentricism** A part of Piaget's preoperational stage; a term used for seeing the self as the central focus.

**ejaculation** Discharging of seminal fluid.

**electroencephalogram** A recording or tracing of the electrical output of the cortex of the brain.

**electroencephalograph** The device or machine that produces the electroencephalogram.

**electrolyte** A charged particle capable of conducting an electrical impulse. Specific electrolytes are essential to body function.

**elemental feeding (enteral feeding)** A formula composed of simple food substances that can be absorbed directly without the need for digestion. Vivonex is a common brand name.

**embolus** An object moving in the bloodstream; for example, a moving blood clot.

**emesis** Vomiting.

**encouraging comparisons** A facilitating response in which the person is asked to compare current experience with other experiences.

**enema** A procedure whereby a fluid, usually for the purpose of cleansing, is instilled into the colon through the rectum.

**enteric coating** A coating on a tablet that is resistive to gastric juices and is broken down by enzymes in the small intestine.

**entry into practice** The issue focusing on what the basic educational requirements should be to begin practice as a nurse.

**enuresis** Involuntary urination during the nighttime hours.

**epidermis** The thinner, outer layer of the skin.

**epilepsy** A condition characterized by seizures.

**epithelial cells** Those cells of the surface of the skin and mucous membranes.

**equilibration** A process described by Piaget for making thought consistent.

**erection** The enlargement and hardening of the penis due to filling with blood.

**erogenous** Areas of the body capable of being sexually aroused.

**erythrocyte** Red blood cell.

**esteem needs** In Maslow's hierarchy, the middle level of the nonphysiological needs.

**ethics** The study of the moral choices to be made by an individual.

**etiology** The source or cause of a problem.

**eupnea** Normal breathing.

**eustress** A level of stress in the body that tends to make it more able to protect itself.

**euthanasia** (1) *Active*: the use of toxic substances or other methods to end life. (2) *Passive*: the withdrawal of or the decision not to use extraordinary means to prolong life.

**evaluation** (1) The process of examining or judging to decide the value of something. (2) Examining the result and ascertaining the success of the nursing intervention; the fourth step in the nursing process.

**evaporation** Heat loss or cooling of the skin by evaporation of perspiration or moisture.

**expectorant** Drugs that promote secretion of respiratory fluids and coughing them up.

**expectorate** To eject from the mouth; to spit.

**expiration** Exhaling of air from the lungs.

**exploratory responses** A variety of facilitating responses that help a person to understand the current situation.

**expressive responses** Behavior that gives overt evidence of pain, such as crying, moaning, grimacing, swearing, and screaming.

**expressive role** The collection of behaviors that serves to assist others to express feelings.

**external cardiac massage** A method for circulating blood by intermittent pressure over the heart.

**external influences on learning** Those factors outside the person that decrease or increase learning.

**external respiration** The exchange that takes place when room air reaches the alveoli.

**extracellular fluid compartment** The fluid found in the circulating blood and lymph and interstitial spaces.

**facilitating responses** Verbal replies that tend to encourage another individual to communicate.

**Fallopian tubes** Slender tubes connecting the region of the ovaries to the uterus.

**false imprisonment** Holding people, either physically or through threats, against their will.

**false reassurance** A blocking response in which general statements that "all will be well" are made.

**fat** A compound composed of glycerol and fatty acids used for energy in the body; may be either plant or animal in origin.

**fear** A feeling of distress due to an objective danger or threat.

**fecal incontinence** Involuntary passing of stool.

**feces** Waste excreted from the bowels.

**feedback** (1) Information provided to the source of a process on the process itself. (2) Information provided to an individual regarding progress.

**feedback theory of sleep** A theory that sleep is caused when, after a period of neuronal activity during which electrical impulses are relayed throughout the system, fatigue takes place.

**fever** Abnormally high body temperature.

**fiber** Undigestible cellulose in vegetables and fruits that provides bulk and prevents constipation.

**fibrin** A protein formed from fibrinogen by the action of thrombin, which creates a fibrous network for clotting and for wound healing.

**filtration** A process of passing a liquid or a gas through a substance to remove certain particles; pressure is required to move the substance.

**filtration pressure** The pressure created by the blood pressure that causes fluid to move out of the capillary into the interstitial space.

**first intention** Healing of wound with edges approximated and no evidence of inflammation.

**"five rights"** A safety measure used to ensure the correct drug administration process. (1) The right drug is given (2) in the right dosage (3) by the right route (4) to the right patient (5) at the right time.

**flatus** Gas generated in the stomach or intestines.

**flow sheet** A chart or graph used to record specific factual information.

**fluid overload** An excessive amount of fluid in the circulatory system characterized first by distended neck veins and delayed emptying of hand veins and then by accumulation of fluid in the chest.

**focusing** A facilitating response in which the person is helped to concentrate on pertinent factors.

**force fluids** A term meaning to encourage a person to drink a large amount of fluid.

**formal operational** Piaget's cognitive stage of the eleven-year-old at which time abstract thought is possible.

**free foods** Those foods that have a minimal number of calories and therefore can be eaten without limit when on a weight-reduction diet. Examples are celery, lettuce, and diet carbonated beverages.

**frequency** The need or desire to void at more frequent intervals than usual.

**frigidity** Inability of the female to become sexually aroused.

**fungus** A moldlike low form of plant life that makes it difficult to subdue pathogens.

**gait** A way of moving on foot or a particular fashion of walking or running.

**gastric** Pertaining to the stomach.

**gastrostomy** A surgical opening directly into the stomach through the abdominal wall. A gastrostomy tube is placed into the opening for the purpose of instilling fluid.

**"gate control theory"** A theory, first proposed by Melzack and Wall, of how pain impulses are transmitted.

**gay** Homosexual.

**General Adaptation Syndrome (G.A.S.)** The common response to all stressors as described by Hans Selye; composed of the alarm reaction, the stage of resistance, and the stage of exhaustion.

**general leads** Facilitating responses that are single words or noncommital sounds.

**generativity** Erikson's task of the middle years; forming ideas and plans for the next generation.

**genitals** The external organs of the reproductive system.

**geriatrics** The specialty in health care dealing with the aged patient.

**gerontology** A broad field of study of old age.

**glycosuria** Sugar or glucose in the urine.

**gout** A systemic, metabolic illness whose most common symptom is swollen and inflamed joints due to uric acid deposits.

**grand mal seizure** A seizure characterized by stages of clonus and tonus and unconsciousness.

**guaiac** A natural resin used as a reagent to test for blood in specimens.

**guilt** (1) A feeling of remorse over having done something wrong. (2) Erikson's unsuccessful outcome of early childhood; being remorseful for having done something wrong.

**gustatory** Pertaining to the sense of taste.

**hair follicle** The cavity out of which a hair grows.

**halitosis** Unpleasant mouth odor.

**hallucinations** The experiencing of sounds, sights, or smells that do not exist.

**healing** Restoring to health.

**health** Being in an optimum state of homeostasis.

**health-care team** All those individuals of a variety of health occupations who work together to provide care to individuals.

**health maintenance** Actions to preserve a state of health.

**health maintenance organization (HMO)** An organization that provides all health care for a set prepaid fee.

**health systems agency (HSA)** An agency established through federal legislation to serve as a focal point for communitywide planning to meet health-care needs.

**heat loss** Loss of heat from the body by any of four processes: radiation, conduction, convection, or evaporation.

**Heimlich maneuver** An emergency procedure devised to expel foreign bodies from the air passageways.

**helminthic infections** Infections caused in a person by the infestation of parasitic worms.

**hematocrit** A measurement of the percentage of red blood cells in whole blood expressed as a volume per 100 ml.

**hematuria** Blood in the urine.

**hemiplegia** Paralysis of one side of the body.

**hemodialysis** The process of circulating a patient's blood through a kidney machine for the purpose of removing wastes and excess fluid.

**hemoglobin** The iron-containing, oxygen-carrying component of the blood; measured as the weight of the hemoglobin contained in the red blood cells in 100 ml of blood.

**hemolytic reaction** An adverse reaction to a blood transfusion in which red blood cells are broken down (hemolyzed).

**hernia** The protrusion of an organ from its normal position through the wall that contains it.

**heterosexual** Pertaining to sexual preference for the opposite sex.

**hierarchy of needs** Maslow's ascending ranking of needs, primary or physiological needs at the bottom and secondary or nonphysiological needs at the top.

**high-level wellness** A term used by Dunn to describe a state of optimum balance and energy within an individual.

**Hispanic** Descriptive of several groups of people who speak Spanish or Portuguese.

**histamine** A protein product found in all tissues of the body that is active in the inflammatory process through dilating blood vessels. It also causes constriction of bronchioles and increases secretion of gastric acid. Histamine production is increased when the body comes into contact with products to which it is sensitive.

**holistic healing** Restoration of total or holistic health.

**holistic health** Optimal functioning of all body systems including psychological well-being.

**Holy Communion** A sacrament of Christians in which bread and wine (or grape juice) are taken as symbols of Christ's death and resurrection.

**homeostasis** The tendency of all living tissue to restore and maintain itself in a condition of balance or equilibrium.

**homosexual** Sexual preference for members of the same sex; gay.

**hospice** A philosophy of care and a system of delivery of care for the terminally ill and their families.

**host** The person in or on whom a pathogen lives.

**hostility** A feeling of antagonism toward another in which the other is perceived as an opponent.

**human dignity** A belief that each individual has intrinsic worth.

**humidification** Increasing the amount of water vapor in the air.

**hunger** A physical sensation of discomfort in the stomach indicating a need for food.

**hydrating solution** An intravenous solution that provides primarily water with dextrose or sodium chloride added for tonicity.

**hygiene** Those practices that bring about personal cleanliness, comfort, and feelings of well-being.

**hypalgesia** Decreased perception of pain.

**hyperalgesia** Increased perception of pain.

**hyperalimentation** A method of providing complete nutrients via an intravenous line, usually into a subclavian vein.

**hypercalcemia** An excessive amount of calcium in the serum; greater than 5.5 mEq/l.

**hyperesthesia** Increased sensation.

**hyperglycemia** High blood sugar; above 120 mg/100 ml.

**hyperkalemia** An excessive amount of potassium in the blood; greater than 5 mEq/l.

**hypernatremia** An excessive amount of sodium in the blood; greater than 145 mEq/l.

**hypertension** An elevated blood pressure; usually considered a pressure above 160 systolic and/or 100 diastolic.

**hypertonic** (1) Designating excessive muscle tone. (2) Having an osmolality (number of particles per liter) greater than blood; greater than 300 mOsm/l.

**hyperventilation** Deep, rapid respiration.

**hypesthesia** Decreased sensation.

**hypnosis** A process of inducing a passive state in which the usual objective abilities are decreased and the person is abnormally suggestible.

**hypnotic** Drug used to induce sleep.

**hypocalcemia** A deficit in calcium in the blood; less than 4.5 mEq/l.

**hypokalemia** A deficit of potassium in the blood; less than 3.5 mEq/l.

**hyponatremia** A deficit of sodium in the blood; less than 136 mEq/l.

**hypostatic pneumonia** Pneumonia occurring due to lack of movement.

**hypotensive** Having a blood pressure lower than normal; in the adult, a systolic below 100.

**hypothermia** A condition in which body temperature is lower than that necessary for body processes to function adequately.

**hypotonic** (1) Designating lessened muscle tone. (2) Having an osmolality (number of particles per liter) less than blood; less than 300 mOsm/l.

**hypoventilation** Shallow respirations.

**hypoxia** An oxygen deficiency of body tissues.

**identification** The adoption of attitudes and behaviors of an admired or cared-for person.

**identity** Erikson's task of the adolescent; to become independent as a person and begin setting goals.

**illusion** The misinterpretation of real sights, sounds, or smells.

**immobility** Inability to move.

**immune response** The reaction of the body to substances identified as nonself.

**immune system** A group of tissues that react to pathogens and defend the body.

**immunity** A condition of heightened responsiveness to an antigen, thus enabling the body to destroy the antigen and not contract the disease; *active*: immunity produced by previous contact with the antigen in which the body develops the ability to produce an antibody against the antigen; *passive*: immunity conferred temporarily by providing the body with an antibody produced elsewhere.

**immunosuppression** Suppression of the body's natural immune system by drugs or other agents.

**impaction** Compressed material in a confined space; for example, hardened feces in the bowel.

**implementation** Carrying out the nursing plan; nursing intervention; the third step in the nursing process.

**impotence** The inability of the male to produce or maintain a penile erection.

**incident report** A form filed with the hospital administration and the insurance carrier to provide information on any untoward incident occurring to anyone in the facility.

**incipient pressure ulcer** An ulcer in an area where pressure has interfered with the blood supply and cell damage has begun.

**incontinence** Involuntary urination or defecation.

**independent** Competent and capable of managing one's own life.

**independent functioning** Actions based on personal decision making.

**indirect contact** The transmission of pathogens from one area to another by means of an object.

**industry** Erikson's task of middle childhood; increasing physical activity, developing competitiveness, and dealing with authority.

**infection** A state in which pathogens multiply to a point where they cause signs and symptoms.

**infectious agent** A pathogen or a disease-causing microorganism.

**inferiority** Erikson's unsuccessful outcome of middle childhood; feeling inadequate.

**infirmity** Disability.

**influence** Power to sway or affect another.

**informed consent** A decision to accept treatment based on knowledge of both the potential benefits and potential risks of the proposed treatment.

**inhibitory ejaculation** The delay or inability to ejaculate semen.

**initial plan** The first comprehensive plan for medical care made by the physician.

**initiation stage** The first stage in the life of a group during which the group members begin to establish a relationship.

**initiative** Erikson's task of early childhood; assertive interaction with family and peers.

**input** Anything put into a system or expended in its operation.

**insomnia** The inability to sleep.

**inspiration** The taking in of air.

**instinctual theory of sleep** The theory that sleep is an instinct of all persons.

**institutionalized racism** Perpetuation of racism within institutions through various practices, including employment.

**instrumental role** The collection of behaviors that serve to assist in the accomplishment of tasks.

**integrity** Erikson's task of the later years; a feeling of being complete and in contact with others in the environment.

**intellectualization** Identifying intellectual reasons for behavior and feelings; also called *rationalization*.

**interaction** The total communication process between two individuals.

**interdependent functioning** Actions based on joint decisions arrived at through consulting with others.

**interferon** A group of small proteins produced by the body that are released by cells invaded by a virus and other agents, thus causing noninvaded cells to form a protein to protect against invasion.

**intermittent fever** One in which the temperature rises each day but sometime during each twenty-four-hour period returns to normal.

**intermittent positive pressure breathing (IPPB)** A treatment performed intermittently by a machine delivering air or oxygen under pressure to cause maximum inflation of the lungs.

**internal girdle** Those muscles of the abdomen, back, and hips that provide support to the abdominal contents and the pelvis.

**internal influences on learning** Those factors within the individual that affect ability to learn.

**internal respiration** Exchange of gases at the cellular level.

**interpreting** A blocking response in which meaning is ascribed to behavior.

**intershift report** A verbal report of the significant information regarding patients given by a nurse finishing a shift to nursing staff beginning a shift.

**interstitial fluid** The body fluid found in the spaces between the cells.

**intervention** Initiating an action.

**interview** A face-to-face conversation in which one person attempts to gain information from another.

**interviewing** A sequenced question-and-answer process.

**intimacy** Erikson's task of the young adult; the ability to establish a close emotional relationship with another.

**intracellular fluid compartment** All the body fluid found inside the cells of the body.

**introductory phase** The time of establishment of a relationship.

**intromission** Insertion.

**ion** An electrically charged particle.

**ischemia** Lack of blood supply to the tissue.

**Islam** A religion based on the teachings of Mohammed who lived in A.D. 600 in the Middle East.

**isolation** (1) Erikson's unsuccessful outcome of young adulthood; to feel separated or set apart from others. (2) A procedure for establishing physical barriers to the spread of microorganisms.

**isometric exercises** Those in which muscles are contracted tightly and held contracted without movement of body parts.

**isotonic** Having the same osmolality as another fluid; fluid (such as normal saline) having the same osmolality as blood, 300 mOsm/l.

**isotonic exercises** Any exercises in which movement results.

**Judaism** The religious beliefs of the Jews based on the Torah and the Talmud.

**keratin** The hard, protein substance that makes up the cells of the nails and the shafts of the hair.

**ketogenic diet** A diet with a high percentage of calories in fats and proteins that produces a mild ketoacidosis.

**kinesthetic feedback** The perception of extent and direction of movement and of the position of body parts.

**kosher** Food prepared and served in accord with Jewish dietary laws.

**Kussmaul's respirations** Deep and rapid respirations that cause a "blowing" sound.

**ladder concept** A general philosophy of providing accessibility from one level of education to another without loss of credit or repetition.

**laissez-faire** A form of group rule in which there is no designated leader and no formal process for decision making.

**lassitude** A feeling of lethargy or exhaustion.

**latency period** Freud's psychosexual stage of persons from six to eleven years of age when sensual needs are satisfied without overt identification with the parent of the opposite sex.

**learning** A change in behavior not due to growth or fatigue.

**learning need** A need for change in behavior.

**leave-taking** The process of terminating an interpersonal relationship.

**lethargy** Sleepiness or somnolence.

**leukocyte** A white blood cell.

**levels of awareness** Levels of responsiveness of an individual, from alert to coma.

**liability insurance** Insurance designed to pay legal costs for defense against a suit and a settlement if awarded.

**libel** Any written, printed, or pictorial statement that damages a person by exposing him or her to ridicule.

**libido** Sexual desire.

**licensed practical nurse (L.P.N.)** An individual with a legal credential attesting to a minimum level of competence and permitting the practice of practical nursing for pay.

**licensure** A legal credential.

**licensure by endorsement** The acquisition of a nursing license in an additional state after licensure by examination in the initial state.

**licensure law** The law that specifies the requirements of obtaining, renewing, and removing a professional license.

**life review** A process of grieving for the patient and family; reflecting about the past and reviewing family events.

**Local Adaptation Syndrome (L.A.S.)** Body responses to localized threats that establish the conditions to restore homeostasis.

**long-term care** Health care for a condition that requires treatment of a less extensive nature for a prolonged period of time.

**love-and-belonging needs** In Maslow's hierarchy, the level of needs just above safety needs.

**lumen** The inner, open space of a needle, tube, or vessel.

**maceration** Softening by exposure to moisture.

*mal de ojo* The myth of the "evil eye" as a cause of illness among Hispanic people.

**malingering** A conscious exaggeration of symptoms to gain rewards.

**malnutrition** A state in which the body is poorly nourished due to dietary lack. It may be a general lack of many nutrients or a specific lack of one essential nutrient.

**malpractice** Failure to act as a reasonably prudent professional person would act in a similar situation.

**mandatory licensure** A legal credential required to practice an occupation.

**mastectomy** Removal of a breast.

**masturbation** Self-stimulation for the purpose of eliciting sexual pleasure.

**maturational crisis** A developmental crisis.

**means of transmission** The route or vehicle by which pathogens move from one person to another.

**meatus** The opening of the urethra onto the surface of the body.

**mediastinum** The group of tissues and organs in the center of the chest including the heart, great vessels, trachea, esophagus, thymus gland, and lymph nodes.

**Medicaid** A federal and state government system for financing care for individuals meeting financial and/or disability requirements.

**medical healing** The cessation of symptoms without surgical intervention.

**medical plan of care** The physician's plan for treating the disease process and its symptoms.

**Medicare** A federal government system for financing care for those 65 or older.

**meditation** A technique for shutting out stimuli and producing the relaxation response by sitting quietly and focusing the mind on a neutral topic.

**menopause** The cessation of menstruation and the end of reproduction in the female; sometimes used broadly to indicate lessening of reproductive ability in both males and females.

**menses** Menstruation.

**mentation** Thinking or cognition.

**message** That which is communicated within the individual.

**microorganisms** Extremely small animals and plants.

**micturition** Urination or voiding.

**migrants** A segment of society who are mobile, primarily farm workers.

**milliequivalent (mEq)** A measure of combining power or electrical charges of a given substance.

**milliosmole (mOsm)** A measure of osmolality (number of particles) in a solution.

**mineral** A nonorganic chemical needed by the body.

**minimum daily requirements (MDR)** The lowest amount of a nutrient for the body to maintain appropriate functioning.

**minority** People who come from diverse social, cultural, and ethnic groups; a group smaller than the main group within a society.

**mistrust** Erikson's unsuccessful outcome of the infant; to fear others or the environment.

**motivation** An internal tendency or desire to learn.

**motor aphasia** The inability to form words due to lack of innervation of the muscles of speech.

**motor impulses** Messages conveyed to the brain regarding movement.

**motor neurons** Neurons that are capable of carrying motor impulses.

**mottled** Descriptive of irregular, discolored blotches on the skin.

**mouth-to-mouth resuscitation** Providing respiration to the nonbreathing individual by blowing into the mouth to inflate the lungs and allowing the natural recoil of the chest to empty them; also called *rescue breathing*.

**Muslim** A person of the Islamic faith.

**narrative charting** A style of patient record in which the nurse records information in a storylike form on the nurses' notes.

**nasogastric tube feeding** A nutritious formula instilled through a tube that passes from the nose through the esophagus to the stomach.

**Native American** American-born Indians or Eskimos.

**nausea** A subjective feeling of discomfort in the stomach that indicates a potential for vomiting.

**nebulization** The producing of a fine spray of moisture in the air.

**necessary but not sufficient** A theory that it is necessary in diseases caused by pathogens to have the pathogen present but that this in itself may not be sufficient to cause the actual disease.

**necrosis** Breakdown or death of tissue.

**need** That which is necessary or required for optimal functioning.

**need to know–understand** In Maslow's hierarchy, one of the higher needs levels in which the person needs to gain knowledge.

**negative feedback** A process whereby a rising level of a substance or increased rate of a process signals the system producing the substance or controlling the process to shut off.

**negligence** The failure to act as a reasonably prudent person would act in a similar situation, resulting in harm to another.

**negotiation stage** The second stage in the life of a group during which members develop a pattern for relating and decision making.

**neuro signs** A brief assessment of neurological status; usually included are pulse, respiration, blood pressure, level of awareness, and pupillary response.

**neurogenic bladder** Partial paralysis of the bladder musculature because of a spinal cord injury that prevents complete emptying.

**neurogenic pain** Pain originating from stimulation or irritation of a nerve.

**neurohormonal theory of sleep** A theory attributing sleep to the increased presence of the neurohormonal substance serotonin.

**nocturia** Urination during the nighttime hours.

**nondirective comments** Facilitating responses that open the conversation but do not direct its flow.

**nonverbal** Relating to communication through body signs and facial expressions.

**normal flora** Beneficial microorganisms that inhibit the growth of pathogens within a certain area of the body.

**normal saline** A solution of sodium chloride with the same osmolality or tonicity as body fluid; usually given as 0.9 percent.

**norms** The standards for behavior within a group.

**nosocomial** Designating hospital-acquired infections.

**Nurse Practice Act** The statutory law that defines nursing and specifies the requirements for obtaining, renewing, and revoking a license to practice nursing.

**nurse practitioner** A registered nurse with special education who provides primary health care.

**nursing care plan** A written, detailed approach to providing nursing care in which problems are identified, desired outcomes or goals are set, and nursing actions are specified.

**nursing diagnosis** A statement of a patient problem that the nurse, by virtue of education and experience, is able to identify and treat; it includes the etiology when known.

**nursing history** A structured interview designed to establish a data base for nursing care.

**nursing orders** Directions for nursing care for a specific patient written by a nurse.

**nursing process** A problem-solving approach to planning care that includes the four steps of assessment, planning, implementation, and evaluation.

**nutrition** All of the processes involved in taking in and using food, including ingestion, digestion, absorption, and metabolism.

**obesity** An excessive body weight; usually considered 20 to 30 percent over average weight for sex, age, height, and bone structure.

**objective** A specific desired outcome; often used interchangeably with goal. However, the term goal is sometimes used to indicate a broader, less specific outcome.

**objective data** Information based on observable phenomena.

**observation** The act of systematically noting phenomena.

**occult blood** Hidden blood, such as blood in the stool, that is not visible.

**Oedipal conflict** Freud's psychosexual stage from four to five years of age, when the parent of the opposite sex is the object of sensual satisfaction.

**olfactory** Pertaining to the sense of smell.

**oliguria** Scanty formation of urine by the kidneys.

**open system** A system in which input comes from a variety of sources and output may occur in different ways.

**operation stage** The third stage in the life of a group during which work is accomplished.

**opisthotonos position** An abnormal positioning of the body in a backward, flexed, bridgelike configuration; it may accompany decerebration.

**oral care** Those actions that cleanse the lips, teeth, tongue, and mucous membranes of the mouth.

**oral irrigator** A device using a high-pressure stream of water, commonly used to clean the teeth.

**orchidectomy** Removal of the testicle in the male.

**orders** Directions for care.

**orgasm** Sexual climax.

**orientation stage** The first stage in the life of a group during which members establish themselves as a group.

**orifice** A body opening.

**orthopnea** Difficulty in breathing that is relieved by sitting up or standing.

**orthopneic position** Sitting upright or standing to relieve difficulty in breathing.

**osmolality** A measure of the number of particles per liter of solvent.

**osmolarity** A measure of the number of particles per kilogram of a solvent. The term is often used interchangeably with osmolality but is exactly the same only when the solvent is pure water at 3.8° C.

**osmosis** The diffusion of water across a semipermeable membrane from an area where there are relatively fewer particles to where there are relatively more particles.

**osteoarthritis** Degeneration and pain of the joints often associated with aging.

**osteoporosis** A metabolic failure to replace bone tissue;

it causes bones to become thin, porous, and easily fractured.

**outcome criteria** Specific standards by which to evaluate results of nursing care.

**output** (1) Anything that results from the operation of a system. (2) The fluid excreted by the body—urine, perspiration, vomitus, and so on.

**outreach** A system whereby care is provided outside of the institutional setting.

**pacing** The rate of speaking and pauses in an interaction.

**pain cocktail** An oral liquid medication containing a pain medication and other agents helpful to the patient such as a tranquilizer or antiemetic.

**pain interpretation** Comparing the sensation of pain to other experiences and identifying type and severity.

**pain perception** Recognition by the brain that the stimulus is pain.

**pain reaction** The response of the individual to pain.

**pain receptor** The nerve ending that receives the stimulus.

**pain threshold** The amount of painful stimulation needed for pain to be perceived.

**pallor** A lack of red color tones given to the skin by oxygen-rich blood.

**palsy** Paralysis.

**panic** A state of overwhelming anxiety in which the individual is unable to function.

**paradoxic sleep** Another name for REM sleep based on the contradiction between the relaxation of the muscles and the extreme activity of the brain.

**paralysis** Loss or impairment of the ability to move or have sensation in a body part as a result of injury to or disease of its nerve supply.

**paraplegia** Paralysis of the lower portion of the body.

**parasitic worms** Long, soft-bodied invertebrates that exist only by feeding off a host.

**parasympathetic nervous system** The division of the autonomic nervous system that decreases stimulation of smooth muscle and glands.

**paresis** Muscular weakness due to partial interruption of stimulus to that muscle or a group of muscles.

**paresthesia** A distortion of sensation such as itching, tingling, crawling, or prickling.

**partial seizure** A seizure during which only certain body parts or areas are involved, with or without unconsciousness.

**passive exercise** Any type of exercise in which another person provides the energy and moves the individual.

**patency** Openness.

**pathogens** Disease-producing microorganisms.

**patient care coordinator** An individual whose job it is to plan for nursing care for those being discharged from an acute-care facility.

**patient outcome** Specific results from the patient's care.

**patients' rights** Those powers or privileges to which the health-care consumer has an established moral claim.

**perception** Becoming aware of the message communicated in an interaction.

**perceptual feedback** Touch as a method of gaining information about the self.

**pericardium** The membrane surrounding the outside of the heart.

**perineum** The portion of the body in the pelvic area that is occupied by urogenital passages and the rectum.

**peripheral nervous system (PNS)** The division of the nervous system that includes all structures and nerves other than the brain and spinal cord.

**peristalsis** Wavelike muscular contractions that propel contained matter along the alimentary canal.

**peritoneal dialysis** Removing waste products from the body by the instillation and removal of a dialyzing solution into the peritoneal cavity.

**permissive license** A legal credential that may be obtained to attest to competence but that is not required for practice.

**petit mal seizure** A seizure characterized by small, short lapses of awareness.

**pH** A measure of the acidity or alkalinity of a solution; 7.0 is neutral, numbers below that are acidic, and numbers above that are alkaline, in a range of 1 to 14.

**phagocytosis** A process by which a leukocyte engulfs another cell in order to destroy it.

**phallic stage** Freud's psychosexual stage of the three- to four-year-old, when the genital region provides greatest sensual satisfaction.

**phantom pain** Pain perceived in a body part that is no longer present, such as an amputated leg.

**phlebitis** An inflammation of a vein.

**physical needs** The external factors necessary for a group to function, including such things as space, light, temperature, and seating.

**physician's assistant** An individual who works with a

physician performing routine aspects of the physician's role such as caring for patients with common illnesses and injuries.

**physiologic status** The status of the body with regard to meeting physiological needs.

**physiological needs** Maslow's lower needs level; those needs essential to life.

**pitting edema** Fluid in the interstitial spaces that can be displaced by pressure from a finger on the surface, thus creating a depression that refills slowly.

**pituitary theory of sleep** A theory that the pituitary, a small gland at the base of the brain, is a sleep regulator.

**placebo** An inert substance given in place of an active agent to which the body reacts as if it were the active agent.

**placebo effect** A positive response to a substance or treatment that is caused by trust and an attitude of expectation rather than a reaction to the substance or treatment itself.

**planning** The second stage in the nursing process that includes setting goals or objectives and establishing a detailed scheme for nursing actions.

**plasma** The liquid portion of the blood after red and white blood cells and platelets are removed.

**platelets** Small disk-shaped elements in the blood that adhere to any damaged surface and begin the clotting process; also called thrombocytes.

**pleural rub** A chest sound of rubbing or grating as the pleurae rub together.

**podiatrist** Specialist in the care of the feet.

**polyuria** Increased formation of urine by the kidneys.

**portal of entry** The portal or opening by which a pathogen enters a susceptible host.

**portal of exit** The place where a pathogen leaves a reservoir or susceptible host.

**postconventional** Kohlberg's level of moral development when moral decision making is based on issues rather than family, friends, or social authority.

**postictal** The final stage of a grand mal seizure with gradual awareness of surroundings. Amnesia, confusion, and drowsiness may also be present.

**postural drainage** A procedure for the purpose of draining secretions from the lungs by placing the person in a variety of positions. Percussion or tapping may also be done.

**postural hypotension** Low blood pressure that occurs when changing from lying to an upright position; also called orthostatic hypotension.

**posture** The position of body parts in relationship to one another.

**power** The ability to exercise control, for example, within a group.

**preconventional** Kohlberg's level of moral development when moral decision making is based on consequences to self, often of a physical nature.

**prejudice** Adverse judgments or opinions without knowledge or facts; bias.

**premature ejaculation** Ejaculation of semen by the male generally within 30 to 60 seconds after intromission.

**preoperational** Piaget's cognitive stage of two to seven years of age and one that incorporates the increasing mastery of symbols and language.

**prescription** A written instruction by a physician, most commonly referring to a medication.

**pressure ulcer** An open sore created by pressure interrupting the blood supply to the tissue; also called decubitus ulcer.

**preventive health care** Intervention that prevents either injury or illness.

**primary care** The initial source of health care through which a person may obtain entry into the health-care system. It includes health examinations, treatment of illness, and referral when necessary.

**principle** A basic rule concerning the functioning of a natural phenomenon that indicates cause and effect.

**priority** That which takes precedence and is established by order of importance or urgency.

**probing** Asking detailed, personal questions not pertinent to current care needs; a blocking response.

**problem list** The combined index and table of contents for the problem-oriented record that identifies all problems and notes and when they were resolved.

**problem-oriented record** A method for organizing the patient's chart around the problems that are present.

**problem-solving approach** An organized, thoughtful method of seeking a solution to a difficulty, usually outlined in steps.

**process** The way a group works to meet its goal, including who speaks, the type of contribution of each person, and the feelings expressed; the "how" of group life.

**process criteria** Specific standards by which to evaluate the methods used in nursing care.

**productivity** Being useful.

**progress notes** An ongoing record of what is happening to the patient in relationship to the problems presented.

**progressive relaxation** A technique for achieving the relaxation response in which parts of the body are relaxed in a gradual manner until the whole body is relaxed.

**projectile vomiting** The forceful expulsion of stomach contents to a distance from the person.

**projection** Placing one's own feelings, ideas, or attributes onto another.

**prophylactic** Preventive.

**proprioception** The ability to know the location of the body parts.

**protein** A complex compound composed of carbon, hydrogen, oxygen, and nitrogen that is essential for building body tissue and that can be broken down to provide energy.

**proteinuria** The abnormal finding of protein in the urine; albuminuria.

**Protestantism** The branch of the Christian church that arose during the Reformation in reaction to what were seen as abuses in the Roman Catholic Church.

**protozoa** Large, single-celled microorganisms.

**pseudoprofessional comments** Inappropriate attempts to use psychological terms or methods in an interaction; a blocking response.

**psychological equilibrium** A state of emotional and mental balance; homeostasis.

**psychological needs** Those internal factors that must be provided for a group to function.

**psychomotor** A type of learning related to acquiring technical skills.

**psychotherapy** Treatment of psychological disorders.

**puberty** Freud's psychosexual stage of the eleven- to fourteen-year-old, when there is integration of sensual tendencies from previous stages.

**pulmonary edema** Fluid accumulating in the interstitial spaces of the lungs.

**pulmonary embolism** An object that moves through the veins to lodge in the lungs.

**pulse deficit** The difference in rate between apical and radial pulses; it represents the number of weak, ineffective heartbeats per minute.

**pulse pressure** The difference between systolic and diastolic blood pressure; it represents the pressure produced by each heartbeat.

**pulse rate** The number of pulse waves per minute.

**pulse rhythm** The pattern of the pulse beats whether regular or irregular.

**pulse strength** The power felt in each pulse beat.

**pyrexia** Fever.

**pyrogenic reaction** A systemic response to a substance, such as a blood transfusion, which causes a fever.

**pyuria** Pus in the urine.

**quadriplegia** Paralysis of all four extremities.

**quiet room** A place in a hospital where individuals may go when a private, quiet atmosphere is desired.

**rabbi** The clergy or teacher in the Jewish faith.

**radiating pain** Pain that spreads from its point of origin to other areas.

**radiation** Heat loss to another object without contact.

**râles** A bubbling chest sound as air moves through moisture or secretions in the lungs.

**range-of-motion exercises (ROM)** Moving joints through the full range or extent to which they can be moved.

**rapid eye movement sleep (REM)** An active stage of sleep during which the eyes move rapidly horizontally.

**rationale** Those definitions, facts, and principles that form the fundamental reasons for nursing action.

**rationalization** Identifying intellectual reasons for behavior and feelings; also called *intellectualization*.

**reaction formation** Adopting ideas and beliefs that are the opposite of those held by an individual or group that one dislikes or wishes to be independent of.

**reader** The individual in the Christian Science Church who provides advice and teaching.

**readiness to learn** The state brought about by the combined effect of internal influences on learning.

**reasonably prudent nurse** A nurse who behaves in accordance with what can be established as the standard for nursing practice in the local community.

**receiver** The person trying to understand the message in an interaction.

**Recommended Dietary Allowances (RDA)** The amounts of foods needed to provide an adequately nutritious diet for activity, growth, and repair in most people as determined by the Food and Nutrition Board of the National Research Council. There are different recommendations for each age group and for pregnant and lactating women.

**referral form** A form used to provide information to another care provider who is being asked to assume responsibility for some portion of the patient's care.

**referred pain** Pain perceived as originating in a place other than where the stimuli occurred.

**reflecting** A facilitating response in which a person's statement is simply repeated as a question.

**registered nurse (R.N.)** An individual who has met the educational and testing requirements for licensure to practice registered nursing as defined in the Nurse Practice Act.

**regression** Acting in a manner characteristic of a younger age.

**rehabilitation** The process of restoring an individual to maximum independence and well-being through education and therapy.

**reinforcement** A reward given to a learner for making the desired responses.

**rejecting** A blocking response in which a person is unwilling to hear feelings or concerns.

**relaxation response** A state characterized by decreased sympathetic nervous system activity, muscle tone, blood pressure, pulse rate, respirations, and pupillary constriction.

**religious medals** Small amulets with religious symbols on the surface.

**REM rebound** A term used for unusually long periods of REM sleep that occur after the discontinuation of many of the hypnotics.

**remittent fever** Rise and fall of a constantly elevated temperature.

**renal failure** Total absence of the formation of urine by the kidneys.

**replacement** Filling or finding a substitute for a loss.

**replacement solution** An intravenous solution containing electrolytes in proportion to those of a body fluid (such as gastric secretions) being lost in excessive amounts.

**report** A verbal or written summary of pertinent information regarding the patient such as that given from one shift to another.

**repression** Unconsciously putting unpleasant or stressful thoughts completely out of awareness.

**reservoir** A place where pathogens, under certain conditions, grow and multiply.

**resignation** Passive submission to a situation.

**resistive exercise** Movement performed against a resistance such as a weight.

**resolution** Taking action to accommodate to a loss.

**respiratory acidosis** A condition characterized by hypoventilation and decreased levels of carbonic acid in the blood resulting in a blood pH of less than 7.35.

**respiratory alkalosis** A condition characterized by hy-perventilation and increased levels of carbonic acid in the blood resulting in a blood pH of greater than 7.45.

**restating** A facilitating response in which a receiver rephrases the statement of the sender.

**restitution** Making life changes or responses to the recognition that a death has occurred.

**retention** The holding of urine within the bladder due to inability to void.

**reticuloendothelial system** The network of tissues and cells throughout the body that are able to phagocytize particles.

**retraction** An abnormal pulling in of soft tissue of the chest on inspiration commonly seen in the supraclavicular, intercostal, and substernal areas.

**reviewing** A facilitating response in which the interaction is reviewed.

**rhonchi** Chest sounds that may be bubbling or wheezing; indicative of moisture in larger airways.

**role** The characteristics and behavior that comprise a function or position.

**role confusion** Erikson's unsuccessful outcome of adolescence; the inability to identify self in relation to others.

**Roman Catholic Church** A branch of the Christian church with a central organization based on the leadership of the Pope in Rome.

**rosary** A specifically patterned chain of beads used in Roman Catholic prayer.

**route of administration** The pathway chosen for giving a drug.

**sacraments** In the Christian church, any of several religious rites instituted by Jesus.

**safety needs** In Maslow's hierarchy, the level just above basic or physiologic needs.

**satiety** A feeling of having eaten a sufficient amount of food.

**scripture** A body of religious writings; for Christians, the Bible; for Muslims, the Koran, etc.

**second intention** Wound healing in which granulation tissue fills in the area between nonapproximated wound edges.

**secondary care** Care provided in a health-care facility, especially an acute-care hospital, to which a person has been referred by the primary care provider.

**seeking clarification** A facilitating response in which one asks the sender to further explain the message.

**seizure** A convulsion.

**self-actualization** The fifth level in Maslow's hierarchy of needs described as "being true to oneself."

**self-centeredness** Preoccupation with and focus on the self.

**self-concept** The total view an individual has of the self.

**self-esteem** The setting of positive values on the self.

**self-hypnosis** A passive state in which the usual objective abilities are decreased and the person is abnormally suggestible.

**self-understanding** The ability to recognize the factors in one's own life that cause feelings and behavior.

**semen** The transport fluid for the sperm.

**semicoma** A condition in which a person shows some spontaneous movement but is difficult to arouse.

**semipermeable membrane** A membrane with openings large enough to permit some particles to pass but too small for the passage of large particles.

**sender** The person in an interaction who is giving the message.

**senility** The state of being old, often used to denote a lack of mental ability due to age.

**sensorimotor** Piaget's stage of cognitive development in which a child learns the properties of things in the environment, primarily through using the senses.

**sensory aphasia** Difficulty with speech due to the inability to receive and understand what others are saying.

**sensory deprivation** A lower level of sensory input than the individual needs for optimum functioning.

**sensory input** All the messages and impressions that are transmitted to the brain by any of the five senses.

**sensory level** The optimum level of sensory input to which we can respond appropriately.

**sensory neurons** Nerves capable of carrying sensory impulses toward the central nervous system.

**sensory overload** The presence of more sensory stimuli during a given period than can be tolerated.

**sensory receptors** Millions of nerve cells in the skin and mucous membrane that send messages of sensation to the brain.

**sequence** The order in which information is taught. The following facilitate learning: known to unknown, normal to abnormal, simple to complex, and wellness to illness.

**sexual awareness** An awareness of one's femininity or masculinity.

**sexual variations** Nontraditional expressions of sexuality.

**sexuality** The aspect of the total person relating to sexual attitudes and behavior.

**shaman** A healing priest of the Native American culture.

**sheltered care** A living environment providing supportive service for those not able to live independently but allowing maximum independence.

**side effect** An effect of a drug or treatment other than that which is the principal reason for its use.

**sign** An objective bodily manifestation that indicates the presence of a health problem.

**signing** A system of communication for the deaf using the position of the hands to convey words or phrases.

**singultus** Hiccoughs.

**skilled nursing facility** A long-term care setting with sufficient licensed personnel (L.P.N.s and R.N.s) to provide skilled care, the kind that demands knowledge and training and is not merely custodial.

**slander** The utterance of defamatory statements injurious to the reputation or well-being of a person.

**sleep cycle** A sequence of five stages during sleep.

**sleep deprivation** Inadequate sleep in the amount needed by a particular individual over a period of time.

**sleep stage** A stage of the sleep cycle with unique characteristics and a distinct electroencephalographic pattern.

**smegma** A thick, whitish substance composed of epithelial cells and mucus that is found around external genitalia.

**SOAPing** The form in which progress notes are written for the Problem-Oriented Medical record: S = subjective information; O = objective information; A = assessment or analysis of data; P = plan for care.

**socializing** Conversation that focuses on nonpersonal social topics.

**somnolence** Lethargy or sleepiness.

**sordes** Accumulation of dried secretions and bacteria in the mouth caused by not eating, mouth-breathing, and inadequate oral hygiene.

**special senses** Hearing, vision, taste, smell, and touch.

**specific gravity** The density of a solution.

**sperm** The male reproductive cell.

**sphincter** A circular muscle that controls an internal or external orifice.

**spinal anesthesia** A process for producing the absence of pain in the lower trunk and legs by injecting an agent into the lower spinal canal.

**spontaneous healing** Healing without obvious intervention.

**spores** Dormant bacteria with thick, resistant walls.

**sputum** Expectorated matter that contains secretions from the lower respiratory tract.

**stage** A period of time in the development of a group, process, or person.

**stage of exhaustion** The third stage of the General Adaptation Syndrome as described by Hans Selye in which the body's resources are depleted by response to stressors and death results.

**stage of resistance** The second stage of the General Adaptation Syndrome during which the body mobilizes its resources and resists the threat.

**starvation** Total intake of calories and other nutrients inadequate to maintain life.

**state board of nursing** The official body appointed by state governments to oversee and administer the Nurse Practice Act.

**statutory laws** Those laws enacted by a legislative body.

**steatorrhea** A condition characterized by stools containing large amounts of fat.

**stereotyped comments** Common social phrases that tend to block communication.

**stereotyping** Presuming a form or pattern often attributed to a group and generalizing or applying it to an individual.

**sterile technique** A technique designed to make areas or objects free of all pathogens and to minimize pathogens on people.

**stimuli** Agents that can evoke a response in the person; *external*: those which originate outside the body; *internal*: those which originate within the individual.

**stoicism** A response to pain or other stressors in which behavior that would demonstrate the distress is suppressed.

**stoma** The surgically created opening onto the body surface of any organ (for example, a colostomy, in which the colon is opened onto the abdomen).

**stool** Feces.

**stress** A generalized body response to a threat.

**stressor** Any agent or stimulus that poses a real or perceived threat to the person.

**stretch reflex** An involuntary reflex that causes the bladder to contract and the internal sphincter to relax, thus releasing urine.

**stridor** A "crowing" sound due to constriction in the larynx.

**structured interview** A question-and-answer interaction in which the questions are preplanned.

**stupor** A condition in which a person may be very drowsy and fall asleep in the middle of a conversation.

**subjective data** Information provided by the patient/client in regard to his or her health status.

**sublimation** Unconsciously redirecting energy from one goal or endeavor toward another.

**substitution** A consciously planned redirection of energy from a blocked goal to another goal.

**sulfonamides** A group of synthetic drugs, with a similar chemical structure (benzene rings), that have an antibacterial effect.

**support system** Those persons and/or groups who offer emotional and physical assistance to an individual.

**suppository** A solid medication that is designed to melt in a body cavity other than the mouth.

**suppressants** Cough medications that eliminate cough by suppressing the cough center in the medulla.

**suppression** Total absence of formation of urine by the kidneys; anuria.

**suppuration** The formation of pus.

**susceptible hosts** Persons who are less able to defend against pathogens and thus will become ill upon contact with pathogens.

**symmetrical** Balanced or even.

**sympathetic nervous system** The division of the autonomic nervous system that increases stimulation of smooth muscle and gland.

**symptom** Another term for subjective data.

**system** A group of interrelated, interreacting, or interdependent elements forming a collective entity.

**tachycardia** An abnormally rapid heartbeat, usually defined as over 100 beats per minute in the adult.

**tachypnea** Very rapid respirations.

**tactile** Pertaining to the sense of touch.

**team conference** A meeting of a health-care team (either nursing or multidisciplinary) in which patient-care problems are discussed, goals set, and plans for action established.

**team nursing** A way of organizing the nursing staff. The team is composed of persons with different levels of education and ability. The team leader organizes the work of the entire team and the team members provide the care that requires their ability.

**terminal pain** Pain caused by an illness that is expected to end in death.

**termination phase** The ending period of an interaction.

**termination stage** The final stage in the life of a group during which the group is ended.

**territoriality** The emotional "space" required for the comfort of an individual or group.

**therapeutic environment** A setting that provides support and an atmosphere conducive to meeting an individual's needs.

**third-party payer** A group or organization that does not receive or provide health care but contracts to pay costs. Insurance companies, Medicaid, and the armed services (CHAMPUS) are examples of third-party payers.

**thrombus** A blood clot.

**tidal volume** The amount of air that can be exchanged with a single breath.

**tonic** Designating the stage of a seizure that involves stiffening of the body and clenching of the jaws.

**tonicity** The osmotic concentration of a fluid. (See *osmolality*.)

**tonus** A state of minimal contraction maintained by an inactive muscle.

**torsion** Twisting.

**tort** A violation of civil law resulting in harm to another individual.

**total parenteral nutrition (TPN)** Providing all essential nutrients via an intravenous line; also called *hyperalimentation*.

**total patient care** A method of organizing nursing care whereby one individual handles all care for a single patient.

**towel bath** A variation of the bed bath using massage with large towels wetted down with warm water and a special antiseptic solution.

**toxic** Poisonous.

**tracheostomy** A surgically devised opening into the trachea from the surface of the neck.

**transcutaneous nerve stimulator (TNS or "tens")** A battery-powered electrical device with electrodes placed on the skin that produces an electrical stimulation that can interfere with transmission of pain impulses.

**trauma** Injury.

**tremor** Involuntary shaking of a part, extremity, or head.

**trust** Erikson's task of infancy; having reliance and a feeling of being safe with others.

**turn sheet** Usually a draw sheet placed under the patient for purposes of turning or moving in bed.

**UA** Urinalysis.

**unstructured interview** A question-and-answer interaction in which the questions arise from the response and are not specifically planned.

**urgency** The inability to postpone urination.

**urimeter** An instrument used for determining the specific gravity of urine.

**urinalysis** The chemical analysis of urine, which commonly includes color, clarity, pH, specific gravity, and checks for the presence of glucose, RBCs, casts, and WBCs.

**urination** The act of excreting urine.

**utilization review** A mechanism for evaluating whether health care was of the right type, in the right setting, and of appropriate length for the needs of the individual patient.

**vaginismus** Pain caused by severe spasm of the vaginal orifice, usually with attempted intercourse.

**validation** Checking with the sender to verify that your understanding of the message is correct.

**vascular theory of sleep** The theory attributing sleep to a periodic drop in blood pressure.

**vasectomy** Surgical interruption of the tubes that carry the sperm.

**vasoconstriction** The narrowing of the lumen of the arteries by contraction of the muscles in the artery wall.

**vasodilatation** The widening of the lumen of the arteries by relaxation of the muscles in the artery wall.

**vectors** Insects or animals that can carry disease.

**vegetarian** Pertaining to a diet containing only plant products; *lacto-vegetarian*: a diet that also includes milk and milk products; *ovo-lacto-vegetarian*: a diet that also includes eggs, milk, and milk products.

**vehicle** An object or substance that can convey pathogens.

**verbal** Pertaining to the words exchanged in an interaction.

**verbal feedback** (1) Explanations from another individual relative to a problem or process. (2) Descriptions of the body and its function from another person.

**virulence** The potency or ability of a pathogen to cause disease.

**virus** A single-celled microorganism, the smallest of all pathogens.

**visceral pain (internal)** Pain originating deep within body tissue.

**visual feedback** (1) Seeing the results of a process. (2)

Visual identification of body parts and their structure to clarify body image.

**vital capacity** The largest possible amount of air that can be exchanged by the lungs.

**vitamins** A group of organic substances that do not contribute calories or building material but are essential to body processes.

**vocabulary level** The level of difficulty of the words and terms used and/or understood.

**voice quality** Loudness or softness of speaking.

**voiding** Emptying urine from the bladder through the urethra; urinating; micturating.

**voluntary association** An organization for the purposes of supporting a specific goal; for example, the American Heart Association.

**vomiting** The ejection of stomach contents through the mouth.

**voting** A formal process for individuals to express their opinion on an issue.

**water soluble** Descriptive of any agent that goes into solution with water.

**working phase** The time during the interaction in which goals are accomplished.

**working stage** The stage in the life of a group during which decisions are made and tasks accomplished; the middle stage of a three-stage process that encompasses negotiation and operation.

**yang** The male, active, dominant, cosmic element in Chinese dual philosophy. Foods designated ''hot'' in terms of healing properties (not temperature) are classified as yang by some Asians.

**yin** The female, passive, cosmic element in Chinese dual philosophy. Foods designated ''cold'' in terms of healing properties (not temperature) are classified as yin by some Asians.

# INDEX

team and, 230−231
   verbal reports and, 216−217
Coordination problems, assessment and intervention in,
   440−441
Coping behaviors, 247
   developing, 251
   *see also* Defense mechanisms
Cortex, 329, 436, 462
   adrenal, 117, 118
Cough, 391
   immobility and, 320
   in older adult, 524
   prevention of, 335
   with respiratory problems, 395
Cough medications, 395−396
   productive and nonproductive, 391
Counseling, 127
   bereavement, 492−493
   rehabilitation, 322
   for sexual problems, 279−280
Counterweight, 309
Cranium, 436
Credé, 372
Credentials, 27
Crimes, 13
Crises, 246
   identifying, 246
   maturational, 246
   situational, 246
Criteria
   for audit of records, 231
   for nursing diagnosis, 141
   outcome, 142
Culture
   body image and, 515
   death and, 491
   diet and, 345−346
   hygiene and, 287
   pain and, 463−464
Cure, miraculous, 259
Cutaneous pain, 461
Cyanosis, 292, 392, 410
Cystogram, 551
Cystoscopy, 548

Dangling, 318
Data
   analysis of, 140
   collection of, 136, 142−143, 270, 335
   objective, 138
   recording, 153
Data base, for problem-oriented record, 220
Davenport Nomogram, 424
Deafness, 444−445, 527
   assessment and intervention in, 445−446
Death, 476
   caring for survivors and, 491
   of child, 485−486
   definition of, 18, 476
   euthanasia and, 486−487

event of, 487−488
   grief and, 488−490
   minority patients and, 78, 81, 82−83, 84, 87
   older adults and, 531−532
   society and, 476
Death care, 488
"Death rattle," 482
Death rites, planning, 485
Decerebration, 439
Decision making
   aids to, 189−190
   in group, 93
   in mental health problems, 251
Decubitus ulcers, 292, 315
   treatment of, 316
Deep breathing
   immobility and, 320
   with respiratory problems, 395
Defecation, 373
   assessment of, 373, 375, 377−378
Defecation problems
   assessment of, 377
   intervention for, 378
   nursing care for, 379−380
Defending, 190
Defense mechanisms, 247
   compensation, 249
   conversion, 250
   denial, 248−249
   displacement, 249
   fantasy, 250
   identification, 249
   projection, 249
   rationalization, 247
   reaction formation, 249
   regression, 247
   repression, 247−248
   restitution, 250
   sublimation, 249
   substitution, 249
   suppression, 248
Delusions, 438
Democratic leadership, 96
Denial, 248−249
   body image integrity and, 513
   dying and, 479
   of patient's statement, 190
Dental floss, 297
Denture care, 297
Denver Developmental Screening Test, 46
Deodorants, 295
Dependency
   illness and, 112
   immobility and, 317
   institutionalization and, 534
Dependent functioning, 28−29
Deposition, 13
Depression, 244
   behavioral signs of, 244−245
   body image integrity and, 514
   cognitive signs of, 244

in-service, 230
learning and, 202–203
Ego, 52
Egocentrism, 53
Ejaculation, 273
Electrical hazards, 155
Electrocardiogram (EKG), 553
Electroencephalogram (EEG), 329, 553
Electroencephalograph (EEG), 329
stages of sleep and, 330
Electrolyte(s), 413
movement of, 414
Electrolyte balance
assessment of, 416–418
control mechanisms for, 415–416
problems of, 418–420
Electromyogram (EMG), 553
Elemental feedings, 350–351
Elimination, 362
organs of, 362
stress and, 120
*see also* Defecation; Urination
Emancipated minor, 15
Emboli, 317
Emergencies, consent in, 15
Emphysema, 388
Enacted law, 12
Endoscopy, 548–549
Enema, 378
barium, 550
Enteral feeding, 350
Enteric coating, 159
Enteric isolation, 178–179
Enuresis, 365
Environment
of group, 90–91
learning and, 204
nausea and vomiting and, 357
safety assessment of, 154–155
sleep and, 335
therapeutic, 515–516
Epidermis, 290
Epilepsy
health teaching and, 451
immediate care in, 450
seizure observations in, 450–451
sexuality and, 275
sleep deprivation and, 333
types of seizures in, 450
Epinephrine, 118
Epithelial cells, 290
Equilibration, 52
Equipment
asepsis and, 173–174
care of, 152–153
gathering, 151
Equivalencies, table of, 547
Erection, 271
Erogenous zones, 279

Errors
of commission, 161
course of action and, 162
of omission, 161–162
Erythrocytes, 404
Esophagoscopy, 548
Esteem needs, 38
Estrogens, 525
Ethical issues, 16
attitudes and, 18
bioethics, 18–19
code for, 16–17
confidentiality and, 17
consumers' rights and, 19
personal behavior and, 17–18
Etiology, 141
Eupnea, 390
Eustress, 117
Euthanasia, 486–487
Evacuation, of patients, 157–158
Evaluation
of activity, 322
audit of records and, 231–232
direct-care audit and, 232
of health-care system, 22
of nursing plan, 136, 144–145
of procedures, 152
Evaporation, heat loss through, 453
Exacerbations, 109
Exchange menus, 355
Exercise, 310
active, 310–314
inadequate, 110
passive, 314
Exhaustion stage, 118
Expectorants, 396
Expectoration, in older adult, 524
Expenses, worry over, 242–243
Experience, learning and, 202–203
Expiration, 386
Exploratory responses, 189
Expressive responses, to pain, 464
Expressive role, 7
Extracellular fluid compartment, 413
Extreme unction, 260
Eye care, 298–299
in unconscious patients, 448
Eye contact, 193

Facial expression, 193
Facilitating responses, 188–190
Facility policies, minority patients and, 76
Falls, preventing, 155, 537
False imprisonment, 15
False reassurance, 190
Family
body image integrity and, 517
minorities and, 79, 82, 83, 86

immobility and, 316
internal, 387
in older adult, 524
stress and, 119–120
in unconscious patients, 448
Respiratory therapy, 398
Rest, 305, 314
assessing, 317
planning, 318
with respiratory problems, 397
*see also* Sleep
Restating, 189
Restitution, 250
death and, 489
Retention, of urine, 364–365
Reticuloendothelial system, 129
Retirement, 529–530
Retirement apartments, 533
Retirement homes, 533
Retraction, 392
Retrograde pyelogram, 552
Reverse isolation, 179–180
Reversibility, 53
Rhonchi, 390
Rickettsia, 169
Role(s)
in group, 95
of patient, 113
Role confusion vs. identity conflict, 62–63
Roman Catholicism, 260
diet and, 346
Rosary, 260
Routines
for hygiene, 290–291
unfamiliar, 242
Rubella, 45
Rules, 12

Safety, 154
blindness and, 446–447
burns and, 155–156
electrical hazards and, 155
environmental assessment and, 154–155
falls and, 155
fire and, 156–158
of older adults, 537
of unconscious patients, 448
Safety needs, 37
Salmonella, 170
Satiety, 344
Sebaceous glands, 290
Secondary health care, 23
Secretions, respiratory, 482–483
Seizures. *See* Epilepsy
Self, as cause of illness, 258–259
Self-actualization, 38–39, 240
Self-awareness, minority patients and, 74
Self-centeredness
illness and, 112
stress and, 120–121

Self-concept, 237–238
feedback and, 238
health and, 106
threat to, 241
Self-esteem, 237
body image and, 238
human dignity and, 238
illness as punishment and, 258
immobility and, 317
need for, 38
self-concept and, 237–238
self-understanding and, 238–239
Self-hypnosis, 125
self-understanding, 238–239
Semicoma, 439
Sender, 185
Senility, 528–529
Sensation problems, assessment and intervention in, 441
Senses, in older adult, 527–528
Sensorimotor stage, 53
Sensory aphasia, 443
Sensory disturbances, 498–499
assessment for, 499–500
intervention in, 501–503
occupations prone to, 503–504
Sensory impulses, 436
Sensory input, 498
Sensory level, 498
Sensory receptors, 436, 438
Sequence, learning and, 206
Serum hepatitis, 429
Seventh-Day Adventists, 261
Sexual assault, 280
Sexual behavior, 269
inappropriate, 270–271
variations in, 269–270
Sexual dysfunction, 273
counseling for, 279–280
in females, 274
in males, 273
Sexual maturing, 62
Sexuality, 269
age and, 272–273
disability and, 278–279
drugs and, 274–275
illness and, 275–276
nursing practice and, 270–272
in older adult, 525
surgery and, 276–277
*see also* Development, psychosexual
Shame and doubt vs. autonomy conflict, 57
Shampooing, 299–300
Shared living, 533
Shaving, 296–297
Sheepskin pads, 321
Sheltered care, 24
Shock
body image integrity and, 513
death and, 489

Showers, 294
Side effects, sexuality and, 274–275
Sighing, 389
Sigmoid, 373
Sigmoidoscopy, 549
Sign(s)
    neuro, 447
    objective, 138
    physical, 119–120, 250
Signing, 445
Silence, 194
Silicone-gel pads, 321
Sitting, 318
Situation, in assessment of mental health, 250
Situational crisis, 246
Size, of group, 91
Skill(s)
    knowledge of, 149
    technical, 149–150
Skilled-nursing facility (SNF), 24–25
Skin, 289–290
    circulation and, 410
    color of, 292–293
    immobility and, 315
    in older adult, 526
    in terminally ill, 481–482
Skin precautions, 179
Slander, 16
Sleep, 328
    REM, 331, 332, 334
    age and, 332
    causes of, 329
    circadian rhythm and, 328–329, 451
    deprivation of, 332–333, 336–337
    drugs and, 334, 335, 336
    inadequate, 110
    insomnia, 332
    of nurses, 336–337
    nursing intervention and, 334–336
    paradoxic, 331
    stages of, 329–331
Small intestine, 372–373
Smegma, 295
Smell
    in older adult, 528
    sensory deprivation and, 503
Smoking, preventing fires and, 156, 537
Snoring, 389
Soap(s), 295
SOAPing, 220
Social distance, 192
Social needs, of terminally ill, 483
Social relationships, 6, 7
    see also Interaction
Social stressors, 122
Socializing, 195–196
Society, death and, 476
Sodium imbalances, 419–420
Solutions, for fluid therapy, 424–426

Somnolence, 439
Sordes, 297
Space
    group need for, 90
    personal and intimate, 192
Specialization, 9–10
Specific dynamic action, 453
Specific gravity, of urine, 366
Specimen, care of, 152–153
Speech, development of, 58–59
Spinal cord, 436
Spine
    torsion of, 307
    see also Posture
Spiritual beliefs. See Religion
Spiritual needs
    assessing, 262–263
    meeting, 263–265
    role in illness, 258
Spores, 169
Sputum, 391
Staff education, 12
Stagnation vs. generativity conflict, 64
Staph infection, 171
Staphylococcus, 170
Starvation, for weight loss, 356
State Health Coordinating Councils (SHCCs), 23
State board of nursing, 12
Statutory law, 12
Steatorrhea, 375
Stereotyped comments, 190
Stereotyping, 73
    of older adults, 537–538
    sexual, 269
Sterile technique, 172
Sterilization, ethics of, 18–19
Stoicism, 464
Stoma, 277
Stool. See Feces
Strengths
    body image integrity and, 515, 516
    in terminally ill, 485
Stress
    behavioral signs of, 121
    cognitive changes due to, 120
    feelings associated with, 120–121
    illness and, 110–111, 123
    nature of, 117
    nausea and vomiting and, 357
    physical signs of, 118–120
    resistance to, 124
    sleep and, 336
    see also Adaptation
Stress management, 123
    basic life skills and, 125
    biofeedback and, 127
    eliminating stressors and, 124
    increasing resistance and, 124
    physical activity and, 124